W0111345

IMMUNOLOGICAL ASPECTS OF ALLERGY AND ALLERGIC DISEASES

VOLUME 1

Basic Concepts in Experimental Immunology

# IMMUNOLOGICAL ASPECTS OF ALLERGY AND ALLERGIC DISEASES

Edited by E. Rajka and S. Korossy

---

VOLUME 1
Basic Concepts in Experimental Immunology

VOLUME 2
Methods in Experimental Immunology

In preparation:

VOLUME 3, 1975

VOLUME 4, 1975

# IMMUNOLOGICAL ASPECTS OF ALLERGY AND ALLERGIC DISEASES

Edited by

E. RAJKA

and

S. KOROSSY

Department of Dermatology
István Municipal Hospital
Budapest, Hungary

VOLUME 1

## Basic Concepts in Experimental Immunology

Springer Science+Business Media, LLC

Originally published by Plenum US London and New York in 1974
Softcover reprint of the hardcover 1st edition 1974

ISBN 978-1-4615-7233-6 ISBN 978-1-4615-7231-2 (eBook)
DOI 10.1007/978-1-4615-7231-2



Library of Congress Catalog Card Number 74–7089

# LIST OF CONTRIBUTORS
# TO VOLUME 1

MIKLÓS BENCZÚR, M.D.

Research Officer, Laboratory for Transplantation Immunity, National Institute of Haematology and Blood Transfusion, Daróczi út 24., 1113 Budapest, Hungary

BÉLA CSABA, M.D., D.Sc. (med.)

Professor of Immunology, Department of Pathophysiology, Debrecen University Medical School, Nagyerdei körút 98., 4032 Debrecen, Hungary

ZOLTÁN CSIZÉR, M.D.

Chief, Vaccines Department, Institute for Serobacteriological Production and Research 'Human', Szállás u. 5., 1107 Budapest, Hungary

JÁNOS GERGELY, M.D., D.Sc. (med.)

Professor and Head, Department of Immunochemistry, National Institute of Haematology and Blood Transfusion, Daróczi út 24., 1113 Budapest, Hungary

GEORGE JÁNOSSY, M.D., Ph.D.

Assistant Professor, Clinical Research Centre, Division of Immunology, Watford Rd., Harrow, Middlesex HA1 3UJ, England

LÓRÁND KESZTYŰS, M.D.

Corresponding Member of the Hungarian Academy of Sciences
Professor and Head, Department of Pathophysiology, Debrecen University Medical School, Nagyerdei körút 98., 4032 Debrecen, Hungary

Miklós Koltay, M.D., C.Sc. (med.)

Late Assistant Professor, Department of Paediatrics, Szeged University Medical School, Hungary

Sándor Korossy, M.D., C.Sc. (med.)

Head, Department of Dermatology, István Municipal Hospital, Nagyvárad tér 1., 1096 Budapest, Hungary

Åke Nilzén, M.D.

Professor of Allergology, Head, Clinic of Allergology, Karolinska Institutet, Karolinska Sjukhuset, Stockholm, Sweden

Karel Nouza, M.D., C.Sc. (med.)

Head, Laboratory for Transplantation Immunology, Institute of Experimental Biology and Genetics of the Czechoslovak Academy of Sciences, Budejovická 1083, Prague 4, Czechoslovakia

Pál Osváth, M.D., C.Sc. (med.)

Senior Lecturer, Department of Paediatrics, Szeged University Medical School, Korányi rakpart 118., 6725 Szeged, Hungary

Győző G. Petrányi, M.D., C.Sc. (med.)

Head, Laboratory for Transplantation Immunity, National Institute of Haematology and Blood Transfusion, Daróczi út 24., 1113 Budapest, Hungary

Edmund Rajka, M.D.,

Late Corresponding Member of the Hungarian Academy of Sciences
Late Dermatologist-in-Chief, István Municipal Hospital, Budapest, Hungary

Georges Sándor, M.D.

Head, Department of Protein Physicochemistry, Institut Pasteur, 25, rue du Docteur Roux, Paris XV$^{e}$, France

Ilona Szeri, M.D., C.Sc. (med.)

Senior Research Officer, Department of Microbiology, Semmelweis University Medical School, Hőgyes E. u. 9., 1092 Budapest, Hungary

Tibor Szilágyi, M.D., D.Sc. (med.)

Professor of Pathophysiology, Department of Pathophysiology, Debrecen University Medical School, Nagyerdei körút 98., 4032 Debrecen, Hungary

# PREFACE

A monograph in German, entitled *Allergie und allergische Erkrankungen,* edited by the late Edmund Rajka, Corresponding Member of the Hungarian Academy of Sciences, was published in 1959. The second edition, revised and completed according to contemporary advances in allergology and immunology, was published in Russian seven years later, in 1966. Both volumes dealt with the theoretical and clinical aspects of allergology and allergic diseases on the basis of the information emerging from fundamental immunological research.

Demand for an English version of the monograph was realized immediately after the second edition. Advances in the discipline of molecular biology, accumulating immunological knowledge and changes in outlook had by then affected the entire view of clinical medicine. Allergology, recently also known as clinical immunology as it provides clues to practically all branches of clinical medicine, has ceased to be the chosen field of specialists. A knowledge in this field is now an essential prerequisite of modern clinical practice and research.

It was in view of these facts that the compilation of this volume was begun; unfortunately, having already done the greater part of the work, Professor Rajka died suddenly. Regrettably, he did not live to see the publication of this book, to the editing of which he devoted so much time and energy. Thus his co-workers undertook the task of completion in the spirit of his instructions and with all due respect to his scientific legacy.

Allergology is primarily a clinical discipline and allergic diseases occur in all fields of medical practice. It might even be stated that allergic processes play a major or minor role in practically every disease, thus specialists are expected to scrutinize every case from the allergic standpoint. Clinicians should make adequate use of the theoretical information available on the recognition, interpretation and treatment of allergic diseases. Immunologists, for their part, are expected to be well versed in clinical allergology in order to be prepared for the solution of various problems posed by everyday practice.

The combination of both theoretical and practical aspects was, therefore, our leading principle in discussing the clinical and research problems of allergy in the present work.

When this book was originally conceived, it fell into two volumes but for the convenience of the reader, it has subsequently been arranged in four volumes. (Thus please note the details set out after the Preface when making cross-references.) The general, theoretical, volumes include chapters summarizing the most recent immunological information indispensable for the understanding of various clinical syndromes. The topics discussed are: the immunochemistry of antigens and antibodies (immunoglobulins); theories of antibody formation; the role of thymus, lymphoid system, etc.; classification and terminology, description of immediate-type and delayed-type reactions; pathomechanism of sensitization and autosensitization; anaphylaxis; immunological tolerance; transplantation immunity; tumour immunity; etc.

In the third and fourth volumes clinical aspects are summarized. Special care has been devoted to the description of advances in research of several informative test procedures and of newer methods of diagnosis. It was thought to be important to pay due attention to the most significant recent literature even if opinions are occasionally controversial or difficult to accept. It is felt, therefore, that this book should not only serve as a manual for the clinical allergologist, but it should also stimulate research in specialized fields of allergology and immunology.

The editors are glad to acknowledge the assistance of all who helped in the immense task of compiling these volumes. We are indebted to the President of the Department of Medical Sciences of the Hungarian Academy of Sciences and to the Immunology and Allergology Research Commission for suggesting the idea of this work, and to Akadémiai Kiadó, Publishing House of the Hungarian Academy of Sciences, for the beautiful presentation.

L. KESZTYŰS, M. D.
Corresponding Member
of the Hungarian Academy of Sciences
S. KOROSSY, M.D., C.Sc. (med.)

March 1974

Chapters 20–33 are contained in Volume 2; Chapters 34–52 in Volume 3; and Chapters 53–80 in Volume 4.
for Chapter 39 on page 51, read Chapter 69
for Chapter 64 on page 52, read Chapter 49
for Chapter 73 on page 59, read Chapter 51
for Chapter 71 on page 62, read Chapter 72.

# CONTENTS OF VOLUME 1

## PART I

## GENERAL ASPECTS



## PART II

## FACTORS PARTICIPATING IN ANTIGEN–ANTIBODY REACTION

PART I

# GENERAL ASPECTS

# INTRODUCTION

by

E. RAJKA

Completed by

L. KESZTYŰS

Allergology as a medical discipline is in the process of an enormous expansion and has already become a pathogenetic principle in practically all branches of medicine. An incredible number of data has accumulated, which are closely linked with certain fundamental problems of biochemistry, genetics, pathology and molecular biology. According to different statistics, in recent years immunological and allergological problems, or the use of immunological methods, have been the subject of 10–20 per cent of all reports from the fields of biology and theoretical and practical medicine [5, 10]. The findings of this new discipline have penetrated all the traditional fields of medicine. In the meantime, the methods of allergy testing, antigen research and antibody detection have become more numerous and complicated. Specialization in allergology has differentiated into branches of allergic manifestations in the respiratory tract, digestive apparatus haemopoietic system, skin, kidney, etc. In addition to traditional methods and newer *in vivo* procedures, *in vitro* tests are increasingly gaining ground; the exact performance of the latter requires extensive serological experience which can only exceptionally be demanded from the practitioner.

It would be, of course, advantageous, if the allergologist were familiar with all details of present knowledge in his field, at least in the clinical context. Attempts at meeting this requirement are reflected by the recently founded allergology research institutes, postgraduate training courses in allergology and educational specialization in independent departments of immunology and allergology of the medical universities. These university departments are in charge of the training of specialists versed in all branches of immunology and theoretical and practical allergology. If, however, the fact is considered that specialists of allergology are supposed to possess a similarly profound knowledge of internal, paediatric, dermatologic and other diseases as well, the learning to be mastered almost seems to be beyond the human reach. For the time being it seems more reasonable that appropriate groups of highly specialized allergologists handle the field in collaboration [1, 3, 4, 7, 9, 11*a*, *b*]. We have followed this system ourselves in compiling this monograph.

The precise nature of the relationship between allergy and immunity is still a matter of dispute. The teleological school of thought still prevailing in medical science is reluctant to give up the obsolete idea that the immunological processes of vertebrates represent a useful biological adaptation to eliminate special pathogenic agents and their products from the body. It has become clear, however, that this view which, due to historical reasons, confronts immunology with allergology is a generalization of the extreme and unreasonably limits the scope of both disciplines. Immunological processes as are understood today imply much more; having developed in the course of evolution, they provide for the chemical identity and stability of the tissues and cells of vertebrates and prevent or reduce variation and mutations in the inherent self-reproductive code system of animal cells induced by macromolecules or by various endogenous or exogenous factors. In other words, the immunological processes protect the species- and sex-specific as well as individual code systems which have become selected from the possible phylo- and ontogenetic variations.

From the point of view of the code protecting immune processes it is irrelevant whether the exogenous or endogenous macromolecule or cell is in itself pathogenic or not. The immune processes protect the code system of the host even at the cost of pathological responses (disease) or destruction of the organism (death). It is still hard to imagine the genetic consequences endangering the species and the individual of the incorporation of 'not self' macromolecules or cells, were they not hampered by the immune mechanism. It is therefore important to detect those molecular mechanisms which in the course of vertebrate evolution have been responsible for the establishment of such an immune system. Reinforcement of heterozygotism by favourable fertilization, prevention of somatic mutation and protection against oncogenic viruses are all methods helping in persuing the above research objective [2].

If this new concept of immunity is accepted, any further discussion of the correctness and conformity of Pirquet and Schick's definitions become superfluous; the same applies to the problem of whether animal anaphylaxis and true (protective) immunity belong in the scope of allergy. Regardless whether the specific, antibody-induced alteration in reactivity is referred to as allergy, anaphylaxis or immunological reaction, clinical medicine is in need of a collective term covering the entire group and the generally accepted term for this is now allergy, and allergology for the entire discipline. Kabat [6] has pointed out that, e.g. any artificial and speculative differentiation between anaphylaxis and clinical allergy should be avoided, because they differ quantitatively rather than qualitatively. Thus the borderline between allergology and immunology tends to vanish. This does not mean that immunologists show generally more interest than before in allergology; it is rather that the allergologists have increasingly adopted the term 'immunopathologic' to designate allergic, above all autoallergic, processes. For the time being it should be accepted that the designations 'allergic' and 'immune' are often used synonymously, especially in the clinical sense. This is in accord with the practical observation that, in addition to altered reactivity, resistance may also develop in a single disease, i.e. in response to the same complex antigen. This occurs most frequently in infectious diseases.

Formerly it was believed that except for certain, e.g. bactericidic, antibodies, serologically demonstrable circulating antibodies as well as the skin sensitizing antibodies (reagins) participating in immediate hypersensitivity reactions usually play no role in the pathogenesis of allergic diseases and are only formed as by-products of the allergic reaction. An increasing body of practical observations and experimental evidence, however, suggests that—like cell-fixed reagins or antigen–antibody complexes—certain humoral and cell-mediated 'antibodies' are essential prerequisites of the allergic process. For instance, the Arthus reaction can be regarded as a necrotic inflammation induced by the interaction of circulating precipitins with the fixed antigen. A still more convincing example is the pathomechanism of immunohaematological diseases, when circulating antibodies exert their pathogenic action at their encounter with blood corpuscular elements or with antigens bound to the latter.

Clinically, allergic events should not only be distinguished with regard to pathologically increased (normal versus pathologic) or pathologically decreased (pathologic versus normal) reactivity, but also with regard to immediate-type and delayed-type reaction forms (see later). The main criterion of allergy is the antigen–antibody reaction, and its demonstration should therefore be the primary aim. It should be pointed out that the state brought about by allergization (sensitization) and allergic disease are different conditions. Antigen–antibody reactions will regularly occur in sensitization, even in connection with a skin test, but in the development of an allergic disease further profound changes are involved, which may be related to genetic predisposition, hereditary and acquired (environmental) factors, functional disturbance of the neuroendocrine system, etc. Allergology in not a universal clue to pathologic processes, but the results of immunology and allergology are utilized in elucidating the pathogenesis, in making the diagnosis, and in the effective treatment of various diseases.

Our intention has been to offer the reader a modern book on allergy, allergic diseases and their immunological aspects. Emphasis has been laid on the pathological conditions throughout because, as already noted, all diseases should be scrutinized for the possible involvement of allergic factors in their pathomechanism. The doctor who disregards allergic events in judging the pathogenesis may deprive himself of a valuable support; increasing knowledge of allergy has disclosed allergic components of major or minor importance in the pathomechanism of several diseases, which had formerly been thought to be entirely unrelated to allergy (e.g. pernicious anaemia, malignant tumours, etc.). This does not, of course, imply that all diseases might be allergic. It would be undue exaggeration to look for allergy where even the slightest sign of its involvement is lacking, but its possibility should always be borne in mind.

## REFERENCES


1. Bach, F. H. and Good, R. A. (Eds): *Clinical Immunobiology.* Vol. I. Academic Press, New York 1972.
2. Ceppellini, R., In *Blood and Tissue Antigens.* Ed. by Aminoff, D. Academic Press, New York 1970.
3. Freedman, S. O. (Ed.): *Clinical Immunology.* Harper and Row, New York 1971.
4. Gell, P. G. H. and Coombs, R. R. A. (Eds): *Clinical Aspects of Immunology.* Blackwell, Oxford 1963.
5. Humphrey, J. H. and White, R. G.: *Immunology for Students of Medicine.* 3rd ed. Blackwell, Oxford 1970.
6. Kabat, E. A.: *II. Int. Congr. Allerg. Rio de Janeiro* 1955.
7. Montagna, W. and Billingham, R. E. (Eds): *Immunology and the Skin.* Appleton-Century-Crofts, New York 1971.
8. Pepys, J.: *Clin. Allergy* **1**, 1 (1971).
9. Samter, M. (Ed.): *Immunological Diseases.* Vols I–II. Little Brown and Co., Boston 1971.

10. Waksman, B. H.: *J. Immunol.* **107,** 617 (1971).
11*a*. WHO Scientific Group: Clinical Immunology. *Wld Hlth Org. techn. Rep. Ser.* No. 496. WHO, Geneva 1972.
11*b*. WHO Scientific Group: Cell-Mediated Immunity and Resistance to Infection. *Wld Hlth Org. techn. Rep. Ser.* No. 519. WHO, Geneva 1973.

CHAPTER 1

# THE CONCEPT AND CRITERIA OF ALLERGY

by

E. RAJKA

Completed by

L. KESZTYŰS

Research of allergy stems from the five fundamental discoveries outlined below:

1. Koch [8] reported in 1890 that subcutaneous inoculation of a *Mycobacterium tuberculosis* suspension to healthy guinea pigs resulted in the formation 10 to 14 days later of a hard, ulcerative nodule at the injection site, which persisted until the animal died in tuberculosis. The regional lymph nodes also became involved. If, however, the same suspension was injected into guinea pigs previously infected with tuberculosis, a diffuse infiltration developed at the injection site, followed by necrosis and rejection of the skin area involved. The ulcer then healed without spread of the infection to adjacent lymph nodes. Thus the second infection differed in its course from the first one.

2. Twelve years later Richet and Portier [16] treated dogs with an actinia extract, which caused slight, temporary digestive troubles (nausea, vomiting, etc.). Treatment with a similar second dose after a few weeks resulted, instead of the expected antitoxic immunity, in acute poisoning and lethal shock symptoms. Administration of elevated doses to dogs which were not previously treated never caused death. The phenomenon that sensitivity to a toxin increases after the first application was termed anaphylaxis.

3. In the same year Smith [18] observed that 0.02 ml horse serum elicited a lethal shock in guinea pigs which had been treated two weeks earlier with a 1 ml dose of the same serum. According to later investigations by Otto [10*a*, *b*], this phenomenon corresponded to specific serum hypersensitivity.

4. One year later Arthus [1, 2] demonstrated experimentally that anaphylaxis can be elicited by various heterologous proteins; rabbits responded to the repeated intracutaneous application of heterologous serum not only with an anaphylactic shock, but also with local necrotic inflammation (Arthus reaction).

5. Pirquet and Schick [13] established that the latency period of infectious diseases and serum sickness are required not so much for microbial growth or a 'toxic change' of the serum, as for the alteration of general reactivity, because no symptoms occur until a reaction takes place between the antigen (pathogenic microorganism or heterologous substance) and the antibodies formed to it. This antibody dependent alteration of reactivity was called allergy by Pirquet [12]. In other words by allergy he meant the temporally, qualitatively and quantitatively changed response of the infected or serum treated, i.e. antibody carrying, individual to further infection or readministration of serum. The result is a more rapid appearance of the allergic symptoms, moreover to considerably lower doses

or to substances which had initially been indifferent. In this context the fundamental observations were made that also non-multiplying protein substances of antigenic nature may alter the individual's reactivity and that the symptoms of serum sickness appear when the synthesis of the specific agent has reached an appropriate level. The definition proposed by Pirquet was later extended to designate not only the increase, but also the diminution or absence of reactivity, which can be regarded as allergic phenomena if they arise on an immunological basis.

Such processes arise in humans either 'spontaneously', without an obvious cause, or are induced with exogenous (macromolecules, well-defined simple chemical substances) or endogenous (various cells, proteins, polysaccharides, etc.) factors. The immune response of man and animals is usually designated as sensitization (immunization or allergization) and consists essentially in the induction of specific immunocytes and/or antibodies. Thus two main forms of immune response can be distinguished: (*i*) the humoral response, characterized by the presence in the plasma of circulating immunoglobulin molecules synthesized and secreted by plasma cells; (*ii*) the cell-mediated response, characterized by the specific alteration or 'sensitization' of lymphocytes (immunolymphocytes). The latter are responsible among others for allergic reactions of the delayed type, for resistance to certain infections and for homograft rejection [9]. The cellular immune response is thymus dependent and can develop independently of humoral antibody formation. The cell generation potentially capable of humoral antibody secretion is thymus independent.

It was a particularly important discovery that—apart from the Koch phenomenon—the antibodies participating in the above described anaphylactic phenomena are passively transferable with serum to previously not treated animals and that, depending on the mode of application of the antigen, on intravenous injection shock phenomena, on intradermal injection inflammatory reactions will appear after a certain time that is required for the antibody to fix to the reactive cells. The fixing of anaphylactic antibodies to cells can be demonstrated by adding *in vitro* antigen to a bath containing surviving bloodless smooth muscle containing organs (virginal uterus, piece of ileum) of guinea pig: an abrupt contraction of the organ will be observed (Schultz–Dale test) [17, 4]. In certain animal species it is indifferent whether the serum donor and recipient are homologous or heterologous (homologous and heterologous passive anaphylaxis). Active anaphylaxis results if a substance elicits both anaphylaxis and shock, whereas in passive anaphylaxis the antibody-containing serum of the donor is the sensitizing substance and the antigen used for the sensitization of the donor is the shock eliciting substance.

The success of the passive transfer of anaphylaxis from one animal to another stimulated attempts at the transfer of allergic reactivity change from man to man. Among such experiments, the passive transfer procedure devised by Prausnitz and Küstner (P–K) [14] was of a decisive importance. Antibody containing serum from fish allergic patient (Küstner) or horse asthmatic and hay fever patients (de Besche) [3] was transferred intradermally to non-allergic healthy subjects and application of the corresponding antigen at the injection site after 24 hours resulted in the development of a local weal and flare response. This finding has affirmed the relationship between human allergy and animal anaphylaxis also in respect of passive transferability and has found expression in the common term 'allergy', the criteria of which were then stated precisely by Doerr as follows [5]:

1. demonstration of the antibody,
2. altered reactivity compared with the normergic state,
3. specificity,
4. independence of the symptom complex from the acting allergen.

ad 1. Antibody demonstration has been discussed in the foregoing.

ad 2. Deviation from the normergic state means that prior to sensitization the individual responded to the allergen in a different way, if at all. The kind of the altered reactivity varies with the target organ (shock tissue) in which the allergic reaction takes place. Altered skin reactions are usually manifested as inflammation; certain substances or effects which elicit no response in normal subjects, provoke an inflammatory reaction in sensitized allergic individuals. If the agent also elicits a reaction in normal subjects, its effect will be more pronounced and will last longer in sensitized individuals. Allergic inflammatory reactions are ranging from immediate-type weal and flare response to delayed-type chronic inflammatory infiltration and may occasionally be accompanied by other histological changes, e.g. granuloma formation. Inflammatory reactions may also develop in mucous membranes and internal organs (brain, kidney, liver, etc.), as a rule in association with other changes related with the organ, which then elicit characteristic symptoms.

Deviation from the normal may also take the form of spastic contraction of smooth muscles, which then is manifested in asthmatic attacks if the lung is involved, or in convulsions if the target organ is a visceral organ. Occasionally, e.g. in asthma, the mucosa and the bronchiolar connective tissue may serve as the shock tissue, responding with oedema and hypersecretion of mucosa [6]. Abnormal reactivity may further be signified by various degenerative phenomena, involving chiefly the collagenous tissue (fibrinoid swelling), or by bleeding, necrosis, cytolysis, etc. Clinically many kinds of allergic diseases belong to this category. The allergic symptoms may be accompanied by various general symptoms, ranging from a slight malaise and headache to a severe collapse (minor and major shock).

Sometimes the only symptom of an allergic reaction is pruritus. It is, as a rule, characteristic of all kinds of allergic processes, but may also be the sole sign of an antigen–antibody reaction, taking in such cases place in the afferent nerve terminals responsible for the mediation of itching within the axon-reflectoric area in which the prurigenic substance is liberated [15].

ad 3. The altered reactivity is specific, i.e. it occurs exclusively in response to the substance (allergen) responsible for the development of the cellular and/or humoral immune response (sensitization). As it is well known from *in vitro* serological reactions, in addition to the corresponding allergen, chemically and/or structurally related substances may also elicit the reaction, the extent of which will depend on the degree of the relationship. This does not exclude the possibility of specific reactivity to chemically (structurally) unrelated substances as well, provided that different substances have provoked cellular and/or humoral immune response, i.e. have sensitized the individual, simultaneously or in succession. In inveterate, long-standing allergic processes specificity tends to decline more or less parallelly with the passing of time, while the range of structurally related substances capable of eliciting the reaction tends to widen. This is in good agreement with the rule known from animal experiments that the range of antibodies formed in the course of hyperimmunization is broader, and their specificity is somewhat lower, compared with those formed in response to a single low dose of antigen. For example, rabbits were immunized with a single inoculation of dinitrophenylated bovine $\gamma$-globulin emulsified in Freund's adjuvant. The distribution and heterogeneity of antibody affinity has been then observed. Initially a symmetrical distribution of heterogeneous low-affinity antibody molecules was obtained. Later there was a shift toward high affinity, and the bulk of the antibody population consisted of a sub-population of high affinity and relatively restricted heterogeneity. Still later, the proportion of high-affinity antibodies decreased, and a highly heterogeneous population of antibody molecules was present with a somewhat decreased average affinity [19].

ad 4. The independence of the symptom complex from the nature and chemical as well as pharmacological properties of the provoking agent means that a complex of allergic symptoms may be elicited by different chemical and physical stimuli, whereas a given antigen may elicit different allergic reactions in various individuals, that is, the allergic symptoms are not characteristic of the acting allergen and usually not conclusive of its nature.

It follows from the above considerations that if the pathological process under examination meets criteria 2, 3 and 4 and the mentioned signs of probability are also present, the allergic nature of the disease can well be postulated, although the precise diagnosis requires antibody demonstration. This limitation is important because the range of allergic reactions still tends to widen, and also because the clinical picture and complex symptoms related to allergy may arise from other conditions. Therefore, it is always the allergic or non-allergic origin of the disease which has to be first ascertained.

In the terminology of allergology, the term allergen is used synonymously with antigen or immunogen, and the terms skin sensitizing antibody and reagin are also used for antibody, at least in connection with positive P–K reactions. The implication that apart from the immunological mechanism also other, endogenous or exogenous, factors may play a secondary causative role in the aetiology of allergic diseases, has already been referred to in the Introduction. Due to the overall effect of these influencing factors an allergic state of the individual may develop, which is designated with the general term of allergic diathesis (predisposition) [7].

The explanation of allergic phenomena by antibody formation is for the time being the sole hypothesis that can be held responsible for almost all clinical and experimental observations related to allergy, above all for the specificity of the reactions. It follows from the foregoing considerations that *in vivo* demonstration of antibodies is of fundamental importance. In human allergy, however, direct tests (provocation of anaphylactic shock, Sch–D reaction) are as a rule impracticable, although bronchial muscle specimens obtained during surgical treatment of patients with allergic asthma, have been shown to contract at contact with the allergen, analogously with the Sch–D reaction. In man, the passive transfer of circulating reagins to human or monkey skin is a decisive proof of allergy; such biological tests have, however, recently been successfully substituted by *in vitro* demonstration of the corresponding immunoglobulin (IgE). Circulating humoral antibodies other than IgE can be demonstrated by various serological tests [11].

The demonstration of cellular immune response, i.e. delayed-type cell-mediated sensitization is equally important; this can usually be achieved by passive transfer of the immunolymphocytes, or their carefully prepared extracts (transfer factor). If the lymphocyte transfer fails, certain highly sensitive and specific tests (migration inhibiting factor, rosette formation) which have recently been elaborated for this purpose may be resorted; to these are suitable for the demonstration—with a high degree of probability—of delayed hypersensitivity. Occasionally the examiner has to resort to tests of minor value which can, nevertheless, affirm the suspicion of allergy. To the latter category belong the provocation, elimination and local skin tests, topical, focal and systemic reactions, etc. The positivity of these tests is, however, no proof in itself unless all other criteria of allergy are met.

## REFERENCES


1. Arthus, M.: *C. R. Soc. Biol. (Paris)* **55,** 819 (1903).
2. Arthus, M. and Breton, M.: *C. R. Soc. Biol. (Paris)* **55,** 1478 (1903).
3. Besche, A. de: *Amer. J. med. Sci.* **166,** 265 (1923).
4. Dale, H. H.: *J. Pharmacol. exp. Ther.* **4,** 517 (1913).
5. Doerr, R.: *Allergie.* Springer, Vienna 1951.
6. Halpern, B. N.: *Acta allerg. (Kbh.)* **9,** 208 (1955).
7. Kämmerer, H. and Michel, H.: *Allergische Diathese und allergische Krankheiten.* Bergmann, Munich 1956.
8. Koch, R.: *Dtsch. med. Wschr.* **17,** 101 (1891).
9. Miller, J. F. A. P.: *Folia allerg. (Roma)* **17,** 381 (1970).

10*a*. Otto, R.: *Leutholdische Gedenkschrift* 1 (1905).

10*b*. id., *Münch. med. Wschr.* **54,** 1665 (1907).

11. Ovary, Z. and Biozzi, G.: *Int. Arch. Allergy* **6,** 252 (1955).
12. Pirquet, C. von: *Münch. med. Wschr.* **53,** 1457 (1906).
13. Pirquet, C. von and Schick, B.: *Die Serumkrankheit.* Deuticke, Vienna 1905.
14. Prausnitz, C. and Küstner, H.: *Zbl. Bakter.* I. Orig. **86,** 160 (1921).
15. Rajka, E., Korossy, S. and Gózony, M.: *Dermatologica* **130,** 113 (1965).
16. Richet, C. and Portier, P.: *C. R. Soc. Biol. (Paris)* **54,** 170 (1902).
17. Schultz, W. H.: *J. Pharmacol. exp. Ther.* **1,** 549 (1909/10).
18. Smith, T.: *J. med. Res.* **13,** 341 (1904).
19. Werblin, T. P., Kim, Y. T., Quagliata, F. and Siskind, G. W.: *Immunology* **24,** 477 (1973).

CHAPTER 2

# TERMINOLOGY AND CLASSIFICATION OF ALLERGY

by

E. RAJKA

Completed by

L. KESZTYŰS

The observation that a skin allergic process manifested initially by sudden eruption, then by positive skin test with focal and systemic reactions and improving subsequently either on specific treatment or even spontaneously so that the skin test becomes negative suggests that, in principle, the signs of increased and decreased reactivity are not opposed to one another, but rather represent two phases of a single biological process. Allergic hyper- and hyposensitivity may alternate as two phases of the same process in nearly all allergic diseases. Both hyper- and hyposensitivity are states resulting from immunological reaction.

The task of clinical allergology is to elucidate the aetiology, pathogenesis and fundamental mechanism of allergic diseases and processes with the aid of various immunological methods. As already noted, allergology can be regarded as clinical immunology, if immunity is understood as a state of specific responsiveness to foreign substances, irrespectively of whether the immune reaction is protective or not. Thus allergology can never dispose of immunology and the best allergy experts are those clinicians who have a profound knowledge of immunology.

Immunology is, however, a theoretical discipline which, despite its immense practical bearing on allergology, deals scarcely if at all with allergology or allergic diseases as such. Thus an amalgamation of the two disciplines seems fairly difficult for the time being, although the recognition of the close relationships between them is essential. It seems probable that clinicians engaged in the study of allergic diseases and processes will continue to use the term allergy [16] and that allergology will still be the field dealing with the different pathologic immunological processes.

Correct classification requires above all an exact terminology, because a wide variety of technical terms is used by different authors and in different countries. The generally accepted collective term *allergy* comprises various sub-groups. The name *atopic diseases* has been given after Coca [2] to the group in which allergic predisposition is mostly hereditary, familial occurrence is frequent, the role of the autonomic nervous system, etc. is obvious and sensitization takes place 'spontaneously', in an experimentally not reproducible manner, although clearly on the basis of a previous contact with an agent. These conditions (e.g. asthma bronchiale, hay fever, infantile eczema, urticaria and prurigo group) were earlier called 'idiosyncrasies'; the term 'atopic diseases' is increasingly used although the synonymous terms 'spontaneous allergy' or 'asthma-hay-fever-group' may be encountered in the literature. Hagerman e.g. proposed the name 'spontaneous seroallergy' [8]; anyway, it would be desirable to find a general term for this disease group, which would cover the various clinical forms having several features in common and being generally characterized by immediate hypersensitivity.

*Anaphylaxis* is usually differentiated from the group of atopic diseases. The term anaphylaxis had originally been used to designate in animals a state of species-specific hypersensitivity following administration of antigen to primed subjects. Since, however, human atopic allergy and animal anaphylaxis have several features in common (free circulating antibodies, passive transfer, immediate-type skin reactions, etc.), the designation 'anaphylaxis group' [7] has recently been preferred as a collective term for both; this is the more feasible because spontaneous allergic diseases of an atopic nature also occur in animals [20].

The term *hypersensitivity* is used for the group of allergic conditions in which the inducing antigen is usually known and which is experimentally reproducible by the use of the known antigen. This is the most common form of allergy comprising infectious allergy, allergic contact dermatitis (eczema), drug allergy, etc., and, generally, experimental sensitization, which is also designated as immunization. Part of these reactions are delayed-type (cell-mediated immunity) and another part are immediate-type in which immunity can be passively transferred with the help of circulating antibodies in the serum. The two reaction types may characterize the same allergic condition in different phases of the process. The terms allergization, sensitization and immunization are often used synonymously.

Allergy and immunity had formerly been dealt with separately, because of the different outcome of the respective reactions: sensitization is pathogenic, whereas immunization has a low pathogenic effect, if any. Terms are more difficult to define and to differentiate in hypo- or desensibility reactions (low or no reactivity) compared with high-reactivity reactions, the more because the former essentially come under the category of 'unresponsiveness', the two main subcategories of which had formerly been defined as 'immunotolerance' and 'immunoparalysis'. In the light of present knowledge, the separation of the latter two concepts seems incorrect, because they seem to rest on the same fundamental mechanism [5, 11, 12].

Earlier the Nomenclature Committee [15] appointed in the USA had differentiated immunity from allergy as an essentially quantitative specific state, whereas allergy is, first of all, a qualitatively changed state. In immunity emphasis is on the antigen–antibody reaction, whereas in allergy the tissue damage due to the antigen–antibody reaction is the most important issue. Certain authors have expressed this difference by designating immune reactions as direct and allergic reactions as indirect reactions.

The term *antigen* [3] is in every respect correct for group designation; when dealing with allergic processes the term allergen has been used synonymously. Other terms, such as anaphylactogen, reactogen, atopen, cannot be misinterpreted, but have not been generally adopted in the literature.

In recent literary reports the term *immunogen* is often encountered which is used to convey the idea of immunogenicity, i.e. the capacity to provoke a specific immune response. Earlier such substances had been called complete antigens [1]. For instance, antibodies induced by immunization with *Bacillus anthracis* react with a polymer (poly-$\gamma$-D-glutamic acid) extractable from the cell wall of the organism [9]. No antibodies will, however, form if the animal is parenterally treated with the polymer. Thus poly-$\gamma$-D-glutamic acid is itself not an immunogen, but combines specifically with antibody formed in response to the appropriate immunogen. The immune response inducing capacity has been termed immunogenecity, while the potential of an antigen to combine with its specific antibody or react specifically with immunocytes as antigen specificity. In this sense, poly-γ-D-glutamic acid is not immunogenic, but antigen specific. Such substances are designated with older terms as incomplete or half antigens or haptens, or they may also be called cross-reacting antigens. The *Bacillus anthracis* cell is immunogenic, because it stimulates the formation of specific antibodies to poly-γ-D-glutamic acid [18].

The term *antibody* (Behring) is generally used in all branches of immunology, but in the allergologic context the skin sensitizing antibodies are preferably called reagin (reagenic antibody) for humans and homocytotropic antibody for animals [21]. Certain findings, however, indicate that human reagin and, for instance, the rat homocytotropic antibody are analogous, possessing not only similar biological, physical and chemical properties, but also common antigenic determinants [13]. Against this, other workers hold the view that different animal species synthesize functionally and probably also structurally different homocytotropic antibodies [6, 14].

As to the classification of allergic processes, it should be pointed out that an exact grouping has still not been elaborated. An aetiological classification is impracticable in allergology, because there is no specific connection between clinical picture and the eliciting agent. At our present state of knowledge, the only acceptable grouping can be made on a pathomechanical basis. This again has the difficulty that a sharp differentiation between the various syndromes is not always possible and a number of allergic diseases can be equally well classified into one or another group; this means that there are many transitory, mixed or biphasic forms (Kallós), while grouping should necessarily be based on a single characteristic property.

Gell and Coombs [7] classified the various hypersensitivity reactions corresponding to pathological changes in specific reactivity and the respective pathologic symptoms as follows: 1. anaphylaxis; 2. cytotoxic phenomena; 3. Arthus reaction and serum sickness and 4. delayed-type hypersensitivity. (The first three are immediate-type reactions.)

1. *Anaphylactic response* (*Type I reaction*). Its model is the anaphylaxis of the guinea pig. Antibody formation begins after the first injection of the protein antigen, but the symptoms and shock appear only after the second application of antigen. In certain species the antigen–antibody reaction is due to the encounter of the cell-fixed antibody with the antigen introduced, but free circulating antibodies may also be present. In other species the free humoral antibodies seem to play the decisive role. The antibodies are passively transferable; the main forms of transfer are the passive anaphylactic shock and the Sch–D reaction. The antigen–antibody reaction is followed by the rapid liberation of the mediator.

Gell and Coombs [7] also regarded the atopic and spontaneous allergic reactions and the asthma-hay-fever-group as anaphylaxis. Both cell-fixed and free circulating antibodies are present in these forms, but the symptoms are elicited exclusively by the reaction between fixed (sessile) reagins and the allergen (specific phase); at the same time pharmacologically highly active mediators (histamine, acetylcholine, heparin, plasma chinines, etc.) are released, probably due to enzyme effect (non-specific phase). The active mediators are, in fact, responsible for the lesions consequent upon the antigen–antibody reaction (clinical phase). Since human atopic reagins are passively transferable to human skin by the P–K method and to monkey skin by Layton's technique, they have been termed as skin sensitizing antibodies.

Both Steffen [19] and Rajka [17] prefer the differentiation of anaphylactic responses from atopic allergy, chiefly for clinical reasons.

2. *Cytotoxic, cytolytic (Type II) reactions,* as a rule, need the contribution of complement. Such reactions are the reverse of the anaphylactic response, because in this case it is the antigen (or a hapten) which is attached to the cell surface (e.g. in drug allergy causing purpura, haemolytic anaemia, agranulocytosis, etc.), or the antigen is a cell surface antigen, (e.g., in haemolytic anaemia of newborn, transfusion reaction, autoallergic haemolytic anaemia, granulo- and thrombocytopenias, etc.). The antibody, whether humoral or cell-fixed, is carried to the antigen-containing site by the blood stream or artificially.

3. In *Type III reactions* the tissue damage is mediated by antigen–antibody complexes. Clinical states due to such reactions include the local *Arthus phenomenon* and *systemic serum sickness.* The symptoms are due to the formation of soluble antigen–antibody complexes in moderate antigen excess, depending on their complement-fixing ability. The insoluble antigen–antibody complexes formed if there is an antibody excess are less active, because they rapidly disappear from circulation owing to the phagocytic activity of the RES. In the Arthus reaction, the bivalent complete precipitins formed in the course of sensitization are circulating in the blood and their encounter with the intradermally applied antigen leads to the formation of an irritative complex. A fundamental component of the irritative effect is the impairment of the lysosomal membrane resulting in the liberation of lysosomal enzymes. In the active Arthus reaction, the antigen is administered intradermally to sensitized rabbits, whereas in the direct passive transfer the antibody containing serum is injected intravenously, and the antigen intradermally, into a normal recipient; in the reversed passive transfer, the antibody is administered intradermally and the antigen intravenously. The reaction occurs without latency, because no fixation of the antibody is necessary.

In serum sickness which may arise due to the injection of antiserum, large amounts of protein are circulating in the blood and when the antibodies formed in the lymphoid system gradually enter circulation, they immediately combine with the antigen to form a soluble complex, the properties of which depend on the antibody rather than on the antigen. This complex elicits an immediate-type pathological response according to the mechanism described in the case of type I reactions. Thus in serum sickness, a single injection of antigen stimulates antibody formation and allergic reaction [4]. Serum-sickness-like drug allergy (e.g to penicillin) develops by a similar mechanism.

4. The *delayed-type (Type IV) reactions* are manifested as a tuberculin-trichophytin-type hypersensitivity in bacterial and mycotic allergy, in certain types of drug allergy, in greater part of autoallergic diseases, in transplantation immunity, etc. and as epicutaneous eczematiform responses in contact allergic dermatitis. In delayed hypersensitivity, the antigen is fixed or deposited and reacts with

immunoactive lymphocytes (cell-mediated immunity) gradually accumulating at the antigen-containing site. Antibodies may also be formed but these probably only play the role of an adjuvant.

Apart from pure immediate-type or delayed-type allergic responses, many mixed forms exist. For example, in the Arthus reaction, initially the immediate-type, later the delayed-type response predominates. In most allergic processes caused by bacteria, fungi, insects, enteral parasites or drugs as well as in certain autoallergic diseases, both types of reaction occur independently or simultaneously and at times one, at times the other is dominant.

From the point of view of allergy it is irrelevant which of the two active factors is fixed; in either case, the process can be regarded as allergic, in accordance with the direct and reversed passive transfer experiments. The two main types of reaction, immediate and delayed, also differ in their sites because immediate-type reactions are generally limited to a given tissue (shock tissue) in which the antigen–antibody reaction takes place, whereas in delayed-type reactions the antigen occurs practically everywhere, almost the entire body serving as a shock tissue.

## REFERENCES


1. Campbell, D. H.: *J. Allergy* **19,** 151 (1948).
2. Coca, A. F.: *Hypersensitiveness.* New York 1920.
3. Deutsch (Detre), L.: *Ann. Inst. Pasteur* 710 (1899).
4. Dixon, F. J.: *III. Int. Congr. Allerg. Paris 1958.* Excerpta Medica, Amsterdam 1958, p. 12.
5. Dresser, D. W. and Mitchison, N. A.: *Adv. Immunol.* **8,** 129 (1968).
6. Freeman, M. J.: *Fed. Proc.* **29,** 639 (1970).
7. Gell, P. G. H. and Coombs, R. R. A. (Eds.): *Clinical Aspects of Immunology.* Blackwell, Oxford 1963.
8. Hagerman, G.: *III. Europ. Allergol. Congr. Firenze 1956.* Vol. II. Il Pensiero Scientifico Ed., Rome 1956, p. 189.
9. Ivánovics, G.: *Z. Immun.-Forsch.* **97,** 443 (1940).
10. Layton, L. L.: *J. Allergy* **36,** 523 (1965).
11. Liacopoulos, P., Amstutz, H. and Gille, M. F.: *Immunology* **20,** 57 (1971).
12. Liacopoulos, P., Couderc, J. and Gille, M. F.: *Eur. J. Immunol.* **1,** 359 (1971).
13. Liakopoulos, A. and Perelmutter, L.: *J. Immunol.* **107,** 131 (1971).
14. Mota, I., Sadun, E. H., Bradshaw, R. M. and Gore, R. W.: *Immunology* **16,** 71 (1969).
15. Nomenclature Committee: *Ann. Allergy* **16,** 680 (1959).
16. Pepys, J.: *Clin. Allergy* **1,** 1 (1971).
17. Rajka, E.: *Allergie und allergische Erkrankungen.* Vol. I. Akadémiai Kiadó, Budapest 1959.
18. Sela, M.: *Naturwissenschaft* **56,** 206 (1969).
19. Steffen C.: *Allgemeine und experimentelle Immunologie und Immunpathologie.* Thieme, Stuttgart 1968.
20. Wittich, F. W.: *Fortschr. Allergielehre* **2,** 58 (1949).
21. Zwaifler, N. J. and Robinson, J. O.: *J. exp. Med.* **130,** 907 (1969).

CHAPTER 3

# DEVELOPMENT OF ALLERGIC PROCESSES. PATHOMECHANISM. SENSITIZATION

by

E. RAJKA

Completed by

L. KESZTYŰS

## INTRODUCTION

The antigen cannot normally elicit an allergic process unless the subject is sensitive. Sensitization is understood as the activation, accumulation, cooperation and transformation of immunologically competent, antigen recognizing cells, occasionally followed by antibody (immunoglobulin) formation. Thus the allergic process is the consequence of an antigen–antibody reaction, in which antigen binding lymphocytes may take part instead of the antibody in the conventional sense. This is shown by experimental reversed passive anaphylaxis in which local reaction and shock symptoms are produced by giving antigen first, followed by the antibody containing serum. The reversion of the transfer experiment was initiated by the wish to avoid artificial sensitization. Nevertheless, fixation of the antibody requires a shorter or longer period of latency also in the reversed experiment. The rate and manner of antibody fixation vary with the different kinds of tissues. For instance, rabbits, known as good precipitin formers, fix the antibodies slowly, whence they become sensitized passively less easily than guinea pigs, which are poor precipitin formers, but fix antibodies readily, and are thus more susceptible to passive sensitization.

Unlike animals, humans usually respond easily to reversed cutaneous anaphylaxis, as shown among others by Voss (see Chapter 20). Human reversed allergic reactions also require a few hours of latency before they can be provoked. The reversed procedure is roughly equivalent to sensitization, because the latter depends on the presence of at least one active factor in the organism. Thus normal subjects into whom antigen is injected and sensitized subjects whose tissues contain antibody behave similarly in respect of the anaphylactic reaction. The effect of the antigen–antibody reaction is in certain cases reversible, in others irreversible.

Allergic conditions are either congenital or acquired by sensitization.

## CONGENITAL ALLERGY

Allergic diseases can occur from the very early infant age, but the critical period is the time of weaning. If allergic signs appear at the first encounter with antigen, the allergic reaction is very likely congenital or primary, because the subject had obviously no opportunity for previous contact with and sensitization by the antigen(s). But usually even the very first contact with the antigen cannot be precisely determined, or excluded. The infant may not have had a direct contact with the sensitizing agent, yet exposure may have occurred during foetal life through the maternal circulation, or later during lactation with the mother's milk. The mother lives on a mixed diet and may occasionally take medicaments; thus the access of minimal amounts of the allergizing substance may be sufficient to elicit sensitization by the placental route or through breast feeding.

## SENSITIZATION IN THE UTERUS

The possibility of this kind of sensitization was first observed in animal experiments [310*a*, *b*, 311]. The anaphylactic antibody (IgG) can pass from mother to foetus by the placental route, but it is not transferable by the paternal germ cells [284], whence it is not hereditary.

Both antigen and antibody can pass across the placental barrier; in the former case the sensitization is active, in the latter case it is passive; the state produced by active sensitization is of long duration, whereas the effects of passive sensitization last for a short time only, for several weeks at the most. The duration of passively transferred hypersensitivity varies with the species: e.g. in guinea pigs delivery of sensitive offspring was observed 383 days after sensitization. The young guinea pigs responded with a lethal anaphylactic shock to the first horse serum injection at 2 months of age. The offspring from the second litter of the same female guinea pig were also sensitive to horse serum [222*a*]. After two months, when the guinea pig mother still delivered sensitive offspring, no transferable antibodies could be demonstrated in the maternal serum [84], thus passive foetal sensitization was probably due to the release and placental transfer of fixed antibodies.

Active sensitization in the uterus of humans depends on the presence of maternal sensitization, while this is not necessarily in passive sensitization. Owing to the relative insufficiency of neonatal antibody forming capacity, the allergic reactions or immune state of infants depend chiefly on the passive, *in utero* transferable antibodies, because colostral transfer is negligible. There are, of course, exceptions; even the foetus can produce antibodies to certain antigens. The passage of certain large molecular substances across the placental barrier is facilitated by the circumstance that in humans, only a trilayered haemochorial membrane separates the foetal from maternal circulation and thus the epithelial cells of the chorion have a practically direct contact with the maternal blood [144]. (The membrane is only about 0.002 mm thick at birth [361].)

Nevertheless, the size of the antibody molecule, the anatomical structure of the barrier and simple filtration cannot in themselves account for impermeability to certain antibodies which varies even within the individual species. For instance, in man, staphylococcus-, streptococcus-, diphteria antitoxins, H-(flagellar) type typhoid agglutinins, etc. can pass across the barrier, but O-(somatic or endotoxin) type agglutinins cannot [339*a*, *b*]. The placenta is impermeable to certain substances of small molecular size. It is usually permeable to IgGs conferring immunity to infection upon the infant, to blocking and univalent Rh antibodies, LE factor, etc. [25, 417]. It has been speculated that those maternal IgGs enter into the foetus which pass from the maternal blood into the amniotic fluid [328] and the rest of IgGs are later synthesized by the baby itself. Since reagin could not be satisfactorily demonstrated, certain authors believe that immediate-type allergic diseases are chiefly due to active sensitization by the allergen in the uterus [323]. In certain cases skin reactions can be elicited very early in life, asthma or hay fever occur shortly after birth and the allergic state of the infant takes a longer time to cease compared with passively transferred hypersensitivity. The skin of human newborns accepts passively the atopic adult serum and responds positively to anti-IgE only at a later time (on average after 21.7 days). The time of conversion from negative to positive response varies widely and it is unrelated to the serum IgE level and to a hereditary atopic background. Breast-fed babies show the positive skin reaction later than those fed on cow's milk [372]. Nevertheless, immediate hypersensitivity occurs chiefly in cases of a bilateral familial predisposition [69].

The immunological relations of pregnant mother and developing foetus have not been studied until recently. It is, however, certain that apart from the histo-incompatibility antigens demonstrated in the ovum and in the developing trophoblast [174, 356], the foetus possesses mother-independent embryonic glomerular basement membrane antigens [341], foetal myoglobin [295], transferrin [288], haemoglobin F [161], IgG H-chain [406, 406*a*] and antigens originating from the embryonic digestive system [125]. Some of these antigens may even elicit a maternal immune response. Continuous migration of syncytial trophoblasts, and maternal immune response induced by them, have been demonstrated during pregnancy [172]. Against this, the antigenic function of trophoblasts has been disputed on the grounds that the negative charge of the mucopolysaccharide component of their sialomucin coat pushes the likewise negatively charged immunologically competent maternal lymphocytes [396]. Allotypic serum protein variants may act as antigens also in the foetal circulation and maternal anti-allotype antisera have been shown to suppress foetal immunoglobulin synthesis [165]. Maternal antibodies to foetal Gm antigens have been demonstrated in the haemolytic disease of newborn and anti-foetal maternal InV antibodies have been detected in congenital nephrosis [98, 120].

The majority of pregnancies are, nevertheless, uncomplicated. According to recent investigations, this is greatly due to a fibrinoid layer, above all to its sialic acid component, which separates foetal antigens from the potentially aggressive maternal lymphocytes like a barrier. Placental materno-foetal immune reactions could in fact be demonstrated by immunofluorescence in normal pregnancy. Deposits of IgG, IgE and occasionally of IgM have been detected in an area of fibrinoid necrosis of mature placenta and no IgM deposition has been found in placentas from premature births. The foetal or maternal origin of the IgG could not be clarified [249].

## SENSITIZATION WITH THE MOTHER'S MILK

Pure mother's milk cannot normally be regarded as an allergen [145]. Thus the immediate-type skin responses to egg and cow's milk of exclusively breast-fed eczematous infants had been attributed to a hereditary predisposition of spontaneous nature, because the mother or the lactating nurse had not been sensitive to egg or cow's milk. But such babies responded positively to mother's milk as well, suggesting that the latter may have contained traces at least of egg white or cow's milk; in certain cases, such phenomena can be regarded as evidence of a Prausnitz–Küstner (P–K) transfer [360]. These babies had probably become sensitized by the enteric route for infantile intestinal walls are permeable to certain large molecular weight proteins. If egg and cow's milk had been omitted from the diet of the mother, the urticariogenic effect of the mother's milk ceased.

Certain drugs causing skin eruptions in the infants and other allergen-like substances have also been demonstrated in mother's milk. Cow's milk may contain in addition to milk-protein antigens various food allergens, e.g. components of clover, alfalfa, hemp, ambrosia, etc. [321]. Such milk can elicit allergic symptoms, e.g. in persons sensitive to ambrosia.

If 'congenital' immediate-type allergic reactions are scrutinized on the basis of the foregoing considerations, almost all could be explained by sensitization acquired through contact with the antigen earlier in life, the more so as minimal doses are sufficient to induce hypersensitivity. The sensitizing doses are always considerably lower than those required to elicit allergic symptoms. It is, nevertheless, still unclear whether sensitization takes place by the diaplacentar route or through mother's milk. The former possibility seems doubtful in the light of the observation that if mothers are sensitized with an Ascaris extract during pregnancy, both the blood of the newborn, and cord blood failed to give a positive P–K reaction, as against the successful passive transfer of maternal blood [428*a*, *b*]. The same applies to certain delayed-type conditions. Newborn babies of women sensitized with dinitrochlorobenzene during pregnancy did not respond to the substance even at one week of age [78]. Similar experiments had negative results also in animals.

Intrauterine sensitization does not seem to take place easily, although there are examples of transplacental transfer of pathogenic antibody; such as the occurrence of chinin-induced thrombocytopenic purpura with *in vitro* thrombocyte agglutination in both mother and infant [247].

The first contact with the sensitizing agent is not less problematic in adults than in infants, for it is often unobserved ('cryptogenic allergy'). The same applies to microbial-viral sensitization as well as to drug antigens. A 'congenital' allergy cannot be reasonably postulated unless the symptoms are elicited by some new synthetic drug with which previous contact can be excluded. It has repeatedly been observed [323] in chemical plants that members of the staff handling new basic materials (sulphonamides, antibiotics, etc.) do not develop allergic dermatitis or other symptoms before 1–3 weeks of contact. The situation is often made even more complicated by cross- or group-sensitization due to chemical or immunological relationship. Chemically related substances may substitute one another in eliciting allergic symptoms if the subject is sensitive to any one compound of the group. Thus allergic reactions may occur to substances with which the subject had had no contact, due to exposure to a related compound.

Whether the immune response is due to cell-bound or humoral antibodies, it requires induction by antigen; a limited antigenic stimulus may already occur in foetal life but it becomes fully activated only after birth, as examplified by the germ-free animals, whose Ig-synthesis is retarded. The same applies to the blood group antibodies, which are not a maternal inheritance, because only the factors A and B arise early at 2–3 months of foetal life, antibodies against them (anti-A, anti-B), as antibody synthesis in general, do not appear until a few months after birth. According to Kabat [188] even isoantibody is a result of immunization, developing either unobserved, or in connection with latent infections, or on contact with A- and B-like substances, these being omnipresent in nature. On the other hand, already newborns (even premature babies) can successfully be immunized to smallpox, diphtheria and tuberculosis (BCG used as a vaccine), but the antibodies are formed at a slower rate and at a lower level than in older babies [237]. A more intensive antibody synthesis commences during the third month of life, with the appearance of plasma cells; at this age, reactivity to reinjection (secondary immune responses) is the same as in older babies. These findings suggest that the antibody forming system of the infant is not so much anatomically as functionally underdeveloped. In animals, neonatal immunological reactivity varies with the species: newborn guinea pigs are immediately capable of response, while rabbits do not normally react until 15 days of age [114*a*]. Under appropriate conditions, sheep may develop a secondary immune response to brucellae already in the uterus [316].

Despite the foregoing examples, tolerance to antigen-like substances is generally acquired during foetal life and immunological tolerance also develops to substances entering the body in foetal or early postnatal life; this tolerance then persists during later life. Foetal immunological tolerance gradually gives way to postnatal immune reactivity after birth. This immunologically important turning point takes 1–4 weeks in the case of the human infant (see Chapter 16).

The appearance of self-synthesized antibodies does not in itself signify a clinical allergic process. If, after sensitization, the specific antigen is either not encountered again, or gets there in an insufficient amount, the allergic reactivity may either remain unobserved, or it is detected only by chance, during experimental study. Bloch [34*a*] has characterized subjects with latent allergy as 'potentially allergic'. Latent allergy of this kind occurs fairly frequently, especially to environmental allergens, the number of which is extremely high.

## HEREDITARY FACTORS

Previous sensitization may well be postulated also in atopic allergy, although the mechanism of 'spontaneous sensitization' has not yet been elucidated. Probably hereditary factors play an important, although not decisive role in the pathomechanism. Such factors are not easily identified; the following approaches may be elucidative:

1. *Statistical data.* These indicate a considerable fluctuation of the frequency of allergic diseases in a mixed population. The percentage of hereditary spontaneous—atopic—allergy has generally been assessed as 7–10 per cent, or 15–20 per cent, if all allergic diseases and identified cases of potential allergy are included [397]. The incidence may abruptly rise if exposure to the appropriate allergen occurs in an occupational group of the population, e.g. in certain industrial plants. The frequent occurrence of flour-induced respiratory allergy among bakery workers is well known [304].

Statistical evaluation of sex distribution has shown a considerably higher incidence of Hymenoptera allergy among teenage males than among females of the same age group. Young boys spend much more time outdoors than girls. No such environment-related difference was, however, found between boy and girl scouts aged 11–16 years: the incidence of allergy to bee-sting was roughly uniform, 0.40 and 0.35 per cent, respectively [2, 55, 178]. The sera of rabbits immunized to insect bites showed different antigen and antibody systems in passive cutaneous anaphylaxis (PCA), haemagglutination and gel precipitation tests; similar observations have been made on passive transfer of human sera [19].

The incidence of allergic diseases tends to rise up to a certain age, because different new sites of sensitization may arise during lifetime. The incidence of allergy tends to decline in advanced age, although the absolute number of cases shows a rising tendency in parallel with the increasing level of civilization and organization of society: the widespread use of drugs, increase of occupational exposure, introduction of new chemicals (e.g. plastics, synthetic resins, etc.) may all become sources of allergic diseases. Also, advances in allergology have enabled the detection of a greater number of such conditions, above all of autoallergic diseases. No constitutional, intellectual or characterologic differences have been observed between allergic and non-allergic subjects [143].

2. *Heredity phylogenetic studies.* These have shown that neither the specificity of allergy, nor the type of reaction are inherited, only the predisposition for allergic disease. Namely, the incidence of allergic diseases is higher in the family of allergic parents compared with the descendants of non-allergic individuals. If both parents are allergic, the disease is manifested earlier (or probably detected earlier) in the next generation. The type of inheritance is irregular and not yet elucidated. Predisposition is usually unrelated to constitution, although certain workers held the view that chiefly leptosomal types with pycnic traits are predisposed to allergy [88]. Constitutional factors may be held responsible for atopic allergic diseases and for sensitivity to certain chemical substances if sensitivity to drug, or an allergic disease occur in a family through several generations [150]. Hereditary predisposition has also been observed in animals, e.g. in strains of guinea pigs, which can easily be sensitized with certain chemical substances, whereas other strains do not respond to the same agent [182].

3. *Comparative studies of monozygotic and dizygotic twins* also indicate that not so much the allergic disease itself is hereditary, as the predisposition for it, although monozygotic twins usually suffer from the same allergic disease (e.g. bronchial asthma), occasionally over several generations, suggesting the role of genetic factors [58]. Against this, heredity could be demonstrated in only 50 per cent of the monozygotic twins with atopic dermatitis [307]. Kämmerer [198] used the term allergic diathesis for the designation of a continuous predisposition with a special allergic trend.

It is clear from studies on 7,000 pairs of twins that allergic diseases have both environmental and hereditary components, but environmental factors play a considerably greater role than originally supposed. This was shown by the low concordance rates in the monozygotic twin group (25.3 per cent) and in the dizygotic group (16.1 per cent). Because of the high prevalence rate of allergic disease (asthma, hay fever or eczema) in the general population (18 per cent) and the low penetrance (40 per cent), the distinction between recessive, dominant and multigenic inheritance could not be made. Most allergic children were born in families in which neither parent (67 per cent) or only one parent (30 per cent) had allergy. The risk of the birth of an allergic child to such couples varies between 0.14–0.29. In the group in which both parents had been allergic, the risk rose only to 0.33–0.40 [92]. Extensive studies on monozygotic twins affected by asthma have shown that along with a genetical identity, there are considerable clinical, physiological and biochemical differences apparent and the allergic manifestations are also dissimilar [97].

The difference between hereditary atopic allergy and acquired hypersensitivity is not easily determined. An important distinguishing trait is that spontaneous atopic allergy unlike acquired allergic diseases, cannot be induced artificially. Allergy is, in fact, acquired in both types, because also 'spontaneous' allergy depends on a previous contact with the antigen, but the mechanism of sensitization in hereditary atopic allergy is not known.

## ACQUIRED ALLERGY. ARTIFICIAL SENSITIZATION

The virtual gap between hereditary atopic allergy and allergy acquired by sensitization is to a certain extent spanned by artificial sensitization experiments, because nearly any human or animal subject can be rendered sensitive with antigens of appropriate purity and concentration and with appropriate techniques [34*b*, 222*c*]. Genetic factors may, however, also play a role under experimental conditions [303], because there are exceptions to the general rules of sensitization, and responsiveness to passive transfer of the P–K reaction varies individually (positive and negative reactors). The rate of sensitization depends on the nature of the sensitizing agent. The susceptibility of guinea pigs to anaphylaxis varies not only with the strain, but also with age and season. Strains of guinea pigs genetically sensitive or non-sensitive to chemical mediators have been established; the sensitive strains show much more severe reactions to egg albumen than non-sensitive ones in both active and passive anaphylaxis [386]. Accordingly, an organism with an average reactivity can regularly be sensitized with certain substances, whereas with others only slowly or occasionally. If it is postulated, in terms of the clonal selection theory, that the normal individual possesses a preformed antibody producing capacity in the immunologically competent cells, it seems probable that the aforementioned variations of sensitivity may be explained either with the disturbance, impairment or pathological alteration of the immunological system, or with the chemical structure of the antigen, or with non-specific factors in the neuroendocrine, or autonomic nervous systems, etc. The best sensitizing agents are those which are able to irritate normal skin or mucous membrane and pass easily across the barrier formed by the horny layer. On intradermal application, the sensitizing substance induces, as a rule, delayed-type reaction, which is the prototype of hypersensitivity due to parenteral sensitization. Immediate-type urticarial hypersensitivity is less frequent, and is usually related to protein sensitization. In addition to local sensitization, also a general response may occur manifested by extensive eruptions and systemic symptoms apart from the local reaction.

## FACTORS OF ARTIFICIAL SENSITIZATION

Sensitization can usually be carried out with success using (*i*) proteins or protein containing dissolved substances; (*ii*) pathogenic microorganisms, fungi or viruses in live or killed state; (*iii*) certain low molecular weight substances with known chemical structure, either alone—if 'strong' antigen—or—if 'weak' antigen e.g. hapten—bound to a carrier protein, or with an adjuvant substance. If the sensitizing antigen is applied intradermally, previous conjugation with a carrier substance, e.g. serum, is not necessary, because appropriate carriers are available in the organism to render the antigen complete for sensitization; (*iv*) antigen–antibody complexes; (*v*) autoantigen containing self-substances if these are sequestered (inaccessible), or even accessible substances if there is a structural change. The above substances are active in themselves, but the complete Freund's adjuvant increases their sensitizing effect.

Factors playing a role in artificial sensitization are discussed in the following.

### *The technique applied*

The easiest technique is the painting of the skin, but for this only very active agents having a primary irritative or tanning effect on the skin in high concentrations and able to form large molecular conjugated antigen are suitable [248*c*]. Agents belonging to this group are primin, the juice of various rhus species, formaldehyde, turpentine, mustard oil, Hg compounds, dinitrochlorobenzene (DNCB), etc., all of which display maximum activity on epicutaneous application [80]. Intradermal administration is also effective, while subcutaneous application is less so; intramuscular and intravenous injection even of the most commonly used agent, DNCB fails to elicit sensitization. It is still unclear why the participation of the epithelium is indispensable for cutaneous sensitization by simple chemical substances. It has been established experimentally that if the sensitizing agent has been conjugated *in vitro* with epithelium, it can both sensitize the skin (positive epicutaneous test) and elicit a delayed-type cutaneous response on intracutaneous application [213]. On the other hand, upon combination with various body proteins (serum protein, erythrocyte) or with azoprotein the same agent does not induce skin hypersensitivity, only anaphylaxis-type reactions. The skin as a site of application is nevertheless not exclusive, because delayed-type skin reaction can be induced by intraperitoneal application of the antigen, if the latter is combined with an immunological adjuvant [220]. Raffel's hard wax (peptido-glycolipid) fraction of Mycobacteria is an adjuvant of this kind; this is the reason why Mycobacteria have been included into the complete Freund's adjuvant. Without this component the latter can only raise the humoral antibody level, but does not bring about a delayed-type response. The mechanism of action of the adjuvant is not fully understood; recently it has been shown to enhance the antibody forming capacity of certain cells [212]. Probably the mycobacterial lipid component of Freund's adjuvant completes the antigen in a certain manner and promotes delayed-type hypersensitivity through stimulation of the immunologically activated lymphocytes [248*c*]. The complex role of the complete Freund's adjuvant in immune response is also indicated by the phenomenon that pretreatment with the adjuvant depresses the delayed-type skin reaction which is otherwise the usual consequence of immunization with antigen + Freund's adjuvant [8*a*, *b*, 14]. The suppressive effect of the previously administered Freund's adjuvant is explicable, at least in part, by the anti-inflammatory effect of pretreatment.

Proteins and protein containing mixtures are effective both intracutaneously and subcutaneously; often a single injection is sufficient. Animals can be sensitized by the inhalatory route if the spray is fine enough [191]. Both epicutaneous and cutaneous-intracutaneous sensitization can be facilitated by making use of the depot-effect i.e. by applying the entire sensitizing dose to the same site; in this manner even substances which normally have a weak or no sensitizing effect can be rendered effective.

### *Chemical composition of the sensitizing agent*

Certain substances are 'good', while others 'bad' sensitizers, depending probably on their chemical structure. Hydro-aromatic benzene compounds sensitize more easily than aliphatic or simple aromatic compounds. Addition of amino-, nitro-, oxy- or carboxyl radicals may increase the sensitizing capacity, especially in a given structural configuration, e.g. the para-position. Addition of halogens, e.g. of chlorine, can enhance sensitization still further. DNCB is one of the most active sensitizers. Addition of other elements, e.g. sulphur, reduces rather than enhances the sensitizing capacity. The latter may be closely related with the presence of a labile exchangeable group [219]. In the case of depot treatment, sensitization occurs first in the depot area, spreading therefrom over the entire body in a shorter or longer time [248*a*]. Irritated, inflammed or injured skin (due to alkaline compounds, soap, cement, microtraumata, etc.) is more easily sensitized than normal skin, as affirmed by many practical observations and animal experiments: skin areas pretreated with detergents, soaps, acetone, etc. responded more intensively than normal skin to various concentrations of DNCB in both man and guinea pig [359].

### *Quantity and concentration of the sensitizing agent*

Sensitization requires a given amount in a given concentration of the agent, the decisive factor being the effective amount of antigen. There is a threshold value for each agent, below which hypersensitivity cannot be induced. Sensitization is either done with one large dose or with several small doses adding up to the threshold in due course. For instance, the quantitative requirements and threshold concentration(s) of DNCB sensitization have been determined by Nilzén [277]. The sensitizing capacity of mixed substances, e.g. plant extracts, depend upon the concentration of the active ingredient in them. The extract of primula e.g. had been concentrated until pure primin (a benzoquinone derivative) was obtained, which can sensitize the skin of any subject [35*a*, *b*]. Epicutaneous sensitization further depends on the size of the skin area into which the agent is rubbed [117], but the area is not decisive in itself if the required concentration is not attained. It is generally recommended to use precise quantitative methods.

The factors listed above may ensure sensitization either in themselves, or in combination. A combined effect may result e.g. in delayed hypersensitivity induced by intradermal injection of minimal amounts (1–2 $\mu$g) of protein antigens (diphtheria toxoid, ovalbumin) in the form of an insoluble precipitated antigen–antibody complex, if the corresponding antigen is present in excess [395]. A long-lasting delayed hypersensitivity develops first and humoral antibodies appear only later. Probably many other, partly unknown factors (actual state of body, especially of the skin, neuroendocrine factors, autonomic nervous system, etc.), but above all the normal or abnormal state of the immune system do also influence sensitization [320]. If there is an immunological deficiency state, sensitization is reduced or even impossible, depending on the partial or complete absence of humoral antibody formation (agammaglobulinaemia, hypogammaglobulinaemia, etc.) or a deficiency of cell-mediated immunity of lymphoid tissues (e.g. combined immunodeficiency syndrome) [96].

## ARTIFICIAL SENSITIZATION WITH DIFFERENT ANTIGENS

### *Sensitization with serum and food*

Artificial sensitization can as a rule easily be achieved with proteins or protein-like substances. Such sensitizing agents are possibly pure, probably crystalline serum protein fractions, egg albumen, etc. Basic proteins are, however, generally weakly immunogenic [72, 224]. The first example of artificial protein allergy was the experimental anaphylaxis of the guinea pig, offering an explanation of the serum sensitivity of humans. Experiments with daily intracutaneous serum injections have shown that hypersensitivity is usually manifested after 5–7 days, first in the form of delayed hypersensitivity, later by immediate-type reaction, which increases up to 14 days, then tends to decline [388*a*, *b*]. A single parenteral dose may be sufficient for sensitization, but in such cases the response takes 2–3 weeks to develop and does not disappear until after several months. A certain amount of fixed antibody, or at least an increased capability for antibody production may, however, persist, depending on the species of the serum donor having stronger or weaker sensitizing capacity. Reinjection within a certain period elicits a secondary response, characterized by the earlier onset and accelerated rate of antibody synthesis (booster effect). Later readministration restores the synthesis of antibody by an anamnestic reaction. Intramuscular injection of serum elicits intensive and long-lasting hypersensitivity. Application of blood serum to the same site of rabbit's ear over a long period causes apart from inflammatory infiltration also hyperkeratosis and papillomatosis as manifestations of the local anaphylactic reaction (Reuterwall phenomenon) [315]. If bovine serum albumin is administered on the same schedule, also vesicles and pustules will develop [152].

Hypersensitivity to protein can also be induced through the digestive tract. Although the digestive system can normally destroy foreign substances, above all proteins, functional insufficiency or inflammatory alteration of the system itself and of its glands results in an inadequate degradation and the undecomposed proteins act as antigens on reabsorption. Vitamin deficiency states, inflammations, injury and ulcer make the absorption of native protein and polysaccharide antigens possible by increasing the permeability of the digestive tract. Under certain conditions, guinea pigs can be sensitized with horse serum even by the oral route [323], but the same serum has no sensitizing effect when administered into normal bladder or urethral mucosa [332]. Rabbits immunized orally with bovine serum albumin (BSA) produce humoral antibodies without requiring an immunogenic blood level of BSA [77*a*, *b*]. A similar local immune response has also been observed in hamsters. These findings suggest that during oral immunization, the antigen reactive cells became localized in the well-associated lymphoid tissue [132].

Apart from serum, egg and milk have also been used in most sensitization experiments. Like serum, ovalbumin elicits first a delayed-type, then an immediate-type reaction with a positive P–K transfer when administered daily by intradermal route [338*a*, *b*]. Recrystallized ovalbumin also induces first delayed hypersensitivity transferable with lymphocytes, then an Arthrus-type reaction with humoral antibody formation, when injected into the foot pad of the guinea pig along with Freund's adjuvant [76, 189]. Sensitization of a normal subject can be carried out generally in the above sequence with plant proteins, insect bite or Ascaris extract [111]. If the antigen dose is not high enough, no humoral antibody formation will follow the delayed hypersensitivity, but the antibodies will appear on reinjection [333]. Using the depot technique, the area of the injection site will become sensitive first, already after the third intracutaneous injection (ovalbumin and milk experiments), but a generalized response will follow soon. Focal reactions, such as flare-up of former injection sites, are not infrequent.

The sensitization course in which the delayed-type reaction takes place first and the plasmacytic phasis, including the appearance of plasma cells and humoral antibodies only next, has been regarded by Dienes [79] as a general rule and as characteristic of protein sensitization. The same is indicated by the Jones–Mote reaction (see page 473). It is still disputed whether delayed hypersensitivity and antibody formation each represent a different immune response to one and the same antigen, or only the different phases of the same immune process. The theory that they are in fact two processes which may or may not be coexistent is more probable, because either can occur independently in various clinical and experimental conditions. On the other hand, consideration should be given to the fact that immunolymphocytes or lymphoblasts transforming under the influence of the antigen may develop to plasmablasts or plasma cells, thus making the synthesis of antibody possible.

### *Sensitization with microorganisms or viruses and their extracts*

Sensitization with live virulent or attenuated viruses of microorganisms used as a vaccine (BCG-, smallpox-, poliomyelitis-vaccination, etc.) takes place according to the norms of spontaneous infection.

The viruses impair the cells in two ways during infection. Above all the virus may in itself cause cell destruction. On the other hand, viruses may stimulate in the host an anti-viral immune response, whose products may damage the cells through reacting with the virus or virus-induced antigen fixed to the cell surface. Since infected cells are specifically eliminated, immunologically mediated damage is usually favourable for the host, but may become hazardous as well in the case of excessive cell destruction. Tissue damage is immunologically mediated in lymphocytic choriomeningitis [280*a*]. The precise role of humoral antibodies and/or sensitized cells is nevertheless not known. In mumps and lymphocytic choriomeningitis, virus infected cells are damaged by anti-viral antibodies in the presence of the complement (C) effector system [280*c*]. At the neutralization of herpes virus, C causes immunocytolysis [404]. According to other authors, accumulation of C on the surface of sensitized virus particles renders them inactive [74]. Immune complex processes have been shown to play a role in infections caused by lactic dehydrogenase virus, Moloney sarcoma virus, Coxsackie B-virus, etc. [279, 280*b*]. Trachoma-inclusion conjunctivitis and lymphogranuloma venereum organisms are closely related [406*a*].

Sensitization with killed microbes and their extracts is a more intricate process. It is not easy to induce bacterial anaphylaxis in animals, because bacterial suspension or extracts may develop a primary toxic action, above all on intravenous administration, and there is scarcely any difference between the toxic and the anaphylactic shock inducing doses [270]. Sensitization with microbial or fungal extracts (old tuberculin, trichophytin, etc.) was likewise unsuccessful. Dissolved bacterial proteins (tuberculoprotein, etc.) can only induce immediate hypersensitivity accompanied by humoral antibody formation, which can be elicited in guinea pigs not only with the protein-, but also with the polysaccharide ($\alpha$-haemosensitin) component [40]. A double diffusion precipitation test has recently been elaborated which makes it possible to determine quantitatively in the serum of most human subjects the specific antibodies formed against the carbohydrate component of group A streptococci [427]. Various special techniques applied, such as the depot technique [222*b*]; tuberculin adsorbed onto sheep erythrocytes [338*b*]; pretreatment of skin with acids or bases [59*b*], etc., failed to enhance sensitization with bacterial or fungal extracts.

### *Sensitization by chemical substances of known structure*

Sensitization with certain simple, chemically defined small molecular compounds (mol. wt. $< 1{,}000$) usually requires previous conjugation of the compound with a large-molecular carrier substance, above all with protein. Such conjugates, in which the species specificity of the original protein is markedly reduced, are known as chemospecific antigens, whereas the small molecular chemical substances which require protein support for sensitizing action, as haptens (*Halbantigens*). The association of hapten + protein antigen has been called by Forssman complete antigen.

Hapten is characterized by a lack of sensitizing ability if applied in itself, but can specifically combine with antibody, thus being the carrier of immunological specificity. The importance of hapten has been affirmed by Avery and Goebel's experiment [16] in which the binding of two different carbohydrates to one and the same protein resulted in immunologically different combinations, whereas binding of the same carbohydrate to different proteins in immunologically identical conjugates.

The effect of the carrier is, nevertheless, often decisive. It has been demonstrated by means of 2,4-dinitrophenylovalbumin that the transfer of immunologically competent lymphoid cells from inbred guinea pigs to allogeneic hosts activates the antibody forming cell precursors of the host through a specific immunologic attack of donor cells (so-called allogeneic phenomenon) [197]. On the other hand, immunization with 2,4-dinitrophenyl–Ascaris conjugate resulted in the formation of both dinitrophenyl-specific and carrier-specific antibodies. On application of a 2,4-dinitrophenyl–Ascaris conjugate, the titres of both the hapten and carrier specific antibodies will be significantly higher than on immunization with 2,4-dinitrophenylhaemocyanine or 2,4-dinitrophenylbovine-$\gamma$-globulin conjugates [375]. For further information on the carrier effect, see p. 473. Recent experiments with L-tyrosine-azobenzenearsonate and poly-$\gamma$-D-glutamic acid have even shown that the antigen reactive cells of the guinea pig recognize the former, about 400 mol. wt. substance, which acts as a carrier of poly-D-$\gamma$-glutamic acid (35,000 mol. wt. !), playing the role of the hapten [7].

The hapten role of the various substances varies with the species of the animal; e.g. the capsular polysaccharide component of Streptococcus pneumoniae acts on rabbits as a hapten, while in humans it occasionally acts as a complete antigen, indicating that certain polysaccharides are capable of sensitizing in themselves (e.g. the polysaccharides of pneumococci and certain helminths) [52, 390]. Type specific pneumococcal polysaccharides have therefore generally been regarded as weakly immunogenic substances. The anti-type-specific-polysaccharide response can, however, be augmented if the animal is preimmunized with the non-conjugated carrier molecule [292]. A surprisingly intensive anamnestic response is obtained if the rabbits are pretreated with type III pneumococci as the primary antigenic stimulus, then immunized with bovine $\gamma$-globulin and finally given the covalent conjugate of type specific polysaccharide + bovine $\gamma$-globulin [291]. The evolution of the immune response to types III and VIII pneumococcal polysaccharides has been examined by Chen et al. [60*a*].

Binding of the hapten to protein was formerly regarded as indispensable for sensitization, as judged from the formation of humoral antibodies on provocation with the hapten, and delayed hypersensitivity on provocation with the carrier to simple chemical substances (Hg, Cr, formaldehyde, etc.) can be elicited by a single intradermal injection, if the chemical agent has previously been mixed with horse serum [157*a*, *b*]. In this procedure, which probably rests on an antigenic cooperation, sensitization can only be induced with proteins or other antigens as accompanying substances. In such cases, as well as with certain hapten + protein bonds, also the carrier protein plays an active role in sensitization as the humoral antibodies produced against the conjugate are also directed against the protein component [95, 399*a*, *b*].

DNA-reactive antibodies can be induced by coupling purines, pyrimidine bases, nucleosides, oligonucleosides or polynucleotides with proteins or synthetic peptides, using the conjugate thus formed for immunization [302*a*, *b*]. The antibodies arising in response are specific for the hapten and cross-reactive, without being specific for the nucleic acid applied. Nucleic acid-specific antibodies can only be stimulated by immunization with phage DNA [226], because such DNA-preparations contain a unique pyrimidin base. Thus the high specificity of anti-protein and anti-polysaccharide antibodies is generally not characteristic of anti-nucleic-acid antibodies.

The role of the secondary structure of polynucleotides in immunochemical reactions can, however, clearly be seen if immunization is carried out with synthetic polynucleotide complexes adsorbed to methylated bovine serum albumin [340]. Polyguanylic (Poly-G) or polycytidylic (Poly-C) acid complexes adsorbed onto methylated bovine serum albumin induce a kind of antibody which reacts exclusively with ribosomal RNA from animal cells and with RNA from certain viruses, thus being able to distinguish not only between rRNA and tRNA, but also between viral and host RNAs. Such antibodies have failed to react with DNA [256, 271]. Recently, evidence has accumulated suggesting that simple, synthetic polyribonucleotides, especially polyinosinic-polycytidylic acid, can elicit an antibody response in the absence of carrier protein or adjuvant [100*a*, 287*a*].

The sensitizing agents find the complementary protein also in the body itself, especially in case of a preceding or simultaneous skin damage, which enables the release of certain supporter substances. Even chemical sensitization is usually followed first by tuberculin-type or contact-type delayed hypersensitivity and humoral antibodies appear only later, as can be seen from experimental protein sensitization. Contact sensitivity may persist after the appearance of humoral antibodies and Arthus reaction [60]. The observations collected by the above methods have contributed to the understanding of the fundamental mechanism of certain allergic diseases, especially of drug allergy. Experiments with synthetic polypeptide antigens have furthermore affirmed that the genetic control of immune response rests on a cellular basis [350*a*, *b*].

## SENSITIZATION WITH ANTIGEN–ANTIBODY COMPLEXES

Antigen–antibody complexes (also called immune complexes) are particularly suitable for sensitization; usually two types are distinguished:

1. Soluble complexes formed in antigen excess.
2. Insoluble complexes formed in antibody excess.

Soluble antigen–antibody complexes give rise to immediate hypersensitivity; they play an important role in pathophysiological processes of humans and in various natural and experimentally induced diseases of animals [62, 218]. Both the RES and various catabolitic processes can eliminate the soluble antigen–antibody complexes from the circulation *in vivo*. It has been demonstrated by quantitative methods that the RES takes up larger complexes more rapidly than smaller ones forming in conditions of a greater antigen excess. *In vitro* studies have shown that both blood monocytes and fixed macrophages possess receptors for both IgG and C3 [171]. Treatment of normal rabbits with soluble immune complexes prepared from IgG-antibodies of intact rabbits can be characterized by a triphasic exponential elimination curve. Those complexes which leave the circulation in the early, rapid phase, are larger than the rest and fix complement avidly [240]. Reduction and alkylation of antibodies are then followed by disappearance or notable reduction of the rapid elimination phase and the larger complexes fail to fix complement.

According to more recent quantitative studies on normal and C-depleted rabbits, immune complexes which are rapidly eliminated from the circulation are chiefly fixed in the liver, and less than 1 per cent of them is found in the lung, kidneys or spleen. The distribution of the complexes in various tissues remains unaltered in C-depleted rabbits. Complexes prepared with reduced and alkylated antibodies fix C ineffectively. Circulating C components do not mediate the *in vivo* interaction between fixed macrophages and IgG antibodies of the soluble antigen–antibody complex. Against this, it has been concluded from Waldenström's macroglobulin studies that the *in vivo* interaction of macrophages and IgM is C3 dependent. The complexes taken up by the RES during the rapid phase contain more than two IgG molecules. The rapidly eliminated complexes fix C markedly *in vitro* although their *in vivo* uptake by the RES is not C-dependent [13].

Treatment of normal guinea pigs with antigen–antibody complex can elicit asthma-like symptoms [126]; i.v. injection of the complex into mice and rats frequently causes serum-sickness-like symptoms, above all glomerulonephritis [27]. Formerly, the deposition of the antigen–antibody complexes in the tissues had been attributed to a vascular permeability increase [64]; pretreatment of rabbits with histamine did, however, not alter the uptake of the soluble complexes by the tissues [13]. In experimental acute immune complex glomerulonephritis, only a very small amount (less than 1 per cent) of antigen was demonstrated in the kidney in the form of an immune complex; it therefore remains to be clarified how such small amounts of immune complex can cause tissue damage [419].

Serum sickness, on the other hand, has been regarded as an example of the soluble antigen–antibody complex effect. Ado [4] observed that lung and bronchi from guinea pigs sensitized with different antigens responded promptly by an anaphylactic contraction to direct stimulation. The effect of the antigen–antibody complex is unrelated to passive sensitization, being 'toxic' in itself [181].

Application of an antibody-coated collagenous biopolymer membrane has shown that such a model can well explain the accumulation of neutrophils, which then enables the release of various inflammatory mediators and lysosomal enzymes [156]. Neutrophils are generally regarded as essential mediators of immune complex induced tissue damage [164]. If antigen–antibody complex is deposited on a non-phagocytic surface, the exterior of the cell will become degranulated. If the complex becomes phagocyted, degranulation takes place inside the phagocytic vacuoles and enzymes gain access to the surrounding medium. Neutrophils attracted to the site of deposition of the immune complex may liberate proteases, collagenases, elastases as well as permeability factors. It has been shown that human neutrophils exposed to immune complexes release lysosomal enzymes ($\beta$-glucuronidase, acid phosphatase), but no lactate dehydrogenase. Agents capable of elevating the level of cyclic AMP and cyclic cellular AMP (theophyllines, prostaglandin, 2-chloroadenosine) inhibit the selective release of acid hydrolases from the leukocytes [409].

Insoluble antigen–antibody complexes, i.e. precipitates in which the antigen part is protein, induce in conditions of antibody excess first delayed hypersensitivity which is followed much latter by an immediate-type response, including circulating antibody formation. Thus this process is analogous with the usual course of protein sensitization with the difference that—depending on the quantity of the antigen–antibody complex—the initial delayed-type phase lasts much longer, 3–4 weeks or more in guinea pigs treated with 1–2 μg or in humans treated with 50 μg (children with 5 μg). This prolongation of the delayed phase facilitates the study of delayed sensitization [395]. The use of Freund's adjuvant may even enhance the effect.

According to Najjar [272], at the encounter of antigen with antibody, i.e. at the formation of an antigen–antibody complex, both components may undergo a change: new antigenic determinants may arise on the antigen molecule against which structure-specific antibodies may form; the formation of new groups may alter the antibody, too, giving rise to antibody production against these groups. Such antibodies are, in fact, autoantibodies (anti-antibodies). This is also supported by the observation that the antibodies formed in rabbits on immunization with antigen–antibody complex occasionally react only with the complex, more precisely, with its antibody component, but not with the antigen.

## AUTOSENSITIZATION. SENSITIZATION WITH AUTOANTIGENS (SELF ANTIGENS)

Normally the organism's own substances have no antigenic effect, although many of them are antigen-like (Ehrlich's horror autotoxicus). The immunological tolerance developing to *accessible* substances in foetal life persists postnatally. Exceptions to this rule are the *inaccessible* (sequestered) substances (e.g. thyroglobulin, lenticular substance, brain-tissue, etc.) which, having no proper communication with lymph or blood circulation, cannot come into contact with the antibody-forming lymphatic system. Accordingly, no immunological tolerance develops to such substances during prenatal life, whence they can postnatally behave as autoantigens, especially if they become released into the lymph or blood stream in consequence of a pathologic process, inflammation or surgical intervention. But even accessible self substances may become antigenic if undergoing certain changes (e.g. separation of serum from plasma, extravasation of red blood cells into tissues, cellular disintegration, etc.). Similarly, proteins and other high molecular weight constituents of various self substances, e.g. formed elements of the blood, organs (kidney, nerve system, skin, etc.) may be rendered antigenic by various infections, pathological conditions or drugs. It should be noted that the autoantigens playing a role in several autoallergic processes have not yet been fully identified. The qualitative and quantitative changes required to transform a self substance into an autoantigen are not easily understood; observations, nevertheless, suggest that minimal effects may be able to elicit such an alteration as it does not interfere with the physiological function of the affected tissue. This preservation of function is probably due to the fact that antigenic function and physiological function are associated with different determinant groups. As already mentioned in the foregoing, microbial substances, drugs and chemicals form by binding or adsorption to body materials a complete (conjugated) antigen of which the autologous substance is a component. In this kind of complete antigen, the autologous substance may play the role of either hapten or carrier.

Conditions in which both the autologous protein and the exogenous antigen play a functional role have been designated as partial autoimmune reactions [258*a*, *b*]. For instance, guinea pigs sensitized with picrylated homologous thyroglobulin do not show a delayed-type reaction unless the partial antigens are administered into the skin together in a conjugated form [259]. A partial autoantibody may also arise when antibodies are produced against the chemical hapten factor, as e.g. in various forms of contact eczema, in which a given skin protein participates in the process as a partial incomplete antigen, resulting in delayed-type partial autosensitization. In all such processes the tissue change caused by infection, disease or drug, etc. is the primary phase during which the autoantigen is formed, and autoantibodies appear relatively late; the antibodies then give rise to a secondary tissue damage leading to a kind of a vicious circle. Under such conditions the autoantibody plays the role of a synergistic agent rather than of the primary pathogenic factor [399*a*, *b*].

## THE ROLE OF AUTOANTIBODY. PHASES OF AUTOSENSITIZATION

The criterion of regarding an antibody as autoantibody is the antibody induced impairment of an organ of the host. Some authors have attributed a pathogenic role to autoantibody in certain autoallergic diseases (e.g. immunohaematological conditions), while others have regarded it only as an accompanying phenomenon of auto-allergization [163]. The prerequisite of autoantibody action is the loss of immunological tolerance [399*f*]. Autoerythrocytic, autoleukocytic and autothrombocytic autoantibodies are good examples of the pathogenic autoantibody. Autoantibodies are not easily accessible by serological methods and therefore less thoroughly known. Autoantigen is poorly defineable not only because of its complex nature, but also because—apart from some exceptions (e.g. thyroglobulin, intrinsic factor)—tissue- and cell-extracts have many antigen-like components, tissue antigens, in addition to the organ-specific antigen.

The formation of autoantigens and autoantibodies can generally be regarded as a triphasic process: (*i*) an accessible antigen-like substance becomes modified inside the body (modification phase); (*ii*) antibodies are formed which are able to react not only with the modified antigen, but also with the unmodified 'antigen' components (autoantibody formation phase); (*iii*) the autoantibodies react with the autoantigen causing tissue damage (phase of clinical manifestations). The concept that the autoantibodies stimulated by the modified autoantigen can also react with unmodified self substances has little evidence in support. According to Burnet and Holmes [46*a*, *b*, 47], the minimal difference existing between structurally related antigens, e.g. between foreign and self erythrocytes behaving and not behaving as an antigen, respectively, probably depend on a very limited number of determinants. This minimal difference should, however, be sufficient for the protection of self substances, by virtue of some homeostatic inhibitory mechanism. In this light it does not seem probable that the autoantibodies induced by the modified antigen could act against the unmodified antigen. Experience, nevertheless, suggests that altered and unaltered substances have certain antigenic determinants in common, which enable cross-reactions. As already mentioned, induction of autoantibodies by inaccessible (sequestered) autoantigens can probably take place if the latter come into contact with the antibody forming lymphoid system in consequence of trauma, surgery, infectious inflammation, permeability increase or some other abnormal condition.

The earliest known example of autoantigen formation is the pathogenetically unimportant process of the autoantibody (autoantilipids) formation against the autoantigen under the influence of *Treponema pallidum* from self phospholipids. Actually, the pseudopositive Wassermann reaction is also an autoimmune phenomenon. It has been demonstrated that self proteins and polysaccharides may also become autoantigens under similar conditions, e.g. under the influence of β-haemolytic streptococci [130].

The pathomechanism outlined above has been affirmed by autosensitization experiments. The difference between artificial and spontaneous or treatment induced autosensitization processes may be blurred to a great extent. The earlier observation that tissue constituents may behave as autoantigens without evidence of infectious, toxic or other influence, i.e. independently of exogenous factors, has received support from the frequent finding of positive serological (haemagglutination) reactions [207*a*] in atherosclerosis, cardiac infarction, cerebral embolism, although autoantibody formation was occasionally associated with the reparative inflammation even in such conditions. Conjugated complete antigens may also arise from chemically defined self substances, e.g. hormones or vitamins, which then play the role of the hapten, with a self or exogenous protein as the carrier.

Autoantibodies act chiefly against those pathologic self antigens (composite autoantigens) which have been responsible for their formation, or against certain components of the latter, but they may also attack unaltered parts of the cell (cytotoxic effect) due to the presence of common antigenic determinants. This is the direct mechanism of autoimmune reaction. We speak of an indirect mechanism if the reacting autoantibody is adsorbed onto the cell, chiefly erythrocytes, if the antigen is a cell-fixed virus or drug. Evidence of organ-specific or tissue-specific autoantibody action has been obtained from the inhibitory effect of autoantibodies on appropriate cell culture [184]. Since usually homologous organs or tissues are used for experimental study, the *in vitro* demonstrable antibodies formed against them are in fact always homologous 'autoantibodies'—isoantibodies—which, unlike the autologous formed elements of blood routinely used in immunohaematology, do not fully correspond to the originally altered organ. Pfeiffer [298] has termed the *in vitro* demonstrable autoantibodies as panantibodies on the basis that they react with both autologous (self) and allogeneic (genetically dissimilar within the same species) tissue. Cytotoxic autoantibodies may act against cytoplasmic membrane and parts or cell organelles. In intact cells *in vivo* especially the anti-cytoplasmic-membrane autoantibodies find appropriate receptors on the cell surface; autoantibodies against the cytoplasm can less readily penetrate the intact cell, whence they can easily be demonstrated in the blood plasma, while antibodies against the cytoplasmic membrane are fixed [338*c*]. Autoantibodies may also arise to organ constituents other than organ-specific cells (connective tissue, vessels, nerves).

## CONDITIONS RELATED WITH AUTOANTIGEN AND AUTOANTIBODY FORMATION

The spectrum of autoallergic diseases is extremely wide ranging from immunological disturbances related to antigen to those related to antibody. Comparison of the two categories reveals the following differences [87]:

*Disturbances of antigenicity (e.g. Hashimoto's disease)*

1. Autoantigen is not normally present in circulation
2. No immunological tolerance develops to the autoantigen
3. Organ-specific antibodies are formed, which are as a rule also species-specific
4. Autoantigens induce autoantibody formation in normal animals
5. Artificially induced lesions resemble the human disease
6. Relatives of the patient are predisposed to thyroid disorders

*Disturbances of antibody formation (disturbances of tolerance) (e.g. SLE)*

1. The autoantigen is accessible to the lymphocytes
2. Tolerance to the autoantigen develops early in life
3. The autoantibody is not necessarily organ-specific and has a broad species specificity
4. No antibodies arise in animals in response to stimulation with the specific autoantigen
5. Human lesions are scarcely reproducible in animal experiments
6. Relatives of the patient may exhibit disturbance of $\gamma$-globulin synthesis

At the same time a number of similar characteristics may also be found:

1. Circulating autoantibodies against normal constituents of the body
2. Tendency of serum $\gamma$-globulin level to rise
3. Lymphocytic invasion of involved organs
4. Different degrees of damage in autoantigen containing cells
5. Rising incidence among females
6. Autoantigens are organ-(cell)-specific, thus autoantibody synthesis can be elicited by isogeneic, or, occasionally, heterologous antigens of the same organ. Since such antigens also participate in organ function, Voisin [398] has proposed a distinction depending on functional specificity.

After these general remarks, let us consider those artificial or spontaneous sensitization processes in which the sensitizing agent can be regarded with more or less certainty as self. The phenomena of this category can be divided into three groups:

1. Preliminary observations and experiments with self blood and self serum
2. Sensitization with chemically defined and/or polypeptide-like self substances (hormones and vitamins) and with chemical mediators (histamine, etc.)
3. Sensitization with autoantigen-like constituents of various organs and formed elements of the blood.
   *a.* Processes, chiefly experimental, resembling human diseases, which are all inflammatory changes of the delayed type, arising chiefly around small

veins with the participation of humoral antibodies (allergic encephalomyelitis, orchitis with concomitant aspermatogenesis, endophthalmitis phacoanaphylactica, etc.).
*b*. Conditions in which humoral antibodies are the pathogenic factor: acquired haemolytic anaemia, certain types of chronic leukopenia, idiopathic thrombocytopenic purpura, paroxysmal cold haemoglobinuria, etc. These are not inflammatory conditions.
*c*. Various mixed processes with chronic destruction of an organ and production of antibodies, which may or may not be pathogenic [401*a*].

Paroxysmal cold haemoglobinuria, a disease in which haemoglobin appears in urine following exposure to cold, is the prototype of the kind of autoallergy which is due to autologous blood or autologous serum. In this condition there is a biphasic lysis of self erythrocytes elicited by cold-adsorptive Donath–Landsteiner haemolysins in serum which bind to red cells in the cold and exert a lytic action in warm environment, if C is present. Such a biphasic haemolysis is induced among others by infection with *Treponema pallidum*. It has long been known that autologous blood can occasionally induce urticaria with fever and shaking chill, or even an Arthus-like phenomenon [231*a*, *b*, 391]. Whitefield [415*a*, *b*] has proposed the term autosensitization to designate those processes in which the symptoms of hypersensitivity are practically elicited by autologous blood. Intracutaneous administration of autologous serum can, especially by the depot technique, elicit a positive delayed-type response, followed not infrequently by an immediate-type reaction [33]. Thus, injection of self serum may give rise to hypersensitivity to the stroma of autologous erythrocytes, because the intracutaneous administration of autologous red cells was followed by a weal and flare reaction and purpura [140].

A similar autosensitization mechanism can account for the autoerycrocyte sensitization syndrome, i.e. painful bruising syndrome (Gardner-Diamond) [123]. In females, traumata (microtraumata) are initially followed by ecchymosis, then a circumscribed painful inflammation appears which develops to a painful gangrene within a few hours. Intracutaneously administered red blood cells or stroma elicit a haemorrhagic reaction. In one such case, anti-erythrocyte antibodies were demonstrable in the serum of the patient [306]. A similar reaction can also be elicited with phosphatidyl-L-serine (an extract of stroma). Delayed-type reactions occur not only to autoerythrocyte stroma, but also to the stroma of foreign red blood cells [135]. Systemic symptoms may set in. Autologous $\gamma$-globulin can exert an autoantigen-like action with a delayed-type response if it becomes denatured, and heterologous $\gamma$-globulin may have the same effect (native autologous $\gamma$-globulin has no such action); this seems to explain the mechanism of certain tissue lesions [250] (see Ch. 39).

The autosensitization nature of sensitization with *chemically defined and polypeptide-like autologous substances* is lacking sufficient proof, as skin test are occasionally equivocal and difficult to interpret. Also, it should be taken into consideration that apart from frequent impurities, commercial preparations do not always correspond to the physiological substances of the body. The initia hypersensitivity actually enhances the inflammatory action of such substances and if these are originally not inflammatory, they may be rendered such by sensitization. Antibodies formed in response may occasionally suppress the physiological function and pharmacological effects of the above autologous substances by binding the antigen.

Sensitization with *chemical mediators,* primarily with *histamine,* could be temporarily achieved by repeated intracutaneous injection to form a depot; the response was of the delayed-type (otherwise histamine elicits exclusively an immediate-type reaction) and occasionally a flare-up occurred at previous injection sites. Coupling of histamine with protein results in the formation of a chemospecific histamine antigen, *p*-aminobenzene azohistamine azoprotein (Antallerg) [318, 382, 383, 384, 410*c*, *d*]. Following long-term treatment with Antallerg, anti-histamine antibodies could temporarily be demonstrated in the patients' sera; these antibodies neutralize the pharmacological effects of histamine. Animals (rats), however, can be sensitized with 1–2 injections of Antallerg, so that reinjection of the conjugated allergen elicits an anaphylactic shock. Similar experiments have been performed in several other laboratories.

No experimental sensitization with *acetylcholine* has been reported so far, but mention should be made of cholinogenic or cholinoergic urticaria of the systemic warm urticaria group, in which the mediator liberated in consequence of the antigen–antibody reaction is acetylcholine, eliciting on intradermal injection a histamine-type immediate urticarial response and on parenteral application a general attack of urticaria [137, 327] (see Ch. 64 in Volume 2). In such cases urticarial eruptions may also appear in the acetylcholine induced, axon-reflectoric hyperaemic halo, whence such conditions can be regarded as autoallergic.

*Heparin,* too, is a normal blood constituent; it enters circulation from liver and mast cells, forms easily bonds with proteins, binds C and its i.v. injections may occasionally elicit allergic symptoms such as severe attacks of dyspnoea and bronchial spasms occasionally accompanied by urticarial skin eruptions [245]. It remains to be clarified, however, whether the allergic symptoms attributed to heparin sensitization are or are not due to the animal protein from which heparin had been extracted. The patient, nevertheless, occasionally responds only to the polysaccharide fraction of bovine heparin, and does not respond to bovine heart extract or swine heparin. In a similar case, early-type reaction and passive transfer were both positive with heparin preparations from different sources, but there was no response to bovine and swine proteins (to the sources of heparin). It is generally believed that although much remains to be clarified in respect of heparin allergy, a true heparin sensitization may in fact occur in certain cases [308].

Sensitization with *hormones* has been extensively studied in recent time. Judgement of the local reaction due to *adrenalin* (*epinephrine*)—*noradrenalin* (*norepinephrine*) is particularly difficult, because the primary response to intradermal injection is a marked anaemia. Accordingly, data on adrenalin allergy are scarce and problematic. In a case of asthma-urticaria, adrenalin ameliorated the asthmatic fit, but effected a flare-up of urticaria; in another case of asthma, the synthetic adrenalin containing spray caused conjunctivitis, palpebral oedema and eczema with a positive epicutaneous test [66]. In another case, L-epinephrine elicited allergic contact dermatitis, affirmed by a positive epicutaneous test (the stereoisomeric D-epinephrine was ineffective) [128]. Pooled homologous adrenal tissue in complete Freund's adjuvant can elicit isoimmune adrenalitis in animals.

The process can also be elicited by autologous adrenal tissue [274]. Antibodies could be demonstrated not only with homologous, but also with autologous adrenal tissue, whence they can be regarded as true antibodies [401*b*]. In idiopathic Addison's disease, specific circulating antibodies could be demonstrated to adrenocortical components, but a cellular-type anti-adrenal sensitization was simultaneously present in part of the cases [420]. Went and Kesztyűs [410*a*, *b*] coupled adrenalin with protein and immunized rabbits using the adrenalin–azoprotein conjugate, as the chemospecific antigen; although the rabbit antiserum precipitated the conjugate antigen, it did not interfere with the physiological effects of adrenalin.

Scarcely any information is available on sensitization with *adrenocortical hormones* (corticosteroids, deoxycorticosterone). Although there are reports of cortisone induced urticaria and prednisolone induced maculopapular, bullous eruptions with positive provocation tests [39], impurities, preserving agents and solvents have been held responsible rather than the active ingredients. For example in a case of eczema due to hydrocortisone acetate, precursor residues, retained as a contamination were held responsible for the reaction. True contact eczema cases caused by hydrocortisone have, however, also been reported, with a positive epicutaneous response to pure synthetic hydrocortisone acetate, as well as with shock symptoms, urticaria and oedema, and occasional positive immediate-type reactions even to intradermal prednisolone acetate [68]. Anyhow, the allergen role of natural corticosteroids is still unproved. It is certain, though, that chronic asthma patients durably treated with corticosteroids do not develop tolerance to these substances [30]. Protein-conjugated aldosterone has, however, been shown to induce the production of C- and D-ring-specific antibodies in rabbits [6].

Most cases of hormone allergy have been reported in connection with *sex hormones*, but evidence is still lacking that an individual can be sensitized to its own endocrine glands and their products. Certain authors have, nevertheless, postulated the existence of sex hormone autoallergy [289*c*]. Sensitization by parenterally applied sex hormones is in fact not rare. The criteria of sex hormone allergy, which apply to a greater or lesser degree to other hormonal and vitamin allergies as well, can be summarized from the available contradictory data as follows: (*i*) Positive skin reaction to hormones. Aqueous solutions usually elicit immediate-type, less often delayed-type reactions. Positive responses to oily solutions are difficult to judge, as pseudopositive reactions may often occur [423]. (*ii*) Flare-up of skin reactions either on readministration of hormone at another injection site or at menstruation. (*iii*) The periodic, pre-menstrual occurrence of the phenomenon. (*iv*) Passive transfer. (*v*) Possibility of specific desensitization with the patient's serum collected during the eruptive phase. (*vi*) Occasionally positive provocation test during the symptom-free stage with serum of the eruptive phase.

Initially no pure hormones had been used but, especially in females, self serum collected in the eruptive phase, which elicited eruptions in the intermenstrual phase of cyclic urticaria or menstrual herpes patients, or effected desensitization [124]; intermenstrual serum was ineffective. It has been postulated that during menstruation, a pathologically altered sex hormone is probably present in the circulating blood or menstrual blood, eliciting symptoms on sensitization

[330]. Symptoms of hormonal autoallergy are usually associated with menstruation or pregnancy.

Using pure hormones, Zondek and Bromberg [429*a*, *b*] have observed hypersensitivity especially to steroid hormones in 63 per cent of allergic conditions related with the menstrual cycle. In these cases, skin tests and P–K transfer were repeatedly positive also with fractions of the hormone, as established also by others [362]. In pre-menstrual urticaria and erythema cases, positive skin and provocation tests have been obtained chiefly with corpus luteum extracts and progesterone [190, 268]. Certain steroid hormones behave like haptens and on conjugation with proteins they stimulate the synthesis of steroid specific antibodies in animals.

Of the protein-like or, more precisely, polypeptide-like *hormones of the anterior pituitary* (corticotropin, thyrotropin, somatotropin, prolactin and gonadotropins) chiefly corticotropin (adrenocorticotrophic hormone = ACTH) is known to act as a sensitizing agent. The mol. wt. of ACTH is 4,566, that of the other pituitary hormones is generally higher. The ACTH molecule consists of 39 amino acids, of which the first 19 carry the biological activity, whereas the group 25–39 represents the immunological capacity, within which group 25–33 is responsible for species specificity. Many cases of ACTH sensitization have been reported, with symptoms ranging from urticaria-erythema to fits of asthma and shock symptoms of varying severity [289*b*]. Also fatal cases have been described [185], but it was not usually clear whether the lethal allergic process was due to ACTH, or to protein contamination originating from the ACTH donor. Therefore, the next step was to obtain pure preparations. Studies with synthetic ACTH (Synacthen), which corresponds to the native hormone, have shown that true ACTH allergy is relatively rare [225]. In animals, the formation of $\gamma$-globulin-like antibodies could be induced not only with swine and human ACTH, but also with synthetic ACTH consisting of 39 or 24 amino acids; in the latter case ACTH behaved as a hapten [99]. The antibodies neutralized the biological effect of ACTH [107]. Sensitization may be organ-specific, i.e. it can be elicited with ACTH preparation from different animals. It should be noted that sensitivity to ACTH does not affect the therapeutic effect of the hormone. Resistance to ACTH—without clinical symptoms—caused by anti-ACTH antibodies or other inactivating agents has also been reported [347*a*, *b*].

Hypersensitivity due to *gonadotropic hormones* (gonadotropin) is more frequent than that caused by steroids. In a case of amenorrhoea, the existence of an antihormone to gonadotropin was postulated on the basis of inhibition of hormonal effect in frogs. In toxaemia of pregnancy, immediate-type and delayed-type responses could repeatedly be elicited by means of a chorion-gonadotropin solution. Follicle stimulating hormone (FSH) may cause an immediate-type allergic reaction [267], or even an anaphylactic shock [199]. The antigen nature of the luteinizing hormone (LH) can be regarded as an established fact [110]. Immediate-type allergic response to the thyrotropic hormone is relatively rare [352].

The *posterior pituitary hormone vasopressin* is an octapeptide. In allergy, posterior pituitary extracts (pituitrin, glanduitrin, etc.) may give rise to urticaria, purpura, fits of asthma and allergic shock [377], with occasionally positive skin test and P–K transfer [357]. A diabetes insipidus patient, who had been treated parenterally and intranasally with various posterior pituitary extracts, developed urticaria several times and on the day of the 6th nasal treatment, an abrupt fit of cough and severe asthmatic dyspnoea set in, followed by generalized urticaria, irrespectively of the type of the preparation used; skin test and P–K transfer also were positive. By the end of specific treatment, the injection caused no symptom but inhalatory treatment continued to elicit cough and sneeze for a long time [108]. This and similar conditions were probably true cases of hormonal sensitization, because different animal proteins from the source of the hormone preparation did not elicit the skin reaction [148]. This, however, does not exlude the role of a possible contamination [357], as occasionally there was no allergic response to the posterior pituitary preparation Syntocinon [50].

On long-term treatment of animals with *thyroid hormone*, neutralizing 'anti-hormones' appeared in them, which had also been active in other animals [67]. The anti-hormone was supposed to be an antibody, because the antibodies formed in animals treated with synthetic thyroxyl protein inhibited the metabolic effect of thyroxin [63*a*, *b*, *c* 411, 412, 414*a*, *b*]. As a sequestered (inaccessible) autoantigen, thyroglobulin gains access to the circulation chiefly in connection with thyroiditis, thyroid gland operations, etc. and, acting as an antigen, stimulates antibody formation; anti-thyroglobulins have, nevertheless, been found in other auto-allergic diseases and in relatives of patients with thyroid disease as well.

Hypersensitivity to insulin is a frequent problem in clinical practice. The insulin produced by $\beta$-cells of the islets of Langerhans is a crystalline polypeptide of about 6,000 mol. wt. It consists of 51 amino acids of which 21 form the A-chain, 30 the B-chain and two disulphide bridges link them with one another. Forty-eight amino acids of the sequence are identical in the different animal species and only the three terminal amino acids show a sequential variation, responsible for differences in antigenicity. Protein from the insulin donor may also sensitize and this acts as the sensitizing factor in most cases of insulin allergy [44]. Autosensitization, however, is only due to the insulin-polypeptide, which is now available in a synthetic form. According to skin tests with human and synthetic insulin, passive cutaneous transfer, release of histamine from leukocytes and radioimmunodiffusion studies, insulin allergy may develop either to the insulin molecule itself, or to the protein impurity of commercial preparations and it is IgE-mediated. The reagin titre as well as cutaneous sensitivity diminish on desensitization and simultaneously tolerance is developed to insulin [230]. Antibodies formed against insulin can easily be demonstrated by various techniques: reagins, blocking antibodies, antibodies neutralizing the biological effect of insulin, tissue-fixed, C-fixing, anaphylactic and lymphocyte-binding antibodies and transfer factors have been described, some of which are probably identical, while others are clearly unrelated. An antibody of the IgA class was found to agglutinate autologous and homologous leukocytes preincubated with crystalline bovine or swine insulin for one hour [246].

The possibility of autosensitization is supported by the observation that guinea pigs passively sensitized with immune serum to calf insulin responded by an anaphylactic shock exclusively to insulin, while calf protein and calf pancreas were ineffective. Preparations obtained from different animals have an insulin antigen in common (cross-reactions). There were patients who responded to each of the insulin preparations from the different animals, and recrystallized five times, but did not react to proteins from the insulin donors [43]. If symptoms cease on change of the preparation, the allergizing factor is clearly a protein contaminant.

Allergic symptoms occur most often at the injection site. Hypersensitivity induced by insulin or an insulin–protein conjugate is initially of the delayed type and as such is passively transferable with leukocytes. Later the immediate-type response appears with P–K transferability of reagins [201]. The two allergic processes are independent. Generalized urticaria, Quincke's angi oedema, intensive pruritus, gastro-intestinal signs, different shock symptoms, etc. may also occur and even lethal cases of insulin allergy have been reported. Shock treatment with insulin has repeatedly given rise to systemic symptoms, urticaria and scarlatiniform eruptions [73]. Out of 15,000 diabetics 300 (2 per cent) showed allergic symptoms [187]. With P–K transfer insulin can be demonstrated at blood levels as low as 0.0002 U per ml in allergic cases [234]. Sera from patients with insulin allergy have been shown to contain precipitins [153] and insulin binding antibodies, which may neutralize insulin. Both humans and animals can form antibodies against autologous insulin, but this is probably due to structural changes occurring during purification and extraction or to the combination of insulin with protein, thus forming a conjugate antigen [200]. *In vivo* insulin probably undergoes such alterations in the course of its passage through the liver, lungs and capillaries, as indicated by the immunological differences found between insulin isolated from circulation and from pancreas. In animals, even synthetic insulin can induce antibody production if it is administered in Freund's adjuvant, i.e. it may act as an antigen without undergoing a structural change.

Apart from the thermolabile skin sensitizing reagin, a thermostable insulin neutralizing or blocking antibody with anti-insulin action may also appear in certain cases; the thermostable antibody inhibits the action of insulin in diabetic patients causing resistance to insulin [236*b*] and protects albino mice against lethal hypoglycaemic convulsions. A mixture of such serum with insulin does not affect the blood glucose level of rabbits, but a much higher dose is required to obtain insulin effect [160]. The blood plasma of diabetes patients binds normally 10 U per litre, in case of resistance even 1,000 U per litre of insulin [298]. In true insulin resistance more than 2,000 U of insulin may be required daily to prevent attacks of hypoglycaemia. A patient of Lowell [236*a*] responded to human insulin with a positive skin reaction and P–K transfer, and on i.v. administration systemic symptoms appeared in addition to hypoglycaemia. But at the same time the patient was resistant to commercial insulin preparations and his serum protected albino mice against a lethal dose of crystalline animal insulin also in an inactivated state, i.e. after it had lost the passive sensitizing capacity due to inactivation. It appears that only the skin sensitizing factor arose in response to human insulin and both the specific and neutralizing factors were scarce. On the other hand, it may be that the latter two factors combined with different groups of the insulin molecule, one with the group responsible for sensitization, and the other with the one responsible for carbohydrate metabolism, each being localized in different globulin fractions: the reagin in IgE and the neutralizing antibody in IgG [342]; in this the neutralizing antibody resembles the blocking antibody. Resistance to insulin declines earlier than the skin reaction. In animals, resistance to insulin can be artificially induced, especially if insulin is given parenterally in Freund's adjuvant [112].

Determination of the maximum insulin binding capacity by means of $^{131}I$-labelled insulin, and its comparison with the daily insulin requirement of the patient showed that the greater the requirement, the higher the maximum insulin binding capacity. The anti-insulin antibody of diabetes serum—usually a bovine or porcine anti-insulin—can also bind human insulin *in vitro* [81]; it is probably an autoantibody in this case [325].

Resistance being associated with antibody is suggested by the finding that when mixing *in vitro* serum from a bovine insulin resistant patient and $^{131}I$-labelled bovine insulin, paper electrophoretic separation will reveal the fixing of insulin in an inactivated form at the top of the $\gamma$-globulin arch [48]. Anti-insulin antibodies can also be demonstrated by the Coombs test in cases of insulin resistance [368]. The greater part of examinations indicate that the anti-hormone antibody can inhibit the pharmacological action of autologous insulin from the pancreas.

Insulin-free *pancreas* extract can occasionally cause allergic symptoms (urticaria, oedema, asthma) in itself, while both skin test and P–K transfer are positive. In such cases, the allergen has been sought among the *kallikrein*-like substances [71]. The insulin-free angiotropin-pancreas extract can even elicit an allergic shock.

It is not only of practical, but also of theoretical interest that *bovine glucagone*, this small molecule consisting of 29 amino acids, can be divided into two functional orbits: the antigenic determinant localized in the amino-terminal part of the molecule controls the specificity of humoral antibodies, whereas the carboxy-terminal segment is the part recognized by the antigen reactive cells [344*a b*]. The specificity of antibodies induced by glucagone combined with poly-$\gamma$-D-glutamic acid hapten (mol. wt. 35,000) depends on the mode of conjugation [345].

Studies on hormone sensitization suggest the conclusion that although the antibodies formed in response are partly species specific, also organ specific, true antibody-like anti-hormones arise, as postulated probably earliest by Collip [67]. However, certain hormones induce not only antibodies which inhibit their pharmacological action, but also antibodies which are responsible for the appearance of the allergic symptoms.

Sensitization with *vitamins*, i.e. vitamin allergy, occurs much more rarely than is the case with hormones.

Several reports have been published on sensitization with *vitamin* $B_1$ (thiamine). Cutaneous symptoms (oedema of eyelids and lips, urticaria), dyspnoea and asthma-like attacks, major and minor shock symptoms and, after parenteral administration, collapse may set in [223, 369]. Intravenous injection has even been reported to cause death [269]. The question is whether the underlying mechanism of these symptoms is toxic or allergic. Skin tests and passive transfer have yielded both positive and negative results on different occasions. Vitamin $B_1$ is as a rule urticariogenic [192], whence cutaneous tests should be evaluated with care in cases regarded as allergic [186]. Contact sensitization with thiamine giving positive epicutaneous reaction, has also been observed. In certain cases of occupational thiamine eczema, flare-ups occurred on intradermal or parenteral administration of the vitamin [167].

*Vitamin* $B_{12}$ is the anti-anaemic principle of the liver. As initially all liver preparations contained vitamin $B_{12}$, treatment with them was not infrequently followed by allergic symptoms ranging from mild to severe, with positive cutaneous test and passive transfer [142]. In most cases the protein of the liver extract donor or, probably, the preserving agent [217], appeared to be responsible for the symptoms, although occasionally both liver protein and preserver failed to elicit a response and positive reactions were only obtained with extracts having a high anti-anaemic titre. The antibody formed was specific for the anti-anaemic factor, irrespective of the species of the liver extract donor. It was in such cases that vitamin $B_{12}$-sensitization was suspected, but there is still no sufficient proof whether the allergic reaction is in fact due to the vitamin. Sensitivity to synthetic vitamin $B_{12}$ (cyanocobalamine) has nevertheless been observed [232]. In a case even severe allergic shock occurred and positive intradermal reactions to purified cyano- and hydroxycobalamine were obtained [170].

Reports on allergy to other vitamins are scarce. Vitamin A and carotine can elicit asthma and urticaria [122], vitamin C (ascorbic acid) may cause generalized eruptions with positive epi- and intracutaneous tests [329] and in a case of asthma both the immediate-type skin reaction and P–K transfer were positive for vitamin C. Injection with vitamin E (tocopherol) was followed by urticaria [141] and, in another case, inflammation appeared at the injection site and the intradermal test was positive [329]. Intramuscular administration of vitamin K (syncamin) elicited severe shock symptoms in one case [18]. Two patients previously treated with nicotinic acid tablets responded to i.v. administration of the vitamin and one of them also showed a positive skin test [294]. Folic acid allergy was described in one instance as an immediate-type urticaria with a positive provocation test [265], in another case as erythematous eruptions accompanied by respiratory disturbances on oral intake of the vitamin; skin tests performed with various, highly purified folic acid preparations were all positive [56].

Several reports are available on hypersensitivity induced by *proteolytic enzymes* (pepsin, trypsin, etc.) chiefly by the inhalatory route. In a single case, trypsin—like streptokinase and streptodornase—elicited urticaria and general shock symptoms on oral application. Intradermal injection of chymotrypsin is not infrequently followed by severe allergic shock symptoms [251]; in such cases there is usually a history of previous occupational exposure to chymotrypsin or injection treatment with the latter in connection with operation for cataract. Workers of a soap factory became sensitized with the proteolytic enzyme alcalase, used as a component in laundry detergents [349]. The alcalase and maxatase components of washing powders have even elicited asthma on occupational exposure [104]. Reduction of exposure to, and contact with, detergent enzymes has become an important problem of industrial hygiene [121, 314]. A pharmacist working with pepsin had been reported to have an attack of asthma and the skin test for pepsin was positive (239). The antisera collected from rabbits immunized with multiple intradermal injections of pepsin and pepsinogen cross-reacted with one another [49]. In a case of contact sensitivity to vitamin $B_1$, cocarboxylase coenzyme sensitivity developed to the latter [167]. Inhalation of a *Bacillus subtilis* enzyme was followed by a mass incidence of rhinorrhoea, lacrimation, cough, etc. among the workers of a detergent factory; skin tests and passive transfer were positive for the appropriate enzyme preparation [113]. Attacks of acute urticaria, allergic signs including facial oedema and even shock symptoms have repeatedly been observed after the use of histaminase preparations [138], but it could not satisfactorily be clarified whether the symptoms were due to the enzyme itself or to the protein of the enzyme donor. The same applies to allergic symptoms caused by hyaluronidase and penicillinase (neutrapen), and the antibodies arising in response can even paralyse the effect of the enzyme itself.

## HYPERSENSITIVITY TO SUBSTANCES FROM DIFFERENT TISSUES, FORMED ELEMENTS OF THE BLOOD AND INTRACELLULAR SUBSTANCES

There are autoantigens in the organism which, being localized at sequestered (inaccessible) sites, can act as antigens without undergoing a structural change (according to Burnet, these are the 'true' autoantigens). The cellular and intracellular substances at accessible sites require either a structural change or a pathological alteration of the immune system to become autoantigens capable of the induction of autoantibody synthesis. Artificial sensitization with tissues from certain organs has chiefly been made possible by the use of Freund's adjuvant.

### *The skin as autoantigen*

Repeated s.c. implantation of self skin into rabbits gives rise to hypersensitivity and rejection of skin autograft [106]. Guinea pigs can also be rendered sensitive to their own skin (using complete Freund's adjuvant): positive skin reactions occur and also the C fixation test will be positive [418]. In the case of a generalized dermatitis (erythrodermia, exfoliative dermatitis), humoral antibodies may form to self skin, but their *in vitro* demonstration may be difficult owing to the frequent occurrence of certain skin antigens (these are identical with ABO blood group antigens) and the interference of non-specific factors. The reacting antigen is probably a protein composite, which is formed in the stratum granulosum or the underlying layer, perhaps a precursor of keratin. In examinations of human epidermis extract with a heterologous antiserum, 5 epithelial antigens were identified as unrelated to plasma proteins [105]. The specificity of the antibody for epithelium has been affirmed by immunofluorescence test.

These skin antigens may, on the grounds of ABO incompatibility, participate in certain immunopathological processes [139]. Sera from such patients can elicit immediate hypersensitivity (cytotoxic effect) [286] in diseased and even in healthy subjects, when administered intradermally. In localized chronic eczema, the formation of autoantigen may be related with antigen-like potential epithelial components which easily become modified under the influence of chemical agents and microbes [319].

The problem of skin autosensitization is also encountered in cases of physical allergy; it is generally postulated that due to physical effects, endogenous substances are released, metabolites of the skin, which then behave as autoantigens inducing autoantibody formation (see Chapter 73 in Volume 2). Autosensitization is usually suspected in obdurate, therapy-resistant cases of eczema (nummular eczema, housewives' eczema, etc.). It certainly may most easily become predominant in microbial eczema, when the skin tissue may be transformed into autoantigen due to the microbial effect [158]; in such cases generalization of the processes may follow, marked by the appearance of secondary microbids [287]. Immunoglobulins and C have actually been demonstrated by immunofluorescence in dermal-epidermal junctions and walls of skin vessels in the course of various skin diseases, above all in lupus erythematosus [17]. Allergic contact dermatitis has hypothetically been interpreted as a partial autoimmunization, in which the exogenous hapten substance combines with a skin-protein carrier [260].

The main fields of dermal autoantigen formation are the burn disease and the pemphigus group. Burns of second degree associated with vesicle formation can elicit an immune response: different kinds of humoral antibodies (C-fixing, haemagglutinating, HL-A-cell-proliferation-inhibitory) may be produced against the burnt tissue [83, 100, 293]; recently, intracellular immune response could be demonstrated by the immunofluorescence technique in the stratum spinosum of the skin in bullous burns. Burn-specific antigens and burn-specific antibodies were, however, not found in convalescent serum [42]. Antigen demonstration by the immunofluorescence technique was chiefly possible in acantholytic and bullous skin processes, using fluorescein-labelled serum. In the pemphigus group (pemphigus vulgaris, pemphigus foliaceus, Senear-Usher form), the autoantigen was localized in the intercellular substance of the stratum spinosum, while in bullous pemphigoid it was detected in the subepithelial layer.

### *Mucosa as autoantigen*

Infected mucous membranes may also play the role of an autoantigen. Extracts of cultures of bacterial isolates from intrinsic asthma patients grown in media containing oral and pharyngeal mucosa elicit delayed, occasionally immediate, hypersensitivity on i.d. administration [29]. The intercellular and subepithelial antibodies occurring in pemphigus and pemphigoid can also be found in the oral and oesophageal mucosa.

### *Blood and haemopoietic organs*

The autosensitizing mechanism of blood and haemopoietic organs is one of the most widely studied topics of the field. Serological autoantibodies (IgG-type biphasic cold haemolysins) were first detected in paroxymal cold haemoglobinuria; such antibodies lyse the target cell (erythrocyte) after fixing to it in the cold and lyse them on warming in the presence of C. Experiments along this line could serve as models in the study of the pathogenic role of true autoantibodies, although several points are still unclear. There is also evidence as to the importance of the $\varkappa$-type light chain in human monoclonal cold IgM agglutinins [21]. Immunohaematologists usually distinguish 'true' and 'allergic' antibodies. True antibodies are those which act on the formed elements of blood directly, without the participation of an external factor. Thus these are autoantibodies and as such can be held responsible for certain kinds of haemolytic anaemia, thrombocytopenia, purpura, immunoleukopenia and leukoagglutination. The allergic antibodies are not active unless an external agent, as a rule a drug, is present in the reaction

[75]. This mechanism plays a role in certain kinds of haemolytic anaemia, thrombocytopenic purpura and agranulocytosis. Drug-immune haemolytic anaemia is most frequently due to penicillin [364*a*, *b*, 424].

The foregoing classification appears, however, artificial if it is considered that an antigen–antibody reaction takes place in both instances, but while in the case of true antibody a primary haematological abnormality is demonstrable, the formation of allergic antibodies (warm- and cold-type autohaemagglutinins) responsible for the haemolytic anaemia is a secondary process, initiated probably by drug action or a primary disease. It seems, however, highly probable that an external or intrinsic factor (intercurrent disease, infection, transfusion, etc.) plays a role in the formation of the autoantigen–antibody system in the first case, too, except for those processes in which unchanged autologous substances serve as the autoantigen. It seems, therefore, more correct to group the autoantibodies of immunohaematological diseases according to the origin of the antigen, using group *a* for combined complete antigens entirely produced within the body, and group *b* for the incomplete antigens which require some kind of external adjuvant to develop action. Autoantibody response to auto-erythrocytes could not yet be provoked in animal experiments, although autohaemolytic disease is known to occur spontaneously in both dogs [379] and NZB/Bl mice [169]. The immunohaematological antibodies are independent of the ABO blood group substances (panerythrocytary) and part of them are blood group specific [408], which weighs in favour of the autosensitization concept.

Administration of homologous bone marrow suspension along with Freund's adjuvant elicits antibody formation in rabbits; such antibodies inhibit maturation in the leukopoietic system and may occasionally cause agranulocytosis and panmyelophthisis. Certain components of the white blood cells can also stimulate antibody formation, as demonstrated by phagocytosis and agglutination tests. The specificity of the leukocyte antigen is linked with the cytoplasm, above all with the mitochondria, whence neutrophilic, basophilic and eosinophilic leukocytes and lymphocytes may immunochemically differ from one another. In these cells the antigenic structure of nucleoproteids is, however, common. The antigens of the leukocyte, localized in different weak and strong H-loci, have acquired a great importance in transplantation studies; their demonstration is carried out by means of serum from polytransfused persons, multiparous women or probably from leukocyte-treated subjects. Such sera contain a measurable amount of antibodies against leukocyte antigen suitable for agglutination or cytotoxic tests. The related examinations as well as descriptions of the properties of anti-lymphocyte serum (ALS), anti-thymic serum (ATS), and anti-lymphocyte globulin (ALG) used for immunosuppression are outlined in more detail in the chapters on transplantation, histocompatibility test and in the descriptions of certain antisera.

Anti-thrombocytic antibody causes the disintegration of platelets; thrombopenia may be accompanied by a prolonged retraction of clotted blood and by purpura. The same destructive leuko- and thrombopenic process takes place in anaphylactic shock and during the haemoclastic crisis of allergic reactions. The pathomechanism may take three different courses: (*i*) the cells adsorb the antigen first and fix the antibody next, or (*ii*) the other way round, the antibody becomes fixed first, or (*iii*) an antigen–antibody complex is formed and this agglutinates the cells.

Antiplasmatic iso- or autosensitization has rarely been encountered. Out of the diseases belonging to this category, the various forms of immunocoagulopathy resemble hereditary haemophilia, but the former are acquired and can affect both sexes, above all polytransfused persons whose plasma contains humoral anticoagulants (in the IgG fraction) acting as isoantibodies [158]. The diseases due to plasmatic iso- or autosensitization are described in Chapter 71 in Volume 2.

## ORGAN-SPECIFIC AUTOSENSITIZATION WITH 'TRUE' AUTOANTIGENS

Processes in which autologous substances act as potential antigens, inducing autoantibody formation without a structural change belong to this group. Such substances are thyroglobulin, components of the ocular lens, nerve tissue, spermatozoa (sperm cells develop only later in life, thus no prenatal tolerance develops to them and they can always serve as autoantigens). According to Burnet's concept, these substances have no direct contact with blood or lymph circulation during embryogenesis, whence they are not recognized as self by the organism.

### *Autosensitization in the thyroid gland*

Thyroglobulin is one of those inaccessible autologous substances which behave like antigens in various thyroid gland diseases (Hashimoto's struma, multifocal thyroiditis, etc.), stimulating different humoral antibodies which are also active against human thyroid gland extracts. Probably thyroglobulin is the main antigen, because according to immunofluorescence studies, the bulk of autoantibody occurs in the follicular colloid, but autoantigens are also localized in the glandular epithelium (in the microsomal fraction), inducing chiefly the formation of C fixing antibodies [322]. Thyroglobulin can elicit both immediate-type and delayed-type skin reactions (coexistence of reactions) [324]. In experimental studies of thyroiditis, certain animals showed only a delayed-type response [252], others developed only humoral antibodies and a third group showed both reactions. Experimental thyroiditis can also be induced with thyroglobulin partially digested with papaine, suggesting the possibility that unfamiliar polypeptides (thyroglobulin fragments) arising due to a genetic or hormonal aberration may be directly responsible for inducing autosensitivity in man [9]. Passive transfer with serum from patients with Hashimoto's disease to monkeys failed to induce thyroid gland lesions in the animals. Anti-thyroglobulin antibodies can also occur in patients manifesting no clinical thyroid disorder, chiefly in women in the 5thdecade of life [166, 179*b*]. Since Hashimoto's disease can simultaneously occur in monozygotic twins, this autosensitization process is probably related with a genetic defect [180] (see Chapter 44 in Volume 2).

Thyroid diseases as organ-specific alterations can be induced experimentally with the aid of an adjuvant. In the early stage of experimental thyroiditis, skin sensitizing antibodies appear [255], which are passively transferable to normal rabbits with spleen and lymph node cells, if the donor rabbits are previously treated with homologous or heterologous thyroglobulin without adjuvant but they have not shown thyroid lesion.

Spontaneous autoimmune thyroiditis occurs frequently among White Leghorn chickens of the Obese strain. Bursectomy on the day of hatching reduces significantly the frequency of thyroiditis and the occurrence of humoral antithyroglobulin antibodies as well. Neonatal thymectomy has no influence on the incidence of thyroid lesions, although it keeps the humoral antibody level low. Welch et al. [409*a*] have shown recently, however, that neonatal thymectomy of Obese strain chickens significantly increased the severity of spontaneous autoimmune thyroiditis. The balance between bursal function (which promotes the autoimmune disorder) and thymic function (which suppresses it) is thus apparent. On reinjection of autologous bursa cells to bursectomized and X-ray irradiated chickens, the incidence of thyroiditis rises again, but the synthesis of humoral anti-thyroid antibodies is not restored. Thus it seems probable that in respect of thyroid autoimmunity, the bursa has a dual function, one humoral, probably hormonal, as this is essential for anti-thyroglobulin antibody formation, the other cellular, as required for the development of inflammatory thyroid gland lesions [276]. In accordance with this implication, turkey antisera formed against chicken bursal cells can also reduce the incidence of spontaneous autoimmune thyroiditis, while turkey antisera formed against chicken thymocytes have no such effect [416].

### *Autosensitization in the eye*

Embryonic lens tissue has species-specific properties which gradually disappear with age, and organ-specific antigenic properties become predominant [381]. If bovine lens substance is completed with staphylotoxin adjuvant to enhance its antigenicity, it will induce the formation of anti-lens antibodies in the rabbit, allergic changes in the rabbit's eye [45*a*, *b*]. The ocular lens of animals sensitized with lens tissue responds with autoantibody formation only if the lenticular substance has been rendered accessible by incision of the capsule or if there is an increased permeability due to some reason. Antibody formation to the homogenized ocular lens of adult animals can be greatly enhanced by the use of Freund's adjuvant or with preceding *in loco* injection of streptolysin O. Haemagglutination is a more sensitive method for the demonstration of such antibodies than gel precipitation. The lenticular substances of different animals cross-react with one another, but ocular lenses from foetal and newborn rabbits do not cross-react until after 10 days [146]. Phacoanaphylactic endophthalmitis is a pure example of delayed-type autosensitization: in the first stage the lenticular substance released from its capsule sensitizes the organism as an antigen; in the second phase, if lenticular substance is released again, e.g. by surgery, an intensive allergic reaction takes place in the sensitized organism. In sympathetic ophthalmia, uveal pigment acts as an autoantigen sensitizing the eye. Uveal pigment injected into guinea pigs in Freund's adjuvant elicits a diffuse inflammation of the choroid.

Two tissue-specific antigens have been detected in the retina of the guinea pig, but only one of them caused allergic uveitis in the species, although antibodies formed against both antigens reacted with the autologous retina. The frequency and severity of the disease depend on the quantity of antigen, but the quantitative relationship between the mycobacterial and antigen components of the immunizing emulsion also plays a role. If the proportion of the two components is appropriate in the inoculum, close to 100 per cent of the guinea pigs will develop uveitis [53], but even a slight rise in the proportion of mycobacteria above the optimum will suppress the immunological and pathologic reactions elicited by the antigen [400].

Corneal tissue can induce hypersensitivity on allogeneic transplantation, but only if the entire cornea is transplanted to the vascular sclera or, in the case of central and partial transplantation, if the corneal tissue becomes vascularized due to some disease. The corneal stroma is much less antigenic than the corneal epithelium. If the epithelium is transplanted to one eye and stroma to the other eye after an appropriate time interval, the immune reaction will take place unless the graft to the first eye was free of epithelium [229]. Extract of the whole eye can also sensitize. If rats are treated with anti-rat-eye serum prepared in rabbits, the overwhelming majority develop panophthalmitis. If these animals are coupled with normal ones using the parabiosis technique many of the normal animals will also develop panophthalmitis by a so far not fully understood mechanism (see Chapter 42 in Volume 2).

### *Autosensitization with testicular tissue and seminal fluid*

Experimental sensitization of animals with seminal fluid has been performed by Landsteiner, Metalnikov and others. Parenteral administration of testicular tissue or sperm cells in complete Freund's adjuvant may elicit delayed hypersensitivity in the course of which the autologous sperm cells become distinctly degenerated (aspermatogenesis) and testicular atrophy occurs [196*b*]. The same can be achieved with purified testicular tissue, but only if it is homologous or autologous, thus the phenomenon is not only organ-specific, but also species-specific [115, 116]. Autoantibodies also develop to sperm cells; such phenomena are known as the earliest examples of autosensitization. Injection of homologous testicular extract into guinea pigs induced the formation of serum antibodies, which reacted *in vitro* not only with homologous, but also with autologous seminal fluid. Long-lived cultures of testicular cells contain appropriate sensitizing antigens [196*a*]. Guinea pigs treated with sperm cells or testicular tissue develop anaphylactic hypersensitivity giving a positive Sch–D test and, if C is present, sperm cell immobilizing antibodies will also develop, localized chiefly in the acrosomal part, as demonstrated by immunofluorescence. Furthermore, the i.d. injection of antigen extracts elicit also an intensive delayed-type response (coexistence of immediate- and delayed-type reactions) [325]. Two different kinds of lesions have been described in guinea pigs immunized with testicular antigens [20]. A characteristic peritubular accumulation of mononuclear cell infiltration in the seminiferous tubules is followed by degeneration of the germinal epithelium. Sperm cells localized in the seminiferous tubules contain neither IgG nor C3. Lesions of the rete testis, efferent ducts and epididymis are characterized by infiltration of neutrophils. Occasionally IgG and C3 are present in the sperm cell acrosome. Thus lesions of the seminiferous tubules are reminiscent of a cell-mediated immune reaction, whereas tissue damage in the seminal passages can be attributed to humoral antibodies. The occurrence and distribution of the lesions depend on the kind of testicular antigen used for immunization [393]. By the indirect immunofluorescence technique three distinct guinea pig spermatozoal autoantigens named S, P and T have been localized. These three autoantigens are testis-specific since they were not found in other organs in guinea pigs; moreover, S was detected on the acrosomal apparatus in rabbits, rats and mice [390*a*].

The serum of rabbits treated with homologous testicular tissue causes testicular tissue disintegration in the host [85]. The testicular hyaluronidase enzymes of various animals act as species-specific antigens, whence they neither cross-react nor cause aspermatogenesis [195*c*]. The aspermatogenic factor is localized in cells from which the secondary spermatocytes originate [195*b*]. Sensitization by seminal fluid may occasionally occur after copulation. If a strong enough sensitivity develops and copulations are repeated, this circumstance may, under given conditions, affect the fertility of the female, as e.g. in guinea pigs, the uterus contracts during the positive Sch–D reaction, rendering the implantation of the blast cell difficult [195*a*, *d*]. Immobilizing antibodies to homologous sperm cells can also develop in the human female after injection of seminal fluid, but as yet there is no evidence whether these antibodies can actually reduce conceptibility. Sperm cell agglutinins have occasionally been encountered in the serum and seminal fluid of infertile males, suggesting that in such cases sperm cells probably gain access to the blood, and lymphatic circulation. Apart from the sperm cell, also the seminal plasma contains 8–9 antigens. There is a case report of a female who developed a severe allergic response to human seminal fluid after coitus; skin test with the fluid was positive even at a high dilution, but there was no response to washed sperm cells [148].

The vesicular fluid of guinea pigs could be separated into 6 components of which 3 were of major importance. The component designated as II—an ellipsoid molecule—proved to be a powerful antigen in heteroimmunization, showing distinct tissue, and species specificity. It stimulated antibody formation under conditions of isoimmunization. Immunized guinea pigs responded positively to the skin test and the seminal vesicle showed microscopic lesions, indicating that an experimental autoimmune disease of the seminal vesicle could be induced [282]. A rare occurrence of seminal vesiculitis is also known among humans [421]. The newer trends of reproduction immunology have been reviewed by Shulman [354].

### *Autosensitization with ovarian tissue*

It has generally been postulated that the endocrine organs are much less subject to the transplantation immune mechanism than other tissues, i.e. that they survive much longer. For instance, chicken ovary allogeneic grafts survived in completely or partially castrated cock 280 days or longer and some of the grafts even maintained function (ovulation); occasionally, prolonged survival of skin grafts in the same animal could be thus achieved. On simultaneous transplantation, the ovary survives longer than the skin [215]. Some birds even produced antibodies to the ovary of the donor [65].

### *Autosensitization with adrenal tissue*

Rabbits inoculated with bovine adrenal tissue (in Freund's adjuvant) developed organ-specific thermostable antibodies, which were localized chiefly in the medulla (steroid inhibition in adrenal cortex?). Rabbits and guinea pigs sensitized in a similar manner with isologous adrenal tissue also produced organ-specific, but thermolabile antibodies demonstrable by C-fixation, haemagglutination and gel diffusion. The antiserum reacted not only with adrenal tissue from homologous species, but also with autologous adrenal tissue (autospecificity) and guinea pigs could also be sensitized with the autologous adrenal (obtained by unilateral adrenalectomy) [262*a*, *b*]. The adrenal lesion is more distinct if the animals are treated with autoantigen [371].

### *Sensitization with cardiac and vascular tissue*

The possibility of autosensitization is suggested by the success of producing infiltrative endocardial lesions in dogs and rabbits by treatment with endocardium-toxic serum [228]. This abacterial endocarditis favours the establishment of *Streptococcus viridans*, which then can give rise to septic endocarditis. Endocardium-toxic serum would often cause a more destructive change of the cardiac and valvular system than normal horse serum + *Streptococcus viridans*. It follows that bacterial antigens do not affect the heart and valve unless a certain degree of hypersensitivity has developed, e.g. in rheumatic tissue reactions. Both antibacterial and anti-endomyocardial antibodies may be produced. The occurrence of an antigen–antibody reaction is suggested by the absence of cardiac lesions and persistence of C after treatment with nitrogen mustard and X-ray [399*c*, *d*, *e*]. These antibodies represent an additional rather than a new pathogenic factor, e.g. in rabbit experiments, non-inflammatory cardiac processes (myocardial infarction induced by adrenalin) act as aseptic degenerative changes causing autosensitization and can be enhanced by means of Freund's adjuvant [89]. This is signified by the frequent positivity of the haemagglutination reaction and the appearance of precipitation lines against cardiac tissue in the gel diffusion test [183]. The materials serving as autoantigens can be isolated by immunoelectrophoresis from the necrotic myocardial tissue in cardiac infarction; these substances may even enter blood circulation. If the serum from an infarction patient is injected into rabbit, an additional precipitation line will appear in the gel diffusion test [208]. Humoral antibody detected in various cardiac processes should, however, be regarded as the product rather than causative factor of the pathological process.

Allergic vascular reactions also play an important role in the pathogenesis of myocardial infarction [370]. The vascular wall itself is of antigenic nature, but only the endothelium and adventitia (no antibody formation against the media has been observed in rabbits). An autoallergic mechanism can well be postulated in certain forms of vasculitis [301]. Feeding of cholesterol can induce atherosclerosis in rabbits and cocks [263]. If normal rabbits or cocks are sensitized with the antigen-like $\beta$-lipoprotein isolated from the hypercholesterolaemic blood of the treated animals or birds and are subsequently fed cholesterol, only slight changes will appear on the aorta in comparison with the controls, indicating that sensitization with β-lipoprotein inhibits the establishment of experimental atherosclerosis [127*a*, *b*]. If, however, homogenates of homologous aorta and large vessel wall are used as antigen, aortic and coronary lesions will develop without feeding of cholesterol [380] (see Chapter 38 in Volume 2).

### *Autosensitization with lung tissue*

In pulmonary tuberculosis, autoantibodies are formed against lung tissue; these are demonstrable in the serum and react specifically with normal lung tissue *in vivo*. Injection of such serum along with mycobacterium tuberculosis into normal animals causes pulmonary tuberculosis [338*a*], as shown by Vorlaender [399*d*] in the experimental renal tuberculosis of the rat.

### *Autosensitization with liver tissue*

A similar autosensitization mechanism can be postulated in various liver diseases in which the affected parenchymal cells serve as the antigen [336]. Organ-specific antibodies are produced against the cytoplasm of such cells, while the anti-mesenchymal antibodies of the 'hepatotoxic' serum react in a non-specific manner and can elicit serous hepatitis [399*e*]. The autoantibody-like serum factors encountered in liver diseases do not behave uniformly some of them react with corpuscular and soluble tissue antigens, some with IgG molecules and they may be formed simultaneously against several subcellular liver antigens (cytoplasmic membrane, mitochondria, microsomes, lysosomal membrane) [82*a*, *b*]. Delayed hypersensitivity may be reduced in certain liver diseases [109]. Antibodies also reacting with autologous liver antigens are formed in the rat after injection of homologous or heterologous liver tissue [317]. Guinea pigs repeatedly inoculated with a homologous whole liver extract in Freund's adjuvant develop degenerative and necrotic changes of the liver as a result of the formation of specific anti-liver antibodies [24]. It is, nevertheless, probable that immunological reactions are more problematic in inflammatory diseases of the liver than in such conditions of other organs, because different non-specific factors (altered serum proteins, lipoproteins, etc.) appear additionally in the affected organs [399*e*]. Antibody-forming cells, reacting with purified specific lipoproteins of the liver have recently been demonstrated in lymphoid aggregates collected by needle biopsy from the portal tract of certain patients suffering from chronic aggressive hepatitis. The formed humoral liver-specific antibodies are only exceptionally demonstrable in patient sera, because they become adsorbed *in vivo* by excess antigen [86].

Hepatitis virus is transferable by blood transfusion; this commonly occurring viral agent found in sera from patients in the acute phase of serum hepatitis has recently been named Australia serum hepatitis virus with Australia antigen or Au SH antigen [36]. This antigen is sometimes found in infectious hepatitis. About one tenth of polytransfused persons posses this antigen without showing signs of hepatitis and about half of the antigen carriers possess antibody as well, which has also been demonstrated in healthy persons [363], e.g. in 1–20 per cent of the normal population of South-West Asia and of the tropics in general. Its occurrence is rare among the population of the USA (0.1 per cent). Two hypotheses have been advanced to explain the true nature of the Australia antigen. According to one hypothesis, it is an infectious agent, causing hepatitis in man, and it is associated with acute viral hepatitis, serum hepatitis and infectious hepatitis as well as with the various forms of chronic hepatitis. It is visible on electron micrographs as a particle of 200 Å diam. It is transferable from man to man and, by passage, to infant African green monkey. It is demonstrable by immunofluorescence in liver cell nuclei and/or blood from hepatitis patients and can replicate in cultures of human liver cells. According to the other hypothesis, the Australia antigen shows the characteristics of a hereditary serum protein polymorphism. Recently, the two hypotheses have been combined and the possibility has been considered that the Australia antigen is not uniform [37, 214]. In 6 patients with histologically verified polyarteritis nodosa and chronic Australia antigenaemia, a circulating immune complex composed of Australia antigen and immunoglobulin was demonstrated. In two cases Australia antigen, IgM and C were detected in the vascular wall of the patients by immunofluorescence [131].

### *Autosensitization with kidney tissue*

Renal sensitization can occur in experimental nephritis, such as Mashugi's nephrotoxic serum nephritis, foreign protein nephritis and autoimmune nephritis (e.g. that elicited in rats by intraperitoneal administration of autologous kidney suspension in complete Freund's adjuvant). Sensitivity to renal tissue is tissue-specific. In the course of nephritis, nephrotoxic autoantibodies are formed, the effect of which can be assessed *in vitro* from the toxic effect of the serum on renal cell culture, or *in vivo* by transfer of blood from patients having nephritis or by parabiosis experiments. In this manner tissue lesions could be transferred from the parabiont having nephritis (due to treatment with anti-rabbit-kidney serum) to the healthy partner (lymphocytotoxic effect). The same experiment was performed with success on genetically identical and immuntolerant animals, even if the time interval between injection of cytotoxic rabbit serum and establishment of parabiosis was prolonged. The experimental results suggest that the inflammatory renal reaction of the normal partner was due to a secondary nephritis inducing factor, arising after the establishment of nephrotoxin nephritis (autosensitization). Species-specific antigens localized on the surface of nucleated cells stimulate the formation of nephrotoxic antibodies. Antibodies to superficial specific antigens of nucleated cells could also be demonstrated in anti-renal-tissue heteroimmunization [193].

The situation is similar in the case of human kidney transplantation with the difference that while in animal parabiosis the blood of the nephritic partner has a continuous access to the kidney of the normal partner, in man the normal kidney is placed into an affected renal circulation so that glomerulonephritis may also involve the originally healthy kidney. This suggests the presence of a humoral nephritis inducing factor, capable of attacking the kidney, also in human nephritis. Probably also the nephritogenic Streptococcus strain plays a role in this mechanism. The immunopathogenesis of post-streptococcal glomerulonephritis is still not fully understood. It has been postulated that the plasma membrane of the nephritogenic Streptococcus cells and the human glomerular basement membrane have determinant groups in common [425]. According to analytical studies, only a small portion (12 per cent or less) of the soluble glycoproteid of the nephritogenic streptococcal plasma membrane cross-reacts with the glomerular basement membrane as the immunogen [242]. Immunofluorescent staining revealed the presence of immunoglobulin and C in the basement membrane during acute glomerulonephritis; this weighs in favour of an immunological process [221]. The pathogenic factor is probably produced by the diseased organ [299]. Several authors, however, failed to demonstrate autoantibodies in either acute or chronic glomerulonephritis [326] and there is no proof whether the specific humoral anti-renal antibodies are causative or concomitant factors in the pathogenesis of renal disease.

### *Autosensitization with nerve tissue*

Experimental allergic encephalomyelitis (EAE) has been classified as a true autoallergic disease in which autoantigen-like tissue components play a role which are separated from circulation by the blood-brain barrier, analogously with the blood-aqueous humour barrier, the basement membrane of the seminiferous tubules and the acinar epithelium of the thyroid follicles. Lymphoid tissue can be regarded as an isolated 'foreign' tissue in the brain, because the cerebral antigen had no previous contact with the lymphoid tissue. Autologous lymph node tissue survives for several months if transplanted into the brain, behaving there like a foreign tissue by eliciting an allergic inflammatory reaction [133]. Such antigens are most suitable for the provocation of experimental autoallergy and such experiments serve as models of demyelinization and inflammatory processes in the central nervous system. This weighs in favour of the concept that the immune response, i.e. the allergic reaction is responsible for the development of the experimental disease. The encephalitogenic factors are substances present in extracts of brain or their tissues which, when injected together with complete Freund's adjuvant are capable of eliciting EAE in experimental animals. A basic protein resembling histone, associated with myelin, is probably the most important of these factors which are organ-specific, but not species-specific [133].

Human myelin contains 23 per cent protein, 30 per cent of which is a strongly basic protein consisting of 169 amino acids [218]. Like other basic proteins, it is weakly immunogenic. According to immunofluorescence and radioimmunological studies, the antibodies specific for the basic protein occur chiefly in the myelinated fibre containing areas. The determinant groups of the basic protein molecule responsible for the induction of antibody production have not yet been identified, probably because they could occur in a molecular region other than that containing the main encephalitogenic determinant [224]. The latter is localized at the molecular site where a single tryptophane residue is present. Modification of the single tryptophane residue of basic protein isolated from bovine brain resulted in loss of encephalitogenic activity in guinea pigs. The same modified preparation did, however, cause EAE in Lewis rats, indicating a variation of the encephalitogenic determinant with the species [378].

Injection of a heterologous encephalitogenic emulsion produces EAE in cats; the picture resembles human encephalomyelitis. The cells involved in the vascular reaction arise locally, through proliferation of the perivascular histiocytes [54].

The cerebrospinal fluid of hydrocephalic children contains a special basic protein, minimal amounts of which cause an acute neurological disease in guinea pigs when injected together with Freund's adjuvant. A margin composed of polymorphonuclear leukocytes appears in the cerebral vessels. This special basic protein and that of human myelin give a weak cross-reaction with each other [253].

EAE has been regarded as a kind of delayed hypersensitivity, whence it is passively transferable with lymph node cells, e.g. from rats sensitized with spinal cord tissue to isologous recipients which had already been treated neonatally with spleen cells from the prospective donor. In animals possessing this kind of acquired tolerance, the donor cells survive and maintain function longer than in unprepared animals [290]. Animals treated with homologous nerve tissue also show cutaneous and corneal reactions of the delayed type. Antibodies formed against various nerve tissue constituents appear in the blood stream and probably have a pathogenic role. It has been shown that apart from the cell-mediated process a demyelinization factor is also involved [12]. The observations that removal of the regional lymph nodes or total body X-ray irradiation inhibit the development of EAE weigh in favour of delayed hypersensitivity. EAE and human autoimmune diseases are, in fact, histologically similar: inflammatory lesions develop chiefly around the small veins and mononuclear, lymphoid and plasma cells enter the parenchyma, causing its destruction (demyelinization). Electron microscopically, the first changes are detected in the mitochondria of the myelin-sheathed nerve fibres. Repeated injection of an aqueous brain extract confers a substantial protection against EAE [156].

Anti-cerebral antibodies induced a transitory psychotic state in normal human volunteers [159] and the majority of acute-stage schizophrenic patients responded positively to skin tests performed with extracts of human cortical grey matter [273]. Nuclear, mitochondrial and microsomal fractions of rat brain in complete Freund's adjuvant induced the production of thermostable, C-fixing and haemagglutinating antibodies. The microsomal fraction was the most effective of the three [351].

Like the tissues of the central nervous system, also peripheral nerve tissue extracts can induce experimental allergic neuritis in rabbits and other laboratory animals when administered along with complete Freund's adjuvant [226*a*, 402].

## NON-ORGAN-SPECIFIC FORMS OF AUTOSENSITIZATION

### *Autosensitization with placental tissue*

Apart from antibodies to foetal erythrocytes and leukocytes, antibodies to the foetal part of the placenta (syncytiotrophoblast) may occasionally appear in the maternal blood [173]. The foetal placenta can be regarded as a syngeneic graft, because it usually differs in composition from the maternal tissue with which it keeps close contact through the maternal circulation. The placenta of $F_1$ hybrid mice induces transplantation immunity only in the male parent, but not in the female, which thus can tolerate hybrid skin grafts [154].

### *Sensitization with mesenchymal tissue*

Mesenchymal tissue, especially that of the joints, may be transformed by trauma, infection, etc. to an autoantigen and thus induce the formation of autoantibodies which may initiate a rheumatoid arthritis-like process after reaction with the connective tissue antigen. The process affects chiefly the arthritic connective tissue and may result in the continuous formation of anti-connective-tissue antibodies. This chain reaction is probably responsible for maintaining the process and for the development of 'rheumatoid arthritis' [389]. The possibility of this mechanism is suggested by the observation that in rabbits sensitized with synovial membrane extract (in Freund's adjuvant), synovial proliferation and hypertrophy of the joints occur in addition to positive skin reactions [38].

The continuous activity lasting longer than two years is explained, on the one hand, by the action of a microbial agent, and on the other, by persistence of the antigen plus autoimmunity induced by components of the inflamed tissue [129].

Non-species-specific collagenous autoantibodies have been demonstrated in a high percentage of severe rheumatoid arthritis cases [366]. Fractions of antibody species specific for human collagen as well as non-species-specific collagen antibodies were demonstrated by means of haemagglutination and immunofluorescence technique in rabbit immune sera produced against acid-soluble human collagen [367]. Helical antigenic determinants which require an intact triple-helical structure of the collagen molecule are mainly recognized by rat antisera [25*a*].

### *Systemic lupus erythematosus (SLE), lupus erythematosus disseminatus (LED)*

Phagocytosis of homogeneous nuclear material or nucleoproteids under the influence of an opsonizing factor indicates an autosensitization mechanism: such a reaction occurs in connection with SLE as an *in vitro* LE cell phenomenon. Patients diseased in SLE possess an abnormal $\gamma$-globulin which induces the formation of LE cells on contact with neutrophil leukocytes as a result of *in vitro* phagocytosis of the antinuclear-factor-coated nuclear substance. Rabbits sensitized with the abnormal $\gamma$-globulin produce antibodies which, along with SLE serum, inhibit the formation of LE cells [209]. Since nuclei from all kinds of species or organs show this phenomenon, the factor appears to be nucleus-specific rather than species or organ-specific, i.e. it seems to depend on the presence of nucleoprotein.

Apart from the specific antinuclear factor, also other kinds of autoantibody are produced against formed elements of blood or against various organs; these autoantibodies are, however, not specific for SLE. Various observations, such as the *in vivo* LE cell formation at the base of natural vesicles, and in synovial fluid, as well as fluorescence of the capillary walls in the renal glomeruli (after treatment with fluorescein labelled antihuman-globulin) suggest the pathogenic role of the different antinuclear factors. Since, however, SLE also occurs in agammaglobulinaemia, the humoral factors alone can hardly be held responsible for the process, because, as a rule, delayed hypersensitivity is dominant [216]. Delayed-type of hypersensitivity is produced by i.d. administration of leukocyte suspension from the patient [118]. The fact that SLE cannot be elicited by a direct immunological reaction suggests the background of a genetic predisposition, characterized by the absence of immunological self-recognition [90].

SLE also occurs in dogs, with simultaneous or successive development of haémolytic anaemia, thrombocytopenic purpura and glomerulonephritis. Occasionally symmetrical polyarthritis, dermatitis, and thyroiditis may occur as intercurrent processes. Breeding experiments have suggested also in this instance that the pathological process is explicable by vertical transmission of an infectious agent in genetically predisposed animals [227].

The LE factor can be regarded [258*d*, 261] as an antibody, because (*i*) passive haemagglutination with LE serum is positive if nucleoprotein or DNA are used as antigen (no reaction takes place with RNA) and C-fixation is also positive with these active factors [343]; (antihistone antibodies play only a subordinate role); (*ii*) LE sera lose activity on saturation with nucleoprotein or DNA; (*iii*) LE factor adsorbed onto, and eluted from, human cell nucleus can bind anti-human-globulin serum, to judge from the fall of serum titre toward D(Rh)-antibody-coated erythrocytes; (*iv*) The properties of the experimental anti-nuclear serum resemble those of the LE serum.

Another argument in support of the antibody property of the LE factor is that nuclei from fresh, untreated SLE tissue and leukocytes show fluorescence on contact with fluorescein labelled anti-human-globulin when pretreated with LE serum [168]. The LE factor is transferable to dogs. There are two factors, one thermostable, transferable and capable of passing across the placenta, the other thermolabile, non-transferable and not capable of passing across the placenta [28].

The serological study of glomerular eluates, immunofluorescence studies and immunochemical analysis have shown that several antigen–antibody systems may be involved in the pathomechanism of various tissue lesions occurring in SLE. Native DNA + anti-native-DNA complex occurs in most SLE patients. Antibodies against single-stranded DNA are frequently demonstrable in sera and glomerular eluates. The problem is whether these antibodies combine with the native DNA which becomes denatured after deposition in the glomerule or whether single-stranded DNA + anti-DNA complexes are deposited from the very beginning. Native DNA is demonstrable both in serum and in glomerular depositions and the latter also contains single-stranded DNA determinants [210]. Anti-native-DNA antibodies are closely associated with the SLE activity [211].

## MIXED AUTOSENSITIZATION PROCESSES

There are many pathological processes in which an autoimmune mechanism can be postulated on the basis of autosensitization; of these only the most important conditions are briefly discussed.

An autoimmune mechanism probably plays a role in the so-called idiopathic form of Addison's disease (adreno-cortical atrophy with hypofunction). Injection of adrenal tissue in complete Freund's adjuvant elicits immunological adrenalitis in the guinea pig (lymphocytic infiltration of the atrophic cortex). Patients' sera contain autoantibodies against cytoplasmic antigens of cortical steroid hormone producing cells (adrenocortical tissue-specific antigen); the former are demonstrable by various serological reactions and immunofluorescence. Coexistence with other autoimmune diseases is frequent; antibodies against thyroid and gastric wall cells are not infrequently encountered [275].

### *Pernicious anaemia*

This is characterized by an atrophic gastritis with achlorhydria and lack of gastric intrinsic factor which leads to failure of absorption of dietary vitamin $B_{12}$ and consequent megaloblastic anaemia. The condition is caused by antibodies formed against two constituents of the gastric mucosa:

(*i*) the microsomal fraction of gastric parietal cells and (*ii*) the intrinsic factor (50 per cent of cases) [387]. These antibodies are not species specific. The gastric antibody can react with autologous gastric mucosal and glandular cell components of the patient [179*a*]. Antibodies to both intrinsic factor and parietal cell can be demonstrated in the serum and gastric secretions of anaemia perniciosa patients, whereas the serum of simple atrophic gastritis patients does not contain antibodies to the intrinsic factor. Parietal antibodies arising in simple atrophic gastritis belong to the three main immunoglobulin classes and IgA is demonstrable in the gastric juice. Parietal antibodies occur in 5 per cent of the normal population; such subjects do not show symptoms, but gastric biopsy indicates a superficial, pre-atrophic gastritis. The sera of patients affected with autoimmune thyroiditis contain markedly high levels of parietal cell antibodies, whereas thyroid antibodies do not show an increased frequency of occurrence in simple atrophic gastritis patients [346].

Atrophic gastritis can be induced immunologically: the gastric secretion of dogs can be inhibited by intravenous injection of human gastric fluid or with autologous gastric fluid in complete Freund's adjuvant [162]. Similar results have been obtained in rhesus monkeys by means of antibodies produced against parietal mucosal cells. Experimental autoimmune gastritis responds to cutaneous provocation with gastric antigen by a delayed-type reaction [11].

### *Ulcerative colitis*

The sensitization mechanism of this disease has been attributed to a nutritive allergy, but occasionally inhalatory allergens (pollens) may also play a role. The autoantibodies produced in this condition react with the mucosa of the colon and with the goblet cells of the ileum; colon mucosa from foetal or germ-free rats can be used as antigen [297]. The autoantibodies associated with ulcerative colitis may arise due to immunization with enteric microorganisms, because the ubiquitous antigen of Enterobacteriaceae is related with the colon antigen. Symptoms reminiscent of the disease can be elicited in rats by injection of certain *E. coli* strains [149]. Cross-reacting antigens between *E. coli* and colonic epithelium have been described and an immune response to such antigens has been postulated as an aetiological factor although this is still in dispute. This kind of hypersensitivity has been regarded as cell-mediated because there is no parallelism between antibody titres and clinical signs [296]. Patients' lymphocytes show cytotoxicity for colon epithelial cells. The process may be associated with other autoimmune diseases. High incidence of carcinoma of the colon has been observed.

### *Myasthenia gravis*

It is often associated with the presence in serum of a number of autoantibodies, to skeletal muscle as well as to thyroid microsomes. Recent data suggest that myosin contains the antigenic sites related to humoral antibody induction in myasthenia gravis [327*a*]. This condition is a manifestation of chronic thymitis and probably represents the immune response of thymic and motoric nerve ending antigens to a common antibody [243]. It is possible that in autoimmune thymitis a substance is released which inhibits neuromuscular transmission. A component combining with the cross striation of skeletal muscle has been demonstrated by immunofluorescence [374].

### *Pemphigus group*

Autoantibodies of IgG nature are demonstrable by immunofluorescence in both serum and vesicular fluid of pemphigus and bullous pemphigoid patients [32, 70]. These antibodies act in acantholytic pemphigus against the intercellular substance of the epidermis and against stratum spinosum antigens [61], whereas in bullous pemphigoid against the basement membrane, by formation of subepidermal bullae. The autoantibodies have a cytolytic effect and affect also the mucosa [1]. Acantholysis can be induced experimentally, using a high level of anti-epithelial autoantibodies and, for provocation, a mucosal antigen [177].

### *Sjögren's syndrome*

Various antibodies can be demonstrated in diseases associated with the chronic inflammation of the salivary, lacrimal, and other glands, with reduced secretion, exsiccosis and, often, with rheumatoid arthritis [10, 358]: antibodies against the duct epithelium of the salivary and lacrimal glands, thyroid antibodies to thyroglobulin and microsomal antigens, gastric antibodies to gastric parietal cells and, of non-organ-specific antibodies, anti-nuclear factor, rheumatoid factor, etc. Association of such antibodies with various autoimmune diseases speaks for an autoimmune mechanism.

# CHARACTERISTICS OF SENSITIZATION

## DIFFERENCES BETWEEN NATURAL AND ARTIFICIAL SENSITIZATION

Comparison of natural with experimental sensitization has shown that the incidence of allergic symptoms increases parallel with increased exposure to antigen and with the number of factors facilitating hypersensitivity in the individual. This is especially true for occupational diseases, many of which are due to sensitization (chromium sensitivity of builders, nickel eczema of galvanizers, etc.). Coating of the various metal instruments with liquid polyurethane can protect the sensitized subject [266]. Frugoni and Ancona [119] described asthma cases caused by flour infected with *Pediculoides ventricosus* larvae (this is reminiscent of inhalatory sensitization by house dust containing mites, among others flour mites). Prausnitz [305] observed asthma bronchiale cases in the cotton industry; he isolated from cotton powder a primary toxic protein, of which 1 mg (i.d.) caused inflammation also in healthy subjects and 0.01–0.001 mg was sufficient to elicit a typical immediate-type reaction in diseased subjects. An epidemic-like occurrence of asthma bronchiale has repeatedly been observed in ricinus seed processing plants and in their neighbourhood; the spread of ricinus-seed dust was identified as the cause [151, 285]. A total of 150 asthma cases, 9 of them lethal, with positive skin test and passive transfer occurred in a small town within a few days after the opening of a new ricinus-seed mill; symptoms subsided when the mill was put out of operation and the dust was removed [57, 254]. In an asbestos mill, 34 per cent of the workers and 15 per cent of the inhabitants of a nearby village were found to be latently sensitized [91]. Out of a total of 20 bakers, millers and pastry makers 11 had bronchial asthma due to flour dust [422].

Accordingly, a substantial part of the population is liable to become sensitive to certain environmental allergens if exposure is lasting long enough [331]. Thus sensitization is a physiological process which can affect all human beings, but only about 20 per cent are predisposed to its clinical manifestation. It follows from the general nature of allergic predisposition that allergens can penetrate even normal skin and mucosa to a certain degree. This is supported by experiments on absorption of allergen: monkeys showed an immediate-type response at the passively sensitized site, regardless of whether the specific allergen was administered into urinary bladder, peritoneal and pleural cavity, mammary gland, cerebrospinal canal or intravenously; even the antigen instilled onto the nasal mucosa became immediately absorbed. On the other hand, agents dissolved in an appropriate vehicle can penetrate the skin via the intact horny layer, but especially through the hair follicles and sebaceous glands; this process can be promoted by physical or chemical agents increasing cutaneous permeability, such as sodium laurylsulphate and, still more, dimethylsulphoxide, under experimental conditions.

Since the schedule of medication is usually regular and the doses of the drug are precisely defined, allergic reactions to drug form a transitory type between natural and artificial sensitization. Artificial sensitization nevertheless differs from natural in certain respects: it takes a more rapid course and the cutaneous reactions associated with it are relatively less intensive. Spontaneous allergy usually persists for a long time, not infrequently throughout lifetime (e.g. sensitivity to turpentine, chromium, as well as certain drug allergies). It can be demonstrated by quantitative epicutaneous tests that in contact dermatitis, skin sensitivity may persist with an unchanged intensity for several months or even years, even if further contact with the allergen has more or less been prevented [377]. In part of the cases, however, sensitivity may vanish after elimination of the allergen and often also drug sensitivity, (e.g. penicillin allergy) ceases after several years. Persistence of sensitivity for several years can also occur in artificial sensitization, (e.g. experimental primula allergy) [235]. In general, the more intensive the sensitization, the longer it may last: individuals unresponsive to concentrations lower than 1 per cent of DNCB lose increased reactivity after one month, whereas those responsive to concentrations as low as 0.1–0.01 per cent, are still sensitive after one year [407*a*, *b*].

A further difference between natural and artificial sensitization is the less frequent occurrence of focal and systemic reaction in the latter. The probable cause is that in the case of a natural exposure, usually larger amounts of the sensitizing agent are active over a larger area and for a longer time compared with the relatively smaller amount of allergen used for experimental sensitization.

## DIFFERENCES BETWEEN SENSITIVITY OF HUMANS AND ANIMALS

In the overwhelming majority of the cases, artificial sensitization has been performed on animals. The findings of animal experiments can, however, not always be transferred to humans. The relation is closest in the case of contact sensitization, e.g. the agent which sensitizes the skin of the guinea pig will behave similarly in man in most of the cases; thus its use is not recommended for humans [248*b*]. Even this analogy cannot be generalized, though, because the mode of action may be different and agents sensitizing the guinea pig do not necessarily affect man; this applies especially to enteral use. The findings of autoimmunization experiments in animals, nevertheless, may give some information about human autoallergic mechanism (EAE, etc.).

The Forssman (heterophilic) shock of guinea pigs, this little-studied immunopathological reaction, deserves special mention. A single i.v. injection of rabbit antiserum to sheep erythrocyte stroma can provoke a lethal response in the guinea pig. Animals in the state of shock show a distinct oedematous-haemorrhagic change of the lungs and occasionally a foamy, sanguinolent fluid fills the trachea and nasal cavity [312]. No histamine release or mast cell degranulation can be observed during the Forssman shock [175]. The components of serum C are used up during the reaction and animals deficient in these factors are protected against lethal shock [365]. It has been postulated that true anaphylaxis and the Forssman shock differ in mechanism [41]. It has been shown by means of fluorescein labelled antibody that the Forssman antigens occur in the vascular endothelium and perivascular connective tissue. It is generally supposed that the interaction of the Forssman antigens with these sites brings about vascular damage through the activation of C [22]. There is electron-microscopic evidence that the vascular endothelium is the primary target of Forssman shock, and thrombocytes and polymorphonuclear leukocytes are pathogenic determinants in the development of this shock [385].

## THE THREE PHASES OF SENSITIZATION

1. *Period of exposure* when the organism comes into contact with the sensitizing agent but behaves indifferently, i.e. shows no sign of even a latent sensitivity. This phase may be observed when in chemical plants production of a new chemical compound is started or in the agriculture new plants are introduced. The duration of the phase of exposure varies from short to very long; it may even be life-long without resulting in manifestations of hypersensitivity, e.g. in the industry.

2. *The period of sensitization* is, in fact, a period of latency, lasting from the beginning of sensitization till the time when changed reactivity can be demonstrated by cutaneous tests (end of biological latency) or till the appearance of clinical symptoms (end of clinical latency). Biological latency—e.g. in serum sensitivity—lasts not so long as clinical latency, as sensitization is demonstrable by cutaneous tests prior to the clinical manifestation of serum sickness. The factors responsible for the switch-over from exposure to sensitization, i.e. to the recognition of the originally indifferent substance as an antigen, are still mostly unknown. Among others, intercurrent diseases may probably play a role.

The period of sensitization is fairly constant under experimental conditions, lasting from 5–6 to 10–14 days, regardless whether the sensitizing agent is serum, a chemical substance, a contact sensitizer or a microorganism. Thus, independently of the antigen, the establishment of delayed skin hypersensitivity may take 5–6 days in animals and 8–10 days in man, and that of immediate hypersensitivity as much as 10–14 days. Natural and artificial sensitization hardly differs in this respect, e.g. newly introduced drugs or chemicals (sulphonamide, penicillin, plastics, etc.) do not cause eruptions until after 7–14 days of application or exposure. Following the appearance of hypersensitivity, the latency of response to the specific antigen becomes much shorter (2–24 h). Sensitivity may remain latent if there is no further contact with the antigen.

3. *In the period of clinical manifestation,* encounter with the antigen elicits clinical symptoms. This phase, too, is fairly constant: in case of immediate-type reactions weal-and-flare response or shock develop within a few (5–10) min, depending on the time required for antigen absorption; delayed-type reactions usually require 24–48 h for the development of contact eczema or other cell-mediated processes. The clinical phase of sensitivity is always shorter than the latency phase and depends on the time of appearance and aggregation of the immunologically active lymphocytes.

## ROUTE OF SENSITIZATION

Apart from the skin also the digestive tract may serve as the starting point of sensitization (enteral sensitization). The gastric mucosa becomes permeable to proteins—antigens—on the slightest impairment, e.g. overfeeding with easily absorbable substances [334], but even the intact intestinal wall may be permeable to antigen if the subject is allergic [405*a*]. Indigestion, particularly in association with hypo- or anacidity, epithelial damage by purgation, inflammations, etc. may all promote the intestinal absorption of proteins. Drug absorption can usually take place through the mucous membrane of other organs as well.

Resistance of the mucous membrane to antigen passage probably varies with the species: serum administered into intact ureter or urinary bladder of guinea pigs does not elicit an anaphylactic shock unless a mucosal inflammation is induced [332]; whereas antigen is promptly absorbed from the urinary bladder of the monkey [405*b*].

The respiratory system is another important route of sensitization, through which inhalatory allergens may enter the body. Damage or inflammatory lesions of the lungs and airways promote the development of hypersensitivity. Many industrial chemicals sensitize through the airways [289*a*]. Guinea pigs sensitized with aerosol horse serum or horse scale spray (according to Kallós of less than 5 m$\mu$ particle diam.) may develop anaphylactic shock on re-application of the spray. Intranasal administration of the allergen to similarly sensitized rabbits elicits acute exudative inflammation in the lungs [51]. Nevertheless, similarly to other true allergic conditions (allergic enteritis, colitis, urticaria, atopic dermatitis), true asthmatic changes and hay fever cannot be induced experimentally.

Parenteral sensitization, above all by intradermal, subcutaneous and intramuscular injection of proteins, or intramuscular and intravenous drug therapy, tends to increase in frequency with the spread of injection treatment. Proteins sensitize by practically all routes of application and if injected intravenously, the lung is the main site of antibody formation.

If antibodies are limited to a circumscribed area of e.g. the skin, sensitivity, too, is limited to this particular area. In this case we may speak of local sensitization. Topical fixed eruptions, chiefly due to drugs such as barbiturates, phenophtalein, tetracyclines, acetylsalicylate belong to this group [335]. There are also transitory cases, in which a circumscribed area reacts first and later hypersensitivity spreads to a continuously increasing area. This suggests that a sharp distinction cannot be made between fixed eruptions and more or less extensive drug allergy eruptions. In experiments using the secretory surface of the lower respiratory tract of guinea pigs, the concept that local cellular immunity may commence independently of systemic cellular immunity has been established [403].

The corneal hypersensitivity concomitant with Wessely's phenomenon has also been interpreted as a local immune reaction. It is known that on injection of antigen into rabbit cornea, the dramatic inflammatory reaction of the corneal periphery will not start until after 10 days of latency. The inside of the cornea becomes oedematous and infiltrating immune precipitations and polymorphous leukocytes appear in it, but later its transparency becomes restored without the development of fibrosis. The latter is the so-called Wessely's phenomenon which can be attributed to humoral antibodies. If the cornea is treated with a second dose of antigen 2–4 weeks or even 11 months after Wessely's reaction has occurred, a distinct ring-like precipitate, enclosing a disc-like opacity, will appear in the cornea within 15 min after the injection. Later on fibrosis and vascularization develop. Immunofluorescence examinations have shown that in such cases the tissue damage is due to the presence of tissue-fixed antibodies in the cornea and/or leukocytes persisting at the site of the original Wessely's reaction. The role of humoral antibodies in the corneal hypersensitivity seems unlikely [348].

## THE ROLE OF THE AUTONOMIC NERVOUS SYSTEM IN SENSITIZATION

The possibility has been considered that the antigenic stimulus is mediated and initiated by the autonomic nervous system, probably via the coordination reflex arising in the lymph nodes [257]. This could account for antibody formation on spot-like antigen effect throughout the organism, without requiring humoral transport of the antigen. If, however, the tip of rabbit ear is treated with a bismuth isotope labelled typhus vaccine and severed 3–10 sec after injection, both isotope and agglutinin will appear in the blood. Isotope and agglutinin will be absent only if the blood and lymph vessels of the ear are compressed to such an extent that not even minute quantities of the antigen can enter circulation. This experiment suggests that no antibody formation can take place reflectorically via the nervous system [202].

According to Ado [3], both the sympathetic and parasympathetic parts of the autonomic nervous system change functionally during protein sensitization. Although the sensory nerve terminals of the carotid sinus receptors can be rendered sensitive to foreign protein, events taking place in the entire organism differ from those occurring in the carotid sinus, because the antigen acts also centrally [5]. The reflectoric mechanism cannot in itself offer a satisfactory explanation of the anaphylactic shock [426]. Similarly contradictory observations have been made in other experimental studies on the role of the autonomic nervous system [26, 134]; in these attempts have been made to explain antibody production by the tone of the autonomic nervous system or, more precisely, by the action of adrenergic and cholinergic substances (adrenalin, pituitrin, atropine, pilocarpine) which, however, had no notable influence on antibody formation. The direct role of the autonomic nervous system is contradicted by the finding that sensitized cats, whose autonomic nervous system had been removed 'in toto' and whose adrenals had been ligated, developed anaphylactic shock much in the 'normal' manner and neither sympathetic nor vagal paralysers had an effect on the process; nor did the normal antibody level of the serum show any change [233, 413]. The neurovegetative reflex theory of sensitization seems improbable in the light of these findings.

This approach offers no resolution of the problem, because according to studies on sympathectomized subjects the autonomic nervous system cannot be fully eliminated, whence its influence persists at least in part. Interpretation is rendered difficult by the many contradictory experimental results.

According to certain authors, no DNCB contact eczema, i.e. delayed hypersensitivity, can be induced on a skin surface in which the sensory radicals have been transfixed or have become degenerated [59*a*], while according to others, semilunar circumcision and denervation of the skin area by Mansfeld's technique [241] does not interfere with DNCB sensitization unless large doses of ganglion paralysers are administered [281, 373], but in such cases the effect is general, not being limited to the dissected flap of skin. Unilateral sympathectomy or transfixion of the boundary bundle in guinea pigs does not affect DNCB sensitization according to one group of authors [283], while according to others it does [239]; a third view is that the degree of the allergic skin reaction depends on the actual state of the central nervous system [136*a*, *b*]. In cases of paralysis of the brachial plexus, the epicutaneous reaction remains unchanged at the sites of sensory and motoric paralysis and sensitivity to DNCB can be induced in the paralysed skin area [376]. In man, drug hibernation had no influence on contact (DNCB) sensitization, nor on reactions to tuberculin, trichophytin and on Frey's reaction [265]. Agents acting on the central nervous system, such as morphine and barbiturates, effected a delay in the DNCB sensitization of guinea pig, and schizophrenic humans either developed only a low sensitivity to DNCB or responded only to high provoking doses [23*a*, *b*].

Patients claimed to be allergic to local anaesthetics responded differently to the intracutaneous test, sometimes by false positive, sometimes by false negative results [355]. Important observations have been made on patients with leprosy [309]: in skin areas in which both the sensory and the autonomic nerve fibres had degenerated (absence of sweat gland activity !), epicutaneous sensitization was possible in the same manner as in sound skin areas. Adults and children with asthma bronchiale showed a decreased response to some, but not all, effects of epinephrine. The $\beta$-adrenergic receptors can be divided into types $\beta_1$ and $\beta_2$ based on pharmacological criteria. Asthma affects only the $\beta_2$-type adrenergic response. The degree of abnormal bronchial reaction to acetylcholine correlates with that of the abnormal metabolic response to epinephrine. It has been postulated that decreased responsiveness to epinephrine is due to the reduced activity of $\beta_2$-receptors. Epinephrine is known to suppress both total and homocytotropic antibody production, but it may stimulate lymphoid cell activity under different conditions of experiment [313]. Sympathicomimetic amines inhibit the antigen induced release of histamine in both actively and passively sensitized tissues; the favourable influence of these compounds on bronchial asthma is at least in part explicable by this circumstance—the effect is mediated by the cyclic AMP [15]. Certain observations suggest that apart from the histamine sensitizing factor, *Bordetella pertussis* vaccine enhances sensitization also by a propranolol-like blocking of the $\beta$-adrenergic receptors of the autonomic nervous system. The $\beta$-adrenergic blocking effect of pertussis vaccine has been found to vary with the species of laboratory animals: it is important in mice, but not in the guinea pig [300].

## THE ROLE OF THE AUTONOMIC NERVOUS SYSTEM IN HUMORAL ANTIBODY PRODUCTION

The course of horse serum sensitization in rabbits kept in prolonged barbiturate anaesthesia and in non-narcotized rabbits did not show any difference; the level of humoral antobodies (precipitins) was probably lower in the former, but the cutaneous Arthus reaction on rabbit skin was retarded [205, 206]. Chemotherapeutic hibernation had no influence on the Arthus phenomenon or on antibody formation [394]. If barbiturate anaesthesia was commenced simultaneously with active sensitization, a blocking of the anaphylactic shock occurred [203, 204]. Thus complete anaesthesia may influence the production of immunoglobulin (antibody), but not the antigen–antibody reaction; lethal anaphylactic shock due to passive sensitization will occur even if it is carried out in barbiturate anaesthesia.

The experiments of Filipp et al. [102, 103], too, failed to resolve the problem: although in the overwhelming majority of their cases the anaphylactic shock of guinea pigs could be inhibited by bringing about a hypothalamic lesion, and also antibody production decreased to a certain degree, neither the Arthus phenomenon, nor the Shwartzman phenomenon had been inhibited. The mechanism of the blockade following electrolytic injury of the tuberal region has not yet been elucidated [100*b*]. The lesion probably blocks thyroid activity, thereby reducing considerably the level of thyrotropin, (thyroid stimulating hormone: TSH). Thyroidectomized animals cannot be sensitized [101]. A similar partial or complete inhibition of anaphylactic shock was observed in dogs after destruction of different hypothalamic nuclei [353]. Ether anaesthesia involving the mesencephalon when applied during sensitization inhibits the development of reinjection shock, but once sensitivity has become established, neither narcosis, nor surgical disconnection of brain centres will affect the reinjection shock, suggesting that the nervous system can only interfere with the induction of sensitization [394]. According to recent observations, focal hypothalamic lesions which cause profound metabolic alterations are not able to reduce antibody production, and do not affect in any way the peripheral reactivity of the animal to the interaction of exogenous antibody and antigen. Similarly no decrease of antibody production takes place after hypophysectomy [392].

### *The role of psychic factors*

It should be noted right at the beginning that psychic effects can neither sensitize, nor elicit allergic symptoms unless in a state of established hypersensitivity or allergic disease. In such cases the allergic symptom complex is probably induced via an established conditioned reflex path, e.g. coincidence of the psychic trauma with an allergic attack builds up a conditioned reflex. This correlation has been demonstrated experimentally in guinea pigs with allergy or histamine induced asthma, using a sound signal as the conditioning stimulus [278]. Although in such cases there is no antigen–antibody reaction, because one active factor, the antigen, is absent, the mediators participating in the non-specific phase of the allergic response which are actually responsible for the symptoms, may be released by the psychic factor, the more so as the autonomic nervous system plays a role in their release also normally. Thus this mechanism corresponds with Pavlov's concept that the physiological functions controlled by the autonomic nervous system can be elicited, and influenced, by conditioned reflexes. Not infrequently, however, the process initiated by an environmental allergen or a drug is attributed to nervous factors. Such cases should, therefore, be carefully scrutinized. No statistically significant difference has been found between the immune responses of schizophrenics and normal subjects [176].

Some cases originally regarded as psychosomatic are described in the following.

A patient of Török [391] developed erythematous skin eruptions every Monday, which had been attributed to the excitement associated with taking up work at the beginning of the week until it was discovered that the patient had regularly taken laxative every Sunday evening after the rich Sunday meals. A similar case is that of a commercial traveller, who always developed rashes on the train and these had been attributed to the excitement connected with travelling until it was traced to the Aspirin tablets which he had regularly taken for the headache caused by coal smoke. A woman regularly developed a severe dermatitis on her birthday; this, too, had been attributed to the emotional and psychic upheaval connected with the day until it was identified as sensitivity to primula, which was presented to her by her husband each year as it happened to be the flower of the season.

It is, nevertheless, clear that psychic factors cannot be disregarded in any process in which the autonomic nervous system is involved; psychic factors may considerably influence established allergic states, e.g. through peripheral circulation, the increase of which may promote the absorption of the antigen. The qualitative and quantitative relationships between psychic and somatic factors is not yet fully understood. One of the main mistakes made in this field is to disregard the fundamental rules of immunology in the analysis of psychosomatic events.

The effect of hypnosis on allergic symptoms and their hypnotic prevention can also be explained by the role of the autonomic nervous system. Kartamyshev [194] reports that a patient with chinin allergy developed urticaria when the sugar given during hypnotic sleep was suggested to be chinin and *vice versa*, no urticaria occurred if the chinin given in the same state was suggested to be sugar. Kleinsorge [207*b*] was able to elicit strawberry urticaria by hypnotic suggestion, but the symptoms subsided on antihistamine treatment even in this instance, and lasted for several hours without medication. The cause of psychically induced allergic responses may obviously be sought in the release of chemical mediators under the influence of the autonomic nervous system. Also attacks of asthma and hay fever can be provoked by hypnosis which, however, has no influence on the skin test [31]. In another case the symptoms improved, but the P–K transfer continued to be positive [244]. Also, intracutaneous injection of distilled water failed to elicit a positive skin reaction under the hypnotic suggestion that it had been the specific allergen. The threshold of skin sensitivity could not be influenced either by deep hypnosis, or by posthypnotic suggestion [377].

These experiments and observations which, on the one hand, deal with allergic reactions occurring despite the elimination of the nervous system and, on the other hand, affirm the limited influence of the central and autonomous nervous system on allergic events, are probably neither irreconcilable nor contradictory if the allergic phenomena are analysed phylogenetically. Scrutiny of the most frequent allergic phenomenon, inflammation, reveals that the organism may respond in different manners to inflammatory allergic stimuli. All living beings, and also non-innervated tissues are capable of an appropriate response to inflammatory stimuli; even the chicken amnion having no innervation can be sensitized with proteins to the degree of an organic 'shock' (Schultz–Dale reaction) [94]. In phylogenetically higher animals and man, the inflammatory response is organized and coordinated chiefly by the neurohormonal system and probably also directly by the autonomic nervous system. But even the highly developed organisms are still capable of the primordial mechanism the function of which had been taken over by the nervous system in the course of phylogeny; if the nervous system is rendered incapable of organizing function by disease, experimental trauma, etc., an appropriate response will nevertheless be given to the inflammatory stimulus without the participation of the nervous system. Accordingly, although paralysis, lesion, transfixion, partial extirpation, etc. of the nervous system may prevent its intact function, but the allergic reactions of the body, i.e. reponse to sensitizing agents with hypersensitivity will not be prevented. According to Lunedei [238], too, sensitization and allergic reaction can occur without the controlling function of the nervous system. This, however, does not mean that sensitization would always take place independently of the nervous system, because the latter very probably participates in the mechanism if it is intact.

Thus, the various nerve-eliminating, and blocking experiments seem to suggest the conclusion that the nervous system is neither indispensible, nor superfluous in sensitization; sensitization *can* take place with or without the participation of the nervous system. It is, therefore, useless to dispute which of the two theories is true, because both of them may be right and can well be reconciled with one another.

## REFERENCES


1. Ablin, R. J. and Beutner, E. H.: *Int. Arch. Allergy* **33,** 227 (1968).
2. Abrishami, M. A., Boyd, K. G. and Settipane, G. A.: *Acta allerg. (Kbh.)* **26,** 117 (1971).
3. (Ado, A. D.) Адо, А. Д.: *Данные по патологии аллергических реакций.* Казан. 1947.
4. Ado, A. D. and Abrossimow, W. N.: *Allergie u. Asthma* **7,** 22 (1961).
5. Ado, A. D. and Ishimova, L. M.: *Allergie u. Asthma* **5,** 93 (1959).
6. Africa, B. and Haber, E.: *Immunochemistry* **8,** 479 (1971).
7. Alkan, S. S., Nitecki, D. E. and Goodman, J.: *J. Immunol.* **107,** 353 (1971).

8*a*. Allwood, G. G. and Asherson, G. L.: *Clin. exp. Immunol.* **9,** 249 (1971).

8*b*. ibid., **9,** 259 (1971).

9. Anderson, C. L. and Rose, N. R.: *J. Immunol.* **107,** 1341 (1971).
10. Anderson, J. R., Beck, J. S., Bloch, K., Buchanan, W. W. and Bunim, J. J.: In *Autoimmunity*. Ed. by Baldwin, R. W. and Humphrey, J. H. Blackwell, Oxford 1965, p. 26.
11. Andrada, J. A., Andrada, N. R. and Andrada, E. C.: *Clin. exp. Immunol.* **4,** 293 (1969).
12. Appel, S. H. and Bornstein, M. B.: *J. exp. Med.* **119,** 303 (1964).
13. Arend, W. P. and Mannik, M.: *J. Immunol.* **107,** 63 (1971).
14. Asherson, G. L., Allison, A. C. and Zembala, M.: *Immunology* **22,** 465 (1972).
15. Assem, E. S. K. and Schild, H. O.: *Int. Arch. Allergy* **40,** 576 (1971).
16. Avery, O. T. and Goebel, W. F.: *J. exp. Med.* **47,** 379 (1928).
17. Baart, E. H. and Cormane, R. H.: *Acta derm.-venereol.* **48,** 578 (1968).
18. Barker, H. E.: *J. Amer. med. Ass.* **163,** 410 (1957).
19. Barr, S. E.: *Ann. Allergy* **29,** 49 (1971).
20. Baum, J., Boughton, B., Mongar, J. L. and Schild, H. O.: *Immunology* **4,** 95 (1961).
21. Bayghioni, C. and Williams, R. C., jr.: *Immunochemistry* **8,** 265 (1971).
22. Becker, E. I. and Austen, K. F.: In *Anaphylaxis. Textbook of Immunopathology I.* Ed. by Miescher, P. A. and Müller-Eberhard, H. J. Grune-Stratton, New York 1968, p. 76.

23*a*. Bednenko, P. F.: *Abstr. Sov. Med. B. (Moscow)* **4,** 230 (1960).

23*b*. ibid., **5,** 590 (1961).

24. Behar, A. J. and Tal, C.: *III. Int. Congr. Allergol. Paris,* Flammarion, Paris 1958.
25. Beickert, A.: *Klin. Wschr.* **39,** 251 (1961).
25*a*. Beil, W., Timpl, R. and Furthmayr, H.: *Immunology* **24** (1973).
26. Belák, S.: *Immun. Forsch.* **100,** 264 (1941).
27. Benacerraf, B., Potter, J. L., McCluskey, R. T. and Miller, F.: *J. exp. Med.* **111,** 195 (1960).
28. Bencze, G.: *Acta med. Acad. Sci. hung.* **17,** 215 (1961).
29. Bergquist, G.: *Acta allerg. (Kbh.)* **10,** 187 (1956).
30. Bernecker, C., Krause, R. and Roetscher, I.: *Acta allerg. (Kbh.)* **26,** 363 (1971).
31. Bernstein, A. E.: *I. Int. Allergol. Kongr. Zürich 1951.* Karger, Basel 1952. p. 839.
32. Beutner, E. H. and Jordon, R. E.: *Proc. Soc. exp. Biol. N. Y.* **117,** 505 (1964).
33. Bizzozero, E.: *Arch. Derm. Syph. (Berlin)* **173,** 342 (1936).
34*a*. Bloch, B.: *Arch. Derm. Syph. (Berlin)* **145,** 34 (1924).
34*b*. id., *C. R. VIII. Congr. Int. Derm. Copenhague* 1930. Ed. by Lombolt, S. Engelsen and Schroeder, Copenhague 1931, p. 101.
35*a*. Bloch, B. and Steiner-Wourlisch, A.: *Arch. Derm. Syph. (Berlin)* **152,** 283 (1926).
35*b*. ibid., **162,** 349 (1930).
36. Blumberg, B. S., Alter, H. J. and Visnich, S.: *J. Amer. med. Ass.* **191,** 541 (1965).
37. Blumberg, B. S., Millman, I., Sitnick, A. I. and London, W. T.: *J. exp. Med.* **134,** 320 (1971).
38. Bocking, D.: *IX. Int. Congr. Rheum. Dis. Toronto* **2,** 140 (1957).
39. Bonner, C. D. and Homburger, F.: *New Engl. J. Med.* **256,** 131 (1957).
40. Boyden, S. V.: *Int. Arch. Allergy* **10,** 65 (1957).
41. Broder, I.: In *Inflammation, Immunity and Hypersensitivity.* Ed. by Movat, H. Z. Harper-Row, New York 1971, p. 334.
42. Brown, H. C., Woolhouse, F. M. and Williams, H. B.: *Plast. reconstr. Surg.* **46,** 588 (1970).
43. Bryce, L-M.: *Med. J. Austr.* **1,** 371 (1933).
44. Bukantz, S. C. and Klingberg, W. G.: *J. Allergy* **25,** 74 (1954).
45*a*. Burky, E. L.: *Arch. Ophthal.* **12,** 536 (1934).
45*b*. id., *J. Allergy* **5,** 466 (1934).
46*a*. Burnet, F. M.: *Brit. med. J.* **2,** 720 (1959).
46*b*. id., *New Engl. J. Med.* **264,** 24 (1961).
47. Burnet, F. M. and Holmes, M. C.: *J. Path. Bact.* **88,** 229 (1964).
48. Burrows, B. A., Peters, T., Lowell, F. C., Trakas, A. N. and Reilly, P.: *J. clin. Invest.* **36,** 393 (1957).
49. Bustin, M. and Conway-Jacobs, A.: *Europ. J. Immunol.* **1,** 421 (1971).
50. Bütikofer, E., De Weck, A. L. and Scherrer, M.: *Schweiz. Med. Wsch.* **100,** 97 (1970).
51. Cannon, P. R., Walsh, T. E. and Marshall, C. E.: *Amer. J. Path.* **17,** 777 (1941).
52. Campbell, D. H.: *Fortschr. Chem. Org. Naturstoffe* **9,** 443 (1952).
53. Campinchi, R., Faure, J., Bloch-Michel, E. and Haut, J.: *L'Uvéite. Phénomènes immunologiques et allergiques.* Masson, Paris 1970.
54. Cazullo, C. L., Businco, Lino, Giordano, P. L., Businco, E. and Businco, Luisa: *Acta allerg. (Kbh.)* **25,** 178 (1970).
55. Chaffee, F. H.: *Acta allerg. (Kbh.)* **25,** 292 (1970).
56. Chanarin, I., Fenton, J. C. B. and Mollin, D. L.: *Brit. med. J.* **1,** 1162 (1957).
57. Charpin, J. and Zafiropoulo, A.: *Acta allerg. (Kbh.)* **9,** 314 (1955).
58. Charpin, J., Zafiropoulo, A. and Roccaserra, J. P.: *Rev. franç. Allerg.* **2,** 117 (1962).
59*a*. Charpy, J.: *Le mécanisme physio-pathologique de l'eczéma.* Masson, Paris 1954.
59*b*. id., *Symp. sur les tests cutanés et humoraux de l'allergie.* Lyon 1956.
60. Chase, M. W.: In *III. Int. Congr. Allergol. Paris* 1959. Ed. by Halpern, B.-N. and Holtzer, A. Flammarion, Paris 1958, p. 193.
60*a*. Chen, F. W., Strosberg, A. D. and Haber, E.: *J. Immunol.* **110,** 98 (1973).
61. Chorzelski, T. and Jablonska, S.: *Derm. Wschr.* **153,** 558 (1967).
62. Christian, C. L.: *New Engl. J. Med.* **280,** 878 (1969).
63*a*. Clutton, R. F., Harington, C. R. and Yuill, M. E.: *Biochem. J.* **31,** 764 (1937).
63*b*. ibid., **32,** 1111 (1938).

63c. ibid., **32,** 1119 (1938).
64. Cochrane, C. G.: *J. exp. Med.* **118,** 503 (1963).
65. Cock, A. G.: *Immunology* **5,** 169 (1962).
66. Colldahl, H. and Fagerberg, E.: *Acta allerg. (Kbh.)* **10,** 77 (1956).
67. Collip, J. B.: *Ann. intern. Med.* **8,** 10 (1934).
68. Comaish, S.: *Brit. J. Derm.* **81,** 919 (1969).
69. Cooke, R. A. and van der Veer, A.: *J. Immunol.* **1,** 201 (1916).
70. Cormane, R. H.: *Lancet* **i,** 534 (1964).
71. Criep, L. H.: *J. Allergy* **12,** 154 (1941).
72. Crowle, A. G., Hu, C. C. and Patrucco, A. J.: *J. Allergy* **42,** 140 (1968).
73. Dahl, L.: *Acta allerg. (Kbh.)* **3,** 26 (1950).
74. Daniels, C. A., Borsos, T., Rapp, H. J., Synderman, R. and Notkins, A. L. *Proc. nat. Acad. Sci. (Wash.)* **65,** 528 (1970).
75. Dausset, J.: *Presse méd.* **65,** 1482 (1957).
76. Davidson, A. G., Baron, B. A. and Walker, M.: *J. Allergy* **18,** 359 (1947).
77a. Dayton, D. H., jr., Small, P. A., jr., Channock, R. M., Kaufman, H. E. and Tomasi, T. B., jr.: *The Secretory Immunologic System.* U.S. Government Printing Office, Washington 1971, p. 293.
77b. ibid., p. 317.
78. Depaoli, M.: *Minerva derm.* **29,** 207 (1954).
79. Dienes, L.: *J. Immunol.* **20,** 333 (1931).
80. Dienes, L. and Simon, F. A.: *J. Immunol.* **28,** 321 (1935).
81. Ditschuneit, H. and Federlin, K.: *Dtsch. med. Wschr.* **91,** 853 (1966).
82a. Dóbiás, G.: *J. clin. Path.* **16,** 441 (1963).
82b. id., *Dtsch. med. Wschr.* **91,** 1836 (1966).
83. Dobrkovsky, M. et al.: *I. Int. Congr. Res. in Burns.* Washington 1960, p. 41.
84. Doerr, R. and Seidenberg, S.: *Z. Immun.-Forsch.* **71,** 242 (1931).
85. Dogo, G.: *Minerva derm.* **33,** 76 (1958).
86. Doniach, D.: *Folia allerg. (Roma)* **17,** 435 (1970).
87. Doniach, D., Roitt, I. M. and Holborow, E. J.: *Brit. med. J.* **2,** 909 (1961).
88. Dorn, H.: *Haut- u. Geschl.-Kr.* **23,** 5, (1957).
89. Dornbusch, S.: *Int. Arch. Allergy* **11,** 206 (1957).
90. Dörner, M., Enderlin, M., Spiegelberg, H. and Mischer, P.: *Dtsch. med. Wschr.* **86,** 431 (1961).
91. Duričić, J.: *Med. Pregl. (Belgrad)* **7,** 177 (1954); cited by *Zbl. Haut-Geschl. Kr.* **91,** 303 (1955).
92. Edfors-Lubs, M. L.: *Acta allerg. (Kbh.)* **26,** 249 (1971).
93. Eickhoff, W.: *Virchows Arch. path. Anat.* **301,** 264 (1938).
94. Engelhardt, G. and Lendle, L.: *Arch. exp. Path. Pharmakol.* **5,** 402 (1955).
95. Epstein, S.: *Ann. Allergy* **10,** 633 (1952).
96. Epstein, W. L.: *J. invest. Derm.* **30,** 31 (1958).
97. Falliers, C. J., Cardoso, A. R. R. de, Bane, H. N., Coffey, R. and Middleton, E.: *J. Allergy* **47,** 207 (1971).
98. Faulk, W. P., Ellefson, R. D. and Stickler, G. B.: *J. Pediat.* **72,** 587 (1968).
99. Felber, J. P., Ashcroft, S. H. J., Villanueva, A. and Vannotti, A.: *Nature* **211,** 656 (1966).
100. Feodorov, N. A.: *I. Int. Congr. Res. in Burns.* Washington, 1960, 41.
100a. Field, A. K., Tytell, A. A., Lampson, G. P. and Hilleman, M. R.: *Proc. Soc. exp. Biol. (N. Y.)* **139,** 1113 (1972).
100b. Filipp, G.: *Ann. Allergy* **31,** 272 (1973).
101. Filipp, G. and Mess, B.: *Ann. Allergy* **27,** 500 (1969).
102. Filipp, G. and Szentiványi, A.: *Ann. Allergy* **16,** 306 (1958).
103. Filipp, G., Szentiványi, A. and Mess, B.: *Acta med. Acad. Sci. hung.* **3,** 163 (1952).
104. Findt, M. L. H.: *Lancet* **i,** 1177 (1969).
105. Fisher, J. P.: *J. invest. Derm.* **47,** 336 (1966).
106. Flarer, F. and Chieregato, G.: *Dermatologica (Basel)* **127,** 1 (1963).
107. Fleischer, N., Givens, J. R., Abe, K., Nicholson, W. E. and Liddle, G. W.: *Endocrinology* **78,** 1067 (1966).
108. Forró, E. and Lendvai, J.: *Orv. Hetil.* **77,** 801 (1933).
109. Fox, R. A., James, D. G., Scheuer, P. J. and Sharma, O.: *Lancet* **i,** 959 (1969).

110. Franchimont, P.: *Acta allerg. (Kbh.)* **22,** 231 (1967).
111. Frankland, A. E.: *Allergie u. Asthma* **1,** 229 (1955).
112. Franklin, W. and Lowell, F. C.: *J. Allergy* **20,** 400 (1949).
113. Franz, T., McMurrain, D., Brooks, S. and Bernstein, I. L.: *J. Allergy* **47,** 170 (1971).
114*a*. Freund, J.: *J. Immunol.* **18,** 315 (1930).
114*b*. id., *J. Allergy* **28,** 18 (1957).
115. Freund, J., Lipton, M. M. and Thompson, G. E.: *J. exp. Med.* **97,** 711 (1963).
116. Freund, J., Thompson, G. E. and Lipton, M. M.: *J. exp. Med.* **101,** 591 (1955).
117. Frey, J. R.: *Dermatologica* **102,** 1 (1951).
118. Friedman, E. A., Bardawill, W. A., Meril, J. P. and Hanan, C.: *New Engl. J. Med.* **262,** 486 (1960).
119. Frugoni, C. and Ancona, G.: *L'asma bronchiale.* Torino 1927.
120. Fudenberg, H. H. and Fudenberg, B. R.: *Science* **145,** 170 (1964).
121. Fulwiler, R. D.: *Amer. industr. Hyg. Ass. J.* **32,** 73 (1971).
122. Garcia, J. M.: *Brasil-méd.* **56,** 6 (1942).
123. Gardner, F. H. and Diamond, L. K.: *Blood* **10,** 675 (1955).
124. Geber, H.: *Derm. Z.* **32,** 143 (1921).
125. Geld, P. and Freedman, S. O.: *Cancer* **20,** 1663 (1967).
126. Germuth, F. G., jr. and McKinnan, G. E.: *Bull. Johns Hopk. Hosp.* **101,** 13 (1957).
127*a*. Gerő, S., Gergely, J., Jakab, L., Székely, J., Virág, S., Farkas, K. and Czuppon, A.: *Lancet* **ii,** 6 (1959).
127*b*. ibid., **i,** 1119 (1961).
128. Gibbs, R. C.: *Arch. Derm.* **101,** 92 (1970).
129. Glynn, L. E.: *Folia allerg. (Roma)* **17,** 433 (1970).
130. Glynn, L. E. and Holborow, E. J.: *Lancet* **ii,** 449 (1952).
131. Gocke, D. J., Hsu, K., Morgan, C., Bombardieri, S., Lockshin, M. and Christian, C. L.: *J. exp. Med.* **134,** 330 (1971).
132. Goldberg, S. S., Kraft, S. C., Peterson, R. D. A. and Rothberg, R. M.: *J. Immunol.* **107,** 757 (1971).
133. Good, R. A. and Condie, R. M.: *III. Int. Congr. Allergol. Paris.* Flammarion, Paris 1958, p. 485.
134. Goreczky, L.: *Dtsch. med. Wschr.* **67,** 114 (1942).
135. Gottlieb, P. M., Stupniker, S., Sandberg, H. and Woldon, I.: *Amer. J. med. Sci* **223,** 196 (1957).
136*a*. Graciansky, P., Israel, L. and Cohen-Solar, J.: *Sem. Hôp. (Paris)* **36,** 1451 (1960).
136*b*. ibid., **36,** 1461 (1960).
137. Grant, R. T., Pearson, B. R. S. and Comeau, W. J.: *Clin. Sci.* **2,** 253 (1936).
138. Greenbaum, S. S.: *J. Amer. med. Ass.* **115,** 847 (1940).
139. Griffith, C. O., jr. and Crickelair, G. F.: *Nature* **193,** 186 (1962).
140. Grigs, R. C. and Dowdell, W. F.: *Arch. Derm.* **80,** 486 (1959)
141. Grubb, E.: *Acta derm.-venereol.* **32,** 256 (1952).
142. Grün, G.: *Wien. klin. Wschr.* **47,** 751 (1934).
143. Gutmann, M. J.: In *I. Int. Allerg. Kongr. Zürich* 1951. Ed. by Grumbach, A. S. and Rivkine, A. Karger, Basel 1952, p. 414.
144. Gyöngyössy, A. and Lampé, L.: *Allergie u. Asthma* **4,** 14 (1958).
145. György, P.: In *Hdb. Kinderheilk.* Bd. X. Ed. by Pfaundler, M. and Schlossmann, A. Vogel, Berlin 1935.
146. Halbert, S. P., Locatcher-Khorazo, D., Swick, L., Witmer, R., Seegal, B. and Fitzgerald, P.: *J. exp. Med.* **105,** 439 (1957).
147. Hale, R.: *Ann. Allergy* **12,** 294 (1954).
148. Halpern, B.-N., Ky, T. and Robert, B.: *Immunology* **12,** 247 (1967).
149. Halpern, B.-N., Zweibaum, A., Oriolpalou, R. and Morard, J. C.: In *Immunopathology.* Vol. 5. Ed. by Miescher, P. and Grabar, P. Schwabe, Basel 1968, p. 161.
150. Hanhart, E.: *Int. Arch. Allergy* **3,** Suppl. (1952).
151. Hanson, K.: *Allergie.* Thieme, Leipzig 1943.
152. Hard, S.: *Acta derm.-venerol.* **36,** 303 (1956).
153. Harten, M. and Walzer, M.: *J. Allergy* **12,** 72 (1940).
154. Haskova, V.: *Nature* **193,** 278 (1962).
155. Hatcher, V. B. and MacPherson, C. F. C.: *J. Immunol.* **102,** 877 (1969).

156. Hawkins, D.: *J. Immunol.* **107,** 344 (1971).
157*a*. Haxthausen, H.: *Acta derm.-venereol.* **21,** 158 (1940).
157*b*. ibid., **24,** 286 (1943).
157*c*. ibid., **35,** 271 (1955).
158. Hässig, A. and Stirnemann, H.: In *Immunopathologie in Klinik und Forschung.* Ed. by Miescher, P. and Vorlaender, K. O. Thieme, Stuttgart 1957, p. 369.
159. Heath, R. and Krupp, I. M.: *Arch. ges. Psychiatr.* **161,** 10 (1967).
160. Heinsen, H. A. and Scheffler, H.: *Ärztl. Wschr.* **10,** 878 (1955).
161. Heller, P., Yakulis, V. J. and Josephson, A. M.: *J. Lab. clin. Med.* **59,** 401 (1962).
162. Hennes, A. R., Sevelius, H., Lewell, Y. N., Joel, W., Woods, A. H. and Wolf, S.: *Arch. Path.* **73,** 281 (1962).
163. Hennig, W.: *Allergie der Atmungs-Verdauungsorgane und der Haut.* Bd. I. Barth, Leipzig 1957, p. 31.
164. Henson, P. M.: *J. exp. Med.* **134,** 114 (1971).
165. Herzenberg, L. A., Gordlin, R. C. and Rivera, E. C.: *J. exp. Med.* **126,** 701 (1967).
166. Hill, O. W.: *Brit. med. J.* **1,** 1793 (1961).
167. Hjorth, N.: *J. invest. Derm.* **30,** 261 (1958).
168. Holborow, E. J. and Weir, D. M.: *Brit. med. J.* **2,** 732 (1957).
169. Holmes, M. C. and Burnet, F. M.: *Ann. intern. Med.* **59,** 265 (1963).
170. Hovding, G.: *Brit. med. J.* **3,** 102 (1968).
171. Huber, H., Douglas, S. D. and Fudenberg, H. H.: *Immunology* **17,** 7 (1969).
172. Hulka, J. F. and Brinton, Y.: *Amer. J. Obstet. Gynec.* **86,** 130 (1963).
173. Hulka, J. F., Hsu, K. C. and Beiser, S. M.: *Nature* **191,** 510 (1961).
174. Hulka, J. F. and Mohr, K.: *Science* **161,** 696 (1968).
175. Humphrey, J. H. and Mota, I.: *Immunology* **2,** 31 (1959).
176. Hussar, A. E., Cradle, J. L. and Beiser, S. M.: *Brit. J. Psychol.* **118,** 91 (1971).
177. Inderbitzin, T. M. and Grob, P. J.: *J. invest. Derm.* **49,** 642 (1967).
178. Insect Allergy Committee of the American Academy of Allergy. *J. Amer. med. Ass.* **193,** 115 (1965).
179*a*. Irvine, W. J.: In *Autoimmunity.* Ed. by Baldwin, R. W. and Humphrey, J. H. Blackwell, Oxford 1965, p. 74.
179*b*. id., *Practitioner* **199,** 180 (1967).
180. Irvine, W. J., MacGregor, A. G., Stuart, A. E. and Hall, G. H.: *Lancet* **ii,** 850 (1961).
181. Ishizaka, K., Ishizaka, T. and Campbell, D. H.: *J. exp. Med.* **109,** 127 (1959).
182. Jacobs, J. L., Kelley, J. J. and Sommers, S. C.: *Proc. Soc. exp. Biol. (N.Y.)* **48,** 639 (1941).
183. Jaffé, R., Jaffé, W. G. and Kozma, C.: *Frankfurt. Z. Path.* **70,** 235 (1959).
184. Jahn, B.: *Virchows Arch. path. Anat.* **324,** 65 (1953).
185. Jamar, J.: *Acta allerg. (Kbh.)* **11,** 178 (1957).
186. Jaros, S. H., Wnuck, A. L. and de Beer, E. J.: *Ann. Allergy* **10,** 291 (1952).
187. Jorpes, E.: cited by 73.
188. Kabat, E. A.: *Fortschr. Allergielehre* **2,** 11 (1949).
189. Kailin, E. W., Davidson, A. G. and Walzer, M.: *J. Allergy* **18,** 373 (1971).
190. Kaiser, W. and Schmidt, H. H.: *Münch. med. Wschr.* **99,** 1072 (1957).
191. Kallós, P. and Kallós-Deffner, L.: *Ergebn. Hyg.* **19,** 178 (1937).
192. Kalz, F.: *J. invest. Derm.* **5,** 135 (1942).
193. Kano, K. and Milgrom, F.: *Int. Arch. Allergy* **40,** 471 (1971).
194. Kartamyshev, A. I.: *Vestn. Vener. Derm. (Moscow)* **25,** 7 (1951).
195*a*. Katsh, S.: *J. exp. Med.* **107,** 95 (1958).
195*b*. id., *Int. Arch. Allergy* **16,** 241 (1960).
195*c*. ibid., **17,** 70 (1960).
195*d*. id., *Ann. Allergy* **24,** 615 (1966).
196*a*. Katsh, S. and Jordan, R. T.: *Nature* **192,** 770 (1961).
196*b*. id., *Int. Arch. Allergy* **21,** 163 (1962).
197. Katz, D. H., Paul, W. E. and Benacerraf, B.: *J. Immunol.* **107,** 1319 (1971).
198. Kämmerer, H. and Michel, H.: *Allergische Diathese und allergische Krankheiten.* Bergmann, München 1956.
199. Keitel, W., Gutschmidt, H. J. and Rosam, W.: *Münch. med. Wschr.* **110,** 707 (1968).

200. Kerp, L.: *Dtsch. med. Wschr.* **90,** 841 (1965).
201. Kerp, L., Steinhilber, S., Kieling, F. and Creutzfeldt, W.: *Dtsch. med. Wschr.* **90,** 806 (1965).
202. Kesztyűs, L.: *Immunität und Nervensystem.* Akadémiai Kiadó, Budapest 1967.
203. Kesztyűs, L., Csaba, B., Csernyánszky, H. and Kocsár, L.: *Acta physiol. Acad. Sci. hung.* **14,** 167 (1958).
204. Kesztyűs, L., Csernyánszky, H., Koller, M. and Salánki, J.: *Acta microbiol. Acad. Sci. hung.* **2,** 343 (1955).
205. Kesztyűs, L., Szabó, E., Gyulai, F. and Szatai, I.: *Acta microbiol. Acad. Sci. hung.* **3,** 277 (1956).
206. Kesztyűs, L., Szilágyi, T. and Gyulai, F.: *Acta microbiol. Acad. Sci. hung.* **1,** 359 (1954).
207*a*. Kleinsorge, H.: *III. Europ. Congr. Allergol. Firenze, 1956.* Vol. I. Ed. by Lunedei, A. and Serafini, U. Il pensiero scientifico, Roma 1956, p. 69.
207*b*. id., *Allergie u. Asthma* **2,** 36 (1956).
208. Kleinsorge, H., Dornsbusch, S. and Römer, R.: *Int. Arch. Allergy* **16,** 200 (1960).
209. Koelsche, G. A.: *Ann. Allergy* **19,** 511 (1961).
210. Koffler, D., Agnello, V., Thoburn, R. and Kunkel, H. G.: *J. exp. Med.* **134,** 169 (1971).
211. Koffler, D., Carr, R., Agnello, V., Thoburn, R. and Kunkel, H. G.: *J. exp. Med.* **134,** 294 (1971).
212. Koga, T., Ishibashi, T., Sugiyama, K. and Tanaka, A.: *Int. Arch. Allergy* **36,** 233 (1969).
213. Korossy, S.: *Acta med. Acad. Sci. hung.* **4,** 87 (1953).
214. Koscielak, K., Madalinski, K., Brzosko, J., Nowoslawski, A. and Kloczewiak, M.: *Nature* **229,** 92 (1971).
215. Krohn, P. L.: In *Biologic Problems of Grafting.* Ed. by Albert, F. and Medawar, P. B. Blackwell, Oxford 1959, p. 146.
216. Kunkel, H. G., Holman, H. R. and Deicher, H. R. G.: In *Ciba Found. Symp.* Ed. by Wolstenholm, G. E. W. Churchill, London 1960, p. 429.
217. Lagerholm, B. Lodin, A. and Gentele, H.: *Acta allerg. (Kbh.)* **12,** 295 (1958).
218. Lambert, P. H. and Dixon, F. J.: *J. exp. Med.* **127,** 507 (1968).
219. Landsteiner, K.: *Schweiz. med. Wschr.* **71,** 1359 (1941).
220. Landsteiner, K. and Chase, M. W.: *J. exp. Med.* **71,** 237 (1940).
221. Lange, K., Treser, G., Sagel, I. and Wasserman, E.: *Ann. intern. Med.* **64,** 25 (1966).
222*a*. Lehner, E. and Rajka, E.: *Derm. Wschr.* **81,** 1731 (1925).
222*b*. id., *Krankheitsforsch.* **5,** 57 (1927).
222*c*. id., *Z. ges. exp. Med.* **71,** 123 (1930).
223. Leitner, Z. A.: *Lancet* **i,** 474 (1943).
224. Lennon, V. A., Wittingham, S., Carnegie, P. R. McPherson, T. A. and Mackay, I. R.: *J. Immunol.* **107,** 56 (1971).
225. Leövey, A.: *Rheum. Balneol. Allerg. (Budapest)* **10,** 51 (1969).
226. Levine, L. and Stollar, B. D.: *Prog. Allergy* **12,** 161 (1968).
226*a*. Levine, S. and Sowinski, R.: *J. Immunol.* **110,** 139 (1973).
227. Lewis, R. M. and Schwartz, R. S.: *J. exp. Med.* **134,** 417 (1971).
228. Levkova, N. A.: *Ref. Abstr. Sov. Med.* **1,** 475 (1957).
229. Lieb, W. A. and Lerman, S.: *Klin. Mbl. Augenheilk.* **132,** 31 (1958).
230. Lieberman, P., Patterson, R., Metz, R. and Lucena, G.: *J. Amer. med. Ass.* **215,** 1106 (1971).
231*a*. Linser, P.: *Arch. Derm. Syph. (Berlin)* **138,** 175 (1922).
231*b*. ibid., **138,** 198 (1922).
232. Lipton, M. M. and Steigman, A. J.: *J. Allergy* **34,** 362 (1963).
233. Lissák, K. and Hodes, B. R.: *Amer. J. Physiol.* 124, 637 (1938).
234. Loveless, M.: *J. Immunol.* **38,** 25 (1940).
235. Low, R. C.: *Anaphylaxis and Sensitization.* Green, Edinburgh 1924.
236*a*. Lowell, F. C.: *Proc. Soc. exp. Biol. (N.Y.)* **50,** 167 (1942).
236*b*. id., *The Nature and Significance of the Antibody Response.* Columbia Univ. Press, Washington 1953, p. 145.
237. Lukács, J.: *Acta med. Acad. Sci. hung.* **15,** 267 (1960).

238. Lunedei, A.: *III. Europ. Congr. Allergol. Firenze 1956*. Vol. I. Ed. by Lunedei, A. and Serafini, K. Il Pensiero Scientifico, Roma 1956, p. 116.
239. Maisel, F. E.: *J. Allergy* **11,** 607 (1940).
240. Mannik, M., Arend, W. P., Hall, A. P. and Gilliland, B. C.: *J. exp. Med.* **133,** 713 (1971).
241. Mansfeld, G.: *Experientia (Basel)* **5,** 188 (1949).
242. Markowitz, A. S., Horn, D., Novak, R. and Battifora, H. A.: *J. Immunol.* **107,** 504 (1971).
243. Marshall, A. H. E. and White, R. G.: *Brit. J. exp. Path.* **42,** 379 (1961).
244. Mason, A. A. and Black, S.: *Lancet* **i,** 877 (1958).
245. Massona, G.: *Minerva ginec.* **7,** 491 (1955).
246. Mathov, E.: *Folia allerg. (Roma)* **17,** 418 (1970).
247. Mauer, A. M., De Vaux, W. and Lahey, M. E.: *Pediatrics* **19,** 84 (1957).
248*a*. Mayer, R. L.: *Fortschr. Allergielehre* **4,** 79 (1954).
248*b*. id., *J. Allergy* **26,** 133 (1955).
248*c*. id., *Int. Arch. Allergy* **8,** 115 (1956).
249. Mc. Cormick, J. N., Faulk, W. P., Fox, H. and Fudenberg, H. H.: *J. exp. Med.* **133,** 1 (1971).
250. McKluskey, R. T., Miller, F. and Benacerraf, B.: *J. exp. Med.* **115,** 253 (1962).
251. McLaren, W. R. and Aladjem, F.: *J. Allergy* **28,** 89 (1957).
252. McMaster, P.R. B., Lerner, E. M. and Exum, E. D.: *J. exp. Med.* **113,** 611 (1961).
253. McPherson, T. A., Robson, G. S. M. and Carnegie, P. R.: *Int. Arch. Allergy* **39,** 566 (1970).
254. Mendes, E. and Cintra, A. V.: *J. Allergy* **25,** 253 (1954).
255. Metzgar, R. S. and Buckley, R. H.: *Int. Arch. Allergy* **31,** 174 (1967).
256. Michelson, A. M., Lacour, F. and Nahon-Merlin, E.: *C. R. Acad. Sci. Serie D.* **272,** 669 (1971).
257. Miescher, G.: *Schweiz. med. Wschr.* **71,** 1360 (1941).
258*a*. Miescher, P.: *Schweiz. med. Wschr.* **87,** 426 (1957).
258*b*. id., In *Die Immunpathologie in Klinik und Forschung*. Ed. by Miescher, P. and Vorlaender, K. O. Thieme, Stuttgart 1957, p. 79.
258*c*. ibid., 260.
258*d*. id., *Hautarzt* **8,** 502 (1957).
259. Miescher, P. and Jackson, F. W.: *Schweiz. med. Wschr.* **92,** 384 (1962).
260. Miescher, P. and March, H.: *Proc. 12th Int. Congr. Derm. Washington* **2,** 1048 (1962).
261. Miescher, P. and Strassle, R.: *Vox Sang. (Basel)* **2,** 283 (1957).
262*a*. Milgrom, F. and Witebsky, E.: *Immunology* **5,** 46 (1962).
262*b*. ibid., **5,** 67 (1962).
263. Minnick, R., Murphy, G. E. and Campbell, W. G., jr.: *J. exp. Med.* **124,** 635 (1966).
264. Mitchell, D. C. and Vilter, R. W.: *Ann. intern. Med.* **31,** 1102 (1949).
265. Mom, A. M., Ubalton, S. P. and Clerc, N. A.: *Arch. Derm.* **75,** 562 (1957).
266. Moseley, J. C.: *Arch. Derm.* **103,** 58 (1971).
267. Mosonyi, L., Csiky, Th. and Oblatt, E.: *Allergie u. Asthma* **2,** 215 (1956).
268. Mosonyi, L., Halmy, L. and Csiky, Th.: *Hautarzt* **18,** 412 (1967).
269. Mouriquand, G., Edel, V. Mlle and Chighizola, Mlle: *Presse méd.* **63,** 1193 (1955).
270. Muller, P. T.: *Infektion und Immunität*. Fischer, Jena, 1909, p. 319.
271. Nahon-Merlin, E., Michelson, A. M., Verger, C. and Lacour, F.: *J. Immunol.* **107,** 222 (1971).
272. Najjar, V. A. and Robinson, J. P.: *Immunity and Virusinfection*. Wiley, New York 1959, p. 71.
273. Nazarov, K. N.: *Fed. Proc.* **23.** (Translation suppl.) 375 (1964).
274. Nerup, J., Andersen, V. and Bendixen, G.: *Clin. exp. Immunol.* **4,** 355 (1969).
275. Nerup, J., Søborg, M. and Halberg, P.: *Acta allerg. (Kbh.)* **22,** 182 (1967).
276. Nilsson, L. A. and Rose, N. A.: *Immunology* **22,** 13 (1972).
277. Nilzén, Å.: *Acta derm.-venereol.* **32,** Suppl. **29,** 231 (1952).
278. Noelpp-Eschenhagen, I. and Noelpp, B.: *Fortschr. Allergielehre* **4,** 361 (1954).
279. Notkins, A. L.: *J. exp. Med.* **134,** 41 (1971).
280*a*. Oldstone, M. B. A. and Dixon, F. J.: *J. exp. Med.* **131,** 1 (1970).
280*b*. ibid., **134,** 32 (1971).

280c. id., *J. Immunol.* **107,** 1274 (1971).
281. Ormea, F. and Zina, G.: *Minerva derm.* **28,** 26 (1953).
282. Orsini, F. and Shulman, S.: *J. exp. Med.* **134,** 120 (1971).
283. Ott, F. and Storck, H.: *Derm. Wschr.* **142,** 1102 (1960).
284. Otto, R.: *Z. ges. Hyg.* **95,** 378 (1932).
285. Panzani, R.: *Int. Arch. Allergy* **11,** 224 (1957).
286. Parish, W. E.: *Brit. J. Derm.* **73,** 10 (1961).
287. Parish, W. E., Rook, A. J. and Champion, R. H.: *Brit. J. Derm.* **77,** 479 (1965).
287*a*. Parker, L. M. and Steinberg, A. D.: *J. Immunol.* **110,** 742 (1973).
288. Parker, W. C., Hagstrom, J. W. C. and Bearn, A. G.: *J. exp. Med.* **118,** 975 (1963).
289*a*. Pasteur Vallery-Radot, L.: *Précis des maladies allergiques.* Flammarion, Paris 1949.
289*b*. id., *Acta allerg. (Kbh.)* **7,** 14 (1954).
289*c*. ibid., **11,** 203 (1957).
290. Paterson, P. Y.: *J. exp. Med.* **111,** 119 (1960).
291. Paul, W. E., Katz, D. H. and Benacerraf, B.: *J. Immunol.* **107,** 685 (1971).
292. Paul, W. E., Katz., D. H., Gridl, E. A. and Benacerraf, B.: *J. exp. Med.* **132,** 283 (1970).
293. Pavkova, L. and Dolezalova, J.: *Symp. Plast. Surg. and Burns. Marianske Lazne* 1960.
294. Pelner, L.: *Ann. intern. Med.* **27,** 290 (1947).
295. Perhoff, G. T.: *J. Lab. clin. Med.* **67,** 585 (1966).
296. Perlman, P.: *Folia allerg. (Roma)* **17,** 434 (1970).
297. Perlman, P., Hammarstrom, S., Lagercrantz, R. and Gustafsson, B. E.: *Ann. N. Y. Acad. Sci.* **124,** 377 (1965).
298. Pfeiffer, E. F.: *Dtsch. med. Wschr.* **91,** 314 (1966).
299. Pfeiffer, E. F. and Merrill, J. P.: *Dtsch. med. Wschr.* **87,** 934 (1962).
300. Pieroni, R. E., Bundealby, A. E., Amdur, M. O. and Levine, L.: *Int. Arch. Allergy* **41,** 637 (1971).
301. Piomelli, S., Stefanini, M. and Mele, R. H.: *J. Lab. clin. Med.* **54,** 241 (1959).
302*a*. Plescia, O. J. and Braun, W.: *Advanc. Immunol.* **6,** 231 (1967).
302*b*. id., *Nucleic Acids in Immunology.* Springer, Berlin 1968.
303. Polak, L. and Turk, J. L.: *J. invest. Derm.* **52,** 219 (1969).
304. Popa, V., George, S. A. and Gavanescu, O.: *Acta allerg. (Kbh.)* **25,** 159 (1970).
305. Prausnitz, C.: *Med. Res. Council.* His Majesty's Stationary Office Sp. Rep. ser. 212. London 1936.
306. Pudlak, P. and Horak, J.: *Čas. Lék. čes. (Prague)* **108.** 649 (1969); cit. in *Excerpta med. (Amst.) Sect. XIII.* **24,** 64 (1970).
307. Rajka, G.: *Acta derm.-venereol.* **40,** 285 (1960).
308. Rajka, G. and Skog, E.: *Acta derm.-venereol.* **42,** 27 (1967).
309. Ramos e Silva, J.: *Dermatologica (Basel)* **111,** 1 (1955).
310*a*. Ratner, B.: *Amer. J. Dis. Child.* **36,** 277 (1928).
310*b*. id., *Proc. Soc. exp. Biol. (N.Y.)* **30,** 88 (1932).
311. Ratner, B. and Greenburgh, B. A.: *J. Allergy* **3,** 149 (1932).
312. Redfern, W. W.: *Amer. J. Hyg.* **6,** 276 (1926).
313. Reed, C. E.: *Folia allerg. (Roma)* **17,** 393 (1970).
314. Reinheimer, W. and Utz, G.: *Dtsch. med. Wschr.* **96,** 246 (1971).
315. Reuterwall, O.: *Acta derm.-venereol.* **36,** Suppl. 36 (1956).
316. Richardson, M., Conner, C. H., Beck, C. H. and Clark, D. T.: *Immunology* **21,** 795 (1971).
317. Richter, M., Sargent, A. U., Myers, J. and Rose, B.: *Immunology* **10,** 211 (1966).
318. Richter, P. and Szőr, A.: *Ann. Immunol. Hung.* **10,** 225 (1967).
319. Rock, A.: *Brit. J. Derm.* **73,** 1 (1961).
320. Rockwell, E. M.: *J. invest. Derm.* **24,** 35 (1955).
321. Rockwell, G. E.: *J. Allergy* **13,** 404 (1942).
322. Roitt, I. M., Doniach, D. and Couchman, K.: In *Mechanism of Antibody Formation.* Ed. by Holub, M. and Jarošková, L. Publ. House of the Czechoslovak Academy of Sciences, Prague 1960, p. 70.
323. Rokstad, J.: *Nord. Med.* **56,** 982 (1941).
324. Rose, N. R. and Witebsky, E.: *J. Immunol.* **76,** 408 (1956).

325. Rosselin, G., Bricaire, H., Dérot, M., Hamburger, J. and Pequignot, H.: *Presse méd.* **76,** 463 (1968).
326. Rother, K. and Sarre, H.: *Klin. Wschr.* **40,** 429 (1962).
327. Rothman, S.: *Psychosom. Med.* **7,** 90 (1945).
327*a*. Roule, A. H., Bartlett, Y. P. and Osserman, K. E.: *J. Immunol.* **110,** 401 (1973).
328. Roulet, D. L. A. and Muralt, G.: *Schweiz. med. Wschr.* **91,** 74 (1961).
329. Rust, S.: *Z. Haut- u. Geschl.-Kr.* **17,** 317 (1954).
330. Salén, E. B.: *Acta med. scand.* **59,** Suppl. 494 (1933).
331. Salén, E. B. and Juhlin-Dannfelt, C.: *Acta med. scand.* **86,** 505 (1935).
332. Salvin, S. B.: *J. exp. Med.* **107,** 109 (1958).
333. Salvin, S. B. and Smith, R. F.: *J. exp. Med.* **111,** 465 (1960).
334. Savić, V., Savić, V. L., Djuričić, I., Mojanović, M. and Gavrilović, Z.: *Acta allerg. (Kbh.)* **14,** 271 (1959).
335. Savin, J. A.: *Brit. J. Derm.* **83,** 546 (1970).
336. Scheiffarth, F. and Berg, G.: *Verh. dtsch. Ges. inn. Med.* **60,** 282 (1954).
337. Schleyer, E.: *Brit. med. J.* **1,** 255 (1944).
338*a*. Schmidt, H.: *Behringwerke Mitt.* **29,** 47 (1954).
338*b*. id., In *Allergie.* Ed. by Hansen, K. Thieme, Leipzig 1943.
338*c*. id., *Int. Arch. Allergy* **9,** 341 (1956).
339*a*. Schneider, L. and Szatmáry, J.: *Z. Immun.-Forsch.* **98,** 24 (1940).
339*b*. ibid. **99,** 275 (1941).
340. Schur, P. H. and Monroe, M.: *Proc. nat. Acad. Sci. (Wash.)* **63,** 1108 (1969).
341. Scott, D. G. and Rowell, N. R.: *Ann. rheum. Dis.* **26,** 10 (1967).
342. Sehon, A. H., Kaye, M., McGarry, E. and Rose, B.: *J. Lab. clin. Med.* **45,** 765 (1955).
343. Seligmann, M. and Milgrom, F.: *C. R. Acad. Sci.* **245,** 1472 (1957).
344*a*. Senyk, G., Nitecki, D. E. and Goodman, J. W.: *Science* **171,** 407 (1971).
344*b*. id., *J. exp. Med.* **133,** 1294 (1971).
345. Senyk, G., Nitecki, D. E., Spitler, L. and Goodman, J. W.: *Immunochemistry* **9,** 97 (1972).
346. Serafini, U., Masala, C. and Pala, A. M.: *Folia allerg. (Roma)* **17,** 433 (1970).
347*a*. Serafini, U. and Pieri, A.: *Presse méd.* **65,** 2220 (1957).
347*b*. id., *Acta allerg. (Kbh.)* **12,** Suppl. 5, 319 (1958).
348. Sery, T. W. and Nagy, R. M.: *J. Immunol.* **106,** 226 (1971).
349. Shapiro, R. S. and Eisenberg, B. C.: *J. Allergy* **47,** 76 (1971).
350*a*. Shearer, G. M., Mozes, E. and Sela, M.: *J. exp. Med.* **132,** 613 (1970).
350*b*. ibid., **133,** 216 (1971).
351. Shek, R. P. N. and MacPherson, C. F. C.: *Immunology* **21,** 333 (1971).
352. Sherman, W. B. and Werner, S. C.: *J. Amer. med. Ass.* **190,** 244 (1964).
353. Shibusava, K.: *Abstr. Jap. Med.* **1,** 2075 (1961).
354. Shulman, S.: *Dtsch. Ärzteblatt* **67,** 3342 (1970).
355. Sidon, M. A. and Aldrete, J. A.: *J. Amer. dent. Ass.* **82,** 369 (1971).
356. Simmons, R. L. and Russel, P. S.: *Nature* **208,** 698 (1964).
357. Simon, F. A.: *J. Amer. med. Ass.* **104,** 996 (1935).
358. Sjögren, H.: *Acta ophthal. (Kbh.) Suppl.* **2,** 187 (1933).
359. Skog, E.: *Acta derm.-venereol.* **38,** 1 (1958).
360. Smyth, F. S. and Bain, K.: *J. Allergy* **2,** 316 (1930).
361. Snoeck, J.: *Triangel* **4,** 178 (1961).
362. Solari, M. A., Moreno, G. R. and De Fernandez, M. N. G.: *Int. Arch. Allergy* **4,** 415 (1953).
363. Soulier, J. P., Courouce-Pauty, A. M., Benamon–Djiane, D.: *Presse méd.* **78,** 487 (1970).
364*a*. Spath, P., Garrathy, G. and Petz, L.: *J. Immunol.* **107,** 854 (1971).
364*b*. ibid., **107,** 860 (1971).
365. Spear, G. S. and Kihara, I.: *Johns Hopk. med. J.* **126,** 210 (1970).
366. Steffen, C., Carmann, H., Schuster, F., Tausch, G., Bosch, J., and Freilinger, G.: *Z. Rheumaforsch.* **30,** 92 (1971).
367. Steffen, C., Dichtl, M., Knapp, W. and Brunner, H.: *Immunology* **21,** 649 (1971).
368. Steigerwald, M. and Spielmann, W.: *Klin. Wschr.* **34,** 80. (1956).
369. Stein, W. and Morgenstern, M.: *Ann. intern. Med.* **20,** 826 (1944).

370. Steinborn, J.: *Allergie u. Asthma* **6,** 250 (1960).
371. Steiner, J. W., Langer, B., Schatz, D. L. and Volpe, R.: *J. exp. Med.* **112,** 187 (1960).
372. Stevenson, D. D., Orgel, H. A., Hamburger, R. N. and Reid, R. T.: *J. Allergy* **48,** 61 (1971).
373. Storck, H. and Koella, W. P.: *Hautarzt* **3,** 509 (1952).
374. Strauss, A. J. L.: *Proc. Soc. exp. Biol. (N.Y.)* **105,** 184 (1960).
375. Strejan, G. H. and Marsh, D. G.: *J. Immunol.* **107,** 306 (1971).
376. Stuttgen, G. and Neveling, R.: *Allergie u. Asthma* **1,** 32 (1955).
377. Sulzberger, M. B.: *Hautarzt* **5,** 520 (1954).
378. Swanborg, R. H. and Amesse, L. S.: *J. Immunol.* **107,** 281 (1971).
379. Swisher, S. N.: In *Henry Ford Hosp. Int. Symp. Detroit, 1958. Mechanism of Hypersensitivity.* Ed. by Shaffer, J. H., LoGrippo, G. A. and Chase, M. W. Little-Brown, Boston 1959, p. 349.
380. Szigeti, I., Ormos, J., Jákó, J. and Tószegi, A.: *Acta allerg. (Kbh.)* **15,** Suppl. 7. 374 (1960).
381. Szily, A.: *Klin. Mbl. Augenheilk.* **49,** 150 (1911).
382. Sző̋r, J., Aberle, L., Csernyánszky, H. and Sző̋r, A.: *Ann. Immunol. Hung.* **14,** 63 (1970).
383. Sző̋r, A., Richter, P., Csernyánszky, H., Kesztyűs, L. and Went, I.: *Allergie u. Asthma* **11,** 50 (1965).
384. Sző̋r, A., Richter, P. and Hámori, L.: *Ann. Immunol. Hung.* **11,** 221 (1968).
385. Taichman, N. I., Creighton, M., Stephenson, A. and Tsai, C. C.: *Immunology* **22,** 93 (1972).
386. Takino, Y., Sugahova, K. and Horino, I.: *J. Allergy* **47,** 247 (1971).
387. Taylor, K. B.: *Brit. med. J.* **2,** 1347 (1962).
388*a*. Tezner, O.: *Jb. Kinderheilk.* **142,** 69 (1934).
388*b*. id., *Arch. Derm. Syph. (Berl.)* **170,** 293 (1934).
389. Thulin, K. E.: *IX. Int. Congr. Rheum. Dis. Toronto* **2,** 45 (1957).
390. Tomcsik, J. and Kurotchkin, T. J.: *J. exp. Med.* **47,** 379 (1928).
390*a*. Toullet, F., Voisin, G. A. and Nemirovsky, M.: *Immunology* **24,** 635 (1973).
391. Török, L.: In *Handbuch der Haut- und Geschlechtskrankheiten.* Bd. VI/2. Ed. by Jadassohn, T. J., Springer, Berlin 1928, p. 145.
392. Trasher, S. G., Bernardis, L. L. and Cohen, S.: *Int. Arch. Allergy* **41,** 813 (1971).
393. Tung, K. S. K., Uannue, E. R. and Dixon, F. J.: *Amer. J. Path.* **60,** 313 (1970).
394. Tusch, E.: *III. Europ. Congr. Allergol. Firenze, 1956.* Vol. 1. Ed. by Lunedei, A. and Serafini, U. Il Pensiero Scientifico, Roma 1956, p. 238.
395. Uhr, J. W., Salvin, S. B. and Pappenheimer, A.M., jr.: *J. exp. Med.* **105,** 11 (1957).
396. Urbach, G. I.: *Fertil. and Steril.* **21,** 356 (1970).
397. Vaughan, W. T.: *Allergy and Applied Immunology.* Mosby, St. Louis 1935.
398. Voisin, G. A.: In *Henry Ford Hosp. Int. Symp. Detroit, 1958. Mechanism of Hypersensitivity.* Ed. by Schaffer, J. H., LoGrippo, G. A. and Chase, M. W. Little-Brown, Boston 1959, p. 408.
399*a*. Vorlaender, K. O.: *Acta allerg. (Kbh.)* **8,** 1 (1954).
399*b*. ibid., **8,** 224 (1954).
399*c*. id., In *Immunopathologie in Klinik und Forschung.* Ed. by Miescher, P. and Vorlaender, K. O. Thieme, Stuttgart 1957, p. 143.
399*d*. ibid., p. 376.
399*e*. ibid., p. 417.
399*f*. id., *Dtsch. med. Wschr.* **87,** 887 (1962).
400. Wacker, W. B. and Lipton, M. M.: *Int. Arch. Allergy* **41,** 370 (1971).
401*a*. Waksman, B. H.: *Int. Arch. Allergy* **12,** Suppl. 14 (1959).
401*b*. id., *Cellular Aspects of Immunity.* Churchill, London 1960.
402. Waksman, B. H. and Adams, R. D.: *J. exp. Med.* **102,** 213 (1955).
403. Waldman, R. H. and Henney, C. S.: *J. exp. Med.* **134,** 482 (1971).
404. Wallis, C. and Melnick, J. L.: *J. Immunol.* **107,** 1235 (1971).
405*a*. Walzer, M.: *J. Immunol.* **23,** 99 (1932).
405*b*. id., *J. Allergy* **13,** 554 (1942).
406. Wang, A. C., Faulk, W. P., Stuckey, M. A. and Fudenberg, H. H.: *Immunochemistry* (In press).

406*a*. Wang, S. P., Grayston, J. T. and Gall, J. L.: *J. Immunol.* **110,** 873 (1973).
407*a*. Wedroff, N. S. and Dolgoff, A. P.: *Arch. Derm. Syph. (Berl.)* **171,** 641 (1935).
407*b*. ibid., **171,** 647 (1935).
408. Weiner, W., Battey, D. A., Cleghorn, T. E., Marson, F. G. W. and Meynell, M. J.: *Brit. Med. J.* **2,** 125 (1953).
409. Weissman, G., Zurier, R. B., Spieler, P. J. and Goldstein, I. M.: *J. exp. Med.* **134,** 149 (1971).
409*a*. Welch, P., Rose, N. R. and Kite, J. H., jr.: *J. Immunol.* **110,** 574 (1973).
410*a*. Went, S. and Kesztyűs, L.: *Naunyn-Schmiedebergs Arch.* **193,** 312 (1939).
410*b*. ibid., **195,** 721 (1940).
410*c*. id., *Schweiz. med. Wschr.* **78,** 1276 (1948).
410*d*. id., *Acta med. Acad. Sci. hung.* **2,** 89 (1951).
411. Went, S., Kesztyűs, L. and Piribauer, K.: *Arbeiten der II. Abt. der Wiss. Gesellschaft in Debrecen* **7,** 1 (1940).
412. Went, S., Kesztyűs, L. and Szilágyi, T.: *Naunyn-Schmiedebergs Arch.* **202,** 143 (1943).
413. Went, S. and Lissák, K.: *Z. Immun.-Forsch.* **99,** 215 (1941).
414*a*. Went, S., Piribauer, K. and Kesztyűs, L.: *Naunyn-Schmiedebergs Arch.* **193,** 312 (1939).
414*b*. ibid., **193,** 609 (1939).
415*a*. Whitefield, A.: *Lancet* **i,** 122 (1921).
415*b*. id., *C. R. VIII. Congr. Int. Derm. Copenhague, 1930.* Engelsen and Schrøder, Copenhague 1931, p. 142.
416. Wick, G., Kite, J. H. and Cole, R. C.: *Int. Arch. Allergy* **40,** 603 (1971).
417. Wiener, A. S.: *Ann. Allergy* **10,** 535 (1952).
418. Wilhelm, C. M. jr., Kierland, R. R. and Owen, C. A.: *Arch. Derm.* **86,** 161 (1962).
419. Wilson, C. B. and Dixon, F. J.: *J. Immunol.* **105,** 279 (1970).
420. Witebsky, E. and Milgrom, F.: *Fed. Proc.* **19,** 210 (1956).
421. Witherington, R. and Rinker, J. R.: *J. Urol.* **104,** 463 (1970).
422. Woitowitz, H. J., Woitowitz, R. H. and Schacke, G.: *Dtsch. med. Wschr.* **92,** 276 (1971).
423. Wolf, A. F., Bailey, H. A. and Coleman, J. M.: *Ann. Allergy* **11,** 78 (1953).
424. Worlledge, S. M.: *Semin. Hemat.* **6,** 181 (1969).
425. Zabriskie, J. B., Lewshenia, R., Moller, G., Wehle, B. and Falk, R. E.: *Science* **168,** 1105 (1970).
426. Zdrodowszkij, P. F.: *Vestn. Akad. med. Nauk* **3,** 3 (1953).
427. Zimmerman, R. A., Auernheimer, A. H. and Tarante, A.: *J. Immunol.* **107,** 757 (1971).
428*a*. Zohn, B.: *Amer. J. Dis. Child.* **57,** 1067 (1939).
428*b*. id., *J. Allergy* **13,** 153 (1942).
429*a*. Zondek, B. and Bromberg, Y. M.: *J. Allergy* **16,** 1 (1945).
429*b*. id., *J. Obstet. Gynaec. Brit. Emp.* **54,** 1 (1947).

CHAPTER 4

# IMMEDIATE-TYPE AND DELAYED-TYPE ALLERGY

by

E. RAJKA

completed by

L. KESZTYŰS



The distinction between the two types of hypersensitivity deserves discussion in a separate chapter because of its importance, although it has already been dealt with in the foregoing. Immediate-type and delayed-type immune reactions are relatively easily differentiated on clinical, morphological and histological grounds, but their pathomechanism is still not fully understood.

## HUMORAL AND CELL-MEDIATED IMMUNITY

The two types of hypersensitivity are in relation with the two principal categories of immune response, humoral and cellular. The lymphoid system can roughly be divided into primary and secondary lymphoid tissues. The primary lymphoid tissue of all vertebrates is the thymus and, in birds, the bursa of Fabricius. The thymus plays the essential role in the differentiation of those stem cells from which the cells participating in cell-mediated immunity (T cells = thymus cells) arise. The bursa of the avian species and the not yet fully identified bursa-equivalents of mammals (probably the tonsils, intestinal lymphoid aggregates, etc.) are the sites of differentiation of the so-called thymus-independent stem cells (B cells = bursa cells), which are capable of synthesizing the known classes of antibodies (immunoglobulin molecules) and of secreting them into the blood stream. Antigens do not play a role in stem cell differentiation taking place in the thymus or bursa (bursa equivalents), but the further differentiation of lymphocytes migrating from thymus or bursa (bursa equivalent) into the secondary lymphoid tissue (lymph nodes, spleen, Peyer's patches, etc.) is antigen dependent.

Specific receptors related with the structural components of immunoglobulin molecules responsible for antigen affinity have been demonstrated on the surface of B lymphocyte membranes. Experimental findings indicate that these receptors are precise replicas of antibodies which the cell or its successors would produce and secrete on appropriate antigenic stimulation [25].

Since in immediate hypersensitivity, apart from antigen, antibodies produced by thymus-independent B cells are involved, it may as well be termed as 'hypersensitively mediated by antibodies' [19].

Experiments have recently been undertaken to characterize the antigen-recognizing receptors of T cells [29]. Avian lymphocytes from thymus and bursa of Fabricius can easily be differentiated from one another by immunoadherence, using rabbit antiserum on the basis of their antigen specificity [14]. The T lymphocytes of mice contain the so-called $\theta$-alloantigen [32, 33, 39]. The percentage of $\theta$-bearing lymphocytes have been assessed in thymus, thoracic duct, blood, lymph nodes, spleen, peritoneal fluid and Peyer's patches as 100, 80, 70, 65, 35, 30 and 20 per cent, respectively, but as yet they could not be demonstrated in the bone marrow. They are probably the long-lived small [11] and recirculating lymphocytes [45].

The delayed-type reaction is unrelated to circulating antibodies, because immunity cannot be passively transferred with serum, only with lymphoid tissue, inflammatory exudation, or leukocytes. Since the T cells play a leading role in this type of reaction, recently it has often been referred to as specific cell-mediated hypersensitivity.

The differences between B and T cells can be characterized as follows: (*i*) B cells are less radiosensitive than T cells. (*ii*) Unlike T cells, B cells are not affected by thymectomy and anti-lymphocyte serum. (*iii*) Stimulation of B cells requires an at least tenfold antigen dose as compared with T cells [31]. (*iv*) Stimulation of T cells by Concanavalin A or phytohaemagglutinin (T-cell-specific mitogens)

TABLE 4-I

*Distiguishing characteristics of T and B lymphocytes* [44*a*]

| Membrane markers | T lymphocytes | B lymphocytes |
|---|---|---|
| IgG | — | + |
| Receptor for C3 (erythrocyte — antibody — complement rosettes) | — | + |
| Receptor for Ig or antigen–antibody complexes (Fc) | — | + |
| Thymus-specific antigens ($\theta$, mouse thymocyte leukaemia antigen, etc.) | + | — |
| Receptors for sheep red blood cells (erythrocyte rosettes) | + | — |
| *In vitro* stimulation of DNA synthesis by mitogens[a] | | |
| Phytohaemagglutinin | + | —[b] |
| Concanavalin A | + | — |
| Lipopolysaccharide (bacterial endotoxin)[c] | — | + |
| Anti-Ig | — | + |
| Specific binding to antigen-coated beads | — | + |
| Mixed lymphocyte culture reactivity | + | — |
| Graft-versus-host reaction inducing capacity | + | — |

[a] These data derive mainly from experiments in mice, and their extrapolation to man is questionable.
[b] Some B lymphocytes may be recruited to divide secondarily by factors elaborated by activated T lymphocytes. B cells may also be stimulated when the mitogen is attached to a solid support.
[c] In mice.

*in vitro* induced the appearance of lymphoblasts; endotoxin (B-cell-specific mitogen) stimulated B cells developed plasmablast features [19*a*, *b*, *c*]. The properties of T cells and B cells have recently been summarized in a WHO Scientific Group Report as shown in Table 4-I [44*a*].

Historically, the delayed-type hypersensitivity phenomenon had first been recognized in connection with chronic infectious diseases, whence it had formerly been known as 'bacterial allergy' or 'allergy of infection'. The classical form of delayed hypersensitivity is the skin response of tuberculotic man or animal to the protein of *Mycobacterium tuberculosis*.

Differentiation was based on immediate-type and delayed-type skin reactions.

## WEAL AND FLARE REACTIVITY

Immediate-type skin reactions are usually characterized by the weal and flare response, appearing immediately after administration of the antigen, reaching its maximum within 15–30 min and disappearing completely within a few hours. Thus the immediate skin reaction corresponds to a superficial serous inflammation with few infiltrating cells, chiefly eosinophils, and is of a transitory nature (Figs 4-1 and 4-2).

## DELAYED REACTIVITY

Delayed-type reaction may, among others, be of the tuberculin-trichophytin type. At the site of antigen administration (usually intradermally), a hyperaemic inflammatory reaction develops after 6–12 h (Fig. 4–6*b*) or occasionally earlier, which soon becomes oedematous and often assumes a papular form gradually infiltrated by cells, reaching its maximum 24–48–72 h after antigen administration. Less often the local change is vesicular (Fig. 4-3) or haemorrhagic-necrotic (Fig. 4-4), if sensitization has been more vigorous, and may persist for several days or weeks.

Originally Gell and Coombs' type IV reaction (see p. 28) included only the tuberculin-trichophytin-type reactions [9], but Storck [40] has reasonably extended it to eczematous skin reactions, which is a prototype of delayed-type allergic response. This eczema-type reaction corresponds to the eczematiform inflammation developing in response to the epicutaneous patch test; it appears only several hours after application of the antigen and is characteristic of allergic contact dermatitis (eczema) (Fig. 4-5).

## DIFFERENTIATION BETWEEN THE TWO TYPES OF REACTIVITY

Immediate-type skin reactions generally correspond to early clinical symptoms, whereas delayed-type skin reactions usually signify symptoms appearing later. There are, of course, many exceptions to this rule and no sharp differentiation can be made. Immediate and delayed-type reactions may also occur on normoreactive skin. Allergic inflammation is not in every respect different from the inflammatory process of the normal skin. Essentially the same phlogogenic substances, effects or factors are involved in both processes, except that in allergic inflammations an additional specific factor, the antibody and/or the immunolymphocyte, play a role.

The problem of the differences between immediate-type and delayed-type reactions should be approached from two angles, viz. from those of the antigen and of the immune response. Analysis of the causes of the difference between the two reaction types has shown that these should be sought on the one hand in the nature, quality and quantity of antigenic substances, and on the other hand, in the variousness of the immune response. Earlier it had been believed that also the chemical composition, dose and mode of application of the antigen and its fate and localization in the body, as well as the species of the animal play a role.

There are certain urticariogenic substances which if applied to the skin cause an urticarial inflammation without delayed response in both normal and allergic skin. For instance, both the normal and allergic skin responds to histamine or

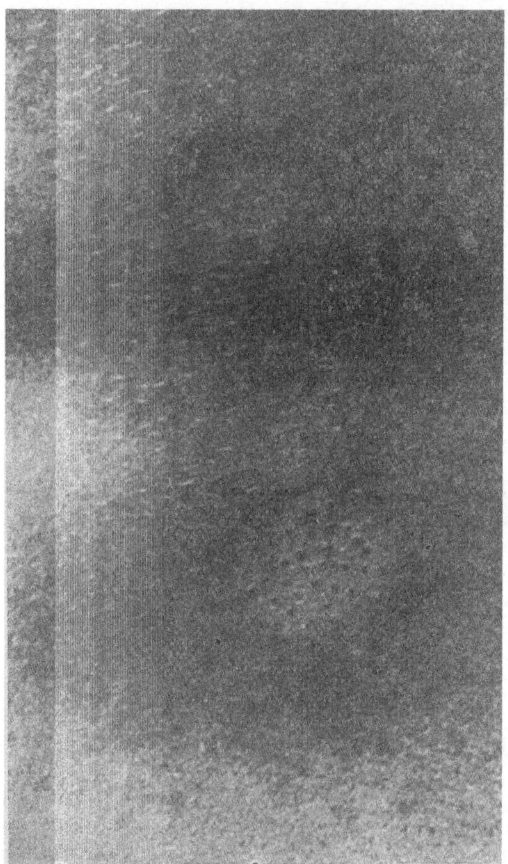

Fig. 4-1. Immediate-type reaction, weal and flare response. Wheat-flour allergy. Bottom: farina tritici; top: control (isotonic NaCl)

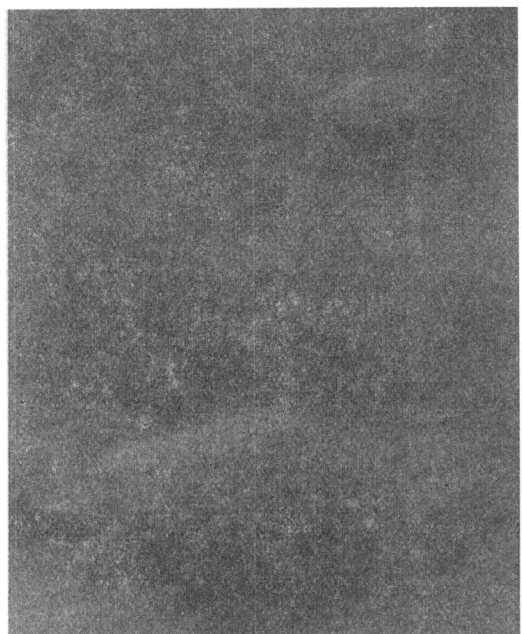

Fig. 4-2. Immediate-type reaction; weal and flare response with pseudopodia. Bottom: trichophytin 1 : 50, intradermally; top: control (isotonic NaCl)

Fig. 4-3. Delayed-type vesicular reaction. Trichophytin 1: 50 intradermally, after 48 hours

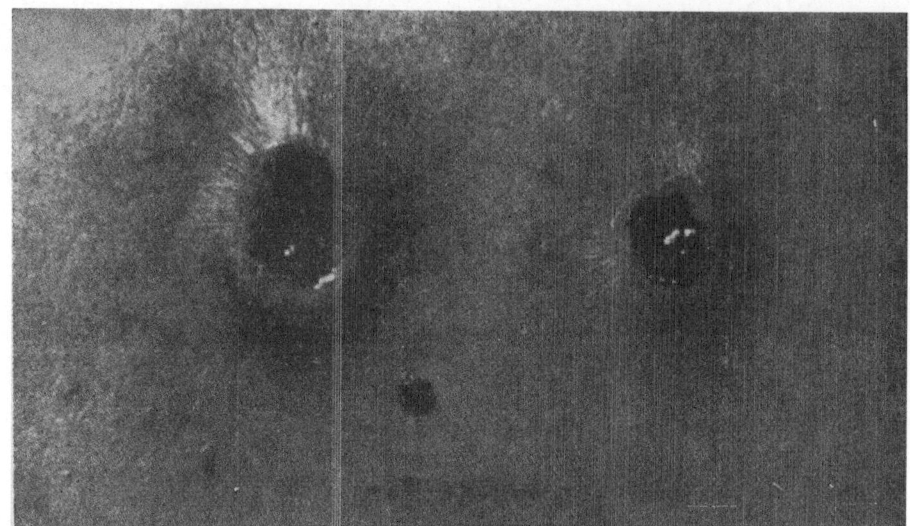

Fig. 4-4. Delayed-type haemorrhagic-necrotic reaction. Tuberculin ($10^{-4}$ and $10^{-5}$) intradermally; after 48 hours

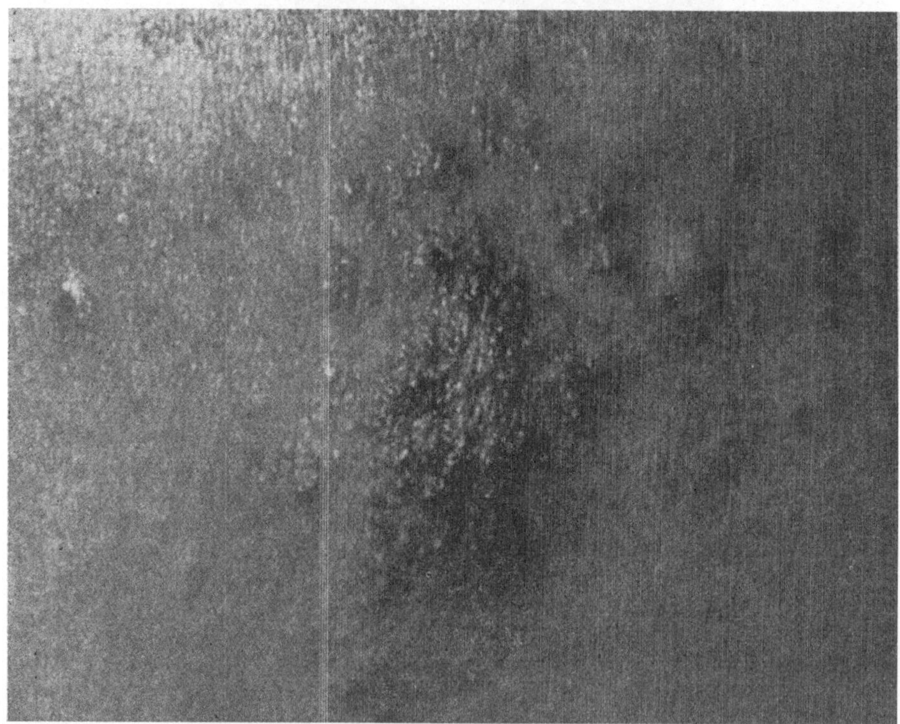

Fig. 4-5. Delayed-type eczematous reaction. Epicutaneous patch reaction: camomile allergy, 24 hours after application of the leaves

histamine releasers with urticarial inflammation of roughly equal intensity, although it may occasionally be stronger if the subject is allergic. The urticariogenic property is an inbuilt capacity of such substances. The situation is, however, different if the subject has been specifically sensitized to the urticariogenic substance; in such cases the effect is much more intensive and a response is given to very strong dilutions which have no effect on normal skin. This form of increased reactivity is rare; a more frequent case is that also a delayed-type reaction develops in addition to the immediate urticarial response. Morphine administered intradermally in the usual concentration elicits an urticarial inflammation in all subjects, which is followed by a delayed-type reaction if the subject is morphine sensitive. Certain complex substances, e.g. blood serum, which is slightly urticariogenic in both normal and allergic skin and causes only a very slight papular form of delayed response, if any, may elicit a score of reactions ranging from an intensive weal and flare response to an intensive delayed reaction with necrosis and papillomatosis if the subject is serum sensitive [4].

There are so-called eczematogenic, primary irritant substances, which on external contact cause an eczematiform inflammation corresponding to the delayed reaction. The allergic subject either responds to low concentrations with greater intensity, or the allergic skin displays an eczematiform response to such substances or effects to which the normal skin is unresponsive (Fig. 4-5). Also, certain antigens (drugs) elicit an eczematiform reaction in sensitive subjects even on oral application of low doses.

Certain substances elicit a delayed tuberculin-type reaction on intradermal administration into normal skin. Unlike eczematogenic substances, the delayed-type reaction involves chiefly the corium.

If the subject is allergic, the inflammatory response islmuch more intensive and the allergic skin will react to substances which are toerated free of symptoms by the normal skin.

Finally there are substances which elicit both immediate-type and delayed-type reactions on normal skin (Fig. 4-6*a* and *b*). To this category belong certain urticariogenic substances (e.g. peptone) and certain drugs (e.g. penicillin). Both types of skin reaction are more intensive if the subject is allergic.

But like the time of onset as well as the intensity of immediate or delayed responses are not always conclusive of the nature of the reaction, neither would morphological findings attest at first sight to a primary irritant or allergic background. The difference between the two effects is clear if it is considered that the irritant effect results in direct damage which determines the polymorphous clinical picture, the effect is obligatory and has a well definable threshold, whereas the allergic effect is mediated by the immune response, thus being to a greater or lesser degree independent of the damage, whence the reactive picture is fairly monomorphous and the threshold varies considerably.

The mode of exposure, viz. the route by which the antigen gains access to the body is usually decisive. Certain drugs or chemical substances cause an eczematous delayed-type inflammation on external contact if the epidermis is sensitized; if the corium is also sensitized, the same reaction is elicited by the parenteral administration of the antigen. There are, of course, exceptions to this rule. If the mucous membranes of the respiratory and gastro-intestinal tracts are sensitized, immediate hypersensitivity reactions (asthma, hay fever) occur due to the allergen

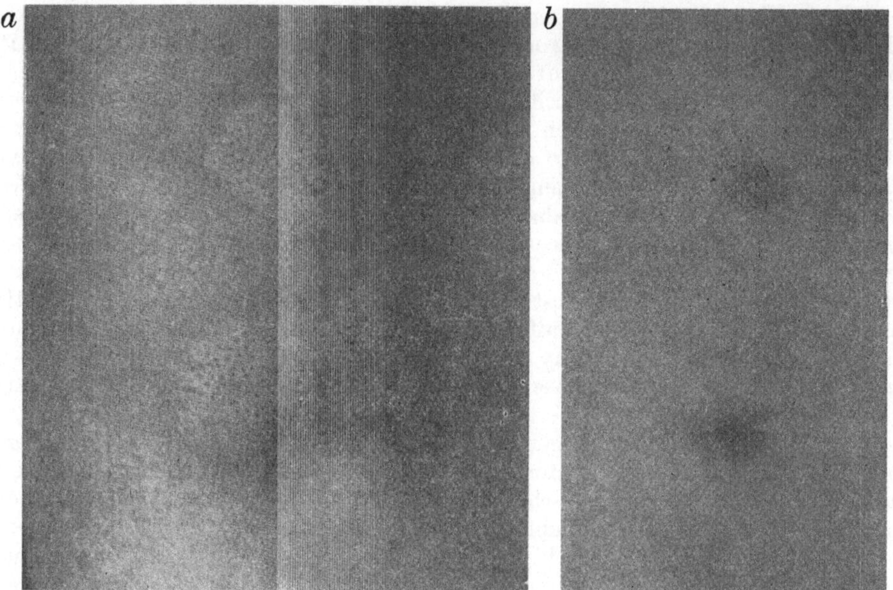

Fig. 4-6. *a)* Immediate-type weal and flare response; *b)* Delayed tuberculin-type infiltrative inflammatory reaction after 4 days. Trichophytin 1: 50, intradermally: 0.05 ml (top); 0.1 ml (bottom)

and even anaphylactic shock may develop if the allergen is administered parenterally. Other organs sensitized by the allergen, probably in a protein-combined complex form, respond chiefly by delayed-type reactions. Autoantigens always act by the internal route, either in the blood stream or in the viscera. Thus the various substances may cause different clinical syndromes depending on the mode of their application and the site of their entry into the body.

In immediate-type reactions, the antibody is fixed to cells and the allergic response occurs when the antigen reaches the cell-fixed antibody. In delayed-type reactions, however, the antigen is fixed and thymus derived lymphocytes approach its site of deposition. Thus in the former case, the antigen–antibody reaction can occur as soon as the antigen or antigen–antibody complex reaches the shock tissue, whereas in the latter case, the thymus derived lymphocytes are not yet present in sufficient numbers when the antigen comes into contact with, or deposits in, a tissue; such cells reach the antigen only later carried by the blood stream as infiltrating lymphocytes. It appears as if the antigen would exert a chemotactic effect on antigen reactive lymphocytes. Nevertheless, it takes some time until their number will be sufficient to elicit the reaction.

Formerly it was generally accepted that corpuscular antigens and insoluble protein complexes elicit a delayed-type reaction if there is an antibody excess, whereas high molecular-weight soluble antigens elicit an immediate-type reaction usually in the presence of antigen excess. It was further concluded from experiments with hapten-protein conjugates that immediate hypersensitivity is primarily hapten specific [1], while delayed-type reactions are characterized by carrier protein specificity. But it was later shown that all kinds of soluble proteins can provoke a delayed-type reaction when applied in Freund's adjuvant; also recent findings on the interaction between specific antibody forming cell precursors and specific helper cells have thrown an entirely new light on the hapten and protein specificity of antibodies formed to hapten-protein conjugates [26]. Multiple injections of bovine serum albumin without adjuvant stimulate production of large amounts of antibody but no detectable delayed-type hypersensitivity in guinea pigs. In contrast, single or multiple injections of bovine serum albumin heavily conjugated with dodecanoic acid, without adjuvant stimulated sustained delayed-type hypersensitivity but no detectable antibody production. The delayed-type hypersensitivity produced was specific for native bovine serum albumin and no detectable immune response was produced against the fatty acid groups [9*a*]. The analysis of humoral and cellular immune responses of guinea pigs to induction with synthetic oligopeptides suggests that the cell population participating in the cellular immune response and eliciting delayed-type hypersensitivity distinguishes even between the minutest details of the chemical structure. Humoral antibodies, in contrast, cannot differentiate between peptides of dissimilar immunogenicity, whence their specificity is comparable with that of the receptors of antibody forming cell precursors. On this basis it seems probable that the cells involved in the cellular immune response participate as helper cells in the stimulation of antibody synthesis, their role being to recognize those delicate differences which are not detected by the precursors of antibody producing cells [29, 41]. Conjugates of *p*-azobenzearsonate with different proteins and polypeptides produced hapten-specific delayed-type skin reactions [22, 23, 27]. According to Parish [30], in adult animals both B and T cell populations possess cell surface receptors reflecting the specificity of the immune response. Intercellular interaction of B and T cells is essential for the induction of antibody formation, but the precise nature of this interaction is still unclear. It probably involves the transfer of non-specific factors, or the translocation of specific genetic material; the latter situation would, however, mean that B cells acquire their receptors passively. Thus, given that the antigen binds exclusively to the T cell and this binding provides the latter with an appropriate threshold energy, the cell will become activated, will proliferate and give rise to delayed hypersensitivity. If, however, the interaction of the two cell lines with the antigen, which acting as a molecular bridge is responsible for transfer or translocation, results in antibody formation and inhibition of the cellular response, an immediate-type allergic response will occur. Thus the affinity of the antigen to the receptors of the two kinds of cells is the decisive factor which determines the type of the immune response, i.e. the immediate or delayed type of the allergic reaction. Accordingly, although B and T cells collaborate in the process of antibody formation, a competition of humoral and cell-mediated immunity may easily occur in various immunological processes, especially if the affinity, or applied dose, of the antigen is extremely high or low. Antigen administered in adjuvant failed to elicit delayed hypersensitivity if the animal had previously been treated with the same antigen in saline [5]. Extremely low doses of antigen were found to elicit a delayed hypersensitivity [36] without antibody production [13]. Intravenous injection of rabbit anti-chicken immunoglobulin (IgG and IgM) resulted in inhibition of delayed hypersensitivity reactions in bursectomized agammaglobulinaemic chickens [42*c*].

## COEXISTENCE OF IMMEDIATE AND DELAYED HYPERSENSITIVITY

Apart from extreme cases, it has long been known from artificial protein sensitization experiments that the two types of allergic reaction would almost regularly occur in combination; Dienes [12], Jones and Mote [20] but earlier also others [42*a*, *b*] reported that intradermal application of the antigen usually elicited first delayed, and later immediate hypersensitivity. The same has been observed, e.g. during the specific treatment of mycoses with trichophytin [34]. Rabbits sensitized with streptococcus whole cells respond by a delayed-type reaction to the nucleoproteid fraction (M-protein); if, however, they are sensitized with the nucleoproteid only, the reaction will be immediate [21], analogously with individuals sensitive only to the polysaccharide fractions of streoptococci and pneumococci. The coexistence of immediate- and delayed-type reactions has been demonstrated in various other types of allergy (drug-, insect-, physical allergy, etc.), being a far more frequent phenomenon than generally supposed.

The analysis of the Arthus reaction presents additional evidence to the coexistence of immediate- and delayed-type reactions. The phenomenon can be divided into three phases [15, 35]: (*i*) initially, soon after the intradermal administration of the antigen, vascular processes predominate over a neutrophil leukocytic infiltration and necrosis. Increased capillary permeability and the formation of leukocytic microthrombi are also characteristic of this phase (no Arthus reaction occurs in the case of leukocyte depletion) [8]. (*ii*) After 24 h, cell proliferation involving mononuclear elements is the most important symptom, which is already a delayed-type reaction. (*iii*) From the 3rd day, first plasma cell precursors (immunoblasts, plasmablasts), then plasma cells appear around the vessels marking the further synthesis of free circulating antibodies, which process reaches its maximum in about one week. (Circulating precipitins already appear in response to the first immunizing antigen injection.) Many factors do in fact influence the occurrence of immediate- and delayed-type reactions which often appear simultaneously. This is in good agreement with the three characteristics of adaptive immunity, as they appeared in vertebrates in the course of evolution: (*i*) specific immunoglobulin production; (*ii*) graft rejection, and (*iii*) delayed allergic reaction involving mononuclear cell proliferation, as elicited by antigen + adjuvant.

## ENCOUNTER OF ANTIGEN WITH ANTIBODY AND ITS CONSEQUENCES

Cell-mediated immunity (delayed hypersensitivity) is believed by many to be essentially a 'protection' against cellular mutation, above all against neoplasia and viral infections [43], termed by Burnet [6, 7] as 'immunological surveillance'.

Some of the circulating humoral antibodies become fixed to certain cells of the shock tissue—in immediate-type atopic processes chiefly to mast cells—and when they encounter the antigen transported by the blood stream, an antigen–antibody reaction occurs along with its secondary consequences. At the same time the circulating antibodies form an antigen–antibody complex with the antigen in the blood stream and after this act in the complex form. It seems, however, that there are circulating antibodies with no apparent pathogenic role, which are probably only by-products of sensitization.

Immediate-type reactions are mediated by a temperature-dependent and Ca-dependent mechanism involving also enzyme effects. The biochemical effect is characterized by a temperature optimum of 37–40 °C and it is inhibited by heating (43 °C) and cooling (28 °C); of the bivalent cations it requires Ca, but no Mg. The SH- and S-S groups play an important role, but complement is not indispensable [18].

Cell-mediated immunity is characterized by a monocytic infiltration, in which lymphocytes are the major cell with only very few granulocytes, if any. In delayed hypersensitivity induced with protein antigen, the lymphocytes of the animal release on contact with the antigen a number of factors of which the one called migration inhibition factor is the best known. This factor characteristically alters the properties of normal macrophages *in vitro* [3, 10, 16, 37]. Phenomena associated with this factor are production of inflammation on skin of normal animal [2]; cytotoxicity and cytolysis, i.e. the specific antigen either inhibits the growth of target cells preincubated with the factor or lyses them in the presence of complement [17]; blastogenesis, i.e. antigen induced transformation of lymphocytes cultured with the factor [28]; chemotaxis [44]; aggregation [24]; reduction in the interfacial energy of the cell surface [43*a*] and, finally, inhibition of migration of macrophages and leukocytes *in vitro* upon the factor's reaction with the specific antigen. The *in vitro* effect of the migration inhibition factor on normal macrophages corresponds essentially to the *in vivo* effect on normal macrophages of the interaction between lymphocytes of animals with delayed hypersensitivity and homologous antigen. Thus at exposure to the antigen, the lymphocytes of animals with delayed hypersensitivity release a soluble factor or factors influencing certain properties of macrophages [38]. There is reason to suppose on this basis that reaction with the antigen of a few specifically sensitized lymphocytes can activate numerous effector cells through these mediator(s). This mechanism may account for the fact that so many cells participate in the delayed-type allergic reactions.

## REFERENCES


1. Benacerraf, B. and Levine, B. B.: *J. exp. Med.* **115,** 1023 (1962).
2. Bennett, B. and Bloom, B. R.: *Proc. Nat. Acad. Sci. (Wash.)* **59,** 765 (1968).
3. Bloom, B. R. and Bennett, B.: *Science* **153,** 80 (1966).
4. Bloom, B. E. and Chase, M. V.: *Progr. Allergy* **10,** 1 (1967).
5. Borel, Y. and David, J. R.: *J. exp. Med.* **131,** 603 (1970).
6. Burnet, M. F.: *Lancet,* **i,** 1171 (1959).
7. Burnet, M. F.: *Self and Not-Self.* Univ. Press. Melbourne (1969).
8. Cochrane, C. G.: *Ann. Inst. Pasteur* **99,** 329 (1960).
9. Coombs, R. R. A. and Gell, P. G. H.: *Clinical Aspects of Immunology.* Davis, Philadelphia 1963.

9*a*. Coon, J. and Hunter, R.: *J. Immunol.* **110,** 183 (1973).

10. David, J. R., Al-Askari, S., Lawrence, H. S. and Thomas, L.: *J. Immunol.* **93,** 264 (1964).
11. Denman, A. M., Denman, E. and Embling, P. H.: *Lancet* **i,** 321 (1968).
12. Dienes, L.: *Proc. Soc. exp. Biol. (N.Y.)* **28,** 75 1930.
13. Dresser, D. W. and Mitchison, N. A.: *Advance Immunol.* **8,** 129 (1968).

14. Forget, A., Potworowski, E. F., Richer, G. and Bordnas, A. G.: *Immunology* **19,** 465 (1970).
15. Gell, P. G. H.: *Int. Arch. Allergy* **6,** 326 (1955).
16. George, M. and Vaughan, J. H.: *Proc. Soc. exp. Biol. Med.* **111,** 514 (1962).
17. Granger, G. A., Schacks, S. J., Williams, T. W. and Kolb, W. P.: *Nature* **221,** 1155 (1969).
18. Greaves, M. W.: *Acta derm. venereol.* **50,** Suppl. 64 (1970).
19. Humphrey, J. G. and White, R. G. (Eds): *Immunology for Students of Medicine.* 3rd ed. Blackwell, Oxford 1970.
19*a*. Janossy, G. and Greaves, M. F.: *Clin. exp. Immunol.* **9,** 483 (1971).
19*b*. ibid., **10,** 525 (1972).
19*c*. Janossy, G. Shohat, M., Greaves, M. F. and Dourmashkin, R. R.: *Immunology* **24,** 211 (1973).
20. Jones, T. D. and Mote, J. R.: *New Engl. J. Med.* **210,** 120 (1934).
21. Kahn, M. C.: *J. Allergy* **22,** 237 (1951).
22. Krüger, J., Wayland, J. S. and Waksman, B. H.: *Immunochemistry* **8,** 319 (1971).
23. Leskowitz, S., Jones, V. E. and Zak, S. J.: *J. exp. Med.* **123,** 299 (1966).
24. Lolekha, S., Dray, S. and Gotoff, S. P.: *J. Immunol.* **104,** 296 (1970).
25. Miller, J. F. A. P.: *Folia allergol.* **17,** 381 (1970.)
26. Mitchison, N. A.: *Eur. J. Immunol.* **1,** 18 (1971).
27. Nauciel, C. and Raynaud, M.: *Eur. J. Immunol.* **1,** 257 (1971).
28. Oppenheim, J. J., Wolstencroft, R. A. and Gell, P. G. H.: *Immunology* **12,** 89 (1967)
29. Paul, W. E., Stupp, Y., Siskin, G. W. and Benacerraf, B.: *Immunology* **21,** 605 (1971).
30. Parish, C. R.: *J. exp. Med.* **134,** 21 (1971).
31. Playfair, J. H. L. and Purves, E. C.: *Immunology* **21,** 113 (1971).
32. Raff, M. C. and Owen, J. J. T.: *Eur. J. Immunol.* **1,** 27 (1971).
33. Raff, M. C. and Wortis, H. H.: *Immunology* **18,** 929 (1970).
34. Rajka, E.: *Acta allerg. (Kbh.)* **7,** 326 (1954).
35. Rothlin, E. and Bircher, R.: *Fortschr. Allergielehre* **3,** 434 (1952).
36. Salvin, S. B.: *J. exp. Med.* **107,** 109 (1958).
37. Salvin, S. B. and Nishio, J.: *Cell Immunol.* **1,** 62 (1970).
38. Salvin, S. B., Sell, S. and Nishio, J.: *J. Immunol.* **107,** 655 (1971).
39. Schimpl, A. and Wecker, E.: *Eur. J. Immunol.* **1,** 305 (1971).
40. Storck, H.: *Fortschr. prakt. Dermat. Venerol.* **5,** 134 (1965).
41. Stupp, Y., Paul, W. E. and Benacerraf, B.: *Immunology* **21,** 583, 595 (1971).
42*a*. Tezner, O.: *Jahrb. Kinderheilk.* **142,** 69 (1934).
42*b*. Tezner, O.: *Arch. Derm., Syph. (Berl.)* **170,** 293 (1934).
42*c*. Theis, G. A. and Thorbecke, G. J.: *J. Immunol.* **110,** 91 (1973).
43. Thomas, L.: in Lawrance, H. S.: *Cellular and Humoral Aspects of Hypersensitive States.* Hoeber, New York 1959.
43*a*. Trasher, S. G., Yoshida, T., van Oss, G. J., Cohen, S. and Rose, N. R.: *J. Immunol.* **110,** 321 (1973).
44. Ward, P. A., Remold, H. G. and David, J. R.: *Cell. Immunol.* **1,** 162 (1970).
44*a*. WHO Scientific Group: Cell-Mediated Immunity and Resistance to Infection. *Wld. Hlth. Org. techn. Rep. Ser.* No. 519. WHO, Geneva 1973, p. 16.
45. Zalz, M. M. and Lanee, E. M.: *Cell Immunol.* **1,** 3 (1970).

CHAPTER 5

# IMMUNOLOGICAL UNRESPONSIVENESS

by

E. RAJKA

completed by

L. KESZTYŰS



Immunological unresponsiveness is characterized by failure to respond to contact with antigen. It may be specific for a given antigen, as in immunological tolerance or in desensitization, or generalized inasmuch as there is non-specific unresponsiveness to many antigens, as, for example, in immunological deficiency states or following therapy with an immunosuppressive agent.

## IMMUNOLOGICAL TOLERANCE. IMMUNOLOGICAL PARALYSIS

These special forms of immunological unresponsiveness are at present difficult to define precisely. Nevertheless, a more or less arbitrary distinction can be made as follows. Immunological tolerance is a specific nonreactivity of lymphoid tissues to a given antigen which may be either natural or acquired, and immunological paralysis is a state of unresponsiveness induced by very small or very large doses of antigen. Nevertheless the synonymous use of the terms 'immunological tolerance' and 'immunological paralysis' is now generally accepted, because the fundamental mechanism of these phenomena, i.e. a central failure of responsiveness in which the immunologically competent cells are unable to form specific antibodies, appears to be identical [38].

### FOETAL AND NEONATAL FORMS

In the case of a normal, natural tolerance, the developing foetus recognizes all accessible antigen-like substances as its own (self recognition), because the predeterminant potential immunologically competent cells (ICC) capable of reacting with these antigenic substances become destroyed or eliminated during foetal life. No tolerance develops, however, in sequestered (inaccessible) sites, i.e. to substances not coming into contact with the antibody forming organs, whence such substances may become sources of auto-antibody formation in postnatal life [16].

Thus immunological tolerance may either be (*i*) natural, preexisting, related with the genetic constitution of the species, or (*ii*) acquired.

*Artificial* (*'foreign'*) *immunological tolerance* develops if the body recognizes foreign antigenic materials as self, tolerating it without reaction (foreign tolerance). This phenomenon occurs when the foreign material is administered to the recipient either during prenatal life, or immediately after birth, i.e. at a stage when the postnatal immune apparatus is still undeveloped, the lymphoid system performs hardly any immunological activity and antibody formation has not yet begun. At this stage of development, artificial immunological tolerance can be easily induced, but exclusively to the donor's tissue [12*a*, *b*, *c*]. Different animal species behave dissimilarly in this respect. In cattle and sheep, the phase of tolerance ends well before birth; in man, rabbit and in most rat and mouse strains, the immune period begins either at birth or a few days after it, whereas in dogs, chickens and ducks, immunological tolerance can be elicited up to 7–14 days after birth or hatching [61]. Also adult animals can be rendered tolerant with administration of large doses of the foreign antigen (see later).

If after the beginning of the immune period, tissue is transferred from an animal of the same species, but of a different strain, the usual homograft rejection mechanism will occur, indicating the specificity of immunological tolerance, i.e. that the tolerant organism responds normally to foreign antigens. In other words, foreign cells which are either present or administered during embryonic life, and their progeny, are accepted like the foetus's own cells (self tolerance) [17] and persist also during adult life despite their dissimilar genetic pattern, if their presence as 'self substance' is continuous. The host thus becomes a cellular chimaera [11]. Self and foreign tolerance are probably based on the same mechanism. An intact classical complement pathway is not necessary for tolerance induction; an equal degree of tolerance was induced in C4-deficient and normal guinea pigs with adequate regimens [23*c*].

Immunological tolerance can be induced primarily with living, homologous cells containing nuclei, especially if the donor and host are closely related, i.e. if the antigenic difference is minor and exists throughout the body. Induction of tolerance is, however, also successful when RNA from different organs of a related strain is used prior to skin transplantation, e.g. in homograft transplantation experiments, because RNase prevents the development of tolerance [3]. Thus injection of microsome, ribosome or RNA extracts from newborn isogeneic (syngeneic) male mice donors into newborn female mice hosts induced tolerance to transplanted donor skin, suggesting that the biological activity related with the establishment of immunological tolerance is associated with the mRNA-containing ergosomes, which are responsible for the continuous biosynthesis of transplantation antigens [138]. Apart from corpuscular antigens, immunological tolerance can also be induced to soluble antigens and even to homogenous proteins, although somewhat less easily.

Immunological tolerance is strictly individual specific, owing probably to determinant specificity, as shown by experiments in which animals rendered tolerant to serum albumin were incapable of producing antibodies to the azotized part of the same albumin.

The highest number of tolerance experiments have been devoted to cell and tissue transplantation. Mouse embryo recipients, e.g. inoculated prenatally with cells of an adult donor mouse do not reject donor tissue transplants (e.g. skin grafts) after birth or in adult age because they had already developed tolerance in foetal life (active acquired tolerance) [12*a*, *b*, *c*]. Injection of appropriate doses of leukocyte suspension into newborn animals induced partial tolerance to skin graft transplants from the leukocyte donor. Immunological tolerance to histocompatibility antigens as assessed by skin grafts, was induced in hormonally bursectomized chickens that could not form antibody responses or even synthesize immunoglobulins. This demonstrates that the induction of allograft tolerance does not require the essential participation of suppressive humoral antibody [113*a*]. It should be pointed out that injection of any nucleus containing cell into foetus or newborn animals imparts tolerance to all tissues of the donor, because the identical structure of the cell nuclei excludes tissue specificity. This accounts for the fact that animals rendered tolerant to anuclear erythrocytes do not form haemagglutinins, but do respond with an immune reaction to skin transplants [57].

Tolerance can be most effectively induced by injection of live spleen or lymph node cells from the future donor [105*a*, *b*]. Repeated injections of spleen cell suspensions induced tolerance in both newborn and adult mice, above all to transplantation, e.g. of male skin to isologous females. Unlike tolerance to intact spleen cells, tolerance to disrupted spleen cells is not transferable to a syngeneic recipient with spleen cells from an areactive donor [94]. Spleen cells administered intravenously as donor antigen can significantly enhance the effect of anti-lymphocyte serum on the prolongation of skin allograft survival, irrespective of whether the histoincompatibility barrier is weak or strong. The effect depends on the appropriate timing of antigen application and may induce a strong enough tolerance to permit the acceptance of second set grafts. If, however, test allografts are applied 9 days after antigen administration, anti-lymphocyte serum treatment and spleen cell injection either fail to induce tolerance or fail to prolong the survival time of first set grafts. Thus probably the skin allograft itself plays an important role in the induction of tolerance [42]. The phenomenon that owing to passage of maternal cell antigens via the placenta into the foetus, guinea pigs are occasionally more tolerant to maternal than to paternal transplants, is probably related to immunological tolerance [28]. Tolerance may also be induced in experimental autoallergic processes: if newborn rats are treated with autologous and homologous kidney suspension, the animals will not develop glomerulonephritis on treatment with the same suspension in complete Freund's adjuvant after one month [76].

Immunological tolerance also develops to serum proteins, e.g. to bovine $\gamma$-globulin, if mice are treated with it immediately after birth. Absence of immune elimination of subsequently administered $^{131}$I-labelled bovine $\gamma$-globulin is in support of tolerance. The degree of tolerance depends on the time interval between the preparatory and provoking injections. Despite tolerance, precipitins and haemagglutinating antibodies may nevertheless arise to another fraction (split tolerance). The following phenomenon is an example of split tolerance: a single injection of a 100 $\mu$g dose of centrifuged rabbit IgG into mice of an appropriate strain induces tolerance to the entire molecule. Ten $\mu$g rabbit IgG, however, renders the animals tolerant to the Fab fragment of IgG, but they form antibodies to the Fc fragment [134*a*, *b*]. Thus tolerance to one fraction and sensitivity to another fraction may occur at the same time [36*a*, *b*].

Under given experimental conditions humoral antibodies can also exert a protective effect. For instance, it is known that rats sensitized with nerve tissue (in Freund's adjuvant) develop allergic encephalomyelitis which is passively transferable with their lymph node cells, but they also form circulating anti-brain antibodies. If, however, the nerve tissue is inoculated into newborn rats, immunological tolerance develops instead of encephalitis, but C-fixing antibodies to the nerve tissue will also arise. High concentrations of such antibodies prevent encephalomyelitis when administered intravenously to rats, as they induce tolerance to the nerve tissue [109].

Treatment of rabbits with bovine serum albumin (BSA) and other heterologous serum albumins had similar effects as bovine $\gamma$-globulin; BSA applied during the first postnatal days did not stimulate antibody formation, whence readministration of the antigen several months later did not result in antigen elimination [145*a*, *b*]. Simultaneous administration of several antigens may induce tolerance to all. Human organ extracts could also induce tolerance in animals, although in a lesser degree than serum antigens [151], e.g. human $\gamma$-globulin [126]. Precipitated antigen–antibody complexes may also elicit immunological tolerance [66]. The majority of guinea pigs treated with egg albumen when newborn survived for 3–5 weeks after the provoking antigen injection, owing, probably, to a considerable repression or delay of the anaphylactic shock [104]. Filipp [41] made similar observations on anaphylactic shock phenomena in guinea pigs pretreated with horse serum during or following intrauterine life; neonatal horse serum treatment greatly repressed the Arthus phenomenon also in rabbits. These experimental observations clearly indicate that immunological tolerance can also be induced in anaphylactic-allergic processes, regardless whether the sensitivity is of immediate or delayed type.

Immunological tolerance to different tumour tissues has also been described. Among others Radzikovskaya [110] demonstrated that inoculation of various organ extracts (spleen, kidney, testicles, etc.) from normal rabbit into newborn mice is associated with tolerance to Brown-Pearce carcinoma. It seems that the antigen responsible for tolerance is localized in the nuclei and cytoplasm of donor cells. Tolerance phenomena were observed in newborn mice treated with large antigen doses from tumours induced by cancerogenic substances (benzpyrene). It should be pointed out that the immunotolerance induced by live cells not only differs from that induced with chemically defined antigens or soluble proteins, but it is also a much more complex phenomenon [103, 143].

Mention should be made of the fact that bacterial and viral antigens do not as a rule induce immunological tolerance; e.g. BCG and heat-killed *Mycobacterium tuberculosis* elicit delayed hypersensitivity rather than tolerance in foetal mice. Treatment of pregnant mice with tuberculin and stimulation of their newborn offspring with tuberculin accelerates the postnatal maturation of lymphoreticular tissue so that the progeny are capable of a positive response to tuberculin skin test already at 3 weeks of age. Against this, the offspring of untreated control mice do not show a positive skin test until 5 weeks of age, despite neonatal stimulation with tuberculin [77]. This finding is in accordance with the clinical observation that newborn babies of tuberculin sensitive mothers give an immediate response to the cutaneous tuberculin test [79]; the cellular transfer of hypersensitivity from adults to non-exposed newborn is obviously impossible. This may be the reason of Burnet's opinion that the clonal selection theory applies above all to vertebrate antigens. On the other hand, there is evidence that after a non-lethal prenatal infection, the infant does not respond to injection of, or infection with, the same antigen [50]. The purified protein antigen flagellin of *Salmonella adelaidae* (mol. wt. approx. 38,000) easily induced tolerance in rats if they had been treated for 6–9 weeks from birth with a daily intraperitoneal injection of 10 $\mu$g of the cyanogenic bromide digest of flagellin. Thoracic duct lymphocytes are reliable indicators of the immunological status of the animal; lymphocytes from normal donors normalize the antibody response of the irradiated host, whereas cells from a tolerant donor cannot restore the response but transfer adoptive tolerance to the host [121]. The aceto-acetylated derivatives of flagellin induce an even firmer tolerance than its cyanogenic bromide digest. It was demonstrated by means of the acetylated derivatives that in adult rats tolerance can only be induced at the humoral antibody level, whereas in neonatal rats at both humoral and cell-mediated levels of immunity. This indicates a marked difference between neonatal and adult tolerance capacities [108*a*, *b*].

True immunological tolerance, spontaneously acquired during intrauterine life, occurs occasionally also in man if there is a blood group chimaera, e.g. in non-identical twins, when the twins possess, in addition to their own blood group, also that of the other twin. This is due to an intrauterine exchange of haemopoietic cells, because in such cases the two circulations obviously communicate, as occurs with dizygotic twin calves and lambs with a common placenta. This observation of Owen [105*a*, *b*] induced Burnet and Fenner [17] to regard the phenomenon as an antigen induced inhibition of antibody formation and the dissimilar blood group antigen as self antigen.

Immunological tolerance may persist throughout life because the cells responsible for it not only induce tolerance, but they also proliferate, thereby providing a continuous source of inducer antigen. If cell chimaerism ceases in the tolerant animal, immunological tolerance will disappear as well. Apart from the blood group chimaera of non-identical twins, there may be a partial tolerance to mutual skin transplantation, because in addition to the exchange of blood group antigens, polynuclear leukocytes containing female sex chromatin may also be present in the male twin, whence the latter's tolerance to skin of the female twin is only partial (cells of the transplant become almost completely substituted by cells of the host twin) [149]. Sex-related incompatibility, depending on the Y-chromosome, could be controlled by parabiosis in special inbred mice even in adult age (adherence of male skin isotransplant to the female animal) [93].

Blood group tolerance can be induced experimentally in newborn infants; treatment of infants of blood group O with human blood group A antigen protects them from complications arising from transfusion with type A blood.

Newborn babies suffering from foetal erythroblastosis can be rendered tolerant to the donor organism (skin grafts) by exchange transfusion [1], whereas those diseased in neonatal haemolytic jaundice develop only partial tolerance upon this treatment and even that only if blood exchange is performed prior to the 'critical' period of antibody-globulin formation [44].

Artificial blood-group chimaeras can be relatively easily produced, especially in parabiosis experiments, e.g. by conjugation of several eggs [63, 80] or by joining chick embryos or newborn animals (rats), as was first performed by Hasek [56*a*, *b*]. Such parabionts are incapable of antibody formation to erythrocytes or skin grafts from the partner even in adult age. Parabiosis makes the development of immunological tolerance possible not only to homologous, but also to heterologous—although related—species [56*a*, *b*]. Tolerance to homograft transplantation can be induced in allogeneic animals of adult mice strains by parabiosis union or by intravenous injection of large doses of live spleen cells [57].

Leukocyte chimaera arises in newborn mice injected with spleen cells from adult mice if they survive the subsequent graft-versus-host reaction and immunologically active cells from the donor are demonstrable in their spleen, which, however, show no tolerance to lymphoid cells from a third strain. Thus in tolerant chimaeras the spleen cell component originating from the donor organism is immunologically inactive. Simonsen's spleen test (splenomegaly) makes it possible to differentiate between the host and donor components; the latter, i.e. spleen cells from the chimaera, do not elicit splenomegaly when injected into newborn mice of the donor strain [98].

Chromosomal chimaeras are also known in individuals possessing 47, 45, etc. chromosomes instead of the normal 46. False mitoses of this kind probably occur in prenatal life and persist in later life. These 'false' cells are recognized by the antibody producing apparatus as self, because the 'error' had occurred in the phase of immunological tolerance.

Thus chimaeras are characterized by mutual accomodation between donor and host components, because both have acquired a specific tolerance to the other. Homologous tissue, e.g. skin, transplanted in immunologically tolerant state, persists until the immunological tolerance lasts; occasionally, however, the transplant attacks the organism of the host, giving rise to the homologous or runt disease. These observations chiefly apply to animal experiments.

Foetal immunological tolerance is gradually replaced by the postnatal immunological reaction phase, when the cell-surface antibody structures are released extracellularly. The time required for this process, i.e. the 'critical period' (or 'adaptive phase') varies individually. Medawar [97*a*, *b*] has referred to this period as 'zero-phase'. The immune process is reversed during this period, because the elimination of globulin structure cells by the antigen is replaced by binding or decomposition of the antigen by the specific antibody globulin.

Tolerance may diminish or disappear spontaneously and thymectomy may occasionally delay this process [145*a*, *b*], as demonstrated on rabbits rendered tolerant with bovine $\gamma$-globulin and thymectomized [22]. Interference with thymic function facilitates the establishment and maintenance of immunological tolerance [136].

The importance of the thymus has also been affirmed by Flanagan's [43] studies on genetically thymus-less (nude) autosomal recessive mouse mutants. These animals are hairless, sterile, and their viability is very low. Their thymus is completely absent and their leukocyte count is unusually low [106]. Depletion of lymphocytes has been demonstrated in all thymus dependent areas (spleen, lymph node, Peyer's patches) of the animals; the abnormalities of their RES have been regarded as secondary and have been attributed to the absence of the thymus [127]. Genetically thymus-less mice do not reject human malignant tumour and rat skin heterografts [117]. Their reponse to antigenic stimuli is poor; they produce a low level of haemolytic antibody to sheep erythrocytes, but no significant amounts of haemagglutinin or anti-T4 bacteriographage antibody arise and allogeneic skin grafts are not rejected. The thymus dependent 7S haemolysin is not produced, only a low level of thymus independent 19S haemolysin [107]. Thus the genetically thymus-less mice are not altogether incompetent immunologically, but their antibody production is very low, if there is any. The primary or secondary nature of the thymus-less condition cannot be judged, but it is certain that thymic function is not taken over by any other organ or tissue. Intravenous administration of normal thymus cells to nude mutants will not restore the normal immune response unless the transferred cells originate from 'related' animals. 'Relationship' was probably understood as a H-2 compatibility. There is, however, no evidence of the transformation of transferred thymus cells to antibody producing cells [75*a*, *b*].

In neonatally thymectomized mice, the capacity of spleen cells to produce *in vitro* antibodies to sheep erythrocytes can be restored by addition of thymocytes to the culture. This again shows that mice immunized with sheep erythrocytes produce specific antibodies through the B cells, after interaction of antigen with T cells and B cells. The nature of the interaction is not yet known. It has been postulated that the thymus dependent cells bind the antigen at receptor sites specific for certain antigenic determinants, thus concentrating other determinants of the same antigen molecule on specific receptors of the thymus independent cells. In other words, the antigen is bound by the T cells, but local antigen concentrations thus arising at critical sites trigger an antibody synthesis in the B cells [111].

The problem that specific receptors of immunoglobulin nature have generally not been demonstrable on the surface of thymus cells is explicable, on the one hand, by the insufficiency of the methods applied, and on the other, by the structural differences between receptors of thymocytes and thymus independent cells. A third possible explanation might be that although thymocytes and B cells contain the same receptor molecule of immunoglobulin nature, the special steric structure of the thymus cell membrane inhibits the combination of the antigens used as indicators with the receptor molecule. As it has already been mentioned, the spleen cells of neonatally thymectomized mice will produce antibodies *in vitro* against sheep erythrocytes if thymocytes are added to the culture. If, however, the spleen cells have been pretreated with rabbit antibodies formed to mouse serum protein, they will not produce such antibodies even on addition of thymocytes. This shows that mouse-protein-type receptors are located on the surface of the mice spleen cells, which are bound and blocked by the specific rabbit antibody. Treatment of the thymocytes in a similar manner, i.e. with anti-mouse-serum-protein rabbit antibodies, prior to adding them to the culture will not affect the *in vitro* antibody production. Receptor molecules of the kind found in normal serum or on the thymus independent cells are not demonstrable on thymocytes [34] even with such experiments, although recent electron-microscopic studies have detected IgM on thymus dependent lymphocytes [59].

It has generally been postulated that immunological tolerance lasts as long as antigen is present in the organism. This view suggests the dependence of immunological tolerance on the quantity of the antigen. Readministration of antigen may prolong the state of immunological tolerance. There is, however, no satisfactory evidence of antigen persistence during immunological tolerance; the presence of antigen is probably not indispensable [31*a*, *b*]. The fate of labelled antigen can be followed by the elimination test. Immunized animals eliminate the antigen much more rapidly than normal ones. Tolerant animals, however, eliminate the antigen at the same speed as controls. With the elimination test serum antibody concentrations as low as 0.0012–0.0033 $\mu$g antibody-N per ml can be detected [32]. Antibody producing capacity normalizes completely after the spontaneous termination of immunological tolerance.

Immunological tolerance can be reduced or eliminated artificially. Since sensitized but normal lymphocytes can promptly terminate immunological tolerance, there is reason to suppose that the state of tolerance, which involves the entire organism, stems from a central absence of immune response. The fact that the lymphocytes of a protein-tolerant animal do not form specific antibodies to protein when transferred to a normal milieu, is in support of this hypothesis [97*b*]. Thus tolerance is transferable under given conditions. Lethally irradiated mice can be protected by transfer of lymphocytes from normal isologous mice, while the transfer of spleen cells [110] from tolerant donor to irradiated host induces in the latter a specific tolerance to the antigen to which the donor had been rendered tolerant [31*b*], without affecting its capacity for antibody response to other antigens. In syngeneic radiation chimaeras (mice) the animal's own thymus is sufficient to restore reactivity to bacterial antigens, but restoration of responsiveness to tissue antigens requires the additional activity of non-irradiated thymus. In allogeneic radiation chimaeras, implantation of a non-irradiated thymus graft is a precondition of reactivity to bacterial antigens (probably via its humoral function), whereas reactivity to tissue antigens is scarcely restored, because even a non-irradiated thymus is incapable of fulfilling the cellular aspect of its function in an allogeneic environment [64].

Tolerant virus carrier mice were produced by intraperitoneal administration of 1,000 $LD_{50}$ lymphocytic choriomeningitis (LCM) virus immediately after birth [54*e*]. The constant and permanent tolerance thus established lasts throughout lifetime, but it ceases on transplantation of syngeneic sensitized or unsensitized lymphoid cells. Unsensitized thymus cells are ineffective. Syngeneic sensitized lymphoid cells implanted into tolerant animals in a millipore chamber confer an antibody producing capacity upon the host, but do not notably affect viraemia. Life-long tolerance is hard to reconcile with Burnet's classical theory [16], according to which the LCM-reactive stem cells had become eliminated in consequence of neonatal exposure to the virus, because the tolerance had not been an 'all-or-nothing' phenomenon. Incomplete and temporary tolerance can also be produced in the same system. It seems more probable that LCM-reactive cells are also present in the tolerant animal, but the suppressive effect of a homeostatic mechanism keeps them on an inproductive, or low-productive level. Syngeneic sensitized lymphoid cells are insensitive to suppression. This interpretation of the mechanism of tolerance is supported by two feed-back-like phenomena: (*i*) the continuous presence of a certain amount of virus and (*ii*) the continuous presence of a weak immune response which can either be detected only by refined methods or it is restricted to certain organs, e.g. the kidneys [54*d*].

The understanding of the homeostatic mechanism presupposes the knowledge of the fact that passive administration of antibodies prior to [116], simultaneously with [114], or after the antigenic stimulus [147] may uniformly result in a considerable suppression of the immune response. At the same time it has also been shown that even a low level of 7S antibody developed a suppressive action if it had been administered before antigen, whereas simultaneous administration of an equimolar concentration of 19S antibody with the antigen specifically enhanced the primary plaque-forming cell response [60]. On this basis, the physiological regulatory role of antibody in normal immune response seems probable. This antibody effect is not always negative, although it often controls even self-overproduction by suppression; a positive regulatory influence may also develop through promotion of antibody formation. Purified $\gamma\ G_1$ (rabbit anti-sheep-erythrocyte antibody) suppressed the immune response of the mouse to sheep erythrocytes at any concentration, when administered 2 h before the antigen. High doses of $\gamma\ G_2$ partially suppressed 19S plaque-forming cells, but they had no significant influence on the serum haemagglutinin level. Low doses of $\gamma\ G_2$ specifically increased both the number of 19S plaque-forming cells and the serum haemagglutinin level. The Fc fragments are known to differ in the two antibody sub-classes. Thus $\gamma\ G_1$ and $\gamma\ G_2$ antibodies are competitive physiological regulators of the primary immune response of the mouse. The promoting effect of $\gamma\ G_2$ and the suppressive effect of $\gamma\ G_1$ are probably Fc-dependent [102*a*, *b*, *c*] and represent a class function. It is not clear whether the above antigen–antibody interaction is manifested by peripheral or central competition [19, 29]. In inhibiting an *in vitro* immune response to sheep erythrocytes $F(ab')_2$ antibody is 5–100 times less efficient than intact IgG antibody. This observation constitutes further proof that the Fc portion of antibody possesses an immunoregulatory function which is not dependent on its role in renal tubular reabsorption [81*a*]. Pre-existing antibodies may also suppress the secondary immune response and they probably act by blocking the passage of the effective antigenic stimulus from antigen-carrier cells to memory cells; this explanation is, however, chiefly hypothetical [52, 53].

It seems, nevertheless, certain that in mice, there is an antigenic competition between the Fc and Fab fragments of IgG, which can be eliminated by passive immunization with antiserum against the dominant antigen (Fc). In this manner, tolerance can be induced to Fc, resulting in the elimination of the antigenic competition. This procedure markedly enhances the production of anti-Fc, which is normally very poor in response to rabbit IgG; this can be regarded as a proof of antigenic competition. It has been postulated that the dominant antigen stimulates the production of a 'cooperative antibody', acting as an inhibitor of the production of specific antibody against the suppressed antigen [134*a*, *b*, 135].

Mixed lymphocyte culture reaction can be used as a simple test to demonstrate immunological tolerance, as no blast transformation will take place if cells from rats rendered tolerant by neonatal bone marrow injection are cultured with such lymphocytes. The specificity of the phenomenon is affirmed by the fact that mixed cells from the tolerant donor and from an unrelated third strain will undergo blast transformation [115].

## ACQUIRED TOLERANCE

Acquired immunological tolerance can be at least temporarily elicited by total body irradiation, immunosuppressive synthetic drugs and large doses of corticosteroids, which all reduce the number of immunoactive cells, as well as by specific antisera (anti-lymphocyte serum—anti-lymphocyte globulin), which suppress the function of the immune system. It is known that immunological tolerance to polyinosinic-polycytidilic acid can be induced in New Zealand mice with cyclophosphamide [130]; the mechanism is that the antigen stimulates the proliferation of lymphoid cells, which then are destroyed by the antimetabolite (cyclophosphamide). According to the cooperation theory, the source of antibody producing cells is the bone marrow and thymus derived cells act as 'helpers' by a specific interaction with the antigen. The synergism of bone marrow and thymus cells of tolerant mice has repeatedly been observed in connection with the mechanism of tolerance [21*a*, *b*, 91, 100]. Appropriate mouse strains can also be rendered tolerant to sheep erythrocytes by means of cyclophosphamide. In certain mouse strains, tolerance is transferable with both bone marrow and thymus cells, whereas in others only with the bone marrow. In the latter type, the thymus of the tolerant donor completely cooperates with the bone marrow cells of the untreated host. In mice of certain New Zealand strains, cyclophosphamide induced immunological tolerance to sheep erythrocytes is bone marrow dependent, whereas in other strains it depends on both thymus and bone marrow. This difference is probably due to an abnormality of bone marrow and thymus and it may also play a role in the genetic predisposition of New Zealand mice to autoimmune diseases [69]. If the mice are provoked with sheep erythrocytes 4 days after a single injection of cyclophosphamide, the response will be almost normal as far as the number of haemolysin forming cells is concerned. Cell-transfer and *in vitro* experiments, however, suggest that the normal competence of the spleen is not restored even after 30 days. This difference has been attributed to various phases of repopulation after the cyclophosphamide induced depletion [92]. Recent studies indicated that the effect of cyclophosphamide on the B cell compartment was more severe and longer-lasting than the effect on the T cell compartment [130*a*]. Pretreatment with cyclophosphamide and other immunosuppressive agents before sensitization increased the intensity and prolonged contact sensitivity reactions. Pretreatment with cyclophosphamide also caused increased intensity and prolonged Jones–Mote type reactions so that they resembled tuberculin-type reactions. This was associated with a marked reduction in antibody production. It is, therefore, suggested that Jones–Mote hypersensitivity is a further example of a T lymphocyte reaction modulated by a B lymphocyte response [140*a*, *b*, *c*].

## IMMUNOLOGICAL PARALYSIS

Non-sensitized animals can be rendered specifically 'resistant' to an agent by previous treatment with very low or very high doses of the same agent. The Sulzberger-Chase phenomenon [20, 133] is of this type: the DNCB-induced delayed contact hypersensitivity of adult guinea pigs can be inhibited by previous feeding of the compound to the animals. The higher the oral dose, the greater the degree of non-reactivity. The animals can, however, be sensitized with other non-related substances. Oral pretreatment of guinea pigs with DNCB inhibits only active but not passive (parabiosis induced) skin sensitization [124]. Unresponsiveness may last longer than a year and it is shown not only to the pure chemical substance, but also to its protein conjugate (complex antigen). Addition of adjuvants shortens the period of unresponsiveness. Oral DNCB treatment probably results in an *in vivo* conjugate formation with somatic proteins and this determines the basic specificity of immunological tolerance. If DNCB-fed tolerant guinea pigs are later sensitized with a conjugate of the hapten and heterologous protein, the immune response will correspond to that of the control animals, whereas if the carrier part of the conjugate is a homologous protein, the immune response will be weak.

Unresponsiveness can also be elicited epicutaneously, by topical application of different chemical substances [88], e.g. if the nipples of DNCB-sensitive guinea pigs are painted daily with an 1 $^0/_{00}$ DNCB solution over a long period [70]. Rajka and Hård [112] made similar observations on long-term treatment with DNCB. Guinea pigs sensitized epicutaneously with DNCB respond to intravenous injection of the antigen by a temporary increase of unresponsiveness, accompanied by a decrease in the intensity of the reaction [47]. In man, the sensitizing dose of DNCB did not reduce sensitivity, either on oral application, or by painting.

An unresponsive state can also be induced by parenteral application of minimal doses of the hapten. For example, active acquired tolerance could be elicited in newborn guinea pigs by intraperitoneal or subcutaneous administration of DNCB [113] and adult guinea pigs could be rendered refractory to the hapten by injections of picryl chloride into the mesenteric vein [7]. If DNCB or picryl chloride are administered orally or parenterally to pregnant guinea pigs and their offspring are sensitized with both agents when mature, they will show a lowered specific reactivity to the homologous allergen owing to the foetal exposure [4, 113] without losing sensitivity to it [146]. Pretreatment depresses chiefly the delayed hypersensitivity response, but not antibody production, which may even increase under the stimulus of sensitization [144].

Remarkably, non-immunogenic conjugates of the co-polymers of D- or L-glutamic acid and lysine with 2-4,dinitrophenyl (DNP) induce in guinea pigs a hapten-specific tolerance, to judge from the depression of anti-DNP antibody formation and decreased frequency of specific DNP-antigen-binding cells and anti-DNP-antibody secreting cells after treatment of the animals with DNP-ovalbumin [74]. Cellular immune responses (T cell mediated functions) to DNP-guinea pig albumin are normal in guinea pigs pretreated with the DNP conjugate of D-glutamic acid and D-lysine. This finding strongly reinforces the concept that a basic specificity distinction exists between receptors on precursors of antibody secreting cells and those on cells participating in cellular immune responses [23*b*].

Foetal exposure by maternal treatment has recently been preferred to treatment of newborns or foetuses. This method spares the young animals, but care should be taken to treat the pregnant females in proper time. Induction of immunological tolerance, e.g. to human $\gamma$-globulin in rabbits, failed unless the injection treatment was made in advanced pregnancy (optimally 17 days before parturition). The failure of early attempts accounts for the contradictory results of different authors [139].

It was examined whether or not the lymphocytes of hapten (picryl chloride)-fed guinea pigs are immunologically inhibited, i.e. whether or not they retain their capacity to transfer delayed hypersensitivity and antibody formation to the hapten-free milieu of normal animals. The lymphocytes of guinea pigs unresponsive to picryl chloride were not capable of transferring delayed hypersensitivity to normal recipients, although the lymphocytes of picryl chloride-immunized animals can uniformly produce picryl-specific antibodies in picryl chloride-fed and normal guinea pigs [6]. Similar experiments [46] have shown that intravenous pretreatment of guinea pigs with DNCB or with the cross-reacting dinitrobenzolsulphonate inhibits delayed contact hypersensitivity to epicutaneous or intracutaneous sensitization with DNCB. This unresponsiveness is specific and relatively durable, and depends on the quantity of the antigen as well as on the time elapsing between sensitization and antigenic stimulation. Administration of the antigen 2 to 4 weeks before sensitization renders the animals completely tolerant.

According to Hasek [56*b*, 57] the phenomenon of immunological unresponsiveness does not occur if the animal has already been sensitized and passively administered antibodies are eliminated as rapidly as from controls. It has nevertheless been demonstrated [35] that adult rabbits sensitized with small doses of bovine serum albumin which, after the primary response, develop a regular secondary response to the second dose, can be rendered tolerant for several months by intravenous administration of a high antigen dose. The protein induced delayed-type response of the guinea pig can be reduced with a single appropriate dose (25 $\mu$g–2 mg) of the antigen–antibody complex or of the antigen alone; the antigen probably blocks the specific critical intracellular antigen binding sites of the sensitized cells, thus rendering the latter inactive [30, 142]. A similar phenomenon may be held responsible for the fact that daily intraperitoneal treatment of ovalbumin sensitized animals with rising doses of the antigen results in a state which corresponds to unresponsiveness, especially in the context of delayed-type reactions [9].

Medawar [97*b*] holds the view that transplantation tolerance differs from the tolerance induced by non-self-reproductive or chemically defined antigens. In the latter case, reactivity cannot be restored by passive transfer of sensitized lymphocytes [57]. Not even the passive transfer of antibodies can restore the responsiveness of animals rendered tolerant by serum proteins [65]. Studies on non-self-reproductive antigens disclosed that the maintenance of tolerance requires antigen. For instance, in rabbit experiments, $10^{10}$ to $10^{12}$ molecules were required to maintain immunological tolerance towards soluble protein antigens.

Induction of immunological tolerance in adults by antigen overloading, using large doses of protein (polysaccharide, chemical substance) is a phenomenon similar to immunological paralysis which, as is known, may be elicited with very high doses of antigen (mostly polysaccharides which persist for a long time) in immunologically mature individuals [33, 39, 40]; its duration is limited and it depends on the continuous presence of the antigen [30]. Dose dependent tolerance can be induced in adult rabbits by intravenous administration of synthetic poly-L-tyrosine-L-glutamic acid-poly-DL-alanine-polylysine antigen [120]. Other polypeptide determinants with a polyalanyl part induced tolerance in adult rats [119].

Similar tolerance to skin homografts can be induced in rabbits and mice by repeated injection into the recipient of polysaccharide and lipid fractions isolated from the homologous organs [72]. In this case, too, immunological paralysis lasts as long as the antigen is demonstrable in circulation (absence of immunological elimination) [36]. Immunological paralysis can also be elicited by small doses of antigen, e.g. heterologous $\gamma$-globulins, if these are alien enough to the recipient [37]. Appropriate doses of antigen can immunologically paralyse even animals already immunized; in this state, passively administered antibodies disappear more rapidly than normally [57]. The course of immunological paralysis induced with soluble heterologous proteins includes a 10–15-day period during which the animal is incapable of recognizing even the structurally different antigens [85].

Formerly, it was postulated that large quantities of tissue-fixed antigen neutralize the newly formed antibodies, thus giving rise to insoluble antigen–antibody complexes [58]. This theory was, however, not substantiated; inhibition of antibody formation, absence of an intermediary compound in the antibody forming mechanism or an inactive, refractory phase of antibody formation offer more plausible explanations of immunological paralysis. The problem is, nevertheless, still far from clear, because there is no evidence of the specificity of the above processes [49]. Halpern and Liacopoulos [84, 85] demonstrated that under given conditions, adult guinea pigs paralysed immunologically with large protein doses, showed neither immediate, nor a delayed hypersensitivity to other heterologous proteins, if these were applied at an appropriately early time.

Stark [129] has proposed the term immunological masking instead of immunological paralysis with regard to the fact that the absence of responsiveness does not necessarily mean the absence of antibodies as well. Unresponsive animals lose tolerance to, e.g. a skin graft if they are treated with lymphocytes from a responding animal sensitized with the same kind of graft [14]. This absence of responsiveness is regarded as the test of immunological paralysis.

According to Dietrich [31*b*], the above outlined states of unresponsiveness should be summarized under the collective term immunological tolerance.

It depends among other on the quantities of antigen and of cells, whether sensitization or tolerance will develop in the early phases. The importance of quantitative and dose relations is indicated by the fact that gradually rising doses of cells can induce tolerance even in adult age; this procedure essentially corresponds to de(hypo)-sensitization. Accordingly, low and high zones of dosage may result in tolerance ('low- and high-zone tolerance'), whereas the intermediate zone confers immunity [89, 125].

## LOW- AND HIGH-ZONE TOLERANCE

It has been shown that repeated administration of bovine serum albumin induces immunological tolerance at two dose levels, low ($\sim$ 0.1 $\mu$g per injection) and high ($>$ 10 mg per injection) [99]. Monomeric flagellin induces tolerance in newborn rats at both 0.1 pg and 20 ng dose levels, whereas the intermediate dose range (1–100 pg) confers immunity [122]. High-dose induction of tolerance is associated with unresponsiveness to unrelated antigens administered during the inductive phase [86]. Non-specific unresponsiveness is accompanied by intensive cellular proliferation and $\gamma$-globulin hyperproduction in the lymphoid organs [18]. Although no such hyperplastic phenomena could be demonstrated during the inductive phase of low-zone tolerance, mice treated with low doses of bovine albumin showed a competitive effect of immunization with unrelated ovalbumin antigen during induction. The competitive effect was less intensive and less durable, compared with that observed in high-zone tolerance to bovine serum albumin. Conversely, the intermediate immunizing doses of bovine serum albumin hyperimmunized against the unrelated ovalbumin antigen [83]. According to other authors [96*a*, *b*], the competitive effect of bovine serum albumin not only inhibits antibody formation, but also affects the development of delayed hypersensitivity and thyroglobulin induced thyroid lesion. The competition of murine thyroglobulin and bovine serum albumin can also be demonstrated by adoptive transfer [141].

At any rate, in view of the low-zone tolerance, the relation of immunity with tolerance can no longer be explained by an appropriate ratio of the numbers of antigen molecules and immunologically competent cells, viz. that tolerance is induced if the ratio is high, and antibody production if it is low. There is evidence that the biological filtration of the antigens through the rabbit reticulo-endothelial system alters the nature of the antigen from immunogenic to tolerogenic [45]. It seems, therefore, that the passage of the antigen through macrophages is a necessary step of immunization. In this way not easily phagocytable antigens, e.g. monomeric flagellin, can contact the lymphocytes directly and render them tolerant. Accordingly, a high-zone or classical tolerance can be induced if antigen is applied in excess of the macrophages' phagocytic capacity so that the free antigen can contact the competent cells. If the antigen is injected in a low dose ($< 0.01\,\mu g$ bovine serum albumin), the cells will not recognize it. Somewhat larger doses (0.01–1 $\mu$g) elicit a high antigen-cell ratio with resting cells in absence of proliferation, whence they induce a low-zone tolerance. Still higher doses (1 $\mu$g–10 mg) of bovine serum albumin initiate proliferation of immunocompetent cells and owing to the increase of the cell count, the ratio of immunologically competent cells to the antigen molecules will alter in favour of antibody production. Since, however, cell proliferation has its biological limits, further elevation of the antigen dose ($>$ 10 mg bovine serum albumin) will again result in an antigen molecule-cell count ratio which again induces tolerance. Thus, according to this theory, the ratio of antigen molecules to immunologically competent cell count is uniformly too high at antigen dose levels below the threshold required for the induction of cell proliferation and at extreme antigen dose levels in excess of the biological limit of cell proliferation. Other experimental results have even suggested that the antigen binding cell receptors active in the induction of immunity and paralysis are identical and the potential humoral antibody forming cells belong to the B-cell line. The T cells, acting as specific helper cells, can also be analysed [21*a*, *b*], but there is no evidence that they possess constant surface receptors capable of different associations with the antigen [2]. Several other authors [51, 111] have failed to demonstrate on the surface of T lymphocytes immunoglobulins acting as receptors, although according to more recent electron-microscopic findings, both thymus derived (T) and bone marrow derived (B) lymphocytes express IgM. No surface-associated immunoglobulins can be detected in the majority (98 per cent) of thymic cells. It has been supposed that the few T lymphocytes (2 per cent) which carry surface immunoglobulins acquire these either shortly before, or shortly after, their exit from the thymus [59].

Ig-type circulating antibodies do not usually arise in the foetal or newborn periods; there are only cells which carry some antibody-like globulin structure on their surface (potential immunologically competent cells) and become eliminated, destroyed or probably only inhibited (functional elimination) [125] at encounter with the complementary foreign material, owing to an antigen–antibody-reaction-like interaction taking place on the cell surface. Since only cells which have been specialized for the antigen will disappear, the entire process of immunological tolerance is specific. Thus the organism recognizes the foreign material as self (annihilation theory).

In this light, immunological tolerance would be introduced by an immune reaction, and the loss of reactivity would only follow after this early phase, whence it appears to be actually induced by the antigen. The tolerant animal seems to loose a certain kind of immunological capacity, which, however, can be restored by homologous lymph node cells. The introductory immune reaction of the tolerance process is in good accordance with the implication that in highly specific immunological tolerance a kind of interaction takes place between the antigen and the homologous antibody (or its immunological equivalent). According to Burnet [16, 17], animals and tissues are rendered tolerant by the lack of potential immunologically competent cells toward the accessible (self) antigenic substances rather than by the change of such cells to tolerant. Against this Boyden [13] maintained that the clonal selection theory can hardly be reconciled with the observation that animals inoculated at birth with a given antigen, e.g. a hapten + protein conjugate, do not form antibodies to either component. The cells competent for antibody formation to the conjugate may become eliminated in consequence of the early antigen administration; this does not, however, apply to the hapten which, as a small-molecular substance is not capable of inducing tolerance in itself (the induction of immunological tolerance requires macromolecules analogously to antibody formation), yet immunological tolerance will develop not only to the protein component, but to the hapten component as well.

According to Lederberg's stem cell theory [81], prior to maturation the immunologically competent cells react differently with the antigen, i.e. instead of antibody formation they either deteriorate or are changed to such an extent that they remain incapable of antibody synthesis. The reason why the maintenance of tolerance requires the presence of antigen is probably the latter's interference with the structurally similar groups of the maturing stem cells. The individual cells presumably carry different antigen reactive sites including those which induce inhibition, and others responsible for immune response (antibody formation). In very young animals, the site of tolerance is probably more accessible and it persists in adult age [38].

Another view is that the immunity induced in mice by pneumococcal polysaccharide antigen depends on peritoneal cells, probably macrophages, and such cells also play a role in immunological paralysis [150]. The antigen + RNA complex originating from these cells induces antibody formation in lymph node cells or spleen cells, and the macrophage RNA influences both the *in vivo* and *in vitro* induction of antibody even in itself [68]. Following passive transfer, RNA originating from spleen cells of immunized mice induces only a minimal response in the host even at very high dose levels ($> 800\,\mu g$). Against this, spleen cell RNA from 'paralysed' donors is very active already in a $100\,\mu g$ dose. The activity is not sensitive to RNase. Unlike in other preparations, antigen can be detected in RNA preparations from spleen cells of 'paralysed' donors. The pneumococcal polysaccharide antigen is also present in the blood serum of 'paralysed' donors; a concentration of about 0.1 $\mu$g per ml was demonstrated 24 days after the injection of 100 $\mu$g of antigen [148]. Speirs's [128] model suggests that the antigen exerts different effects on cells capable of globulin synthesis. The antigen may combine with the surface globulin receptors, thus inducing an increase in the rate of globulin synthesis. An adaptive enzyme synthesis starts in the organism for the catabolization of the complexes. Fragments of the antigen may react with cellular RNA and may repress globulin synthesis, resulting in the formation of two specific complexes: antigenic determinant+nascent peptide and tRNA + mRNA bound to ribosome. Derepression may occur if almost identical complexes of antigen + peptidyl-tRNA push the repressor molecule away from one of the combining sites. The three levels of immunological activity, high-zone and low-zone tolerance and the effect of the immunity-inducing intermediary antigen dose range can well be explained by the theory of repression and derepression of polysomal units, although the mechanism of this process is still not fully understood.

It has generally been accepted that the first step of the immune response is the combination of the antigen with antibody-like receptors on the surface of potentially reactive cells [8]. According to Cohen [24*a*, *b*, *c*, 25], there are three possible ways for the cell to 'decide' whether it will respond to a given antigen with immunity or with tolerance:

1. The cell may exist in a wide range of time-dependent physiological states; activation by the antigen can only take place if the cell is in an appropriate state, otherwise it will become tolerant.
2. The cellular response is determined by the type of the contacting antigen rather than by the actual state of the cell. For instance, if the antigen requires a chemical transformation to become immunogenic, the unprocessed antigen may be tolerogenic.
3. Cellular response may be determined by the manner in which the antigen contacts the cell, i.e. the geometrical distribution of the antigen-binding cellular receptors on the cell may represent the critical signal of activation or suppression. Based on a mathematical analysis of this possibility, analogously to that of enzymic inhibition, it was postulated that the signal for cellular suppression is the binding of two distinct antigen molecules to two adjacent receptors in the form of a 'doublet', whereas the signal for activation is the binding of a single antigen molecule to a single receptor ('singlet').

These findings and the hypotheses derived from them are, however, not sufficient to elucidate the entire mechanism of immunological tolerance, many aspects of which remain to be investigated.

The central dilemma of the mechanism of immunological tolerance is the existence or non-existence of 'tolerant' cells. Induced tolerance may cease spontaneously, thus if—according to the annihilation theory—death or irreversible inactivation of the potentially immunologically competent cells active against specific antigens is postulated, virgin cells must be recruited during escape from tolerance, whereas if the existence of reversibly paralysed ('tolerant') cells is accepted, these might spontaneously recover from the state of inhibition. A further complication is that antibody responses to different antigens are mediated by two kinds of lymphocytes (T and B) both having a distinct specific antibody recognizing function, which cooperate in a common transfer system, but differ in the kinetics of their tolerance inducing and escape functions [21*b*]. Recently, it has become clear that both cell types may indeed be affected in the tolerant animal [21*b*]. B cells are more refractory than are T cells to tolerance induction requiring higher doses and longer exposure to the tolerogen [145*c*]; thus, low-zone tolerance presumably affects T cells only whereas high-zone tolerance affects both T and B cells [120*a*]. B cell tolerance is short lived compared to T cell tolerance [118*a*]. Recent observations of Iványi and Salerno [67*a, b*] on bursectomized or thymectomized chicks rendered tolerant to bovine serum albumin after hatching suggest that the recovery of the IgG response is due to bursa derived precursors which had previously been in contact with the antigen and kept in a state of reversibly arrested differentiation. This explanation is substantiated by the early and complete restoration and the increased avidity of the antibodies produced. On the other hand, cells at peripheral sites may have concomitantly become immunized during the induction of tolerance and may later have potentiated the response of virgin B cells through the mechanism operative in transfer experiments. In this case the primed cell population may have been thymus derived, which can also explain the increase of antibody avidity [48].

The restoration of the IgM response can be attributed to bursal precursor cells, which probably differentiate from bone marrow derived stem cells. The more gradual restoration of the IgM response compared with IgG reflects the time required for the passage of stem cells from bone marrow to bursa. The nature of these stem cells has not yet been elucidated. Thus the existence of immature precursor T cells within the bursa cannot be excluded; these cells do not acquire receptors during the induction of tolerance and serve later as virgin progenitor cells.

This hypothesis can explain the mechanism of immunological tolerance at the cellular level according to contemporary knowledge, but the interpretation of the subcellular (molecular biologic) processes is still not beyond the stage of a working hypothesis.

## DESENSITIZATION—HYPOSENSITIZATION

Desensitization or hyposensitization is the reduction, or probably elimination, of the state of hypersensitivity and of consequent pathological symptoms by repeated administration of the specific allergen to the allergic patient. Some authors have used the two terms for terminological distinction between mere neutralization of the antibody (desensitization) and decrease of reactivity (hyposensitization), in consequence of the specific treatment, but this differentiation is arbitrary and the synonymous use of the two terms has generally been accepted. The true nature of the process is still not fully understood. Whether the underlying mechanism is immunologic, non-immunologic, or a combination of both, desensitization is often encountered in clinical practice, above all in certain allergic diseases and the decline or disappearance of hypersensitivity can be frequently demonstrated, e.g. by skin tests. The explanations offered by different authors for the origin and fundamental mechanism of desensitization differ greatly.

The prompt disappearance or gradual decline of hypersensitivity (rush or long-run desensitization), although they cannot always be sharply differentiated, generally take place in two ways discussed in the following sub-sections.

## TEMPORARY DECLINE OF ALLERGIC REACTIVITY

Circulating and cell-fixed antibodies diminish in number or disappear temporarily. Their disappearance (or inactivation or neutralization) from the blood does not necessarily imply their disappearance from the tissues as well. The main proofs of antibody disappearance are:

1. Following the macro-shock, in the anti-anaphylactic state (on the average for about 2 weeks), the same dose fails to elicit a shock again, passive transfer with serum is not possible and attempts for challenge of isolated organs often have negative results. The same applies to the Schultz-Dale reaction (Sch-D reaction). If the animal dies in the shock, the positive Sch-D reaction may persist, because immediate death prevents the disappearance of antibodies from the smooth muscle containing organs.
2. Animals 'de-allergized' by the micro-shock method, i.e. by small doses given to prevent the symptoms, are indifferent to the shock dose [71], but the shock tissues respond differently and hypersensitivity may persist in the isolated organs.
3. Apart from binding and neutralization of the antibodies, repeated micro-shock may weaken or depress the function of the antibody producing organs.

It is considerably more difficult to judge the conditions prevailing in human allergic diseases, because information is only available from passive transfer and skin reactions. After sudden shock-like symptoms (minor or major shock associated with an attack of urticaria), humans as well as animals may often show a decline of reactivity, to judge from the absence of both local and general symptoms on readministration of the allergen. The serum antibody level falls parallel with the decline of reactivity and it may even disappear temporarily so that passive transfer with the patient's serum is hardly or not at all possible. The reversion of the skin test to negative is less important in man than is generally believed, because the test often remains positive, especially in partial desensitization, suggesting the persistence of cell-fixed reagins. But the antibody producing capacity of the organism is not lost: the reagins will gradually reappear and after a certain time the organism will respond to the pathogenic allergen in the same manner as originally. Thus desensitization means, in fact, only a temporary decline of allergic reactivity.

If the antigen is applied in low doses or by a route by which it is slowly absorbed (orally, intradermally or subcutaneously), only part of the antibodies will become inactivated or inhibited on readministration, yet there is scarcely any response to the repeated antigenic stimulus. This phenomenon has been named skeptophylaxis, or—after Besredka and Urbach—de-allergization.

## TRUE DE- OR HYPOSENSITIZATION

In this kind of desensitization, fractionated or depot injections of the antigen alter the allergic reactivity in a manner that the symptoms either become weaker or do not develop at all on repeated re-exposure to the antigen (recent clinical observations, especially in connection with allergic rhinitis, argue in favour of pollen or house-dust emulsions in mineral oil, i.e. of depot preparations) [99, 137]. It has been postulated that in such cases new antibodies or antibody-like specific complexes arise, which inhibit the antigen–antibody reaction and weaken or prevent allergic symptoms. Clinically, this mechanism is comparable to classical immunity. Considering that in anti-infection immunity, microbial extracts and vaccines are used to combat not only the infectious diseases, but also the associated allergic processes, e.g. skin reactions, it seems highly probable that desensitization and immunity cannot be sharply delimited [71]. They must represent the same phenomenon if hyposensitization and production of the immune state are based on identical mechanisms. This mechanism is, however, still unknown, at least in the relation of hyposensitization. A further difficulty arises from the fact that even the mechanisms of rush and long-run desensitization (see Chapter 14) differ in certain respects [10].

### *Inhibiting or blocking antibodies*

Several substances in succession had been held responsible for the phenomenon of desensitization, such as 'antiallergen' (Storm van Leeuwen and Kremer) [131*a*, *b*], 'dereagin' (Lehner and Rajka), [82*a*, *b*], 'resistin' (Karády,) [73], etc., but no convincing proof has been found as to their role. Greater interest was aroused by the observation of Cooke et al. [26] that after specific treatment, a blocking or inhibiting substance is formed in the sera of hay fever patients, which may paralyse the effect of the allergen both *in vivo* and *in vitro*, can be passively transferred and differs from Coca-Grove's neutralizing factor [23*a*, 78]. Biologically highly active reaginic and blocking antibody could both be isolated by immunoadsorption from the sera of timothy grass pollen sensitive patients [90].

It was initially speculated on the basis of the inhibition reaction that the desensitization and clinical improvement of specifically treated hay fever patients are due to the blocking antibody even in those cases in which the skin response to the allergen remains positive and circulating reagins persist in the blood [27], although large doses of allergen reduce the intensity of the cutaneous response [55*a*, *b*]. It is known that in hay fever the reactivity of the shock tissue, i.e. of mucosa, decreases first and skin reactivity only later [5]. The allergen dose still capable of eliciting a skin reaction is no longer responded to by the mucous membranes [87]. It was concluded from these findings that in the initial stage of treatment, the reaginic effect is predominant, whereas with the progress of specific therapy the blocking antibodies become prevalent and the inhibitory effect comes to the fore. Clinical observations have, however, not fully justified these speculations: there is no significant correlation between clinical improvement, on the one hand, and the titres of blocking antibodies and of haemagglutinins increasing in the course of the specific treatment, on the other [123]. As apart from a temporary reduction, the reagins do not disappear in the course of desensitization, so far unidentified factor(s) is probably responsible for the suppression of their action.

In conventional desensitization procedures, the dose of the specific allergen is raised gradually with each injection. Some patients, however, do not tolerate the elevation of the dose and respond to one or another injection of the series by a general allergic attack. To eliminate this risk, Japanese authors [95] have proposed a new effective desensitization therapy of bronchial asthma. Sera from desensitized patients and from healthy subjects repeatedly treated with allergen extract, containing blocking antibodies in high titres, were incubated at 56 °C to destroy the reagins. The inactivated sera were then mixed with an extract of the corresponding allergen and repeatedly administered to patients with bronchial asthma. Neither local nor systemic reactions occurred in the patients, their serum blocking antibody titres rose to a significantly high level and they remained free of symptoms for a long time. The method has been applied with success especially in Konnyaku asthma (an inhalatory asthma occurring in Japan) and in silk asthma.

According to an earlier opinion, desensitization always follows a phase of hypersensitivity [118]. The role of the free circulating antibodies is still not fully understood. In rabbit experiments, passively administered homologous 7S antibodies suppressed the formation of reagins (homocytotropic antibodies). In view of this, the dose levels of antigen for human desensitization therapy have recently been so established as to promote the production not only of 19S, but also of sufficiently high levels of 7S [132].

Under certain quantitative conditions of the antigen–antibody reaction, when this takes place between humoral antibodies and allergen rather than between cell-fixed antibody and antigen, the issue is probably neutralization rather than a pathologic alteration. This phenomenon is, however, not likely to account in itself for desensitization.

### *Behaviour of skin tests*

The result of the skin test is not a reliable indicator of desensitization. This applies not only to immediate-type but also to delayed-type reaction [140], which also may decrease or disappear, as shown by the specific treatment of microbial or fungal infections of the skin. The phenomenon has been observed in both therapeutic (parenteral) and experimental (oral or epicutaneous) desensitization. Long-term painting of the nipples of DNCB sensitized guinea pigs with a $1^0/_{00}$ DNCB solution resulted in the weakening of the reaction; similar observations have also been reported by others in connection with long-term DNCB-treatment [112]. The functional changes occurring in the respective immunoactive lymphocytes in connection with the desensitization in delayed hypersensitivity states are still unclear. Both qualitative and quantitative alterations may probably occur along with the depression of cell-mediated immunity and predominance of humoral antibodies which, however, do not seem to play an important role in the desensitization of delayed-type allergic processes.

Nevertheless, the weakening of the skin response does not imply desensitization, nor does the persistence of a positive skin test mean its absence, because reactivity does not decline simultaneously in the different shock tissues, nor do the cell-fixed and circulating reagins disappear simultaneously.

In summary, at our present state of knowledge specific desensitization has two main phases [15]. Initially, a new antibody, the so-called blocking antibody arises in the IgG class. Blocking antibody synthesis is completed relatively rapidly, within a few months, or even few weeks following the application of the desensitizing doses and this phase can be regarded as the period of clinical immunization. The second phase, which may last several years, is the period of true desensitization which can as a rule be demonstrated by intradermal tests.

Other factors are also involved in specific desensitization, such as the influence on basophils, changes in histamine liberation, etc., but clinically the above-mentioned two phases are decisive.

In specific desensitization the dose of the allergen should be raised as high as possible, because large-dose therapy is more efficient than a small-dose regimen. Specific desensitization therapy should be continued until a realistic state of desensitivity becomes established, which can be affirmed by intradermal tests. For this purpose, treatment for 3 to 5 years is usually required. Double blind tests using a placebo drug and specific allergen can verify the effectiveness of specific desensitization. If an allergic shock occurs in the course of treatment, epinephrine should be injected subcutaneously or, if the symptoms are serious, intravenously or intracardially; water-soluble steroids have also been recommended for this purpose. The main fields of desensitization therapy are hay fever, bronchial asthma, vasomotor rhinitis and insect bites [62].

Undoubtedly, the simultaneous presence of the two kinds of antibody, i.e. stimulatory and inhibitory (theoretical distinction), would easily explain the simultaneous presence of desensitization and immunity. The two antibody types do, in fact, exist simultaneously, but they are not necessarily co-existent, because they may also occur independently. Studies of the co-existence of allergy and immunity have chiefly been conducted in infectious diseases, in which both states are usually present, each being induced by another antigenic determinant (e.g. in pneumococcal infections, the antibodies stimulated by the capsular polysaccharides confer immunity, whereas those stimulated by microbial proteins elicit a delayed-type allergic response).

Immunodeficiency states, i.e. any condition in which a deficiency of humoral or cell-mediated immunity exists, e.g. combined immunity deficiency syndrome, Di George's syndrome, Bruton-type hypogammaglobulinaemia, antibody deficiency syndrome, etc. will be discussed in the clinical part of the present work (see Chapter 77 in Volume 2). Immuno-suppression, i.e. the artifical suppression of immune responses by use of drugs (antimetabolites), irradiation or agents such as anti-lymphocyte serum is treated in separate chapters owing to the importance of the subject (Chapters 18 and 19).

## REFERENCES


1. Albert, F., In *Biologic Problems of Grafting*. Ed. by Albert, F. and Medawar, P. B. Blackwell, Oxford 1959, p. 369.
2. Andersson, B. and Wigzell, H.: *Eur. J. Immunol.* **1,** 384 (1971).
3. Ashley, F. L., McNall, E. G., Dutt, N. R., Garcia, E. N. and Sloan, R. F.: *Ann. N.Y. Acad. Sci.* **87,** 429 (1960).

4. Baer, R. L., Rosenthal, S. A. and Hagel, B.: *J. Immunol.* **80,** 429 (1958).
5. Baldwin, L. B. and Glaser, J.: *J. Allergy* **8,** 126 (1937).
6. Battisto, J. E. and Chase, M. W.: *J. exp. Med.* **118,** 1021 (1963).
7. Battisto, J. R. and Miller, J.: *Proc. Soc. exp. Biol. (N.Y.)* **111,** 111 (1962).
8. Benacerraf, B. and Paul, W. E. In, *Cellular Interactions in the Immune Response.* Ed. by Cohen, S., Cudkowicz, G. and McCluskey, R. T. Karger, Basel 1971, p. 298.
9. Benacerraf, B., Potter, J. L., McCluskey, R. T. and Miller, F.: *J. exp. Med.* **3,** 195 (1960).
10. Berg, T. and Johansson, S. G. O.: *Int. Arch. Allergy* **41,** 434 (1971).
11. Billingham, R. E., In *Immunity and Virus Infection.* Ed. by Najjar, V. A. and Robinson, J. P. Wiley, New York 1959, p. 50.
12*a*. Billingham, R. E., Brent, L. and Medawar, T. B.: *Nature* **172,** 603 (1953).
12*b*. id., *Experientia (Basel)* **11,** 444 (1955).
12*c*. id., *Ann. N.Y. Acad. Sci.* **59,** 409 (1955).
13. Boyden, S. V. and Sorkin, E.: *Immunology* **5,** 370 (1962).
14. Brent, L.: *Progr. Allergy* **5,** 271 (1958).
15. Bruun, E.: *Folia allerg. (Roma)* **17,** 439 (1970).
16. Burnet, F. M.: *Brit. med. J.* **2,** 720 (1959).
17. Burnet, F. M. and Fenner, F.: *The Production of Antibodies.* MacMillan, Melbourne 1949.
18. Cerný, J., Viklický, V. and Rymasewka-Kossakowska, T.: *Folia biol. (Prague)* **15,** 41 (1969).
19. Chan, P. L. and Sinclair, N. R. S. C.: *Immunology* **21,** 967 (1971).
20. Chase, M. W.: *Proc. Soc. exp. Biol. (N.Y.)* **61,** 257 (1946).
21*a*. Chiller, J. M., Habicht, G. S. and Weigle, O.: *Proc. nat. Acad. Sci. (Wash.)* **65,** 551 (1970).
21*b*. id., *Science* **171,** 813 (1971).
22. Claman, H. N. and Talmage, D. W.: *Science* **141,** 1193 (1963).
23*a*. Coca, A. F. and Grove, E. F.: *J. Immunol.* **10,** 445 (1925).
23*b*. Cohen, B. E., Davie, J. M. and Paul. W. E.: *J. Immunol.* **110,** 213 (1973).
23*c*. Cohen, B. E., Green, I. and Davie, J. M.: *J. Immunol.* **110,** 608 (1973).
24*a*. Cohen, S.: *J. theoret. Biol.* **27,** 19 (1970).
24*b*. id., *Immunochemistry* **8,** 1099 (1971).
24*c*. id., In *Cellular Interactions in the Immune Response.* Ed. by Cohen, S., Cudkowicz, G. and McCluskey, R. T. Karger, Basel 1971, p. 298.
25. Cohen, S. and Milgrom, M.: *J. Immunol.* **107,** 115 (1971).
26. Cooke, R. A., Barnard, J. H., Hebald, S. and Stull, A.: *J. exp. Med.* **62,** 733 (1935).
27. Cooke, R. A., Stull, A., Hebald, S. and Barnard, J. H.: *J. Allergy* **6,** 311 (1935).
28. Démant, P., Iványi, P., Ivašková, E.: *Ann. N.Y. Acad. Sci.* **129,** 234 (1966).
29. Dennert, G.: *J. Immunol.* **106,** 951 (1971).
30. de Weck, A. L. and Frey, J. R.: *Immunotolerance to Simple Chemicals.* Karger, Basel 1966.
31*a*. Dietrich, F. M.: *Schweiz. med. Wschr.* **94,** 109 (1964).
31*b*. id., *Int. Arch. Allergy* **27,** 365 (1965).
32. Dietrich, F. M. and Grey, H. M.: *Nature* **201,** 1236 (1964).
33. Dixon, F. J., Maurer, P. H. and Weigle, W. O.: *J. Immunol.* **74,** 188 (1955).
34. Doria, G., Agerossi, G. and Dipietro, S.: *J. Immunol.* **107,** 1314 (1971).
35. Dorner, M. M. and Uhr, J. W.: *J. exp. Med.* **120,** 435 (1964).
36*a*. Dresser, D. W.: *Immunology* **4,** 13 (1961).
36*b*. ibid., **5,** 161 (1962).
37. Dresser, D. W. and Gowland, G.: *Nature* **203,** 733 (1964).
38. Dresser, D. W. and Mitchison, N. A.: *Advanc. Immunol.* **8,** 129 (1968).
39. Felton, L. D.: *J. Immunol.* **61,** 107 (1949).
40. Felton, L. D., Kaufmann, G., Prescott, D. and Ottinger, B.: *J. Immunol.* **74,** 17 (1955).
41. Filipp, G.: *Acta allerg. (Kbh.)* **17,** 505 (1962).
42. Fisher, J. C., Davis, R. C. aod Mannick, J. A.: *Immunology* **20,** 901 (1971).
43. Flanagan, S. P.: *Genet. Res. (Camb.)* **8,** 295 (1966).

44. Fowler, R., jr., Schubert, W. K. and West, C. G.: *IV. Tissue Homotranspii Conf. Ann. N.Y. Acad. Sci.* **87,** 403 (1960).
45. Frei, P. C., Benacerraf, B. and Thorbecke, G. J.: *Proc. nat. Acad. Sci. (Washid* **53,** 20 (1965).
46. Frey, J. R., de Weck, A. L. and Geleick, H.: *Dermatologica (Basel)* **129,** 118 (1964).
47. Frey, J. R., and Geleick, H.: *Int. Arch. Allergy* **19,** 409 (1961).
48. Gershon, R. K. and Paul, W. E.: *J. Immunol.* **106,** 872 (1971).
49. Goldstein, D. J.: *Ann. Allergy* **18,** 1081 (1960).
50. Gottlieb, P. M.: *Ann. Allergy* **21,** 187 (1963).
51. Greaves, M. F., Hogg, N. M., In *Third Sigrid Juselius Symposium on Cell Interactions in Immune Response. Helsinki.* Ed. by Mäkelä, O., Cross, A. and Kosunen, T. Academic Press, London 1971, p. 145.
52. Hamaoka, T. and Kitagawa, M.: *Immunology* **20,** 191 (1971).
53. Hamaoka, T., Takatsu, K., Masaki, H., Matsuoka, Y. and Kitagawa, M.: *Immunology* **20,** 871 (1971).
54*a*. Hannover Larsen, T.: Thesis. Copenhagen 1968.
54*b*. id., *Acta path. microbiol. scand.* **73,** 106 (1968).
54*c*. ibid., **77,** 433 (1969).
54*d*. id., *J. Immunol.* **102,** 941 (1969).
54*e*. ibid. **107,** 185 (1971).
55*a*. Harley, D.: *Lancet* **i,** 690 (1933).
55*b*. ibid., **ii,** 1469 (1933).
56*a*. Hašek, M.: *Čsl. Biol. (Prague)* **2,** 265 (1953).
56*b*. id., In *Biologic Problems of Grafting.* Ed. by Albert, F. and Medawar, P. B. Blackwell, Oxford 1959.
57. Hašek, M., Lengerová, A. and Hraba, T.: *Advanc. Immunol.* **1,** 1 (1961).
58. Haurowitz, F., In *Mechanisms of Hypersensitivity.* Ed. by Schaffer, J. H., Lo-Grippo, G. A. and Chase, M. W. Churchill, London 1959, p. 547.
59. Hämmerling, V. and Rajewsky, K.: *Eur. J. Immunol.* **1,** 447 (1971).
60. Henry, C. and Jerne, N. K.: *J. exp. Med.* **128,** 113 (1968).
61. Hildemann, W. H. and Haas, R. In *Mechanisms of Immunological Tolerance.* Ed. by Hašek, M., Lengerová, A. and Vojtisková, M. Publishing House of the Czechoslovak Academy of Sciences, Prague 1962, p. 35.
62. Hosen, H.: *Rev. Allergy* **25,** 265 (1971).
63. Hraba, T.: *Mechanism and Role of Immunological Tolerance.* Karger, Basel 1968.
64. Hrsak, I., Bovanić, M., Slijepčević, M. and Stanković, V.: *Immunology* **20,** 909 (1971).
65. Humphrey, J. H.: *Immunology* **7,** 449 (1964).
66. Humphrey, J. H. and Turk, J. L.: *Immunology* **4,** 301 (1961).
67*a*. Iványi, J. and Salerno, A.: *Eur. J. Immunol.* **1,** 227 (1971).
67*b*. id., *Immunology* **22,** 247 (1972).
68. Jackerts, D. and Drescher, J.: *J. Immunol.* **104,** 746 (1970).
69. Jacobs, M. E., Gordon, J. K. and Talal, N.: *J. Immunol.* **107,** 359 (1971).
70. Jadassohn, S., Brun, R. and Bujard, E.: *Dermatologica (Basel)* **119,** 186 (1959).
71. Kallós, P. and Kallós-Deffner, L.: *Erg. Hyg.* **19,** 178 (1937).
72. Kapichnikov, M. M., Mondrus, K. A. and Sushko, N. G., In *Mechanism of Immunological Tolerance.* Ed. by Hašek, M., Lengerová, A. and Vojtisková, M. Publishing House of the Czechoslovak Academy of Sciences, Prague 1962, p. 363.
73. Karády, S., Gecse, A. and Horpácsy, G.: *Int. Arch. Allergy* **28,** 28 (1965).
74. Katz, D. H., Davie, J. M., Paul, W. E. and Benacerraf, B.: *J. exp. Med.* **134,** 201 (1971).
75*a*. Kindred, B.: *Eur. J. Immunol.* **1,** 59 (1971).
75*b*. id., *J. Immunol.* **107,** 1291 (1971).
76. Kramer, N. C. et al.: In *IV. Int. Congr. Nephrology.* Abstr. 1. Stockholm 1969, p. 17.
77. Krüger, G. and Stolpmann, H. J.: *Z. Immun. Forsch.* **142,** 115 (1971).
78. Langner, P. H. and Kern, R. A.: *J. Allergy* **10,** 1 (1938).
79. Lawrence, H. S.: *Cellular and Humoral Aspects of the Hypersensitivity States.* Hoeber, New York 1959.

80. Lazzarini, A. A., jr.: *IV. Tissue Homotransp. Conf. Ann. N.Y. Acad. Sci.* **87**, 133 (1960).
81. Lederberg, G.: *Science* **129**, 1649 (1959).
81*a*. Lees, R. K. and Sinclair, N. R. St.: *Immunology* **24**, 735 (1973).
82*a*. Lehner, E. and Rajka, E.: *Klin. Wschr.* **8**, 1724 (1929).
82*b*. id., *Krankheitsforsch.* **8**, 85 (1930).
83. Liacopoulos, P., Couderc, J. and Gille, M. F.: *Eur. J. Immunol.* **1**, 359 (1971).
84. Liacopoulos, P., Halpern, B. and Perramant, F.: *Nature* **195**, 1112 (1962).
85. Liacopoulos, P. and Neveu, T.: *Immunology* **7**, 26 (1964).
86. Liacopoulos, P. and Perramant, F.: *Ann. Inst. Pasteur* **110**, 1961 (1966).
87. Loveless, M.: *J. Immunol.* **38**, 25 (1940).
88. Lowney, E. D.: *J. Immunol.* **95**, 397 (1965).
89. Macher, E.: *Hautarzt* **20**, 145 (1969).
90. Malely, A., Baecher, L., Wilson, B. and Perlman, F.: *J. Allergy* **47**, 131 (1971).
91. Many, A. and Schwartz, R. A.: *Proc. Soc. exp. Biol. (N.Y.)* **133**, 254 (1970).
92. Marbrook, J. and Baguly, B. C.: *Int. Arch. Allergy* **41**, 802 (1971).
93. Mariani, T., Martinez, C., Smith, J. M. and Good, R. A.: *Ann. N.Y. Acad. Sci.* **87**, 93 (1960).
94. Martinez, C., Smith, J. M., Blaese, M., Good, R. A.: *J. exp. Med.* **118**, 743 (1963).
95. Matsumuro, T., Tateno, K. and Nakaima, S.: *Folia allerg. (Roma)* **17**, 403 (1970).
96*a*. McMaster, P. R. B. and Kyriakos, M.: *Fed. Proc.* **28**, 425 (1969).
96*b*. id., *J. Immunol.* **105**, 1201 (1970).
97*a*. Medawar, P. B.: *Cellular Aspects of Immunity.* Churchill, London 1960, p. 134.
97*b*. id., In *Mechanisms of Immunological Tolerance.* Ed. by Hašek, M., Lengerová, A. and Vojtisková, M. Publishing House of the Czechoslovak Academy of Sciences, Prague 1962, p. 17.
98. Michie, D., Woodruff, M. F. and Zeiss, I. M.: *Immunology* **4**, 413 (1961).
99. Miller, A. C. M. L.: *Acta allerg. (Kbh.)* **26**, 430 (1971).
100. Miller, J. F. A. P. and Mitchell, G. F.: *J. exp. Med.* **131**, 675 (1970).
101. Mitchison, N. A.: *Immunology* **15**, 509 (1968).
102*a*. Murgita, R. A. and Vas, S. I.: *Fed. Canad. Biol. Soc.* **13**, 640 (1970).
102*b*. id., *J. Immunol.* **104**, 514 (1970).
102*c*. id., *Immunology* **22**, 319 (1972).
103. Nakić, B., Kaštelan, A. and Avdalović, N.: In *Ciba Found. Symp. on Transplantation.* Ed. by Wolstenholme, G. E. W. and Cameron, M. P. Churchill, London 1962, p. 328.
104. Naranjo, P. and Naranjo, E.: *Allergie u. Asthma* **7**, 259 (1961).
105*a*. Owen, R. D.: *Science* **102**, 400 (1945).
105*b*. id., In *Immunity and Virus Infection.* Ed. by Najjar, V. A. and Robinson, J. P. Wiley, New York 1959, p. 31.
106. Pantelouris, E. M.: *Nature* **217**, 370 (1968).
107. Pantelouris, E. M. and Flisch, P. A.: *Immunology* **22**, 159 (1972).
108*a*. Parish, C. R.: *J. exp. Med.* **134**, 1 (1971).
108*b*. ibid., **134**, 21 (1971).
109. Paterson, P. Y. and Harwin, S. M., In *Mechanisms of Immunological Tolerance.* Ed. by Hašek, M., Lengerová, A. and Vojtisková, M. Publishing House of the Czechoslovak Academy of Sciences, Prague 1962, p. 507.
110. Radzikovskaya, R. M., In *Mechanisms of Immunological Tolerance.* Ed. by Hašek, M., Lengerová, A. and Vojtisková, M. Publishing House of the Czechoslovak Academy of Sciences, Prague 1962, p. 211.
111. Raff, M. C., Sternberg, M. and Taylor, R. B.: *Nature* **225**, 553 (1970).
112. Rajka, G. and Hård, S.: *Acta derm. venereol.* **40**, 64 (1960).
113. Rosenthal, S. A. and Baer, R. L.: *J. invest. Derm.* **41**, 351 (1963).
113*a*. Rouse, B. T. and Warner, N. L.: *Eur. J. Immunol.* **2**, 102 (1972).
114. Rowley, D. A., Fitch, F. W., Axelrad, M. A. and Pierce, C. W.: *Immunology* **16**, 549 (1969).
115. Roy Schwarz, M.: *J. exp. Med.* **127**, 879 (1968).
116. Ryder, R. J. W. and Schwartz, R. S.: *J. Immunol.* **103**, 970 (1969).
117. Rygard, J.: *Acta path. microbiol. scand.* **77**, 761 (1969).
118. Schmidt, H.: *Behring-Werke Mitt.* Heft **29**, 47 (1954).

118a. Scibiensky, R. and Sercarz, E.: *J. Immunol.* **110,** 540 (1973).
119. Scott, D. W., Waksman, B., Bauminger, S. and Sela, M.: *Immunochemistry* **7,** 357 (1970).
120. Sela, M., Fuchs, S., Maron, R. and Gertner, B.: *J. Immunol.* **1,** 36 (1971).
120a. Sercarz, E., Cuningham, A. J. and Green, N. M.: *Fed. Proc.* **31,** 773 (1972).
121. Shellam, G. R.: *Int. Arch. Allergy* **40,** 507 (1971).
122. Shellam, G. R. and Nossal, G. J. V.: *Immunology* **14,** 273 (1968).
123. Sherman, W. B.: *J. Allergy* **28,** 62 (1957).
124. Skog, E.: *Acta derm.-venereol.* **35,** 264 (1955).
125. Smith, R. T.: *Adv. Immunology* **1,** 67 (1961).
126. Smith, R. T. and Bridges, R. A.: *J. exp. Med.* **106,** 227 (1958).
127. Sousa, M. A. B. de, Parrott, D. M. V. and Pantelouris, E. M.: *Clin. exp. Immunol.* **4,** 637 (1969).
128. Speirs, R. S.: *Immunochemistry* **8,** 665 (1971).
129. Stark, O. K., In *Mechanisms of Hypersensitivity*. Ed. by Shaffer, J. H., Lo-Groppo, G. A. and Chase, M. W. Churchill, London 1959, p. 519.
130. Steinberg, A. D., Daley, G. and Talal, N.: *Science* **167,** 870 (1970).
130a. Stockman, G. D., Heim, L. R., South, M. A. and Trentin, J. J.: *J. Immunol.* **110,** 277 (1973).
131a. Storm van Leeuwen, W. S. and Kremer, W.: *Z. Immun. Forsch.* **50,** 1 (1927).
131b. ibid., **50,** 462 (1927).
132. Strannegard, O. and Belin, L.: *Immunology* **20,** 427 (1971).
133. Sulzberger, M.-B.: *Arch. Derm.* **20,** 669 (1929).
134a. Taussig, M. J.: *Eur. J. Immunol.* **1,** 367 (1971).
134b. id., *Immunology* **21,** 54 (1971).
135. Taussig, M. J. and Lachmann, P. J.: *Immunology* **22,** 85 (1972).
136. Taylor, R. B.: *Immunology* **7,** 595 (1964).
137. Tees, E. C. and Milner, F. H.: *Acta allerg. (Kbh.)* **20,** 235 (1968).
138. Trakatellis, A. C., Axelrod, A. E., Montjar, M. and Lamy, F.: *Nature* **202,** 154 (1964).
139. Trench, C. A., Gardner, P. S. and Green, C. A.: *Immunology* **7,** 567 (1964).
140. Tuft, L. and Heck, V. M.: *J. Allergy* **27,** 100 (1956).
140a. Turk, J. L. and Parker, D.: *Immunology* **24,** 751 (1973).
140b. Turk, J. L., Parker, D. and Poulter, L. W.: *Immunology* **23,** 493 (1972).
140c. Turk, J. L. and Poulter, L. W.: *Clin. exp. Immunol.* **10,** 285 (1972).
141. Twarog, F. J. and Rose, N. R.: *J. Immunol.* **107,** 738 (1971).
142. Uhr, J. W. and Pappenheimer, A. M., jr.: *J. exp. Med.* **108,** 891 (1958).
143. Voisin, G. A., In *Mechanisms of Immunological Tolerance*. Ed. by Hašek, M., Lengerová, A. and Vojtisková, M. Publishing House of the Czechoslovak Academy of Sciences, Prague 1962, p. 435.
144. Waksman, B. H., In *Mechanisms of Antibody Formation*. Ed. by Holub, M. and Jarosková, L. Publishing House of the Czechoslovak Academy of Sciences. Prague 1960, p. 354.
145a. Weigle, W. O.: *J. exp. Med.* **114,** 111 (1961).
145b. id., *Nature* **201,** 632 (1964).
145c. Weigle, W. O., Chiller, J. M. and Habicht, G. S.: In *Progress in Immunology*. Proceedings of the First International Congress of Immunology. Ed. by Amos, B. Academic Press, New York 1971, p. 331.
146. White, W. A., jr. and Baer, R. L.: *J. Allergy* **21,** 344 (1950).
147. Wigzell, H.: *J. exp. Med.* **124,** 953 (1966).
148. Williams, C. C. and Wu, W. G.: *J. Immunol.* **107,** 163 (1971).
149. Woodruff, M. F. A., In *Biologic Problems of Grafting*. Ed. by Albert, G. and Medawar, P. B. Blackwell, Oxford 1959, p. 83.
150. Wu, W. G., Horve, F. O. and Williams, C. C.: *J. Immunol.* **107,** 154 (1971).
151. Zilber, L. A., In *Mechanisms of Antibody Formation*. Ed. by Holub, M. and Jarosková, L. Publishing House of the Czechoslovak Academy of Sciences, Prague 1960, p. 332.

CHAPTER 6

# THE SHWARTZMAN PHENOMENON

by

L. KESZTYŰS and T. SZILÁGYI



## INTRODUCTION

Sanarelli [73c] made the observation that if he injected intraperitoneally a non-lethal dose of *Vibrio cholerae*, and later followed this with a small quantity of intravenous *E. coli* toxin, the animals perished. He had already reported on similar observations in earlier papers [73*a*, *b*]; this phenomenon was initially called 'epithalaxia' by him, and later 'haemorrhagic allergy'. These results were confirmed by the injection of two small doses of *E. coli* endotoxin at 24-hour intervals [106]. The reaction thus produced is called Sanarelli-Shwartzman phenomenon, or generalized Shwartzman reaction, in current literature.

Shwartzman [77*a*] injected a filtrate of *S. typhi* into the skin of rabbits, and this was repeated 24 h later intravenously, when a haemorrhagic necrosis developed at the site of the injection. Similar observations were made with *B. lepisepticum* [25]. This phenomenon is now termed local Shwartzman phenomenon.

## LOCAL SHWARTZMAN PHENOMENON

This reaction is characterized by oedema, haemorrhage and necrosis occurring at the site of intracutaneous injection of endotoxin. The intensity of the reaction is generally measured by the size of the haemorrhagic and necrotic area (the largest

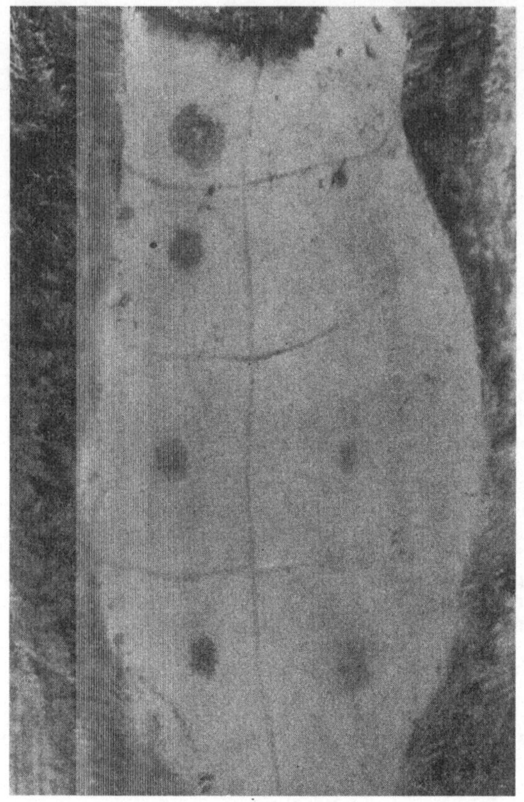

Fig. 6-1. Quantitative Shwartzman phenomenon (Kesztyűs et al.) [39]

and smallest diameter). The accuracy of the evaluation is greatly increased by a quantitative method, described by Kesztyűs et al. [39]: diminishing doses of endotoxin are given intracutaneously (6–8 doses); the ensuing reaction is proportionate with the dose of endotoxin (Fig. 6-1). Histologically, the reaction is characterized by haemorrhage and thrombus formation in the small vessels (Fig. 6-2). The first dose of endotoxin, which is locally used, is named the preparatory ('sensitizing') dose, while the second, which is given intravenously, is termed the provoking dose. The effect of the preparatory dose is a mild inflammatory reaction with oedema and leukocytic infiltration which lasts 1 to 2 days. Haemorrhagic necrosis does not develop if the provoking endotoxin is injected into the same area of skin—even if given repeatedly [77*a*]—although there have been contrasting reports in this respect [64, 82*c*].

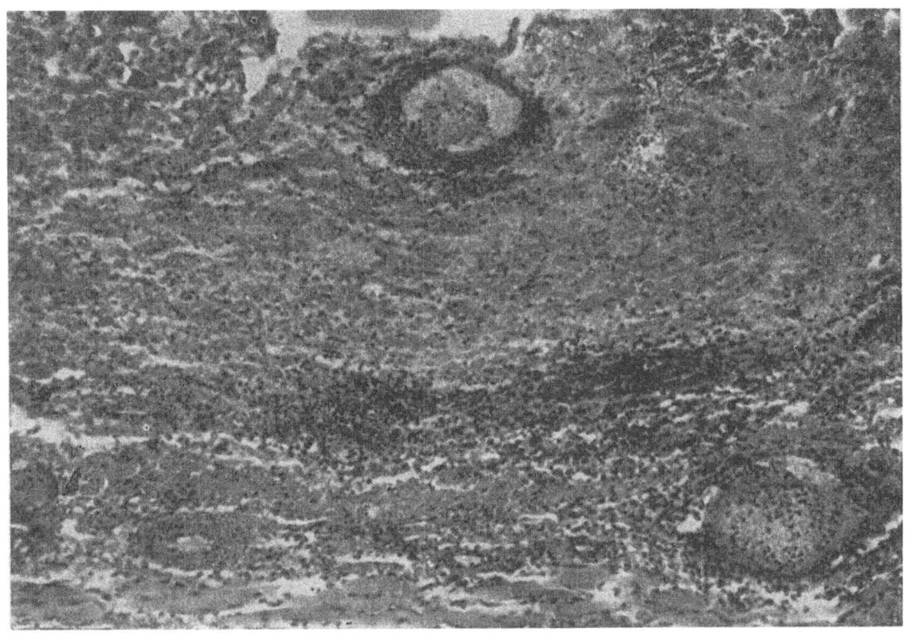

Fig. 6-2. Classical local Shwartzman phenomenon in the skin. ×90; haematoxylin-eosin

## PREPARATORY AND PROVOKING AGENTS

Bacterial, spirochaetal filtrates, viruses, i.e. microorganisms, or agents causing functional disturbances in the affected tissues can be used as the preparatory doses. Leukocyte (polymorphonuclear) granules [24, 94*b*], or monocytes [42] may also be given. Leukotactic substances have also been described as preparatory agents [99]. It was observed in experiments using endotoxin with $^{32}P$ as a tracer [84], that the intradermally introduced endotoxin is evenly distributed in the surrounding tissues within a relatively short time. Irrespective of whether the phenomenon has occurred (provocation after 24 h) or not (provocation after 72 h), there is no significant difference between the activity of the skin samples; thus the production of the phenomenon does not depend upon the accumulation of the preparatory endotoxin. Using tritium labelled endotoxin it was found, that the locally introduced endotoxin, or its decomposition products remain, for the most part, at the site of injection [75].

Beside endotoxin, also glycogen, starch, agar [82*a*] and dextran [5] may be used as the provoking injection, although the resultant reaction is by no means so well developed as in the case of intravenous endotoxin injection. Animal tissues and plant extracts ('Shear polysaccharides') may act as preparatory and provoking doses [48]. The optimal time interval between preparation and provocation is about 24 h, and the possibility of provocation ceases after 2 to 3 days, but t can be extended by the use of intravenous neosalvarsan [70]. The local Shwartzman phenomenon develops 4 to 5 h after the introduction of the provoking dose, and hyperbaric oxygenation greatly accelerates the course of the reaction [90]. Seasonal factors may also affect the intensity of the reaction [47*b*].

## PATHOMECHANISM

The experimental animal used most frequently for producing the Shwartzman phenomenon is the rabbit. In guinea pigs, oral mucous membrane of hamsters [22], and in several strains of mice the reaction can also be produced; in rats it occurs only after pre-treatment with bacteria [42]. The increased sensitivity of rabbits may be due to the fact that endotoxin—in contrast to other animals—does not enhance fibrinolysis in rabbits [49]. The reaction is more regular in full-grown animals, but it can also be elicited in newborn rabbits [14]. It is generally accepted that the local Shwartzman phenomenon cannot be transferred passively. If a passive transfer can, nevertheless, be effected, the reaction should, in fact, be regarded as an immunological (Arthus) phenomenon.

The preparatory injection is usually given intradermally, but the local Shwartzman reaction is, in fact, inducible in several tissues and organs, e.g. in the intestinal tract, liver, spleen, lung, various glands (pancreas, salivary gland) (Fig. 6-3); in the

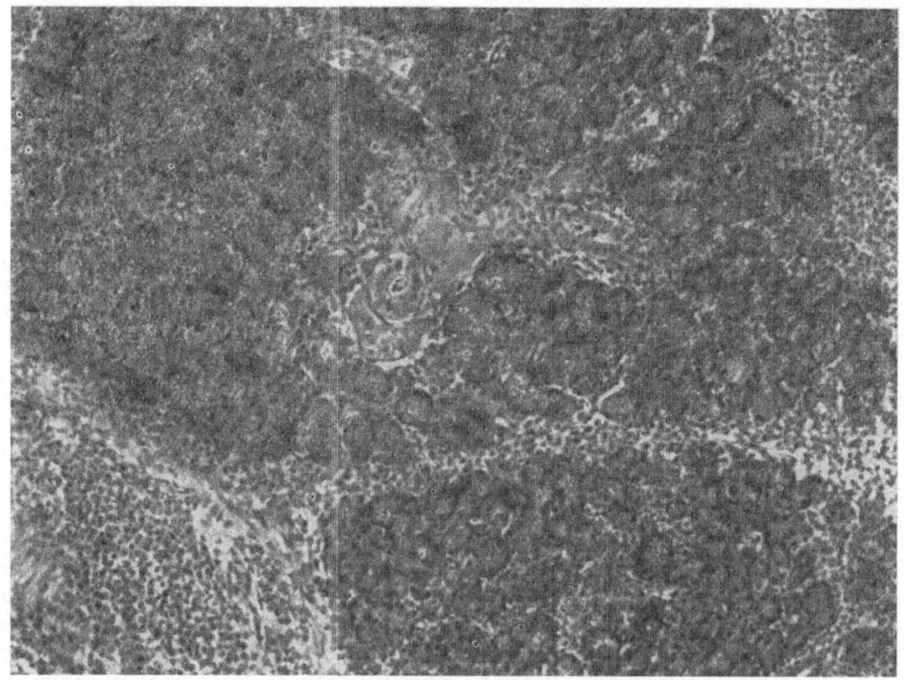

Fig. 6-3. Local Shwartzman phenomenon in a salivary gland. ×90; haematoxylin-eosin. (Szilágyi et al.) [89]

latter, by applying the preparatory dose into the excretory duct [93], or into the gland itself [89]. It is questionable, however, whether such a reaction can be produced in nervous tissue; in the cornea it occurs only after its vascularization [69].

With repeated introduction of endotoxin (i.v., i.c., or i.m.) resistance can be achieved [12], i.e. the local Shwartzman phenomenon cannot be demonstrated. This status, however, is only transient, lasting for about 2 to 3 weeks. The reactivity can be restored if a large provoking dose is given [12], or if RES blockers are used [4]. In rabbits, which have been made resistant, the local reaction can also be produced by the use of heterologous endotoxin [47*b*].

### *Blood coagulation phenomenon*

Several explanations of the local Shwartzman phenomenon have been published; the one suggesting that disturbances of blood coagulation might be involved has many adherents. One of the proofs of this concept would be that various anticoagulant substances prevent the local reaction, e.g. heparin [13, 19*b*], coumarin [67], warfarin [37] and hirudin [29]. However, the haemostatic agent Reptilase vigorously enhances the local Shwartzman phenomenon [97]. It has also been reported that ε-aminocaproic acid prevents the local reaction in mice [68], while others state that antifibrinolytic substances have no protective effect [107]. In thrombocytopenia of rabbits produced by anti-thrombocyte serum local Shwartzman phenomenon occurred unhindered [78, 51].

Fibrin and fibrinoid formation are significant and basic symptoms of the reaction, but the mechanism of their development is still unknown. Cold (+ 4 °C) precipitable fibrinogen (i.e. cryprofibrin) will appear in response to endotoxin combined with heparin [93]. Liquoid (sodium polyanetholsulphonate), which precipitates fibrinogen *in vitro*, also enhances the Shwartzman phenomenon [96]. Recently, it has been reported that the accumulation of heparin precipitable protein is by itself insufficient for producing the reaction [71].

### *Enzymes of the polymorphonuclear leukocytes*

The important role of granulocytes is shown by the fact that the most characteristic sign of the local preparation is the infiltration of polymorphonuclear (PMN) leukocytes. As a result of the considerable anaerobic glycolysis of these leukocytes, lactic acid accumulates, and this enhances the sensitivity of the tissues to cell proteases [82*b*]. In rabbits rendered leukopenic by nitrogen mustard the local Shwartzman phenomenon is less vigorous [3, 83]. Nitrogen mustard has a significant inhibitory effect, but leukopenia produced by total body irradiation hardly affects the appearance of the Shwartzman phenomenon [34]. Leukocytes play a more important role in the pathomechanism than thrombocytes; namely cysteine given i.v. following provocation, enhanced the leukopenia and prevented the thrombocytopenia, resulting in a more vigorous local reaction [35]. On the other hand, when antithymocyte, antigranulocyte, anti-γ-globulin and anti-complement sera were given one hour before provocation to guinea pigs, only the anticomplement and, to a lesser extent, the anti-$\gamma$-globulin sera had any preventive effect [66].

According to experimental evidence, the lysosomal enzymes released from PMN leukocytes, primarily proteases, are responsible for initiating the reaction [94*b*]. Recently, further observations have confirmed this view. Halpern [24] has shown that substances preventing proteolysis inhibit the course of the local Shwartzman phenomenon produced by PMN leukocyte granules (preparation) and endotoxin (provocation). It is possible to enhance the local reaction with trypsin, and to hinder it by means of trypsin inhibitors [11*a*]. It was demonstrated by Szilágyi et al. [90] that hyperbaric oxygenation which renders the lysosomes unstable, has an enhancing effect upon the phenomenon, while local gold treatment, which inhibits lysosomal enzymes and stabilizes the lysosomes, has an inhibitory effect [91]. In this context, it is important to note that endotoxin applied *in vivo* belongs to the most effective lysosome labilizing factors [103]. Following vitamin A treatment, which causes lysosome degranulation, the endotoxin induced dermatitis is greatly reduced [30].

### *Endothelial damage and the altered microcirculation*

These are factors which also have a role in the development of the reaction and of the necrosis. Particularly important is the alteration of the reactivity of the blood vessels to adrenalin. If adrenalin is injected into the skin of animals treated with intravenous endotoxin, a Shwartzman-like reaction can be induced [94*a*]. This phenomenon is also called 'Thomas reaction'; a reaction similar to this was first described by Marcus [54]. On the other hand, the fragility of the capillaries is of no significance [33]. In contrast to immune reactions, dye substances do not accumulate in the affected skin areas [76].

### *Role of the nervous system and hormones*

Investigating the neuro-endocrine regulation, or in other words, the role of the nervous system and of hormones, it was found [100] that if before the preparatory injection, the spinal cord was transected at the level of the 6th cervical vertebra, the local Shwartzman phenomenon could not be provoked. The evaluation of the results of these experiments is made difficult by the thermoregulatory disturbances occurring as a consequence of cord transaction, which also have a bearing on the development of the reaction (see later). According to Kesztyűs et al. [38] there is no difference in the intensity of the Shwartzman phenomenon produced in rabbits on denervated hind limbs and on the dorsal skin area and that produced in animals with non-denervated skin. Unilateral sympathectomy diminishes, while transection of the ischiadic nerve enhances the skin reaction on the hind limb [102], but lumbal sympathectomy has no effect upon the hind limb phenomenon [53]. In contrast, lasting phenobarbital narcosis [38], as well as TEAB, and hexamethonium treatment [85] have inhibiting effects. Numerous drugs acting on the nervous system (atropine, chlorpromazine, ergotamine, procaine, curare) do not inhibit but, in fact, rather enhance the local reaction. In contrast, locally applied dibenamine decreases the haemorrhage [43]. Thus the nervous system, and substances affecting it, have only a modifying effect upon the local Shwartzman phenomenon, and it is probable that they act mainly through blood vessel reactions.

Analysing the effects of the nervous system, it was shown by Szilágyi et al. [87] that if the provoking endotoxin was given to rabbits cooled below 30 °C, the local Shwartzman phenomenon could be fully prevented [101]. If the animals were cooled down and the local sites of injection of the preparatory doses were rewarmed to varying temperatures (30 to 40 °C) prior to provocation, necrosis only occurred if the prepared skin temperature was about 37 °C [10]. It has been proved in more recent experiments that hypothermia also prevents the reaction in which leukocyte granules have been used for preparation, and also those provoked by adrenalin [89].

Among the hormones, apart from adrenalin, the inhibiting effects of ACTH [80] and of cortisone [78] were most often studied. A single i.c. dose of endotoxin caused local haemorrhagic necrosis in cortisone treated rabbits [95*a*], moreover also a generalized reaction may develop from the enhanced toxin absorption due to the glycocorticoid effect. Cortisone also prevents the development of resistance, and extinguishes the already developed endotoxin resistance [6]. The reason for the divergent results may be the difference in methods and doses of cortisone treatment; in appropriate doses, cortisone decreases the local reaction [40].

Several hormones (vasopressin, oxytocin, oestradiol, progesterone, thyroxine, and parathormone) have no significant effect upon the local Shwartzman phenomenon. In rabbits with alloxan diabetes and in glucose induced hyperglycaemia the reaction is greatly diminished, but insulin has a significant enhancing effect [86].

### *Immune reaction theory*

Gratia and Linz [20] and Sanarelli [73*d*] have proposed to term it 'haemorrhagic allergy', others called it 'haemorrhagic heteroallergy' [41] or 'non-specific allergy' [7*b*]. These different names also indicate that some investigators attribute a role to the antigen–antibody reactions in the local Shwartzman phenomenon, i.e. it is regarded as an immunological phenomenon. According to Bordet [7*a*], a local haemorrhage and necrosis can be produced in guinea pigs treated with BCG vaccine when injected with killed *E. coli* (Bordet phenomenon). If to rabbits sensitized with animal proteins bacterial toxin is given i.c. and followed by an i.v. injection of animal protein 24 h later, haemorrhagic skin necrosis develops in the affected skin area [77*b*]. These experiments—with certain modifications—have been repeated by others, too.

Lee and Stetson [50] gave endotoxin of *E. coli* to rabbits i.v. and 6 h later, endotoxin of *E. coli* and *S. typhosa*, respectively. Within an hour an 'accelerated' and intensive cutaneous reaction developed; this reaction could be elicited for up to one month after the i.v. endotoxin injection. Incidentally, the 'accelerated reactivity' of the rabbit treated with i.v. endotoxin could be transferred by serum to untreated animals. The resulting reaction was not identical with the local Shwartzman phenomenon (haemorrhage and necrosis were rarely found) and in certain respects, looked like an Arthus-type reaction. Kováts et al. [45, 47*a*] regard the response given to the preparatory dose as a specific immune reaction.

According to them every animal which is in symbiosis with endotoxin producing microorganisms shows a specific sensitization to the endotoxin and the i.c. preparatory dose reacts with the naturally occurring antibodies producing the alteration of the skin. They substantiate this statement with the following evidence: the reaction is transferable with sera of rabbits hyperimmunized with endotoxin. According to another opinion, the precipitating antibodies may play a part in the local Shwartzman phenomenon [21].

The immune reaction theory concerning the local Shwartzman phenomenon is not acceptable because:

1. There are much more arguments against it than for it. Thus, e.g. the preparatory and the provoking doses can be widely differring substances; the latency period between the introduction of the two doses is rather short; the outcome of desensitization is uncertain; the phenomenon can be elicited in newborn and germ-free animals; separate parts of the endotoxin molecule are responsible for its biological and antigenic properties; in some cases of Hodgkin's disease it is not possible to produce delayed hypersensitivity, but it is still possible to elicit endotoxin phenomena [82*d*].

2. The experiments in support of the immune reaction theory are not convincing, particularly in view of the recent results suggesting that antigen–antibody complexes themselves have an inflammatory effect, and that preparation is possible also without endotoxin, etc.

Of the so-called chemical mediators, i.e. histamine, 5-hydroxytryptamine (5-HT), bradykinin, only the last named enhances the local Shwartzman phenomenon. Local application of the inhibitor substances of the mediators prevents the haemorrhagic skin reaction [1*c*], although only a few of the antihistamines (antistine, promethazine) have some effect, while the others are ineffective. 5-HT and bradykinin and their antagonists interfere with blood coagulation, and fibrinolysis, too [11*b*]. It is also important that in the course of the Shwartzman phenomenon degranulation of mast cells cannot be elicited [21]. Thus chemical mediators seem to have no significant function in the local Shwartzman phenomenon.

The Shwartzman reaction is accompanied and followed by a number of changes in the serum, other than those already mentioned. Some of these are only side-effects, but some may have an important part in the pathomechanism of the reaction. A few hours after provocation, there is an increase in the $\beta$-lipoprotein and free and esterified cholesterol levels of blood, i.e. in its total lipid content. [46]. It is possible that this not only accelerates blood coagulation, but also blocks the RES [61]. Besides the hyperglycaemia [39] the glucoprotein level also rises [44]. At the site of the skin reaction the level of hexose, hexoseamine, and uric acid rises significantly [76], as does also the incorporation of $^{35}$S into mucopolysaccharides [28]. Of the serum proteins the level of $\gamma$-globulin decreases [105], which could be taken as a proof of the enhanced activity of proteases. Of the enzymes—apart from the proteases [1*b*]—an enhanced activity of the characteristic lysosomal enzymes: acid phosphatase, $\beta$-glucuronidase [88] and phosphohexoseisomerase [39] is evident; the increase of the latter is probably related to muscle impairment. As regards the electrolyte content, the decrease in serum K and Ca levels is the most obvious change [39].

*Shwartzman phenomenon-like reaction*

This reaction type has been treated in several reports. Apart from what has been already mentioned [50], e.g. heterologous serum (human serum to dogs), may function as a provoking agent, but if applied with i.c. endotoxin it has an adjuvant effect [1*a*]. When i.c. endotoxin was given to rabbits sensitized with protein and, if 24 h later, the sensitizing antigen was given i.v., a haemorrhagic skin necrosis developed [77*b*]. When hypersensitivity was induced in the skin of guinea pigs with neoarsphenamine, or 2-4-dinitro-chlorobenzene, and then the i.v. sensitizing agent was given, it was observed that a haemorrhagic reaction —specific to the sensitizing agent—developed [15]. In such 'Shwartzman phenomenon-like' reactions the occurrence of thrombi has not been proved though it is a basic criterion; a majority of these reactions are based upon antigen–antibody reactions and any process which is accompanied by leukotaxis and disturbances of blood coagulation, could 'sensitize' to a Shwartzman-like alteration, or could lead to a haemorrhagic-necrotic reaction.

Based upon the foregoing, we may draw the conclusion that the local Shwartzman phenomenon which appears as a haemorrhagic necrosis mostly affecting the skin, is not only a local alteration, but a complex disorder of metabolism, having conspicuous local symptoms which are by no means the only ones.

The preparatory phase most probably corresponds to the development of a leukocyte, or rather lysosome pool which 'explodes' upon provocation when a number of enzymes are released and activated [107]. Two points are obvious:

1. Endotoxin is the most suitable agent both for preparation and for provocation.
2. The complexity of the symptoms which appear following provocation indicates that the Shwartzman phenomenon is open to the enhancing or diminishing effect of several factors.

## GENERALIZED SHWARTZMAN PHENOMENON

The local Shwarztman phenomenon is often regarded as the localized form of the Sanarelli–Shwartzman reaction, or, as it is generally called today, the generalized Shwartzman phenomenon. Undoubtedly, the two reactions have a number of common characteristics, but they also show significant differences. The classical generalized Shwartzman phenomenon may be produced by two injections of endotoxin from Gram-negative bacteria given at 24-hour intervals. A single i.v. or intraaortic injection of endotoxin may also produce the reaction [2*a*, 26], although some authors deny this possibility [8].

The generalized reaction can, in general, be elicited in the same kinds of animals as the localized reaction, the most suitable and most frequently used animal being the rabbit for both. However, unlike for the local Shwartzman reaction, for the generalized reaction young rabbits are more suitable [79]. True passive transfer is not possible; if, however, such a transfer seems to occur it is, in fact, due to endotoxin transfer, or to the adjuvant effect of blood, or simply the transfer of fibrinoid.

The generalized Shwartzman phenomenon consists in the appearance of precipitate rich in fibrin (thrombi) in the small blood vessels of various organs (kidney, adrenals, liver, spleen, heart, lungs). The most important symptom is the renal lesion (Figs 6-4 and 6-5). First of all, hyaline or fibrinoid thrombi, which contain fats, lipids and sulphurated esters of mucopolysaccharides besides fibrin and thrombocytes, are seen in the afferent arterioles. Haemorrhage is visible around the vessels, the renal cortex shows extensive necrosis, the medulla is hyperaemic. Nevertheless, both the localized and the generalized Shwartzman phenomena are also to be elicited after the removal of both kidneys [52].

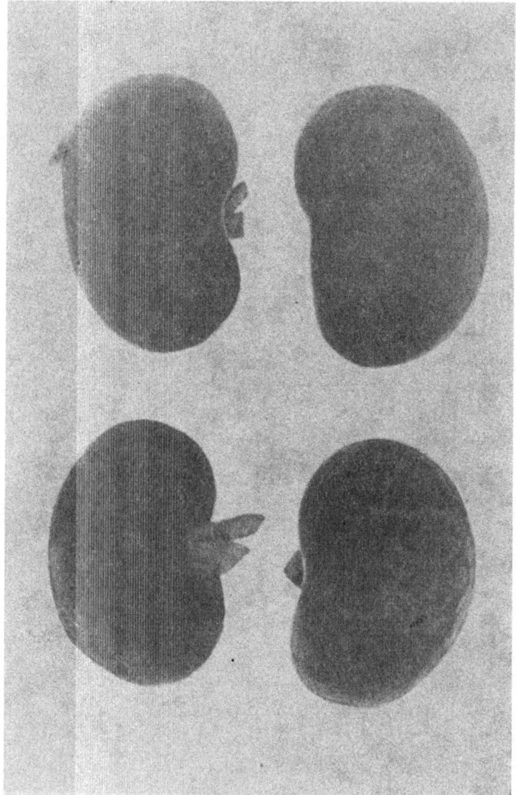

Fig. 6-4. Generalized Shwartzman phenomenon (bottom) and controls (top)

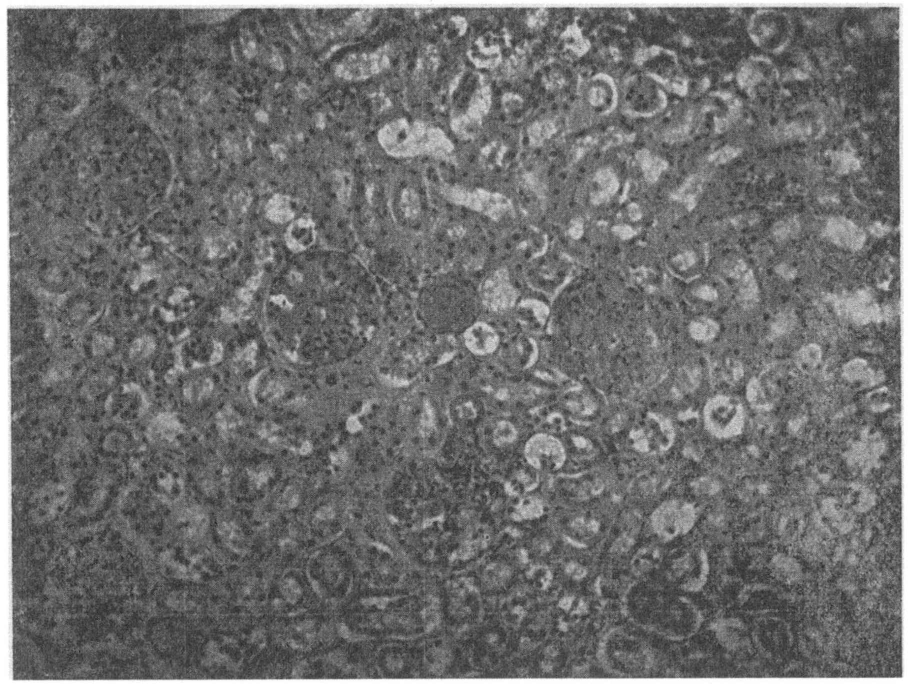

Fig. 6-5. Generalized Shwartzman phenomenon in the kidney. ×90; haematoxylin-eosin

*Consumption coagulopathy with thrombus formation*

The significance of blood coagulation in the pathomechanism of the generalized Shwartzman phenomenon, apart from the formation of fibrin, is also documented by the already mentioned fact that anticoagulants (heparin, warfarin, coumarin) prevent the reaction. Further proof is that a single i.v. injection of liquoid is sufficient to produce a typical generalized reaction [72]. Administration of reptilase promotes the development and increases the intensity of the generalized Shwartzman reaction [98]. Similarity between blood clotting and the Shwartzman phenomenon is also shown by the fact that the activity of blood clotting factors V, VII, IX, and X decrease and severe thrombocytopenia develops following both of them. The massive fibrin precipitation ('disseminated intravascular thrombosis') together with the depletion of some of the clotting factors leads to consumption coagulopathy [58*a*]. A similar renal cortical necrosis can be brought about with the i.v. infusion of thrombin [56]. The importance of thrombocytes is reflected by the experiment in which no generalized reaction could be produced in thrombocytopenic state due to antithrombocyte serum (there was no significant change in the leukocyte count) [57]. Thrombocytopenia—as mentioned—does not prevent the local Shwartzman phenomenon [51].

## *Role of the reticuloendothelial system*

A special significance is attributed to the RES in the pathomechanism of the generalized Shwartzman phenomenon. Generalized reaction has been brought about with a single i.v. endotoxin injection in rabbits previously treated with i.v. Thorotrast [16], or with colloidal silver [45]. The effects of an i.v. injection of thrombin are greatly enhanced if the animal is pretreated with Thorotrast, or denatured albumin [49]. Besides, with two consecutive i.v. Thorotrast injections a 'generalized Shwartzman-like reaction' can be produced [16]. In contrast to the above-mentioned other RES blocking agents, e.g. starch, glycogen, PVP (polyvinylpyrrolidone), tissue extracts and certain antigens have no such effects [19*a*]. The role of the RES is considered to be the elimination of the provoking agents of the Shwartzman phenomenon, even of fibrin. The endotoxin itself —especially the second dose—strongly blocks the RES and hinders the removal of the altered fibrinogen [96] from circulation. However, endotoxin given in increasing doses stimulates the RES and brings about a resistant state, which can be broken through, e.g. with trypan blue. Thus, the actual functional state of the RES is decisive in the pathogenesis of the Shwartzman phenomenon.

## *Granulocytes*

The importance of the role of the granulocytes is shown by the finding that after nitrogen mustard treatment—in granulocytopenic state—the generalized reaction cannot be elicited; but the reaction will appear if a part of the bone marrow is protected against the effects of nitrogen mustard [95*b*]. According to experimental evidence [31], the role of the first endotoxin injection is to produce a granulocytosis: by giving PMN granules the effect of the preparing endotoxin dose can be completely substituted. According to histochemical, isotope $^{35}S$, and autoradiographic experiments [32], the granules contain sulphomucopolysaccharides, which are also present in the fibrinoids blocking the glomeruli. This suggested the concept that this acidic polymer and the altered fibrinogen constitute a complex and play an essential role in the formation of fibrinoid. However, contradicting results also exist, e.g. it was shown that the generalized reaction could be elicited if granulocytopenia was produced with nitrogen mustard, especially four days after treatment, and independently of the granulocyte count [104].

## *Alteration of hormonal balance*

Besides other factors (blood coagulation, RES function), the altered hormonal balance plays certainly a great part in the increased endotoxin sensitivity during pregnancy. In pregnant rabbits a single injection of endotoxin can produce a generalized Shwartzman phenomenon [2*b*], and, in fact, it can be produced also in the usually resistant rat with one i.v. endotoxin dose if applied in the last days of pregnancy [36]; though the alterations are not exactly the same as those normally seen [59]. Oral contraceptive substances have a similar preparing effect as does pregnancy [9]. Using colchicine, one can produce characteristic glomerular changes in pregnant golden hamsters [18]. It is possible that the endotoxin derived from the native bacterial flora has a role in the formation of the reaction (the exogenic endotoxin is ineffective in this case). Pregnant rats kept on a diet of free vitamin E and in excess of oxidized lipids will develop a generalized Shwartzman phenomenon [58*b*]. The sensitizing effect of pregnancy might partly be explained by the fact that following a slow i.v. infusion of thrombin, a massive and lasting glomerular thrombosis develops in the pregnant rats, in contrast to the non-pregnant controls, in which the thrombi are quickly eliminated: consequently, fibrinolysis is considerably decreased in pregnancy [56]. The importance of sex hormones is shown by the fact that if progesterone is given to rats in the late stages of pregnancy, renal cortical necrosis will appear [60]. A further problem is why these different substances produce generalized Shwartzman phenomenon in pregnant animals that otherwise would be resistant to the reaction.

An observation facilitating the distinction between local and generalized Shwartzman phenomena is that in adrenalin tolerant rabbits there may occur a local reaction, whereas the generalized phenomenon cannot be elicited [23]. There are contrasting opinions concerning the effects of ACTH and cortisone, and recently an aggravating effect of the two hormones [8, 55], and that of stress, [17], has been reported. Renal cortical necrosis can be prevented by sympathectomy [65], which suggests the involvement of the adrenergic system similarly to the finding that $\alpha$-adrenergic blocking agents can diminish the thrombosis of the glomerular capillaries [62]. The sympathetic excitement, adrenalin mobilization and inhibited histamine synthesis in response to endotoxin [74], further, the special renal circulatory state may all contribute to the marked necrosis in the kidney.

## CONNECTION OF THE SHWARTZMAN PHENOMENON WITH VARIOUS PATHOLOGICAL CONDITIONS

The question may be asked—and with right—what is the use of research trying to elucidate the pathomechanism of the Shwartzman phenomenon. The local reaction is an excellent experimental tool for the research of inflammation and thrombohaemorrhagic symptoms; furthermore, there is evidence accumulating which supports the view that certain pathological processes can be regarded as generalized or local Shwartzman phenomenon-like reactions, such as e.g. the hyperacute rejection of kidney transplantats [63, 81], toxaemia in pregnancy, acute pancreatitis, purpura fulminans, the Waterhouse–Friderichsen syndrome, appendicitis, etc. [27]. It is interesting that tumours become necrotic due to a single injection of endotoxin, since they are in a state of 'permanent preparation'. It is possible that in the future endotoxin, or endotoxin-like substances, will acquire a significant part in tumour therapy [48].

## REFERENCES


1*a*. Antopol, W. and Chryssanthou, C.: *Fed. Proc.* **18,** 466 (1959).
1*b*. id., *Ann. N.Y. Acad. Sci.* **104,** 346 (1963).
1c. id., *Arch. Path.* **78,** 313 (1964).
2*a*. Apitz, K.: *Virchows Arch. path. Anat.* **293,** 1 (1934).

2b. id., *J. Immunol.* **29,** 255 (1935).
3. Becker, R. M.: *Proc. Soc. exp. Biol. (N.Y.)* **69,** 247 (1948).
4. Beeson, P. B.: *Proc. Soc. exp. Biol. (N.Y.)* **64,** 146 (1947).
5. Bennett, I. L.: *Proc. Soc. exp. Biol. (N.Y.)* **81,** 266 (1952).
6. Bennett, I. L. and Beeson, P. B.: *Bull. Hopkins Hosp.* **93,** 290 (1953).
7a. Bordet, P.: *C. R. Soc. Biol. (Paris)* **106,** 1251 (1931).
7b. id., *Ann. Inst. Pasteur* **56,** 325 (1936).
8. Bouissou, H., Familiadés, J., Fabre, J., Kanoun, T. and Laplanche, A.-M.: *J. Urol. Néphrol. (Paris)* **70,** 785 (1964).
9. Buitrago, B. and Jensen, O. M.: *Acta path. microbiol. scand.* **73,** 323 (1968).
10. Burack, W. R. and Mosimann, W. F.: *Arch. Path.* **71,** 175 (1961).
11a. Chryssanthou, C. and Antopol, W.: *Proc. Soc. exp. Biol. (N.Y.)* **108,** 587 (1961).
11b. id., *Fed. Proc.* **23,** 2 (1964).
12. Cluff, L. E. and Bennett, I. L.: *Proc. Soc. exp. Biol. (N.Y.)* **77,** 461 (1951).
13. Cluff, L. E. and Berthrong, M.: *Bull. Johns Hopkins Hosp.* **92,** 353 (1953).
14. Dachy, A.: *C. R. Soc. Biol. (Paris)* **159,** 1626 (1965).
15. De Weck, A. L., Frey, J. R. and Geleick, H.: *J. Immunol.* **100,** 1 (1968).
16. Fine, J., Rutenburg, S. and Schweinburg, F. B.: *J. exp. Med.* **110,** 547 (1959).
17. Gabbiani, G., Selye, H. and Tuchweber, B.: *Endocrinology* **77,** 179 (1965).
18. Galton, M.: *Proc. Soc. exp. Biol. (N.Y.)* **119,** 1139 (1965).
19a. Good, R. A. and Thomas, L.: *J. exp. Med.* **96,** 625 (1952).
19b. ibid., **97,** 871 (1953).
20. Gratia, A. and Linz, R.: *Ann. Inst. Pasteur* **49,** 131 (1932).
21. Gustafson, G. T.: *Acta path. microbiol. scand.* Suppl. **196** (1968).
22. Gustafson, G. T. and Cornberg, S.: *Acta path. microbiol. scand.* **59,** 21 (1963).
23. Hall, D. L., Broom, J. S. and Brunson, J. G.: *Amer. J. Path.* **44,** 431 (1964).
24. Halpern, B. N.: *Proc. Soc. exp. Biol. (N.Y.)* **115,** 273 (1964).
25. Hanger, F. M.: *Proc. Soc. exp. Biol. (N.Y.)* **25,** 775 (1927–28).
26. Hardaway, R. M.: *Ann. Surg.* **155,** 325 (1962).
27. Hardaway, R. M. and McKay, D. G.: *Rev. Surg.* **20,** 297 (1963).
28. Hauss, W. H. and Junge-Hülsing, G.: *Expos. ann. Biochim. méd.* **24,** 239 (1963).
29. Haustein, K. O., Markwardt, F.: *Thrombos. Diathes. haemorrh. (Stuttg.)* **13,** 6 (1965).
30. Heilmeyer, L., Kerp, L., Kasemir, H. and Günther, E.: *Klin. Wschr.* **45,** 586 (1967).
31. Horn, R. G. and Collins, R. D.: *Lab. Invest.* **18,** 101 (1968).
32. Horn, R. G. and Spicer, S. S.: *Amer. J. Path.* **46,** 197 (1965).
33. Illig, L., Kunich, I. and Paul, E.: *Arch. klin. exp. Derm.* **231,** 221 (1968).
34. Johnstone, D. E. and Howland, J. W.: *J. exp. Med.* **108,** 431 (1958).
35. Jókay, I., Kiss, A., Kassay, L.: *Acta microbiol. Acad. Sci. hung.* **11,** 29 (1964).
36. Kaley, G., Demopoulos, H. and Zweifach, B. W.: *Proc. Soc. exp. Biol. (N.Y.)* **109,** 456 (1962).
37. Kelly, M. G., Smith, N. H., Wodinsky, I. and Rall, D. P.: *J. exp. Med.* **105,** 653 (1957).
38. Kesztyűs, L., Csernyánszky, H., Koller, M. and Salánki, J.: *Acta microbiol. Acad. Sci. hung.* **2,** 343 (1955).
39. Kesztyűs, L., Szabó, E., Bot, G. and Jókay, I.: *Acta microbiol. Acad. Sci. hung.* **5,** 209 (1958).
40. Kesztyűs, L., Szilágyi, T., Kiss, A. and Csernyánszky, H.: *Abhandl. ü. die Pathophysiol. Regul.* **11,** 45 (1966).
41. Kielanowski, T.: *Polska Gaz. Lek.* **14,** 309 (1935).
42. Kováts, T. G.: *Nature* **190,** 177 (1961).
43. Kováts, T. G., Bálint, G. and Végh, P.: *Naturwissenschaften* **51,** 488 (1964).
44. Kováts, T. G., Lázár, G., Reök, A. and Végh, P.: *Kisérl. Orvostud.* **12,** 30 (1960).
45. Kováts, T. G., Lázár, G. and Végh, P.: *Acta physiol. Acad. Sci. hung.* **23,** 169 (1963).
46. Kováts, T. G., Reök, A., Lázár, G., Takáts, S. and Végh, P.: *Z. ges. inn. Med.* **16,** 15 (1961).
47a. Kováts, T. G. and Végh, P.: *Naturwissenschaften* **45,** 111 (1966).

47*b*. id., *Immunology* **12,** 445 (1967).
48. Landy, M. and Shear, M. J.: *J. exp. Med.* **106,** 77 (1957).
49. Lee, L.: *J. exp. Med.* **115,** 1065 (1962).
50. Lee, L. and Stetson, C. A.: *J. exp. Med.* **111,** 761 (1960).
51. Levin, J. and Cluff, L. E.: *J. exp. Med.* **121,** 235 (1965).
52. Lindberg, D. A. B. and Riggins, R. C. K.: *Exp. mol. Pathol.* **2,** 114 (1963).
53. Lukasiak, B., Wnorowski, J. and Rozanski, A.: *Z. Haut- u. Geschl.-Kr.* **40,** 217 (1966).
54. Marcus, H.: *Acta med. scand.* **14,** 413 (1921).
55. Margaretten, W., Elting, J. and Rothenberg, J.: *Fed. Proc.* **23/1,** 251 (1964).
56. Margaretten, W. and McKay, D. G.: *Fed. Proc.* **22/1,** 201 (1963).
57. Margaretten, W. and McKay, D. G.: *J. exp. Med.* **129,** 585 (1969).
58*a*. McKay, D. G.: *Amer. J. Path.* **67,** 181 (1972).
58*b*. McKay, D. G. and Kaunitz, H.: *Metabolism* **12,** 983 (1963).
59. McKay, D. G., Wong, T. and Galton, M.: *Fed. Proc.* **19,** 246 (1960).
60. Moore, H. C.: *J. Obstet. Gynaec. Brit. Cwlth.* **70,** 151 (1963).
61. Müller-Berghaus, G., Huth, K., Krecke, H.-J. and Lasch. H.-G.: *Schweiz. med. Wschr.* **94,** 1519 (1964).
62. Müller-Berghaus, G. and McKay, D. G.: *Lab. Invest.* **17,** 276 (1967).
63. Myburgh, J. A., Cohen, I., Gecelter, L., Meyers, A. M., Abrahams, C., Furman, K. I., Goldberg, B. and van Blerk, P. J. P.: *New. Engl. J. Med.* **281,** 131 (1969).
64. Ogata, T.: *Trans. Soc. path. Jap.* **31,** 512 (1941).
65. Palmerio, C., Ming., S. C., Frank, E. and Fine, J.: *J. exp. Med.* **115,** 609 (1962).
66. Polák, L. and Turk, J. L.: *Nature* **223,** 738 (1969).
67. Rall, D. P., Smith, N. H. and Kelly, M. G.: *Proc. Soc. exp. Biol. (N.Y.)* **88,** 241 (1955).
68. Ramos, A. O., Chapman, L. F., Corrado, A. P., Fortes, V. A. and Fiorillo, A. M.: *Arch. int. Pharmacodyn.* **132,** 270 (1961).
69. Raus, R.: *Ophthalmologica (Basel)* **132,** 137 (1956).
70. Renaux, E. and Alechinsky, A.: *Brux.-méd.* **17,** 149 (1936).
71. Rifkind, D. and Hill, R. B.: *J. Immunol.* **99,** 564 (1967).
72. Rodriguez-Erdman, F., Krecke, H.-J., Lasch, H. G. and Bohle, A.: *Z. ges. exp. Med.* **134,** 109 (1960).
73*a*. Sanarelli, G.: *Presse Méd.* **24,** 505 (1916).
73*b*. id., *Bull. Acad. nat. Méd. (Paris)* **90,** 204 (1923).
73*c*. id., *Ann. Inst. Pasteur* **38,** 11 (1924).
73*d*. id., *C. R. Soc. Biol. (Paris)* **129,** 1049 (1938).
74. Schayer, R. W., Janoff, A., Zweifach, B. W.: *Amer. J. Physiol.* **204,** 369 (1963).
75. Schrader, W. H., Woolfrey, B. F. and Brunning, R. D.: *Amer. J. Path.* **44,** 597 (1964).
76. Schulhof, Ö. and Richter, A.: *Kisérl. Orvostud.* **11,** 496 (1959).
77*a*. Shwartzman, G.: *Proc. Soc. exp. Biol. (N.Y.)* **25,** 560 (1927–28).
77*b*. id., *Science* **76,** 127 (1932).
78. Shwartzman, G., Schneierson, S. S. and Soffer, L. J.: *Proc. Soc. exp. Biol. (N. Y.)* **75,** 175 (1950).
79. Smith, R. T. and Thomas, L.: *Proc. Soc. exp. Biol. (N. Y.)* **86,** 806 (1954).
80. Soffer, L. J., Shwartzman, G., Schneierson, S. S. and Gabrilove, J. L.: *Science* **111,** 303 (1950).
81. Starzl, T. E., Lerner, R. A., Dixon, F. J., Groth, C. G., Brettschneider, L. and Terasaki, P. I.: *New Engl. J. Med.* **278,** 642 (1968).
82*a*. Stetson, C. A.: *J. exp. Med.* **93,** 485 (1951).
82*b*. ibid., **93,** 489 (1951).
82*c*. ibid., **101,** 421 (1955).
82*d*. id., *Bact. Rev.* **25,** 457 (1961).
83. Stetson, C. A. and Good, R. A.: *J. exp. Med.* **93,** 49 (1951).
84. Szabó, E., Csongor, J., Csaba, B., Kocsár, L. and Kesztyűs, L.: *Acta microbiol. Acad. Sci. hung.* **8,** 275 (1961).
85. Szilágyi, T. and Damjanovich, S.: *Acta physiol. Acad. Sci. hung.* **24,** Supp. 11 (1963).
86. Szilágyi, T., Kiss, A. and Csaba, B.: *Acta physiol. Acad. Sci. hung.* **23,** 281 (1963).

87. Szilágyi, T., Kocsár, L. and Csernyánszky, H.: *Acta microbiol. Acad. Sci. hung.* **3,** 327 (1956).
88. Szilágyi, T., Tóth, S., Csernyánszky, H. and Sümegi, J.: *Kísérl. Orvostud.* **24,** 178 (1973).
89. Szilágyi, T., Tóth, S., Lévai, G. and Kassay, L.: *Acta microbiol. Acad. Sci. hung.* **15,** 229 (1968).
90. Szilágyi, T., Tóth, S., Miltényi, L. and Jóna, G.: *Acta microbiol. Acad. Sci. hung.* **15,** 5 (1968).
91. Szilágyi, T., Tóth, S., Muszbek, L., Lévai, G. and Laczkó, J.: *Acta microbiol. Acad. Sci. hung.* **15,** 331 (1968).
92. Taichman, N. S., Uriuhara, T. and Movat, H. Z.: *Lab. Invest.* **14,** 2160 (1966).
93. Thal, A. and Brackney, E.: *J. Amer. med. Ass.* **115,** 569 (1954).
94*a*. Thomas, L.: *J. exp Med.* **104,** 865 (1956).
94*b*. id., *Proc. Soc. exp. Biol. (N.Y.)* **115,** 235 (1964).
95*a*. Thomas, L. and Good, R. A.: *J. exp. Med.* **95,** 409 (1952).
95*b*. ibid., **96,** 605 (1952).
96. Thomas, L., Smith, R. T. and von Korff, R.: *J. exp. Med.* **102,** 263 (1955).
97. Tóth, S., Kassay, L., Barzó, E. and Szilágyi, T.: *Acta microbiol. Acad. Sci. hung.* **14,** 371 (1967).
98. Tóth, S., Lévai, G. and Szilágyi, T.: *Acta morphol. Acad. Sci. hung.* **19,** 123 (1971).
99. Tóth, S., Muszbek, L., Szilágyi, T. and Laczkó, J.: *Experientia (Basel)* **25,** 1085 (1969).
100. Tusch, E. and Moser, H.: *Z. Immun.-Forsch.* **108,** 89 (1950).
101. Uchitel, I. J. and Krimszki, L. D.: *Éksp. Khir.* **3,** 19 (1956).
102. Vrubel, J.: *Rev. Czech. Med.* **4,** 1 (1958).
103. Weissmann, G. and Thomas, L.: *J. exp. Med.* **116,** 433 (1962).
104. Wendt, F., Kappler, C., Bruckhardt, K. and Bohle, A.: *Proc. Soc. exp. Biol. (N. Y.)* **125,** 486 (1967).
105. Yamanaka, M.: *Jinsen Igaku* **8,** 293 (1958).
106. Zdrodowski, P. and Brenn, H.: *Zbl. Bakt. I. Abt.* Orig. **99,** 159 (1926).
107. Zweifach, B. W., Nagler, A. L. and Troll, W.: *J. exp. Med.* **113,** 437 (1961).

PART II

# FACTORS PARTICIPATING IN ANTIGEN–ANTIBODY REACTION

CHAPTER 7

# ANTIGEN (ALLERGEN)

by

L. KESZTYŰS and T. SZILÁGYI



## TERMINOLOGICAL CONSIDERATIONS

Allergens are substances which are capable of sensitizing man or higher animals and, combining with the antibodies of the sensitized organism, produce specific reactions. Therefore, allergens are substances which, upon getting into the organism, have both sensitizing and reaction producing abilities. It is obvious that the function of the allergen is identical with that of the anaphylactogen. The latter also displays sensitizing and shock-producing abilities under other experimental conditions. Undoubtedly, the function of the allergen and the anaphylactogen is identical in principle, and here we only deal with the transfer of the notion of antigen to a special area, that of allergic and anaphylactic diseases.

The above concept is frequently opposed—primarily by clinicians—the objections being as follows: In contrast to anaphylaxis, in allergic diseases it is often difficult to establish when and under what circumstances sensitization occurred, as sometimes the sensitizing and reaction producing agents are not the same; also, the way of entry of the allergen into the organism may have special significance; moreover, allergic symptoms may be produced sometimes also by psychological factors.

It would not be correct, however, to regard, on the basis of the above, allergen and anaphylactogen as completely different concepts. Naturally, the establishing of the circumstances of sensitization will be solved with the spread of more precise and specific diagnostic procedures. With regard to the difference between the sensitizing and provoking agents, we must refer to the fact that the role of the so-called cross-reaction and of determinant groups has been known for a long time. In relation to the way of entry of the allergen, we must stress that, irrespective of the route of introduction of the allergen into the organism, and of the symptoms produced, the basic pathogenic process is the production of antibodies and the reaction of these with the allergen. The so-called 'psychoallergies' have the same connection to allergen produced specific reactions as has the Pavlovian conditioned reflex, e.g. salivary secretion obtained through training, to the unconditioned reflex provoked by direct irritation of the oral mucous membrane [25].

It has been tried to make a distinction between allergens and antigens, maintaining that the concept of allergen is broader, and includes the antigen and many other substances with antigenic effects. This view was based on the fact that certain substances of simple chemical structure which, owing to their simple structures, are not called antigens in the immunological sense, proved to be allergenic in clinical practice, frequently producing sensitization and provoking reactions.

In connection with this, we must refer to the classical experiments of Obermayer and Pick [67] and to the concept of chemospecificity demonstrated by Landsteiner [54*b*], moreover to some most recent investigations to be described later. On the basis of these it is generally accepted today that substances of simple chemical structure may also act as allergens.

Consequently, we have no reason to differentiate between allergen, anaphylactogen, and antigen, but may use those expressions as synonyms. Thus all the knowledge about the antigens established by immunochemistry contributes significantly to the understanding of the allergic processes.

The aim of this chapter is to summarize briefly the most important information available on the structure and function of antigens.

## DEFINITION OF ANTIGEN

The term antigen was first used by the Hungarian author Deutsch (Detre) [26] and was in fact derived from the word 'antisomatogen'. The greatest difficulty in defining the antigen is due to the problem that no definition of validity based on chemical structure can be given. Antigens are substances producing immune response in living organisms (immunogenicity) and reacting specifically with the substance produced as a result of this response (specificity). Antibody production, generally, does not occur in the same individual in which the antigen arises, but in another organism, in which, under physiological conditions, the antigen is not to be found. In the organism containing the antigen under physiological conditions, it is not an antigen, but an immunologically neutral substance like any other chemical component of the organism. The concept of antigen is by no means absolute, i.e. substances having antigenic effect cannot be defined chemically as e.g. carbohydrates or fats. Antigen is a term applied to a functional concept: referring exclusively to the reaction of the organism in which it is present as a foreign substance. It is, however, a characteristic property of antibodies, the specific proteins formed in response to the introduction of antigens, that their molecular surface fits the molecular surface of the antigen, 'like key to the lock'.

On this basis, it is customary to distinguish between the two functions of antigen, i.e. between stimulation of antibody formation (productive antigenic function), and its ability to react with the produced antibodies (binding capacity). This distinction of antigenic functions is justified by the existence of the so-called semi-antigens, or haptens, which, in contrast to complete antigens, cannot in themselves stimulate antibody formation, but can react specifically with antibodies produced by stimulation with a complete antigen. In other words, haptens have only a binding capacity with no productive antigenic function.

To understand the concept of hapten, it should be realized that, in the reaction of the specific antibody with a complete antigen, only a small part of the surface of the antigen molecule, the so-called determinant group, takes part, so that the specificity of the antibody is not directed towards the whole antigen molecule, but only to its determinant group. The structure of haptens is the same as that of the determinant groups of the antigen and so they fit in with the antibody molecules formed upon antigenic stimulation. It has been shown recently that glucose [74], nucleosides [92], glycolipids [49] linked with synthetic antigens, produce antibodies which are hapten specific.

The concept of complete antigen and hapten is relative, and no clear distinction can be made between them. The protein-free capsular polysaccharides used in pneumococcal typing do not cause antibody formation in rabbit or guinea pig, but react specifically with antibodies formed in response to the effects of the complete bacterium. Thus, they have no productive antigenic function in rabbits or guinea pigs, but are capable of being bound, or, in other words, behave like haptens. Man or mouse, however, can be defended against the appropriate type of pneumococcus by immunization with protein-free capsular polysaccharides. Thus, in man or mouse, the purified, protein-free pneumococcal polysaccharide has also a productive antigenic function, i.e. behaves like a complete antigen; this may also be seen with many Salmonella polysaccharides [33, 60, 71].

The antigens may be not only exogenic, but also of endogenic origin. It has been known for a long time that animals will produce antibodies to extracts of their own lens [41]. Certain components of the nervous system, thyroid gland, testicles, and walls of the vessels, being outside the circulation, may become autoantigens, i.e. following their injection produce a humoral or cellular immune response [28, 50, 93*a*]. In response to certain effects, various cells, proteins, etc. may undergo such a change that they become foreign to the host organism (autoantigen transformation) and that they elicit the formation of antibodies. Chapter 11 in this volume deals with this question in more detail.

By administration of special doses of certain antigens the formation of specific antibodies may be arrested for shorter or longer periods. This is termed the tolerogenic function of antigens.

## PROTEIN STRUCTURE

Undoubtedly, the great majority of antigens (allergens) are proteins, or substances linked with proteins, so that a brief description of protein structure becomes necessary. In one of the groups of proteins the polypeptide chains are arranged in thread-like form and these are the so-called fibrous proteins. In the other group, the molecule is spherical or shaped like a rotating ellipsoid and these are known as globular proteins.

Primary protein structure relates to the number of contributing amino acids and the sequence of the amino acids linked to each other by peptide bonds. Secondary protein structure relates to the bonds between the parts of the polypeptide chain of the protein molecule, i.e. intramolecular bonds which stabilize the spatial arrangement of the molecule. These may be the following:

1. *Disulphide bridges.* For example, the SH groups of two cysteine residues each form an S—S bond following oxidation.

2. *Hydrogen bonds* are formed on the same peptide chain, or between neighbouring peptide chains between the —CO— and —NH— groups. As O contains an unbound electron pair, the H atomic nucleus is periodically attached to the N atom and the —CO— group in turn and thus joins two electronegative atoms (Fig. 7-1).

In contrast with peptide and disulphide bonds, hydrogen bonding is rather labile, but still has an important role in the maintenance of the particular three-dimensional structure of the proteins. It is more than likely that the reason for the denaturation of proteins by heat is due to the cleavage of hydrogen bonds. With respect to the forthcoming, it is also significant that e.g. concentrated solutions of guanidine or carbamide denature some proteins. The reason for this is that these chemicals rearrange the molecule, either by forming new hydrogen bonds, or by destroying the existing ones, without affecting the covalent bonds.

3. Native proteins consist of L-amino acids, and it is more than probable that the backbone of the polypeptide chain takes the form of a *helix* (Fig. 7-2). Pauling et al. [69] were the first to demonstrate that one loop of the helix was made up of 3.7 amino acid groups, and this accounts for approximately 5.4 Å in length; according to their hypothesis, this is the most frequently occurring, so-called *α-helix,* running along the surface of a polygonal column, and the single threads are stabilized by hydrogen bonds.

4. *Ionic* or *salt bonds* occur between the free carboxyl and free amino groups, at the end or along the chain, through polar connections. The dissociation relationships of the mentioned groups, and thus the strength and stability of the bonding between them, is, to a large extent, dependent on the pH. This will explain why certain proteins lose their original properties, the shape and structure of the molecules, as a result of rearrangement or alterations of the above bonds, when the pH is slightly altered.

5. It is probable that cohesive forces will appear also between the apolar amino acid side chains contributing to the structure and stability of the protein.

By the *tertiary* structure of proteins we mean the arrangement of the side chains in space and the coiling of the polypeptide chain. The geometrical arrangement of the secondary and tertiary structures gives the conformation of the protein molecule.

The term *quaternary* structure is used only in connection with larger protein molecules built up of two or more, already conforming polypeptide chains; the generally weak bonding of these subunits to each other gives the quaternary structure of the protein molecule.

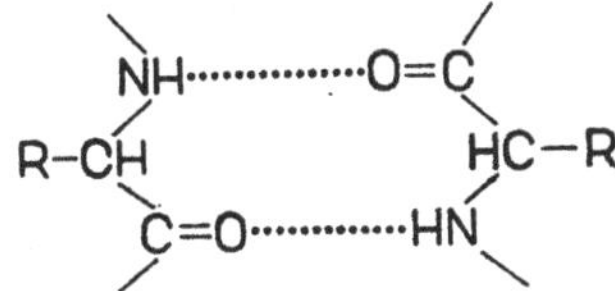


Fig. 7-1. Hydrogen bonding between adjacent —CO— and —NH— groups

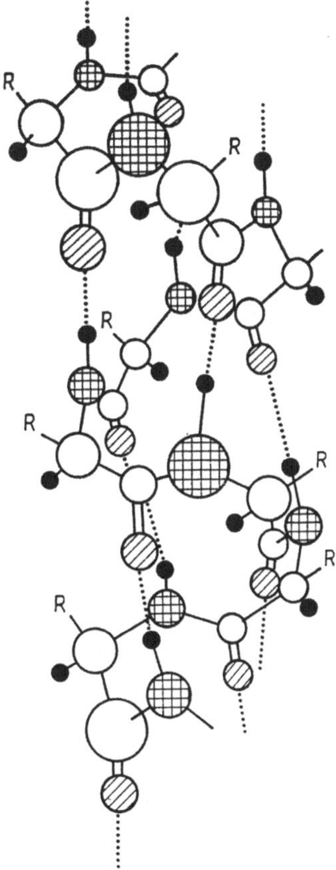


Fig. 7-2. The α-helix of proteins. Empty circles = C atoms; cross-hatched circles = O atoms; squared circles = N atoms; full circles = H atoms; dotted line = H bonding; R = side chain

## IMMUNOGENICITY AND MOLECULAR WEIGHT

Earlier, high molecular weight was regarded as an important criterion which, in general, was decisive from the point of view of antigenicity, but even at that time data contradicting to this concept were known. Thus, e.g. the molecular weights of serum albumin and haemoglobin are similar, but serum albumin is a strong antigen while this could hardly be said about haemoglobin. Gelatin with a molecular weight range between 40,000–80,000 is a weak antigen, while ovalbumin with a molecular weight of 40,000 can be classed among the strongest antigens. Subsequently, experiments showed that compounds with smaller molecular weights also displayed antibody producing ability. The molecular weight of clupein, produced from fish sperm, is 4,470; it is not antigenic for rabbits or guinea pigs, but linked with phenylisocyanate, gives rise to production of precipitins, though the molecular weight of the phenylisocyanate–clupein complex does not exceed 5,000 [4]. Pollen extracts prepared from plants belonging to the genus *Ambrosia*, despite molecular weights of around 4,500, proved to be a good antigen [73]. On the basis of these, the predominant view until the 1960s was that the molecular weight of immunogenic substances had a lowest limit at around 5,000.

In recent years more publications have appeared describing some substances of lower molecular weights, but exerting immunogenic effects. Abuelo and Óváry [1] described that trinitrophenyl-bacitracin-A (mol. wt. 1,928) caused antibody production in guinea pigs. The produced antibodies are specific only to the determinants. Berglund [13] found that human fibrinopeptide-B (mol. wt. about 1,400) is not an antigen in rabbits, but if adsorbed onto methylmethacrylate particles (0.6 $\mu$ dia.) and injected together with incomplete Freund's adjuvant, antibodies could be demonstrated in the rabbit's serum by means of the gel diffusion technique. The antibody did not react either with fibrinogen, or with the acrylate particles.

Experiments using the synthetic aspartylamide valyl$_5$-angiotensin II (Hypertensin®, Ciba) have shown [27] that the linkage of angiotensin to carrier proteins is not a prerequisite of its immunogenicity. The free octapeptide, injected either with adjuvant, or in a salt solution, is capable of sensitizing a guinea pig. The molecular weight of the octapeptide is 1,031. This result is interesting and important, because angiotensin II is a physiologically active substance. Furthermore, the synthetic oxytocin, consisting of eight amino acids, also proved to be antigenic in rabbits [38].

The preparation of synthetic polypeptides made it possible to clarify the role of the molecular size from the point of view of immunogenicity. Sela et al. [81] reported that a linear copolymer of tyrosine, glutamic acid and of alanine (mol. wt. approx. 4,000) exerted an immunogenic effect in rabbits. Schlossman et al. [77] ascertained this with $\alpha$-2-4-dinitrophenyl-hepta-L-lysine (mol. wt. 1,080); *p*-azobenzenearsonate-hexa-L-tyrosine (mol. wt. approx. 1,200) gave rise to antibody production in guinea pig [15*a*] and rabbit [15*b*]. At present, azobenzenearsonate-N-acetyl-D-tyrosine (mol. wt. 451) [58], and azobenzenearsonate-N-acetyl-L-tyrosine amide (mol. wt. 450) [15*a*] are the synthetic polypeptides with smallest molecular weights, still having immunogenic and sensitizing effect in the guinea pig.

It became obvious that many low molecular weight substances can produce long lasting and specific delayed-type hypersensitivity in guinea pigs, as, e.g. neoarsphenamine (mol. wt. 466) [34], nitrohexenes (mol. wt. 129) [51]. Baer et al. [10] established that alkylcatecholes (mol. wt. between 120 and 130) regardless of the position of the alkyl group in the ring, bring about a delayed-type contact hypersensitivity in guinea pigs. The introduction of a carboxyl group either into the ring or into the side chain prevents the sensitizing ability of catecholes.

In relation to the described experiments, the question obviously arises whether the chemicals used are linked to the host animal's proteins and thus they are indirect and not *per se* immunogenic substances. Undoubtedly, no uniform answer can yet be given to this question. Despite all these, we must state that the molecular size has no decisive role in immunogenicity, and it is determined by other factors.

## INVESTIGATION OF THE ANTIGENIC DETERMINANT

Several methods have been used to determine what part of the proteins, i.e. substances with antigenic nature, are responsible for immunogenicity. The oldest method is the chemical alteration of the antigen, to see how its alterations will affect the immunological reactivity. Later, the effects of linking polyamino acids to proteins were studied with respect to immunogenic property. Recently, the immunogenicity and determinant characteristics of synthetic polypeptides composed of several amino acids have been investigated. A valuable and important method is the splitting of the antigen and examination of its active fragments. With reference to the above, we speak today of natural, artificial and synthetic antigens.

## CHEMICALLY ALTERED ANTIGENS

Obermayer and Pick [67] showed that nitric acid treated proteins (xanthoproteins) or iodinated proteins, do not react any more with antibodies, which were produced by immunization with the original protein. Nevertheless, these chemically altered proteins retain their antigenic function; when given parenterally, they will elicit the production of antibodies reacting with the xanthoproteins and iodinated proteins of all animal species, and even with those of plants. Thus instead of species specificity, chemospecificity has been produced as a consequence of chemical intervention. This obviously occurs because the determinant groups responsible for the species specificity of the protein molecule, were pushed to the background, or were destroyed through the chemical manipulation, and by substitution different specificity determining groups were introduced into the protein molecule.

The experimental examination of chemospecificity became possible when Ehrlich [29] demonstrated that diazo compounds react with proteins while pigment is being formed. Pauly [70], on the other hand, established that the diazo compounds are linked to the tyrosine and histidine groups of the protein molecule. Following these preliminaries, Landsteiner [54*b*] linked the most varied diazo compounds to different proteins and established that immunization with these azoprotein compounds results in the production of antibodies which are not species specific, i.e. do not react with the original proteins, though precipitating with proteins of any origin, which contain the same diazo radical. In these cases, the determinant group responsible for the species specificity of the protein is repressed as a result of the combination, and the antigenicity of the azoprotein is determined by the simple diazo radical attached to the protein. Thus, e.g. he linked ortho-, meta-, and para-aminophenylsulphonic acid to horse serum protein. These artificial antigens produced such antibodies which precipitated only with the homologous antigen. In similar experiments, the *cis* and *trans* bondings, the D and L isomers could also be differentiated (Fig. 7-3).

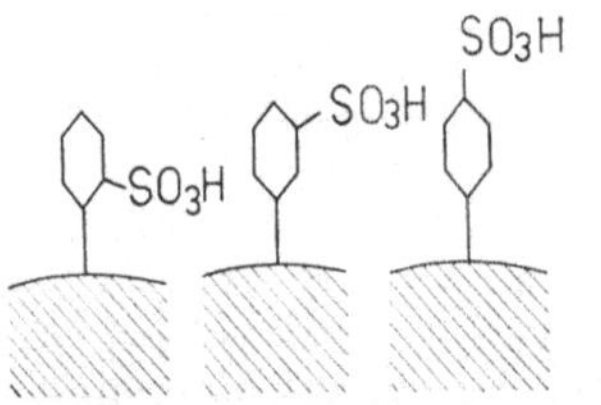

$SO_3H$ $SO_3H$ $SO_3H$

Fig. 7-3. Determinant groups of azoproteins: *o*-aminophenylsulphonic acid (left); *m*-aminophenylsulphonic acid (centre); *p*-aminophenylsulphonic acid (right)

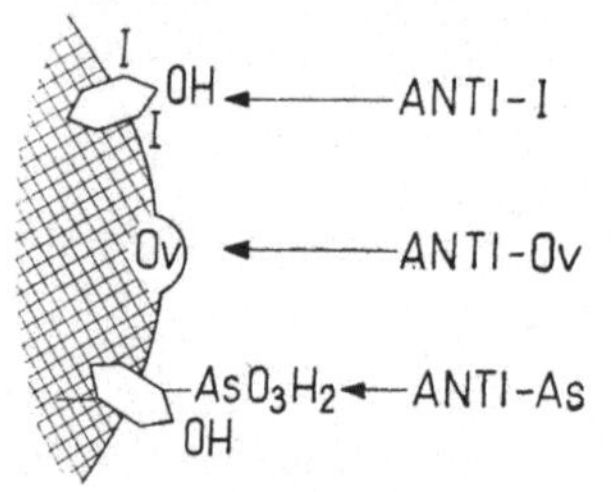

I OH ← ANTI-I
I
Ov ← ANTI-Ov
$AsO_3H_2$ ← ANTI-As
OH

Fig. 7-4. Determinant groups of a conjugated antigen: iodinated tyrosine (above); ovalbumin (species specific group) (centre); aminophenylarsonic acid (below)

With the repeated parenteral introduction of some azoprotein compounds, immune sera may be produced which will, on the one hand, react with the original protein, but on the other, also with the azo compounds of heterologous proteins. Therefore, in these cases chemospecificity was developed, without the repression of species specificity; this might be explained by the fact that the diazo compound containing the new determinant group was bound by leaving the original, species specific determinant group intact, which, therefore, retains its prominent role (Fig. 7-4).

The significance of these diazotized, chemospecific proteins—also called 'complete antigens'—is unusually great, particularly from the point of view of clinical allergology· These model experiments clearly demonstrate that even the most simple chemical substance can be linked with the organism's own proteins. As a results, new determinant groups may arise which will alter the organism's own proteins into chemospecific antigens, which will become foreign to the organism and thus may elicit the production of antibodies directed against the simple chemical compounds and reacting specifically with them.

With the chemical alterations of the antigen valuable observations can be made concerning the role played by single atomic groups in the *in vitro* (precipitation, haemagglutination, complement fixation) and *in vivo* (passive cutaneous anaphylaxis, systemic anaphylaxis) immunological reactions. From this point of view, bovine serum albumin was studied most extensively. Marrack and Orlans [63] had previously established that the amino groups do not play a significant role in reactions with antibodies. The ability to precipitate bovine serum albumin is only slightly diminished by deamination, by guanidine treatment [83] and by acetylation. In contrast, the ability to precipitate the protein is completely lost with succination of the amino groups [66] and with their carboxymethylation [65].

Similarly to horse serum albumin, the phenol groups and the only sulph-hydryl group of bovine serum albumin [88] play no significant role in the reaction with the antibody [89*a*]. The results obtained with esterification of the carboxyl group are very interesting and important [89*b*]. It became apparent that bovine serum albumin esterified in 55–60 per cent does not precipitate with antibodies; though soluble antigen–antibody complexes are formed which fix complement and produce a positive passive cutaneous reaction in guinea pigs. In addition, the antigen regains its precipitating capacity with de-esterification.

## POLYPEPTIDYL PROTEINS

Two objections arise in connection with the above described method of chemical alteration of the antigen, and particularly with the linkage with diazo compounds. One is that all kinds of interference alter the structure of the native protein, and the other is that the compounds bound to proteins are not physiological ones. The method of Becker and Stahmann [12] made it possible to bind large amounts of amino acids and peptides to native proteins. Glycine molecules were attached to bovine serum albumin (mol. wt. 69,000) [62] by this method; in fact, ten times more glycine than contained in the protein originally, and so the molecular weight of the modified protein became approx. 81,000. Chickens were immunized with native and modified protein and it was found that the considerable amount of glycine bound to the surface of bovine serum albumin had only a little quantitative effect on immunogenicity. Subsequently, polypeptides of glutamic acid, lysine, leucine or phenylalanine were bound to bovine serum albumin and rabbits were immunized with these [90]. Three different types of antibodies arose: the first one reacted with the polypeptide, the second one with the carrier protein, and the third one with the polyleucyl and polyphenylalanyl polypeptide and with small part of the carrier protein. The latter is the so-called 'antibonding' antibody. It is quite interesting that the polyleucyl and the polyphenylalanyl rabbit serum albumin has an immunogenic effect in the rabbit itself. In fact, two types of antibodies were produced against this modified albumin: one was toward the polypeptidyl group, the other one was toward the polypeptidyl group plus a part of the rabbit serum albumin; no antibody was produced toward the carrier protein, i.e. against the rabbit's own serum albumin [18].

From these experiments, two important conclusions can be drawn. One is that the various polypeptides can weaken the antigenic property and, from this point of view, the length of the polypeptide chain is more important than the number of polypeptide chains; the other is that the polypeptides can alter the organism's own proteins rendering them antigenic.

Schechter and Sela [76] bound poly-DL-alanine to human and bovine serum albumin and to ribonuclease. The produced antibodies reacted with poly-DL-alanyl as well as with poly-D-alanyl rabbit sera. The homologous reaction could be prevented by as few as four D-alanine tetrapeptides, however, the tetra-L-alanine was completely ineffective. Experiments in which poly-L-, poly-D-, and poly-DL-alanyl bovine serum albumin [75] were used, have shown that the peptides of alanine prevent the homologous reaction and, in this context, the dimers are only slightly, while the pentamers are considerably effective. The antibodies showed marked stereospecificity.

Gelatin was considered for a long time to be a compound having no antigenic properties; later, however, the opinion arose that it is in fact an antigen, but with only a slight immunogenic affect [64]. Cluttonet al. [24] had stated as early as in 1938 that the linking of $o$-$\beta$-glucosido-N-carboxytyrosine to gelatin caused significant antibody formation. Polypeptidyl chains were used in the clarification of this question, too. In guinea pigs sensitized with polytyrosyl gelatin, a characteristic anaphylactic shock was produced by intracardial injection [78]. Polytyrosyl, polytryptophyl, polyphenylalanyl and, to a certain extent, polycysticyl derivatives of gelatin are, in general, powerful antigens; but, polyglutamyl, polysyl and polyalanyl chains do not increase the immunogenic effect of gelatin considerably [79*a*]. Furthermore, the D-tyrosine peptides—similarly to the L-tyrosine peptides—increase the immunogenicity of gelatin [80]. The produced antibodies react fairly specifically with homologous antigens. Later it also became apparent that in addition to the aromatic amino acids, e.g. prepared by hydrogenation of the aromatic ring of phenylalanine could also enhance the immunogenicity of gelatin [79*b*].

It is interesting that peptidization can alter also the solubility properties of proteins. Thus e.g. combining poly-DL-alanine with gliadin makes the latter water soluble [82].

## SYNTHETIC POLYPEPTIDE ANTIGENS

Ivanovics [43], and Ivanovics and Bruckner showed [44] that the immunospecificity of *Bacillus anthracis* was due to the polyglutamic acid isolated from the capsule. The synthesized poly-$\gamma$-D-glutamic acid [17] may be regarded as the first synthetic hapten. In fact, these experiments were the forerunners of the period of synthetic antigens.

Synthetic polypeptides may be:

*Homopolymers*: linear polymers of the same $\alpha$-amino acid (Fig. 7-5, I).

*Copolymers*: the common polymers of two or more amino acids; the amino acids are arranged in a random sequence (Fig. 7-5, II) or following each other in regularly recurring order (Fig. 7-5, III).

*Multichain polyamino acids*: amino acid polypeptide chains attached to the free amino groups of linear homopolymers (Fig. 7-5, IV).

Buchanan-Davidson et al. [19, 20] were the first to examine in detail the immunogenicity of synthetic polypeptides. They prepared numerous linear L-polypeptides; polyglutamic acids of varying molecular weights were used as acidic polymers, various polylysines represented the basic polymers, while neutral polyleucine, polyphenylalanine, and polyproline were also used. They immunized rabbits, guinea pigs, chickens and mice, but a measurable amount of precipitating antibody appeared only to one polyglutamic acid preparation. It is interesting that, with some synthetic homopolymers, antibodies were produced which precipitated the native and modified bovine serum albumins and fibrinogen; homologous synthetic polypeptides failed to prevent the precipitation. Passive anaphylaxis could also be more readily produced with the proteins mentioned than with the homologous synthetic polypeptides. Although poly-L-glutamic acid and poly-L-lysine are not immunogenic in rabbits, when applied separately, given together with complete Freund's adjuvant, they elicited moderate antibody formation [35]. In addition, the polylysine—similarly to other strongly positively charged polymers—causes a non-specific precipitation with the serum [7] and fixes complement [5]. Poly-L-proline (mol. wt. 17,000) is an effective antigen in guinea pig, unlike in rabbits, when given with Freund's adjuvant [39*a*, 48].

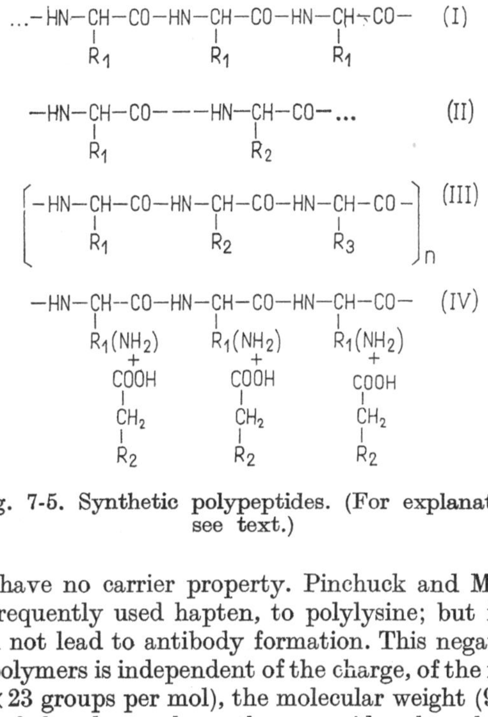

$$\ldots\text{–HN–}\underset{\substack{|\\R_1}}{\text{CH}}\text{–CO–HN–}\underset{\substack{|\\R_1}}{\text{CH}}\text{–CO–HN–}\underset{\substack{|\\R_1}}{\text{CH}}\text{–CO–} \qquad \text{(I)}$$

$$\text{–HN–}\underset{\substack{|\\R_1}}{\text{CH}}\text{–CO– – –HN–}\underset{\substack{|\\R_2}}{\text{CH}}\text{–CO–}\ldots \qquad \text{(II)}$$

$$\left[\text{–HN–}\underset{\substack{|\\R_1}}{\text{CH}}\text{–CO–HN–}\underset{\substack{|\\R_2}}{\text{CH}}\text{–CO–HN–}\underset{\substack{|\\R_3}}{\text{CH}}\text{–CO–}\right]_n \qquad \text{(III)}$$

$$\text{–HN–}\underset{\substack{|\\R_1(NH_2)\\+\\COOH\\|\\CH_2\\|\\R_2}}{\text{CH}}\text{–CO–HN–}\underset{\substack{|\\R_1(NH_2)\\+\\COOH\\|\\CH_2\\|\\R_2}}{\text{CH}}\text{–CO–HN–}\underset{\substack{|\\R_1(NH_2)\\+\\COOH\\|\\CH_2\\|\\R_2}}{\text{CH}}\text{–CO–} \qquad \text{(IV)}$$

Fig. 7-5. Synthetic polypeptides. (For explanation see text.)

Homopolymers have no carrier property. Pinchuck and Maurer [72*b*] linked dinitrophenyl, a frequently used hapten, to polylysine; but immunization with the compound did not lead to antibody formation. This negative hapten carrier property of homopolymers is independent of the charge, of the numbers of dinitrophenyl groups ($3\times 23$ groups per mol), the molecular weight (92,000) and solubility. On the basis of the above, the authors consider that the 'Schlepper' itself must have an immunogenic effect. Recent experiments have verified this opinion [40]. As it was seen previously [76], homopolymers linked to protein carriers behave like haptens.

Unlike homopolymers, copolymers containing two amino acids have an immunogenic effect in rabbits and in guinea pigs. Particularly effective are the copolymers produced between glutamic acid and alanine (e.g. $Ala_{30}Glu_{70}$) and between glutamic acid and lysine (e.g. $Glu_{59}Lys_{41}$). The mouse gives no immune response to dipolymers, but reacts well with terpolymers (e.g. $Glu_{58}Lys_{38}Phe_4$; $Glu_{60}Ala_{30}Tyr_{10}$); the third amino acid may be of any kind and is effective even at a concentration of 4 M% [72*a*]. Terpolymers are thus excellent carriers [72*b*].

It is well known that higher animals can use only the L-amino acids for synthesis; therefore the experiments using polypeptides synthesized exclusively from D-amino acids aroused considerable interest. In the beginning, the investigations failed to yield any results, but in 1964 Gill et al. [37] announced that poly-$DGlu_{55}DLys_{39}DTyr_{6}$ showed immunogenic effects in the rabbit. Janeway and Sela [47] established using 247, *p*(DTyr, DGlu, DAla) (mol. wt. 19,700) that the antibodies produced in mice were strongly stereospecific, and further, that the D-isomer was about 50–1,000 times more effective from the point of view of immune paralysis, than its corresponding L-isomer. The paralysis, in addition, was also specific. Another interesting observation is that the degradation of the D-polymer occurs about 24 times more slowly than that of the L-form, and that

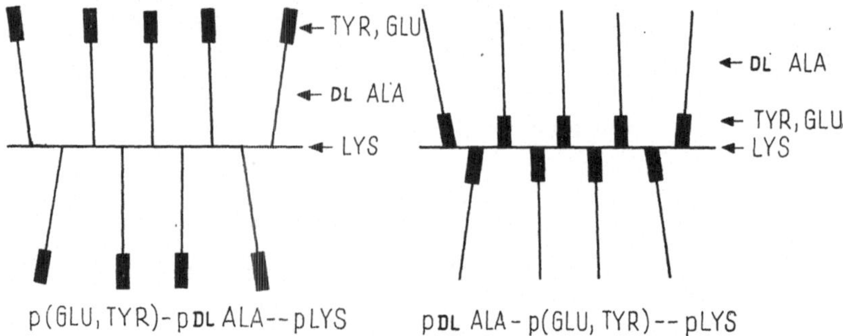


Fig. 7-6. Multichain copolymers. (For explanation see text.) (After Sela, M.: *Adv. Immunol.* **5**, 30, 1966)

a part of the D-polymer is excreted in the urine in an unaltered form; moreover, that the D-polymer accumulates exclusively in the macrophages and does not reach the germinal centres [46]. Janeway [45] demonstrated that a secondary response can also be produced with the D-polymers; the prerequisites for this are (*i*) that the mice must be immunized with small quantities of D-amino acid polypeptides; (*ii*) that a long time interval must elapse between the first and second antigen stimuli.

Sela et al. [82] verified in their experiments with multichain copolymers the significance of the accessibility of the immunologically important parts. To a poly-L-lysine backbone they linked a poly-DL-alanyl side chain which was lengthened with either L-tyrosine or L-glutamic acid (Fig. 7-6). The compounds had pronounced immunogenic effects. If the side chains were reversed, and by this way, the DL-alanyl chain became situated on the outer side, while the tyrosine and glutamic acid to the less accessible parts, the new compound had no immunogenic property at all.

## PARTIAL BREAKDOWN OF THE PROTEIN ANTIGENS

A well-known method for investigating the specific polar groups on proteins is their partial degradation. Depending upon the size of the fragments, various tests may be applied, thus, e.g. *in vitro* tests: precipitation, immunoelectrophoresis, complement fixation, and examination of the fragment's inhibiting effect on antigen–antibody reactions; *in vivo* production or prevention of systematic anaphylaxis and passive cutaneous anaphylaxis, by the fragment being examined. The first investigations of this kind were performed by Landsteiner and Chase [55]. The protein which was investigated in greatest detail was silk fibroin; Landsteiner [53] demonstrated that the fragments obtained by partial acidic hydrolysis, have an inhibitory effect. They established [23] that the octapeptide constituted by Gly ($Gly_3Ala_3$) Tyr already has a pronounced inhibitory action on the silk fibroin–antibody reaction, and that the dodekapeptide fraction was the most effective in this respect. These experiments are also interesting because no smaller, similarly well-defined molecule could be isolated during the breakdown of any protein. Of course, similar experiments involving many other proteins have also been performed. The most significant among these is the fractionation of human serum albumin. By digesting with chymotrypsin two antigen determinants, whereas with pepsin and rabbit spleen extract, three different determinants were obtained [57].

Recently, a tyrosine- and tryptophan-free fragment of 6,600 molecular weight was prepared and used to immunize rabbits. The antibodies produced agglutinated red cells sensitized with both the fragment and complete human serum albumin [56]. These experiments also verify that a peptide of relatively small molecular weight can also elicit antibody production; that tyrosine and tryptophan are not necessary for immunogenicity; and that antibodies formed against a fragment holding only one of the determinant groups may react—under certain circumstances—with the complete molecule.

These experiments also show that in some antigens 'hidden' antigenic determinants may be present [11]. Naturally, the question arises whether these internal antigenic determinants behave in a similar way *in vivo* as they do *in vitro* in the course of digestion [42].

## THE ROLE OF OTHER FACTORS IN IMMUNOGENICITY

It has a great importance in immunogenicity of antigens whether they are suitable for resorption and decomposition. Substances which are poorly or barely absorbed are weak antigens. Collagen fibrils, which are practically insoluble, barely have any immunogenic effect, however, when introduced in soluble form, they elicit antibody formation [91].

A number of observations suggest that the decomposition of the antigen in the immunized animal is an important factor regulating the beginning of antibody production. Substances which are decomposed extremely fast in the organism, are not immunogenic and, likewise, the 'non-digestible' substances fail to give rise to antibody production. Thus, e.g. the naturally occurring gum acacia, or the artificially produced polyvinylpyrrolidone, which hardly undergo any change in the tissues of the organism, are not antigens [21]. The weak immunogenicity of polymers consisting exclusively of D-amino acids may be explained partly by their hard digestibility [46]. According to some experiments [30, 31], in order to produce an immune response, antigens must be incorporated by macrophages and also the antigen or antigen fragment must form a complex with a low molecular weight ribonucleic acid. Treatment with ribonuclease prevents this biological effect of ribonucleic acid, and antibody formation does not occur. Recently, it has been shown that antimacrophage serum diminishes the phagocytic activity of peritoneal macrophages of mice and has a marked immunosuppressive effect [3]. The non-fragmentable foreign molecules are non-antigenic [22], because these block ribonucleic acid completely; this may have two consequences: either a failure of antibody production, or immunological paralysis. On the contrary, antigen fragments of sizes corresponding to the determinants, form complexes with ribonucleic acid and elicit antibody production.

Maurer [64*b*] immunized 120 guinea pigs of the Hartley strain with $Glu_{60}Lys_{40}$ antigen; 57 animals showed no response at all. Others [53] found that a significant number of the treated guinea pigs reacted neither with dinitrophenylpolylysine, nor with $Glu_{60}Lys_{40}$.

From experiments performed with hapten–polylysine conjugates it became obvious that the ability of guinea pigs to give an immune response, is determined by genetic factors and is inherited as a dominant trait [59]. Experiments on mice have shown that a determinant-specific genetic control is also possible [66*a*], e.g. the responders became non-responders, and *vice versa* [61] following the replacement of tyrosine with histidine in a synthetic antigen. Recently, it has been shown [32] that mice which were non-responsive to poly-L-lysine conjugates, and to copolymers of 2,4-dinitrophenyl-L-glutamic acid-L-lysine became responders if the bone marrow, lymph nodes or spleen cells were transplanted from another, responding animal.

Although, it has been described recently that the immune response to bovine serum albumin [85] and to insulin [8] may also be under genetic control, this situation is quite infrequent in relation to the naturally occurring protein antigens. The different behaviour of native and synthetic antigens is explained by the fact that while the native protein antigens have numerous determinant groups, synthetic antigens have only one or a few determinant groups, and are therefore suitable for investigating the phenomenon of genetic control.

Up to 1956 it had been thought that immunoglobulins are isotype specific, i.e. are uniform within individual members of the same species. Oudin [68] first showed in rabbits, and then Grubb [39] in man, that genetically controlled antigens may be present on the surface of the IgG molecule, i.e. the immunoglobulins are allotype specific and can be different in various members of the same species (see Chapter 13). This allotype property, however, involves the possibility of allergization following treatment with immunoglobulins.

The role of electrical charge in antigenicity and in antigen–antibody reactions was emphasized by Landsteiner [54*b*]. Sela and Fuchs [80] investigated this problem in detail; they used synthetic antigens containing atomic groups with positive or negative charge or having no charge at all. They reached the conclusion that an electrical charge is not always necessary for immunogenicity.

Recently, the possibility has arisen that besides (or even above) the primary structure, the conformation of the molecule may have great significance in immunogenicity. There is no doubt that different chemical modifications of the secondary and tertiary structures—as could be seen—frequently have no effect on immunogenicity. Experiments performed with synthetic antigens, have also proved that the helical form of the molecule or whether it contains a helix do not determine the immunogenicity of the antigen [36]. However, there are observations pointing to the importance of conformation. Berson and Yalow [14] used pork and whale insulin in their experiments as the primary structure of the two insulins is identical. They experienced that there are such human antisera which are clearly 'able to distinguish between the two insulins'. The authors regarded the different conformations of the two insulin molecules as an explanation of this phenomenon. Arnon and Sela [6] bound the amino acid group from positions 57–83 on the lysozyme obtained from egg white, to poly-DL-alanine; cysteine residues at positions 64 and 80 are linked by disulphide bridges in this fragment. They established that immunization with these compounds produced such antibodies which were directed against the conformation dependent determinant groups.

Experiments performed with ribonuclease [16], myoglobin [9], tobacco mosaic virus [2], and bradykinin [86], support the significance of conformation. Current investigations prove that molecular conformation influences not so much the immunogenicity, but rather the specificity of the antigen (the so-called immunodominant group) and the antigen–antibody reaction [84].

## CARBOHYDRATES AS ANTIGENS

Carbohydrates play an essential role in the antigenicity of glycoproteins and lipopolysaccharides, and primarily, in the determination of the specificity of the antigen. Thus, e.g. the specificity of the blood group substance A would be determined by N-acetylgalactosamine, that of group B by D-galactose, and of group O (H) by fucose. The frequent occurrence of the heterophil antigens is also explained by the presence of identical or similar, generally small immunodominant carbohydrate groups. Springer et al. [87] reviewed the activity of 282 Gram negative bacteria on blood groups; in response to the bacteria, high titres—primarily of anti-O (H) and anti-B antibodies—were formed.

It has been well known for a long time that certain pure polysaccharides display immunogenic properties and elicit antibody formation, in man and mouse, but not in rabbits and guinea pigs, whose reacting ability to protein antigens is very good. Pneumococci may be subdivided into more than 80 types on the basis of their capsular polysaccharides. The formation of the various capsular polysaccharides is under genetic control. Recently, dextran and laevan have come to the forefront of interest in immunological research. The dextran produced by bacterial enzymes is exclusively glucose, laevan is exclusively a fructose polymer. The linking of carbon atoms in dextran may be: $1 \rightarrow 6$ (isomaltose), $1 \rightarrow 4$ (maltose), $1 \rightarrow 8$ (nigerose), $1 \rightarrow 2$ (kojibiose). Native dextran (doubtful) has a molecular weight of several millions, but this may be degraded by weak acidic hydrolysis. The molecular weight of 'clinical dextran' is about 75,000 ($\pm$25,000). Due to these properties, dextran is very suitable for investigating antigenic determinants and antigen–antibody reactions [52].

## REFERENCES

1. Abuelo, J. G. and Óváry, Z.: *J. Immunol.* **95,** 113 (1965).
2. Anderer, F. A.: *Z. Naturforsch.* **18b,** 1010 (1963).
3. Argyris, B. F. and Plotkin, D. H.: *J. Immunol.* **103,** 372 (1969).

4. Armangué, M., Novel, E. and Dedie, O.: *Z. Path. Bakter.* **7,** 505 (1944).
5. Arnon, R., Levinhar, H. and Sela, M.: *Israel J. Med. Sci.* **1,** 404 (1965).
6. Arnon, R. and Sela, M.: *Proc. nat. Acad. Sci. (Wash.)* **62,** 163 (1969).
7. Arnon, R., Sela, M., Yaron, A. and Sober, H. A.: *Biochemistry* **4,** 948 (1965).
8. Arquilla, E. R. and Finn, J.: *J. exp. Med.* **122,** 771 (1965).
9. Atassi, M. Z. and Caruso, D. R.: *Biochemistry* **7,** 699 (1968).
10. Baer, H., Watkins, R. C. and Bowser, R. T.: *Immunochemistry* **3,** 479 (1966).
11. Bartel, A. H. and Campbell, D. H.: *Arch. Biochem.* **82,** 94 (1959).
12. Becker, R. R. and Stahman, M. A.: *J. biol. Chem.* **204,** 745 (1953).
13. Berglund, G.: *Nature* **206,** 523 (1965).
14. Berson, S. A. and Yalow, R. S.: *Nature* **191,** 1392 (1961).
15. Borek, F., Stupp, Y. and Sela, M.: *Science* **150,** 1177 (1965).
16. Brown, R. K.: *Ann. N. Y. Acad. Sci.* **81,** 524 (1959).
17. Bruckner, V., Weiss, J., Kajtár, M. and Kovács, J.: *Naturwissenschaften* **42,** 463 (1955).
18. Buchanan-Davidson, D. J., Dellert, E. E., Kornguth, S. E. and Stahmann, M. J.: *J. Immunol.* **83,** 543 (1959).
19. Buchanan-Davidson, D. J., Stahmann, M. A. and Dellert, E. E.: *J. Immunol.* **83,** 561 (1959).
20. Buchanan-Davidson, D. J., Stahmann, M. A., Lapresle, C. and Grabar, P.: *J. Immunol.* **83,** 552 (1959).
21. Campbell, D. H.: *Blood* **72,** 589 (1957).
22. Campbell, D. H. and Garvey, J. S.: *Advanc. Immunol.* **3,** 261 (1963).
23. Cebra, J. J.: *J. Immunol.* **86,** 205 (1961).
24. Clutton, R. F., Harington, C. R. and Yuill, M. E.: *Biochem. J.* **32,** 1111 (1938).
25. Dale, H. H.: *Harvey Lectures.* Williams and Wilkins, Baltimore. 1936, p. 220.
26. Deutsch, L. *Ann. Inst. Pasteur* 710 (1899).
27. Dietrich, F. M.: *Int. Arch. Allergy* **30,** 497 (1966).
28. Ehrlich, G., Halbert, S. P. and Manski, W.: *J. Immunol.* **89,** 391 (1962).
29. Ehrlich, P.: *Z. Klin. Med.* **5,** 285 (1882).
30. Fishman, M.: *J. exp. Med.* **114,** 837 (1961).
31. Fishman, M. and Adler, F. L.: *J. exp. Med.* **117,** 595 (1963).
32. Foerster, J., Green, I., Lamelin, J.-P. and Benacerraf, B.: *J. exp. Med.* **130,** 1107 (1969).
33. Francis, T. and Tillett, W. S.: *J. exp. Med.* **52,** 573 (1930).
34. Frey, J. R., De Weck, A. L. and Geleick, H.: *Int. Arch. Allergy* **30,** 288 (1966).
35. Gill, T. J. III and Doty, P.: *Biochim. biophys. Acta (Amst.)* **60,** 450 (1962).
36. Gill, T. J. III., Kunz, H. W., Friedman, E. and Doty, P.: *J. biol. Chem.* **238,** 108 (1963).
37. Gill, T. J. III., Kunz, H. W., Gould, H. J. and Doty, P.: *J. biol. Chem.* **239,** 1107 (1964).
38. Gilliland, P. F. and Prout, T. E.: *Metabolism* **14,** 918 (1965).
39. Grubb, R.: *Acta path. microbiol. scand.* **39,** 195 (1956).
39*a*. Gurari, D., Ungar-Waron, H. and Sela, M.: *Eur. J. Immunol.* **3,** 196 (1973).
40. Havas, H. F.: *Immunology* **17,** 819 (1969).
41. Hektoen, L.: *J. infect. Dis.* **31,** 72 (1922).
42. Ishizaka, T., Campbell, D. H. and Ishizaka, K.: *Proc. Soc. exp. Biol. (N.Y.)* **103,** 5 (1960).
43. Ivanovics, G.: *Zbl. Bakteriol. Parasitenk.* **138,** 211 (1937).
44. Ivanovics, G. and Bruckner, V.: *Z. Immun. Forsch.* **91,** 175 (1937).
45. Janeway, C. A.: *Immunology* **17,** 715 (1969).
46. Janeway, C. A. and Humphrey, J. H.: *Immunology* **14,** 225 (1968).
47. Janeway, C. A. and Sela, M.: *Immunology* **13,** 29 (1967).
48. Jasin, H. E. and Glynn, L. E.: *Immunology* **8,** 95 (1965).
49. Jaton, J.-C. and Ungar-Waron, H.: *Arch. Biochem.* **122,** 157 (1967).
50. Jones, H. E. H. and Roitt, I. M.: *Brit. J. exp. Path.* **42,** 546 (1961).
51. Josephson, A. S.: *J. Immunol.* **96,** 699 (1966).
52. Kabat, E. A.: *J. Immunol.* **97,** 1 (1966).
53. Kantor, F. S., Ojeda, A. and Benacerraf, B.: *J. exp. Med.* **117,** 55 (1963).
54*a*. Landsteiner, K.: *J. exp. Med.* **75,** 269 (1942).

54b. id., *The Specificity of Serological Reactions*. Harvard Univ. Press, Cambridge 1947.
55. Landsteiner, K. and Chase, M. W.: *Proc. Soc. exp. Biol. (N.Y.)* **30,** 1413 (1933).
56. Lapresle, C. and Goldstein, I. J.: *J. Immunol.* **102,** 753 (1969).
57. Lapresle, C., Kaminski, M. and Tanner, C. E.: *J. Immunol.* **82,** 94 (1959).
58. Leskowitz, S., Jones, V. E. and Zak, S. J.: *J. exp. Med.* **123,** 229 (1966).
59. Levine, B. B., Ojeda, A. and Benacerraf, B.: *J. exp. Med.* **118,** 953 (1963).
60. Mac Leod, C. M., Hoodges, R. G., Heidelberger, M. and Bernhard, W. G.: *J. exp. Med.* **82,** 445 (1945).
61. McDevitt, H. O. and Sela, M.: *J. exp. Med.* **122,** 517 (1965).
62. Makinodan, T., Becker, R. R., Wolfe, R. and Stahmann, M. A.: *J. Immunol.* **73,** 159 (1954).
63. Marrack, J. R. and Orlans, E. S.: *Brit. J. exp. Path.* **35,** 28 (1954).
64a. Maurer, P. H.: *J. exp. Med.* **100,** 515 (1954).
64b. id., *Progr. Allerg.* **8,** 1 (1964).
65. Maurer, P. H. and Korman, S.: *Arch. Biochem.* **67,** 145 (1957).
66. Maurer, P. H. and Lebovitz, H.: *J. Immunol.* **76,** 335 (1954).
66a. Mozes, E., Sela, M. and McDeritt, H. O.: *Eur. J. Immunol.* **3,** 1 (1973).
67. Obermayer, F. and Pick, E. P.: *Wien. klin. Wschr.* **17,** 265 (1904).
68. Oudin, J.: *C. R. Acad. Sci. (Paris)* **242,** 2489 (1956).
69. Pauling, L., Corey, B. and Bransson, H.: *Proc. nat. Acad. Sci. (Wash.)* **37,** 205 (1951).
70. Pauly, H.: *Chem. Zbl.* **II.** 1583 (1904).
71. Perlzweig, W. A. and Steffen, G. I.: *J. exp. Med.* **38,** 163 (1923).
72a. Pinchuck, P. and Maurer, P. H.: *J. exp. Med.* **122,** 665 (1965).
72b. id., *J. Immunol.* **100,** 384 (1968).
73. Rockwell, G. E.: *J. Immunol.* **43,** 259 (1952).
74. Rüde, E., Westphal, O., Hurwitz, E., Fuchs, S. and Sela, M.: *Immunochemistry* **3,** 137 (1966).
75. Sage, H. I., Deutsch, G. F., Fasman, G. D. and Levine, L.: *Immunochemistry* **1,** 133 (1964).
76. Schechter, I. and Sela, M.: *Biochim. biophys. Acta (Amst.)* **104,** 301 (1965).
77. Schlossman, S. F., Yaron, A., Ben-Efraim, S. and Sober, H. A.: *Fed. Proc.* **24,** 319 (1965).
78. Sela, M.: *Bull. Res. Counc. Israel* **4,** 109 (1954).
79a. Sela, M. and Arnon, E.: *Biochem. J.* **75,** 91 (1960).
79b. ibid., **77,** 394 (1960).
80. Sela, M. and Fuchs, S.: In *Molecular and Cellular Basis of Antibody Formation*. Publ. House Czech. Acad. Sci., Prague 1965, pp. 43–56.
81. Sela, M., Fuchs, S. and Arnon, R.: *Biochem. J.* **85,** 223 (1962).
82. Sela, M., Lupu, N., Yaron, A. and Berger, A.: *Biochim. biophys. Acta (Amst).* **62,** 594 (1962).
83. Singer, S. J.: *J. cell. comp. Physiol.* **50,** 51 (1957).
84. Slobin, L. I.: *Nature* **225,** 698 (1970).
85. Sobey, W. R., Magrath, J. M. and Reisner, A. H.: *Immunology* **11,** 511 (1966).
86. Spragg, J., Schroder, E., Stewart, M. J., Austen, K. F. and Haber, E.: *Biochemistry* **6,** 3933 (1967).
87. Springer, C. F., Williamson, P. and Brandes, W. C.: *J. exp. Med.* **113,** 1077 (1961).
88. Sri Ram, J.: *Fed. Proc.* **20,** 31 (1961).
89a. Sri Ram, J. and Maurer, P. H.: *Arch. Biochim.* **74,** 119 (1958).
89b. ibid., **83,** 223 (1959).
90. Stahman, M. A., Lapresle, C., Buchanan-Davidson, D. J. and Grabar, P.: *J. Immunol.* **83,** 534 (1959).
91. Steffen, C., Timpl. R. and Wolff, I.: *J. Immunol.* **93,** 656 (1964).
92. Ungar-Waron, H., Hurwitz, E., Jaton, J.-C. and Sela, M.: *Biochim. biophys. Acta (Amst.)* **138,** 513 (1967).
93a. Waksman, B. H.: *Fortschr. Allergielehre* **5,** 349 (1958).
93b. id., *Int. Arch. Allergy* **14,** Suppl. 1 (1959).

CHAPTER 8

# THE CELLULAR BASIS OF IMMUNOLOGICAL PROCESSES* (IMMUNOCYTES AND MACROPHAGES)

by

G. GY. PETRÁNYI and G. JÁNOSSY



* The aim of the following survey is to present a common basis for the sections 'Immunocytes' and 'Macrophages'. For further details, the reader is referred to the following chapters: 'Antibody production and its theories' (Ch. 11), 'Theoretical considerations on 'transplantation immunity' (Ch. 28), 'Lymphocyte transformation test' (Ch. 26) and 'The thymus' (Ch. 9).

## AN OUTLINE OF THE IMMUNE SYSTEM

### THE CONCEPT OF IMMUNOCYTE

The cells participating in various immunological processes and their precursors have been, according to the classical concept of Ehrlich, classified into the following three morphologically distinct categories (evolutionary series) [66, 122, 123]:

1. cells belonging to the reticulo-endothelial system (RES): macrophages, monocytes
2. lymphocytes
3. plasma cell (plasmacyte).

Owing the to circumstance that immunological phenomena could for a long time be detected only by morphological methods the morphological categories were interpreted more rigorously as compared to our present views. Thus, for example, the lymphocytes were regarded a *sui generis* cell type which had no relationship with other types of cells [43]. Classification on a morphological basis has become obsolete because more recent data have unequivocally shown that not infrequently the function of cells involved in immunological processes is not related to their morphology; on the other hand, it has become evident that the fundamental characteristics of immunological reactions are determined by interactions between the various cell types.

Immunocytes begin to differentiate and are transformed under the influence of antigenic stimulus. According to the definition of Rebuck et al. [108], differentiation is a process associated with morphological changes, in the course of which the cell acquires new structural and functional characteristics as regards cell-type and responsiveness, etc. Differentiation means the irreversible acquisition of new characteristics and, consequently, the irreversible loss of some of the original properties of the cell. *Transformation,* on the other hand, is a reversible acquisition of new morphological characteristics and functional properties (functional adaptation, modulation), which does not exclude the possibility of regaining the original characteristics of the cell.

It is generally accepted that one type of the small lymphocytes, which is a morphologically mature cell, can differentiate into antibody producing plasmablast and plasmacyte. Nevertheless, antibody producing immunocytes may exhibit, according to microplaque observations, morphological characteristics of lymphocytes as well as of plasmacytes, blast cells, or even of monocytes. The distinction between 'lymphocyte' and 'plasmacyte' may be confusing if the morphological characteristics are considered together with functional ones. Therefore, in the present chapter, the classification based entirely on the morphological appearance will be deliberately omitted, and the cells involved in immunological processes will be discussed using the collective term 'immunocyte' introduced originally by Dameshek [35]. This term does not include the monocytes and macrophages.

The term *immunocyte* covers all immunologically competent cells, which possess the ability of actively participating in various immunological processes, from the recognition of the antigen to the immunological response. Immunocytes may produce various classes of immunoglobulins (IgM, IgG, IgE, IgA, IgD) which are specific antibodies, they may take part as effector cells in cell-mediated immune responses or in the rejection of transplants. They may also represent or retain the memory of a certain immune response against some antigen (memory cells). Blast cells undergoing transformation or differentiation in the course of clonal division also belong to the group of immunocytes.

The morphologically different immunocytes are continuously moving in the body. In mammals, lymphoid tissue makes up about 1 per cent of the total body weight. In an adult man, the total weight of lymphocytes amounts to 0.5 to 1.0 per cent of the body weight. According to the calculations of Osgood, there are 3 g of lymphocytes in the blood, and the amount of lymphoid cells is 70 g in the bone marrow and 100 g in the lymphoid tissue, while 1,300 g of lymphoid cells are in movement in the organism. This distribution of lymphatic cells indicates that the immunocytes are not restricted to the lymphatic organs but are characterized by a wide, dynamic dispersion which is called the immunocyte pool [36].

The immunocytes and their precursors are formed (*i*) in the bone marrow, (*ii*) in the thymus and in immune organs corresponding to the bursa of Fabricius of young birds (bursa equivalents), and (*iii*) in peripheral lymphatic organs, i.e. lymph nodes and the spleen.

## THE ROLE OF THE BONE MARROW IN THE PRODUCTION OF IMMUNOCYTES

It is commonly accepted now that the precursors or stem cells which are responsible for the self-maintenance of the immune system derive from the bone marrow [87, 88]. These precursor cells are presumably similar to the so-called colony-forming cells which in an irradiated animal or man are capable of repopulating the destroyed myeloid and erythroid elements. The precursors of immunocytes do not produce antibodies, do not participate in cellular immune reactions; thus they are not immunologically competent. In the irradiated animal, however, they induce the regeneration of lymphoid tissue.

Stem cells are produced in the bone marrow throughout life; the rate of production is about ten times higher in the perinatal period than in adults. In the blood of the mouse there are approximately 10 stem cells per ml. It is extremely difficult or even impossible to recognize these cells on the basis of their morphological characteristics; however, there is some speculation that the avian precursor cells are of the blast type with markedly basophilic cytoplasm, while in mammals they resemble monocytes or lymphocytes [36, 88, 96*a*, *b*].

The stem cells pass into the central lymphatic organs (thymus, bursa) and are thereafter distributed among the circulation and the peripheral lymphatic organs (lymph nodes and spleen). They are located in the 'thymus-dependent' or 'bursa-dependent' regions of the peripheral lymphatic organs, depending on which of the central organs have determined their immunological competence.

## THE ROLE OF THE THYMUS AND BURSA IN THE PRODUCTION OF IMMUNOCYTES

The immunological role of the thymus is discussed in a separate chapter, therefore only the most important facts pertinent to the following section will be summarized here.

The *thymus* of newborn and young animals, and the *bursa of Fabricius* which has been most distinctly demonstrated in young birds are the central lymphatic organs. The lymphatic tissue fixed to the intestinal epithelium, i.e. Peyer's patches, the appendix, tonsils, and in the rabbit also the sacculus rotundus, have recently been considered to have a role similar to that of the bursa of Fabricius and have thus been termed *bursa equivalents.*

In the mouse, the thymus retains about 50 per cent of the stem cells originating from the bone marrow. These precursor cells are then induced to proliferate by the large epithelial cells of the thymus, resulting in their differentiation into thymus dependent *T lymphocytes* which are already immunologically competent and responsive to antigens [96*b*]. T lymphocytes, with their marker, theta ($\theta$) antigen [107] have a relatively long life-span [117] and make up the majority (64 per cent) of the circulating small lymphocyte pool [138]. The T lymphocytes get from the thymus into the peripheral lymphatic organs via the blood. There they accumulate in the paracortical area surrounding the follicles; they are involved in cell-mediated immune responses, e.g. delayed hypersensitivity, transplantation immunity and graft-versus-host reaction as well as in the humoral immune response as antigen sensitive co-operating cells [36, 51, 134].

The bursa equivalent lymphatic organs are in part responsible for the antibody producing precursor cells becoming immunologically competent; on the other hand, they are also capable, as primary proliferation centres, to multiply the number of immunocytes [2, 36, 86]. The lymphocytes depending on the bursa equivalent lymphatic organs in mammals are called thymus independent [134] *B lymphocytes* [111]. These cells are accumulated in the follicles of the spleen and lymph nodes and are involved in the production of immunoglobulins, thus playing a significant part in the synthesis of specific antibodies against bacterial, viral toxin and other antigens. The life-span of B lymphocytes is somewhat shorter than that of the T lymphocytes. The B cells constitute the minority (10–35 per cent) of the circulating small lymphocytes of the organism [1*a*]. These cells display a high density of surface immunoglobulins in contrast to the T cells [138] and specific B-lymphocyte antigen (in the mouse) as marker [107].

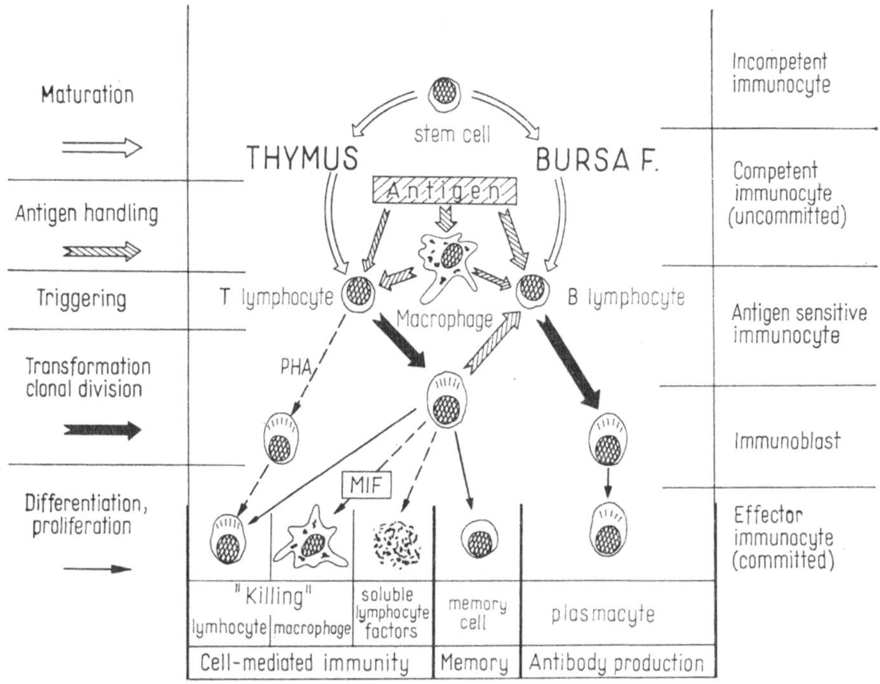


Fig. 8-1. Schematic representation of the functional connections of immunocytes and of their role in immunological processes. Left, main stages of the development of immunocytes; right, characteristic cell groups; bottom, role of the various specific cell forms in immunological processes PHA, phytohaemagglutinin, MIF, migration inhibition factor

The immunologically competent T and B lymphocytes belonging to the above two regulating centres cannot be distinguished morphologically or by histochemical or electron-microscopic methods. These cells are also called *uncommitted* lymphocytes for they are not yet committed to any particular immunological response (Fig. 8-1).

## IMMUNOCYTE PRODUCTION IN THE PERIPHERAL LYMPH NODES

Competent T and B lymphocytes, which are already prepared for immunological functions but are still uncommitted, differentiate in the peripheral lymphatic organs into immunocytes which, in response to specific antigenic stimulus, are able to participate in the specific humoral or cell-mediated immunological reaction as *committed* cells. It is now generally accepted that the small lymphocytes are the primary source of the proliferating cell clones participating in various specific immunological functions [52]. The immunological response is initiated by the contact of the *antigen-responsive cells* present in both T and B lymphocyte populations with the antigen (Fig. 8-1). Due to this *triggering* impact the cells start to become transformed. Transformation is indicated by the appearance of immunoblasts and their proliferation which finally leads to the development of the cell clone committed to the specific immune response to the antigen [84, 100]. The members of this clone are also called *executive cells* or *effector cells* because they are involved in the efferent part of the cell-mediated or humoral immune response. Most probably, the *memory cells* capable of retaining the memory of an immune response are also formed in the course of clonal division. These cells start to proliferate in response to the secondary antigen stimulus.

The transformation of lymphocytes to blast cells can be evoked by aspecific mitogenic stimuli (phytohaemagglutinin, concanavalin-A, pokeweed mitogen, anti-lymphocyte globulin, anti-Ig, etc.); moreover, these substances cause a larger proportion of lymphocytes to undergo blast transformation than the specific antigenic stimulus. The stimulating effect of mitogenic agents, particularly that of the phytohaemagglutinin, can be observed mainly on T lymphocyte populations. Pokeweed mitogen stimulates both T and B cells and it has been recently observed that bacterial lipopolysaccharides are polyclonal mitogens for mouse B lymphocytes.

It is the T lymphocyte population which is involved in cell-mediated immunity and hence in the immunological response following transplantation. Of the antigen-responsive circulating T lymphocytes only those will bind the antigen introduced into the body which have preformed antibody-like surface receptors fitting well to the given antigen (*fitting mechanism*). The antigenic stimulus, by inducing blast transformation, gives rise to the differentiation of the 'killer' effector cells which are directed against the antigen itself. These cells take part in the cellular infiltration of tuberculin hypersensitivity, in the rejection of allogeneic grafts, and in the graft-versus-host reaction. The killer lymphocytes, during their contact with the cells bearing the antigen, or with cell populations of the same antigeneity, i.e. with the target cells, produce toxic substances directed against and finally killing the target cells. The effector cells are also capable of releasing a number of active factors, which promote the aspecific participation in the immunological response of monocytes and macrophages on one hand and of non-stimulated lymphocytes on the other. The exact chemical nature of these factors has hitherto been only vaguely defined; the ones more thoroughly studied include the migration inhibition factor (MIF), the lymph node permeability factor (LNPF), the chemotactic factor, and the mitosis stimulating substances.

*Antibody production* is the function of the cell population of *plasma cells* arising as the result of the differentiation of B lymphocytes. Several antigens are capable to stimulate directly the antigen sensitive cells of the B lymphocyte population. These antigens are called *thymus independent antigens*. Stimulation occurs with or without the interaction of macrophages. Other antigens, on the other hand, are not capable to stimulate directly the B lymphocytes. These antigens, called *thymus dependent antigens* induce antibody production by the B lymphocytes through the interaction of macrophages and T lymphocytes (Fig. 8-1). Cell clones derived from stimulated B lymphocytes produce only a single type of immunoglobulin belonging to the same class or subclass, and it is probable that the immunoglobulin synthetised by a single cell is specific only to one antigen. This holds most likely also for the memory cells. The molecular structure of the antibody formed by the effector cell or memory cell is a genetically determined property of the precursor cell. It is evident thus that with the majority of antigens the induction of specific antibody production requires the interaction of two or three cell types.

Various immunological phenomena can now be analysed at the cellular level in the light of a variety of experimental results. In the development of different immunological processes the quantitative aspects and handling of the antigen play a decisive role. As already mentioned, most antigens stimulate first of all the T lymphocytes through the interaction of the macrophages. However, the T lymphocytes are capable of inducing both humoral and cell-mediated immunity. It seems probable that, at least under certain circumstances, the cell-mediated response is a basic introductory step in the sequence of events leading finally to the production of the specific antibody.

# IMMUNOCYTES

## CHARACTERISTICS OF THE VARIOUS CELL TYPES

### *Lymphocytes*

#### *Morphology*

The lymphocytes are spherical cells, from 7 to 12 $\mu$m in diam., with very scanty cytoplasm. If stained according to Pappenheim, the cytoplasm is hardly stained, it is not basophilic, and occasionally may contain azurophilic granules. The nucleus is round or slightly indented, with a coarse chromatin meshwork. Nucleoli are not recognizable. It is common to distinguish large, medium and small lymphocytes; the distinction between these types is ill-defined. Attempts to demonstrate a triple peak in the distribution curve have failed, therefore the classification according to size of lymphocytes seems to be an artificial one [52]. Lymphocytes cannot be classified on the basis of other morphological characteristics either, although functionally they form a markedly heterogeneous population [36, 88].

By using the phase contrast microscope it was possible to recognize in the cytoplasm of lymphocytes round lipid structures of 0.5 $\mu$m diam. showing double refraction and covering about one-third of the whole area of the cytoplasm, which have been termed Gall's neutral red bodies [36].

According to cytochemical investigations, there is a relatively high lactate dehydrogenase activity in the lymphocytes, while other enzymes, e.g. nuclease, adenosinase, cathepsin, amylase, lysosyme, lipase, are present in varying concentrations depending mainly on the functional state and activity of the cell. RNA content of the lymphocytes is not constant either. High RNA levels and low concentrations of cytochrome are characteristic of the resting lymphocytes termed also hibernating forms [36].

Using electron microscopy, it is possible to recognize a double nuclear membrane, and a scarce Golgi apparatus containing vacuoles. Although the ribonucleoprotein granules are easily recognizable in the small lymphocytes, the ergastoplasm is usually absent. In a small proportion of the cells, however, the ergastoplasm is readily demonstrable. The transition between the plasma cells containing a particularly well-developed ergastoplasm and the small lymphocytes is continuous. Stereo electron-microscopic studies have shown that the entire surface of the lymphocytes is covered with a large number of microvilli which significantly increase the surface area of these cells [27].

While studying the movements of lymphocytes, MacFarland [78, 79] distinguished two main parts of the cells. The so-called pseudopod contains the nucleus surrounded by the major portion of the cytoplasm, while the uropod is the tail portion of the lymphocytes which is formed during migration. The uropod is an important part of the lymphocyte, since by this organ the lymphocyte establishes contact with other cells. There are about 80 microvilli on the surface of the uropod, each 125 to 2,500 Å in diam. and approximately 8,000 Å in length. The microvilli exhibit linear striation. The uropod contains microtubules, mitochondria, pynocytotic vacuoles, and occasionally scanty ergastoplasm.

### *Surface receptors of lymphocytes*

The superficial plasma membrane of the lymphocytes can be regarded as a cell organelle with specific functions, to which certain substances may attach and this attachment initiates the typical response of transformation into blast cell. This reaction, which is largely independent of the kind of substance attached to the cell membrane, is treated in detail in the section 'Blast transformation', and the present heading includes only the functional data concerning the sites of attachment or receptors on the surface plasma membrane of the lymphocyte.

In response to certain substances, about 40 to 80 per cent of the lymphocytes undergo blast transformation *in vitro*. The compounds which aspecifically stimulate the lymphocytes are mitogenic agents; this group comprises substances like phytohaemagglutinin (PHA), staphylococcal filtrate, pokeweed mitogen, anti-lymphocyte globulin (ALG), anti-Ig (in rabbit), etc. The high percentage of transformation indicates that these compounds contain chemical groups which readily combine with the groups normally present on the surface of the lymphocytes constituting an integral part of the cell membrane [191].

A smaller portion (1 to 5 per cent) of lymphocytes derived from sensitized subjects are capable of blast transformation also when stimulated *in vitro* by the specific antigen. The time-course of stimulation by antigen is more protracted lasting 5 to 7 days, in contrast to the stimulation induced by aspecific mitogenic substances taking only 3–4 days. In case of antigenic stimulation the transforming antigen is not attached to the usual structures of the lymphocyte membrane but most likely to preformed receptors specific to the antigen. Transformation in response to antigen is demonstrable both after humoral and cell-mediated immunological reactions.

The functional study of aspecific and specific sites of attachment has been facilitated by the introduction of the so-called *in vitro* restimulation experiments [55]. In this test, the lymphocyte suspension is stimulated with mitogens and thymidine uptake is detected on the 4th day when using PHA, ALG or anti-immunoglobulin serum, and on the 7th day when using specific antigens. The suspension is restimulated by antigen, mitogens, or in mixed cultures. If restimulation results in increased DNA synthesis of the cells, it may be assumed that the stimulants applied in the first and second stimulation procedures were attached to different receptors of the cell surface.

It is now commonly known that PHA is attached to the N-acetylgalactose-amine groups abundantly present on the lymphocyte cell membrane, while ALG combines with the H-2 (transplantation) antigens. Restimulation studies have also shown that the two mitogens attach to different sites of the cell membrane because binding of ALG onto the surface of the lymphocyte does not prevent the stimulating effect of PHA [55]. The receptor sites binding PHA and the mitogenic components of staphylococcal filtrate are not identical either. On the other hand, it has been demonstrated that ALG covers the various receptors recognizing different antigens on the surface of the lymphocyte [55]. Following *in vitro* incubation with ALG the lymphocytes failed to detect either the tuberculin antigen or foreign H-2 antigens in a mixed culture; this process has been termed 'blind folding effect' (see Chapter 19).

Lymphocytes possess surface immunoglobulin molecules or their components [13, 54, 120]. It has become known since the work of Sell [115] that antiserum prepared against rabbit immunoglobulins (anti-Ig serum) is attached to the surface of the lymphocytes stimulating them in a significant proportion.

This stimulation could be shown both with anti-Ig-sera produced in a different species (xenogeneic or heterologous serum) and with sera prepared in animals of the same species but having immunoglobulins of different allotypes (anti-allotype sera). Antiserum prepared against the Ab4 allotype immunoglobulins (anti-Ab4-serum) was potent in stimulating 77 per cent of the lymphocytes of homozygous rabbits with Ab4-Ab4 globulins and only 39 per cent of the cells of Ab4-Ab5 heterozygous rabbits. However, 42 per cent of the latter cell population could also be stimulated with anti-Ab5 serum. These data indicate that in heterozygous animals the lymphocytes bear on their surface only one of the allotypes of the genetically possible two determinants of immunoglobulins. Similarly as it has been shown with immunoglobulin molecules and plasmacytes, in such heterozygous animals the two types of lymphocytes are present in about the same number. On the surface of lymphocytes there are also light chains of the types which make up the immunoglobulins (IgM, IgG, IgA); this has been clearly indicated by the observation that lymphoblast transformation can be induced *in vitro* also by anti-light-chain serum [56].

The fact that constituents of the immunoglobulin molecules are present on the surface of the lymphocytes allows the assumption that in the course of humoral immune reactions committed cells may carry on their surface such immunoglobulin structures which are capable of recognizing the specific antigen, i.e. they are acting as receptors. This assumption seems to be supported by the finding that soluble antigens eliciting the humoral immune response, e.g. tetanus and diphtheria-toxoid, typhoid and pertussis vaccine, streptolysin O antigen, etc., are capable of transforming previously sensitized cells into blast cells *in vitro*. Furthermore, Wigzell and Anderson [135] have shown that immunocytes responsible for the specific immunological reaction are adsorbed on a column made up of antigen-coated glass beads.

There is some evidence indicating that in delayed hypersensitivity (cell-mediated immune response) the cellular antigens are recognized by immunoglobulin receptors on the surface of the immunologically activated lymphocytes. Anti-light-chain serum and its Fab fragment blocked blast transformation both occurring in response to tuberculin antigen and in mixed cultures in restimulation experiments [56]. Thus immunoglobulins, or at least their light chains, participate in the formation of the recognizing receptors of these lymphocytes in cell-mediated immune reactions, too. There is no unequivocal evidence as to whether the antigen recognizing receptors of immunologically activated lymphocytes have IgM, IgG or IgA globulin characteristics, therefore they have been arbitrarily termed IgX [56].

Of the numerous data indicating that the immunoglobulin-like structure of the receptors of lymphocytes does not diminish the justification of distinguishing between cell-mediated and humoral immunological responses let us mention only a few. Benaceraff and Levin [8] succeeded in demonstrating that after immunizing with α-DNP-oligolysines, the serum antibodies were specific for the α-DNP-hapten, while the receptors of committed lymphocytes could immunologically recognize smaller or larger parts of the carrier oligo-lysine molecule, too. Similar results were obtained by *in vitro* experiments with cells of inbred mice [21]. When immunizing C3H mice with cells derived from C57BL/10 mice immunological response may develop against Snell's 2, 6, 14, 22, 27, 28, 29 and 33-type H-2 antigens. Of these eight H-2 antigen specificities, five (6, 14, 27, 28, 29) can be detected on the cells of mice of the strain A. Despite this overlap, immunologically activated lymphocytes derived from C3H animals immunized with cells of C57BL/10 mice failed to attach to cells of strain A and had no cytotoxic effect on them. To achieve attachment of immunologically activated lymphocytes on the surface of cells derived from another strain, the presence on the surface of the target cell of almost the entire antigen complex determining the H-2 antigenic specificity and operating in the sensitization procedure was necessary. This was the case with C57Bl/10 lymphocytes immunized with cells of the B10.D2 strain, which found five of the six sensitizing H-2 antigenic specificities on the C3H target cells. In sharp contrast to the above findings, isoimmune sera obtained after immunization with cells were specific to *single* H-2 antigenic specificities. These isoimmune sera killed, in the presence of complement, cells of the third mouse strain even if they recognized on the cell surface only a single H-2 specificity. All these findings support the view that in cell-mediated immunity the effector cells are responsive to foreign structures more complex than the antigens eliciting humoral immunological reaction. Whether this reflects operational differences between the triggering of cells in cell-mediated reactions and humoral immune responses or the complexity of receptors is different on T and B cells remains to be answered. (For further details, cf. section 'Cytotoxic effects of immunologically activated lymphocytes'.)

On the surface of the B lymphocytes there are also *complement fixing receptors* (C receptors), which can be destroyed by trypsin treatment. These receptors found on the lymphocytes differ from the complement receptor of macrophages in that they are able to fix C–IgM–antigen or C–IgG–antigen complexes even in the absence of $Mg^{++}$ ions, hence also in the presence of Na-EDTA. In the case of macrophages these complexes are bound only if $Mg^{++}$ ions are present [62, 77]. The role and significance of the C receptor is not known at present.

Little is known about the life history of the progenitors of effector T cells [134*a*].

On the basis of studies of graft-versus-host reactions in mice it has been proposed that induction can require co-operation between two different classes of T cell [4*a*, 107*a*]. The two types may belong to different cell lineages or may represent different stages of maturation within a single cell line. The first type of T cell postulated ($T_1$) is normally present in the thymus and spleen and may decrease in number in secondary lymphoid tissue 2–6 weeks after adult thymectomy, i.e. it might be in an early stage of post-thymic maturation in these tissues. The second type postulated ($T_2$) is scarce in the thymus and does not decrease in number in secondary lymphoid tissue after adult thymectomy, i.e. it might be in a late stage of post-thymic maturation. It has been suggested that $T_1$ cells are the progenitors of effector cells and that $T_2$ cells act as amplifiers of the response [29*a*, 121*a*]. Investigations of the cellular requirements for cell-mediated immune response in diverse systems suggest that $T_1$ type cells act as progenitors but $T_2$ amplifiers are not absolutely essential for the response [134*a*].

### *Immunoblasts*

The morphological category of 'immunoblast' comprises all cells which have undergone transformation or differentiation as the result of activation of immunologically competent T and B lymphocytes. Earlier a number of terms were in use for these cells, such as lymphoblast, plasmablast, proplasmablast, large primitive cell, lymphoid plasmacyte, transitional cell, activated reticular cell, large pure reticulum cell, acute splenic tumour cell and large pyroninophilic blast cell [36].

The diameter of the immunoblast may exceed that of the lymphocyte, even three times. In its nucleus having a fine chromatin meshwork a single or a few nucleoli can be well recognized. The cytoplasm is basophilic (pyroninophilic) and does not show granules.

Electron-microscopic studies have revealed that the 'immunoblast' category, as expected, is heterogeneous. Immunoblasts of both T and B lymphocyte origin can express lymphoblastoid character. The cytoplasm of these blast cells is filled with polyribosomes. The ergastoplasm (rough endoplasmic reticulum) is poorly developed, although few lamellae can usually be seen around the mitochondria. The Golgi apparatus is well developed and the abundant mitochondria are frequently swollen. Lymphoblasts of T cell origin use anaerobic glycolysis as the source of energy and glycogen inclusions can frequently be seen in their cytoplasm. Although there is a considerable overlap in the morphology of activated T and B lymphocytes, the latter frequently undergo further morphological changes and develop into 'plasmablast' forms. This type of differentiation is never seen in blasts of T cell origin. Plasmablasts contain large amounts of ergastoplasm (rough endoplasmic reticulum) which is independent of mitochondria and is usually filled with a faint substance (i.e. immunoglobulin). The degree of development of ergastoplasm in plasmablasts is variable and immature plasmablasts are larger than the more mature proplasmacytes with concentrically arranged ergastoplasmic lamellae. The transition between these forms and plasmacytes is continuous. Although plasmablasts do not contain glycogen, other cell organalles such as Golgi apparatus and mitochondria are abundant.

### *Plasmacyte (plasma cell)*

These cells appear in various degrees of maturity and may be regarded as immunoglobulin-producing glands consisting of a single cell. Plasma cells are larger in size than the lymphocytes, their cytoplasm shows basophilic and pyroninophilic staining due to its high RNA content. In the mature cell, the small rounded nucleus is excentrically situated. The chromatin substance is condensed mainly to the nuclear membrane. Similarly to other protein-synthesizing cells, plasmacytes have a well-developed Golgi apparatus. As to their ultrastructure, a parallelly arranged complex system of the endoplasmic reticulum or ergastoplasmic membranes also indicate a high degree of differentiation. In this system, there are numerous saccules and cisternae communicating with each other and more or less filled with protein-like substance. The membranes are 70 Å thick and ribosomes of 150 Å diam. are visible on their surface. Similar granules can be detected in the cytoplasmic matrix, too. Protein synthesis takes place on the surface of these granules. The endoplasmic reticulum is assumed to play a part in the intracellular accumulation and transport of secretion products, i.e. of antibody. The synthesized antibodies are contained in the large cysts of the mature plasmacytes, bounded by the membrane of the endoplasmic reticulum and showing eosinophilic staining like hyalin (Russel's bodies) [66].

Stereo electron-microscopic investigations have failed to reveal microvilli-like formations on the smooth surface of plasmacytes as there are on the lymphocytes and macrophages [27].

Attempts to detect receptors on the surface of plasmacytes have also failed so far; the demonstration of receptors would be of doubtful significance anyhow, since these cells are end-stage mature forms which do not react with antigen and fail to get into interaction with other cells.

## FUNCTIONAL CHARACTERISTICS OF IMMUNOCYTES

### *Life-span*

Some of the small lymphocytes have a remarkably long life-span. Lymphocytes derived from the thoracic duct of rabbits could be kept alive in a diffusion chamber placed into the peritoneal cavity of mice over periods longer than 200 days [121]. Potentially, human small lymphocytes may live even 10 years [23]. Lymphocytes with a long life-span constitute the cellular basis of immunity persisting for longer time [46]. There are also data indicating that certain lymphocyte populations have a short life-span [44]. These are most likely the effector cells arising as a result of differentiation in response to antigenic stimulus. Mature plasmacytes, too, live only two or three days. The two populations of lymphocytes with different life-spans could be distinguished by experiments investigating the biological half-life of $^{32}P$ incorporated into DNA of lymphocytes [101]. In subjects with apparently normal haemopoiesis the average life-span of about 20 per cent of the lymphocytes was found 2 to 3 days, while the larger portion lived longer than 100 or even 200 days. In patients with chronic lymphoid leukaemia there were also two distinct populations of lymphocytes with different life-spans [58].

By all probability the T lymphocytes are those having a longer life-span, and the B lymphocytes those living shorter [111].

### *Motility*

Immunocytes are cells capable of active movement. Motile lymphocytes exhibit clearly recognizable pseudopod and uropod parts. Lymphocytes can migrate distances of 40 $\mu$ per min in cultures [36]. Cinematographic investigations revealed various kinds of amoeboid movements some of which did not result in displacement [83].

### *Migration*

As has been mentioned, 88 per cent of the lymphocyte population is migrating in the body distributed in the interstitial space, blood and lymphatic vessels. This is a continuous migration from the bone marrow towards the thymus, bursa and the peripheral lymphatic tissue on the one hand, and from the thymus and bursa towards the peripheral lymphatic tissue on the other. The direction and rate of migration between the various parts of the lymphoid system and in the entire body are not clear as yet. Lymphocytes of different origin and function are accumulated at distinctly different parts of the various lymphatic organs [76]. It has been supposed that lymphocytes belonging to the same functional type can be sorted out from a mixed population, in the course of serial transfer experiments since they would accumulate in different lymphatic organs. However, very little is known about the factors governing the migration of lymphocytes. Heparin is known to block migration. The spleen is able to filter out the lymphocytes from a heparinized perfusion fluid rich in lymphocytes [20].

### *Pinocytosis*

Investigations of the past few years have unequivocally demonstrated that not only macrophages and microphages are capable of phagocytosing various particles, e.g. those of India-ink, erythrocytes, polystirene, but also lymphocytes, moreover, lymphoid cells of leukaemia and lymphosarcoma cultures [71, 93*b*]. Other observations have indicated that about 10 per cent of the active antibody producing cells are capable of pinocytosis, and such activity can be demonstrated particularly in the initial stage of antibody production [93*b*].

## THE ROLE AND FUNCTION OF IMMUNOCYTES IN THE IMMUNOLOGICAL RESPONSE

### *Antigen recognition by non-committed immunocytes*

In the induction of antibody production two types of lymphocytes are involved in addition to macrophages. One type of these cells, the *antigen-reactive (T) cells* participate in the recognition of the antigen, react by rapid division in response to antigen, but do not give rise to antibody forming cells. The other type, i.e. the *precursors of antibody forming (B) cells* are small lymphocytes which are also capable of establishing specific contact with the antigen by means of their antigen recognition site or receptor structure, and by recognizing the molecular structure of the antigen, give rise to antibody forming cells [4, 86, 111, 112]. Cells of the T type react with thymus dependent antigens (erythrocytes, human and bovine serum albumin, etc.), while the B cells react with both thymus dependent and thymus independent antigens (haemocyanin, polysaccharides, etc.) [111]. Approximately every 50,000th lymphoid cell isolated from thoracic duct lymph is capable of recognizing an antigen, probably each cell only a single antigen [96*c*, 99]. Data concerning their distribution among other lymphatic tissues are inconsistent. Most likely the majority of antigen sensitive T cells are migrating in the body, whilst precursors of antibody forming B cells are mostly accumulated in the spleen, lymph nodes and at sites most exposed to antigen [99, 116].

Macrophages seem to play an important part in the interaction of antigen sensitive cells with antigen. They process the antigen before its encounter with the sensitive cells by partial digestion, and they also attach the antigen to the surface of the lymphocytes [28, 59, 98]. The interaction of the macrophages is a favourable process both when antigens stimulating the T lymphocytes (erythrocytes, various albumins) and B lymphocytes (e.g. polysaccharide antigens) are involved. However, there are some cells among the lymphocytes, which are capable of responding to certain antigens even without the interaction of macrophages [111]. The interaction of the antigen sensitive cells with the antigen is termed triggering, since it switches on the process of immunological response.

### *Blast transformation and clonal division*

In response to the antigenic stimulus the resting cells are transformed into large immunoblasts and begin to multiply. This process leads to the formation of a cell clone the members of which are active participants of the immunological response given to the specific antigen. Forty-eight hours after painting the skin of laboratory animals with oxazolone (2-phenyl-4-ethoxymethylene-5-oxazolone) strongly pyroninophilic immunoblasts have been shown to appear in large numbers in the paracortical area of the regional lymph nodes [128*a*, *b*]. Similar observations were made after skin grafting, when the rate and the dynamics of the appearance of blast cells were proportionalwith the degree of histoincompatibility [73]. Transformation into blast cells, however, is observed not only in cell-mediated and transplantation immune reactions, but is easily detectable also in the initial phases of antibody production [9, 50, 74]. The increase in the number of blast cells is observed not only in the regional lymph nodes but also in other parts of the lymphatic system. The number of large lymphoid cells in the peripherial blood of human subjects has been shown to increase after immunization; 30 per cent of the cells showed DNA synthesis [32, 60].

The *in vitro* methods based on blast transformation proved to be of great practical value in selecting appropriate donors for organ transplantation, using mixed lymphocyte cultures, and in assessing the degree of aspecific immune suppression, based on the determination of PHA-reactivity of lymphocytes. Furthermore, one of the most important fields where transformation test is used is the *in vitro* screening of allergens for diagnostic purposes in autoimmune and particularly in allergic diseases (cf. Chapter 26).

Blast transformation is accompanied by proliferation of the immunocytes. Using mixed cultures or by stimulating peripheral lymphocyte cultures with antigens it was possible after 48 h to separate several cells showing the first signs of transformation and to transfer them by micromanipulation into chambers where their further growth could be followed microcinematographically [83]. The observed lymphoblasts divided and formed during the following days a clone of 64 or more cells. Generation time of the dividing cells was 8 to 13 h, with extremes of 7.5 and 38 h. Others cultivated human lymphocytes in millipore chambers and demonstrated that the period of DNA-synthesis (phase S) averaged 9 to 10 h, the resting ($G_1$) phase 16 to 18 h, while phase $G_2$ amounted to only 2 h [68, 71, 125].

### *Functional morphology of the immunocytes participating in the process of humoral antibody production*

There are only a few well-established facts and a great number of theories available about the precursor cells initiating antibody formation. Precursors are competent, but not yet committed, immunocytes which are capable of recognizing antigen. The morphology of the antigen sensitive precursor cells is not fully known, however, in transfer experiments B cell derived from the bone marrow are essential for the *in vitro* induction of the primary antibody response [25, 119]. It is now established that the antigen sensitive precursor cells are of B lymphocyte origin. There are some data indicating that these precursor cells are present in the bone marrow already differentiated according to the molecular type of the antibody (IgM, IgG, IgA); it has been found that the IgM precursor cells outnumber the IgG-type precursors 15 times [33].

The precursor cells are rapidly converted into antibody forming cells following stimulation with the antigen. The initial maturation process probably does not involve cell division. This is followed by a latency period of 12 h introducing the cell proliferation which occurs simultaneously with the onset of antibody production [114]. Others maintain that precursor cells also multiply but their generation time is twice as long as that of the antibody forming cells [25]. Morphological data are more abundant about the antibody forming immunocytes arising from the precursor cells because more demonstrative methods are available for the morphological examinations.

If cell suspension derived from animals immunized with heterologous erythrocytes is mixed with the sensitizing erythrocytes and incubated at 37 °C in a semisolid medium, the antibodies released by the antibody forming cells cause local haemolysis; (Jerne's haemolytic plaque method) [67]. The immunocytes in the centre of each plaque can be examined by light or electron microscopy (microplaque technique). Several morphologically distinct types of antibody-forming cells could be distinguished by this method [94]. In mice, on the 4th day after immunization with sheep erythrocytes, small, medium and large lymphocytes, various members of the lymphocyte cell series, immunoblasts, basophilic reticulum cells and histiocytes were found to produce haemolysins.

The morphological distribution of the antibody forming cells depends primarily on the actual stage of antibody production at the moment of examination. In the early phase of antibody production immunoblasts predominate, while in the later phase plasmacytes can be detected almost exclusively (cf. Chapter 11).

The method of autoradiography has also been employed for the detection of antibody forming cells [17], based on the finding that the isotope-labelled antigen becomes attached to the surface of the antibody forming cell, since antibody is present there already prior to its release. By this method it has been demonstrated that among the antibody forming cell population approx. 10 per cent are macrophages (monocytes). In animals not immunized previously this ratio has been found to occur up to 85 per cent.

The reliability of the data pointing to the great morphological heterogeneity of the antibody forming cell is made doubtful by a number of methodological problems. Both the microplaque and the autoradiography techniques may have the common error of identifying cells which passively absorbed antibodies on their surface as antibody forming cells [112]; (cf. sections dealing with macrophage). Nevertheless, it seems that the morphological heterogeneity of the antibody forming cells is basically due to the continuous process of clonal division, as a consequence of which the individual cells reach maturity at different times.

There is evidence indicating, based in part on microcinematographic observation of the primary immune response *in vitro,* that proliferation and antibody production are mutually interrelated processes in the case of both IgM and IgG-type antibodies. The generation time of antibody forming cells is 13 h, of which phase S lasts 8 h, phase $G_1$ 3 h, and phase $G_2$ 2 h [74]. The antibody forming daughter-cells usually have a short life-span, which rarely exceeds 2 or 3 days [31]. More recent data have indicated that a single antibody forming cell is only capable of synthesizing immunoglobulin of one light-chain and heavy-chain type. As already mentioned, this property of the cell is inherent already in the stem cell in the bone marrow [14, 132, 140]. This view seems to be supported by the findings obtained in patients with plasmocytoma, nevertheless, the question is still far from being settled.

The amount of immunoglobulins produced by a single cell has been assessed in cultures of myeloma cells: cells produced 3 $\mu$g of IgG in two patients and 20 $\mu$g of light chain in the case of a third patient [85].

### *Functional morphology of the immunocytes involved in cell-mediated immune response*

It is the T lymphocytes which play a primary part in the cell-mediated immunological response. These cells have a long life-span and make up the greater part of the circulating small lymphocytes (30–75 per cent) [5*a*]. The cells are found predominantly in the paracortical region of the lymph nodes.

The formation of effector cells of the cell-mediated immune response is bound to the development and proliferation of pyroninophilic immunoblasts, similarly to the proliferation step in the development of antibody forming cells. These immunoblasts develop from small lymphocytes [52]; the formation of the clone has been observed first in the paracortical area of the regional lymph nodes following heterologous grafting or painting the animal's skin with oxazolone (2-phenyl-4-ethoxymethylene-5-oxazolone) [128*b*] (cf. Chapter 28).

Already on the 5th to 7th day following skin grafting, the draining lymph nodes contain cells showing the morphological characteristics of small lymphocytes, which are capable of specific immunological agglutination with the sensitizing donor cells *in vitro* ('contactual agglutination'). An apparently similar reaction occurs with normal non-immune lymphocytes, however, normal cells can be easily detached from the target cells, while a small fraction of the sensitized lymphocyte population cannot be detached from the target cells after an incubation period of 6 to 8 h. It is an important feature of contactual agglutination that it is relatively independent of temperature, the degree of agglutination being similar at 37 °C and 27 °C [137]. This finding indicates that in the course of immunization specific receptors are formed against the heterologous cells on the surface of lymphocytes, which by attaching to the heterologous H-2 antigen give rise to agglutination (cf. section dealing with the surface receptors of lymphocytes).

The effector lymphocytes possess two very important abilities. First, by means of their cytotoxic or 'killing' potency they kill the cell to which they are attached, second, they are capable of synthetizing soluble factors which activate non-immune lymphocytes and macrophages in a non-specific way.

### *Cytotoxic effect of immunologically activated lymphocytes*

There are several *in vitro* methods available for the detection of the cytotoxic killing effect on various target cells of effector lymphocytes. Some of the techniques allow the assessing of the degree of cytotoxicity by measuring the radioactivity released from $^{51}$Cr-labelled target cells after ther death. Other techniques are based on direct counting of surviving target cells or on estimating their colony forming capacity [11, 22, 103]. Both T cells and non-T cells are able to exert cytotoxic effects. Different target cells vary in their sensitivity to different types of cytotoxicity. For instance, chicken red blood cells, coated with non-lytic amounts of antibody, are particularly sensitive to the cytotoxic effects of a non-T cell line which is presumably a sub-population of non-phagocytic macrophages ('antibody mediated' cytotoxicity [104]). Some tumour cells (e.g. methyl-cholantrene induced sarcoma) are effectively killed by 'classical' macrophages [103]. Nevertheless, in the majority of the cytotoxic systems the effector 'killer' cells are of T lymphoid origin and the data below are mainly relevant to this particular type of cytotoxicity, which could be demonstrated in target cells of various types, e.g. in cultures of fibroblasts, kidney cells and especially on the sensitive mastocytoma target cells [22]. To obtain a marked cytotoxic effect it is necessary to use lymphocytes in numbers 1 or 2 orders of magnitude in excess to the target cells in the culture. The dose-response curves relating to the lymphocyte count have a pattern similar to the 'single hit' inactivation phenomenon, indicating that each target cell is killed by one active lymphocyte and that the proportion of active lymphocytes in the suspension derived from the immunized animal amounts to only 1 to 2 per cent [137].

A direct and close contact, the so-called contactual agglutination, is necessary between the lymphocyte and the target cell for the cytotoxic effect to develop. This contact is probably effected through preformed receptors on the surface of the effector lymphocytes. It seems that the number of active lymphocytes in cell suspensions does not exceed 1 to 2 per cent because this is the proportion of lymphocytes bearing specific receptors on their surface [137]. If the lymphocytes are attached to the surface of the target cells by some aspecific means, for example by utilizing the agglutination caused by PHA, normal non-immune small lymphocytes, or rather the lymphoblasts developing from them, will show cytotoxic properties [91], thus most T lymphocytes have a *sui generis* cytotoxic potency, which, however, is only activated by direct contact with the target cell.

The morphology of 'killing' cells has still a number of unclarified aspects. Most likely, lymphocytes are activated at the time of their attachment to the target cell and their transformation begins. Thus, morphological findings mostly depend on the time of observation. Active cells showing the morphological appearance of lymphocytes have frequently been described [21, 118]; on the other hand, the 'killing' effect has also been reported to be proportional with the number of lymphoblasts [11]. There are lymphoid elements of various sizes involved in the *graft-versus-host* reaction [118] from which it may be concluded that the active cells are in various stages of metabolism and proliferation at any given time of observation [133].

Particulars of the development of the killing effect are not clear as yet. It has been supposed that a so-called *lymphocyte cytotoxic factor* is released, the chemical properties of which are not known but which can be readily demonstrated 30 min after admixing the effector lymphocytes to the suspension of target cells [56, 59, 113]. The cytotoxic effect is more prominent in dividing cell cultures than in cultures of target cells not capable of multiplication (e.g. previously irradiated) indicating that in addition to the cytocidal effect there is also a cytostatic factor involved in the process [137]. Nevertheless, the most likely explanation for the mechanism of cytotoxicity in the majority of the experimental systems is that the close membrane–membrane contact between the activated effector cell and the target cell results in a considerable rearrangement of the molecular structure of the adjacent membrane elements with consequent leakage and, perhaps, osmotic shock of the target cells (A. Allison, personal communication).

The cytotoxic effect of lymphocytes is different from the complement-mediated cytolysis; C is probably not necessary for the 'killing' effect [137]. There are also contradictory findings, but in these cases cytolysis was probably due to antibodies attached to the cell surface and not to effector lymphocytes [104]. However, antibodies may mediate cytotoxic effect to B lymphocytes; moreover by occupying the receptors on the surface of the target cells antibodies may prevent or at least impede the close contact between the lymphocyte and target cell, thereby protecting the latter from the destroying effect of the active lymphocytes [137]. This fact forms the basis of the 'enhancement' phenomenon.

Although only a small fraction of lymphocytes derived from the immunized animal exhibits cytotoxic properties *in vitro*, there is strong evidence that vigorous aspecific cytotoxic reactions occur *in vivo* as a result of the specific immunological reaction between the lymphocytes and target cells. It has been shown that in the presence of RNA preparation from the 8 to 18 S fractions of extracts of active lymphocytes, target cells are killed also by non-immune lymphocytes [15]. The various aspecific factors involved in these aspecific reactions will be the subject of the following section.

*Production of the migration inhibition factor (MIF) in activated lymphocytes*

Inhibition of macrophage migration as the *in vitro* method of studying delayed hypersensitivity was first described in 1902 by George and Vaugham [49]. The method has been improved by David et al. [37*a*, 38, 39], who succeeded in demonstrating that a cell-free substance was released during *in vitro* interaction of activated lymphocytes with antigen, which was potent in inhibiting the migration of macrophages. The phenomenon proved highly specific, since it could be elicited only when the specific antigen was added to the lymphocyte culture. MIF release could in turn be demonstrated in tuberculin and brucellosis hypersensitivity, allergic encephalitis and after skin grafting [37*b*]. While releasing MIF the sensitized lymphocytes undergo blast transformation as well [10]. An RNA-containing fraction could be extracted from human lymph node cells sensitized with tuberculin and histoplasmin; this, too, inhibited the migration of macrophages [126]. It is likely that this fraction is similar [70] to the preparation of Lawrence, who in 1955 succeeded in transmitting delayed hypersensitivity from one subject to another by a cell-free extract prepared from human lymphocytes (transfer factor). (For other problems related with MIF and the clinical aspects see Chapter 27.)

*Other factors produced by activated lymphocytes*

At their encounter with antigen the active lymphocytes release not only MIF but also a number of other substances. Isolation and study of the effect of these factors is still in an early stage. Here only some of the more important factors will be listed together with their biological activities [37*c*, 42, 72, 80, 82, 111, 134*b*].

*A. Affecting macrophages*

| | |
|---|---|
| Migration inhibition factor (MIF) | inhibits the migration of normal macrophages |
| Macrophage aggregation factor (MAF) | agglutinates macrophages in suspension |
| Macrophage chemotactic factor (MCF) | causes macrophages to migrate through micropore filter along gradient |
| Macrophage resistance factor (postulated) | renders macrophages non-specifically resistant to infection with certain bacteria and viruses |
| Cytophilic antibodies | confer on macrophages specific reactivity with antigen |

*B. Affecting lymphocytes*

| | |
|---|---|
| Blastogenic or mitogenic factor (BF or MF) | induces blast cell transformation and tritiated thymidine incorporation in normal lymphocytes |
| Potentiating factor (PF) | augments or enhances ongoing transformation in mixed lymphocyte culture or antigen-stimulated cultures |
| Cell co-operation or helper factor | produced by T cells, increases the number or rate of formation of antibody producing cells *in vitro* |
| Suppressor factor (postulated) | inhibits activation of, and/or antibody production by B cells |

*C. Affecting granulocytes*

| | |
|---|---|
| Inhibition factor | inhibits the migration of human buffy coat cells or peripheral blood leukocytes from capillary tubes or wells in agar plates |
| Chemotactic factor | causes granulocytes to migrate through micropore filter along a gradient |

*D. Affecting cultured cells*

| | |
|---|---|
| Lymphotoxin (LT) | cytotoxic for certain cultured cells, e.g. mouse L cells or HeLa cells |
| Proliferation inhibition factor and cloning inhibition factor (PIF, CLIF) | inhibit proliferation of cultured cells without lysing them |
| Interferon | protects cells against virus infection |

*E. Producing effects* in vivo

| | |
|---|---|
| Skin reactive factor (possibly a combination of several of the above activities) (SRF) | in normal guinea pig skin induces indurated skin reactions that are histologically similar to delayed-type hypersensitivity reactions |
| Macrophage disappearance factor | injected intraperitoneally, causes macrophages to adhere to peritoneal wall |

## MORPHOLOGICAL BASIS OF IMMUNOLOGICAL MEMORY

The two basic forms of immunological response, i.e. the production of antibodies and cell-mediated immunity, involve the development of immunological memory. Whenever the immune system encounters the same antigen repeatedly, the immunological response called *secondary* is elicited which takes a much shorter time to develop than the primary response. On cellular level this may mean that proliferation of the antibody forming cells commences quicker after the connection with the boosting antigen, than during the primary immune response. Alternatively, the number of specific cells interacting in the secondary response could be higher than in the primary response, resulting in a quicker outburst of proliferation. Data supporting both possibilities are mentioned in Chapter 11. The memory cells are most likely long-lived cells differentiated in the course of transformation and clonal division from T lymphocytes after their encounter with antigen. The mature cells appearing as small lymphocytes do not produce antibodies and do not participate in the cell-mediated immune response either; however, they are highly sensitive to new specific antigenic stimuli and are capable of differentiating into effector cells within a very short time: in about 1 h [24, 36, 111].

Furthermore, it has recently been shown that cells of B lymphoid line also develop memory (see Chapter 11). Combining the *in vitro* culture technique with transfer experiments a method has been devised for the study of memory cells [57]. It has been found that in mice cells of IgM and IgG-type memory are independent of each other, and moreover memory related to different IgG subclasses ($IgG_1$ and $IgG_2$) also developed in different cells. The formation of memory cells increases gradually from the 1st to 6th week after the administration of the antigen. First the $IgG_1$, then the $IgG_2$ memory cells differentiate. The various types of memory cells are not capable of taking over one another's function [57].

# MACROPHAGES

## MORPHOLOGICAL AND FUNCTIONAL CHARACTERISTICS OF MACROPHAGES

### *Distribution of macrophages in the body*

Mechnikov was the first to suggest that the cells capable of phagocytosis might play an important part in the defense mechanism of the organism. These cells, like unicellular organisms, are able to ingest various particles. Aschoff termed the system of phagocytes dispersed all over the body as reticuloendothelial system (RES). The RES is composed of macrophages and microphages. The microphages will not be dealt with in this chapter, since the neutrophil and eosinophil leukocytes are not primarily involved in immunological processes.

Cells of macrophage function found in different parts of the body have different names:

1. *Histiocytes.* These are found in the connective tissue of all organs and originate from circulating monocytes. They are found in abundant numbers in the peritoneal cavity, in the 'milk-spots' along the vessels of the omentum and in the alveoli of the lung. About 40 to 70 per cent of the cells of the peritoneal exudate are macrophages the remaining being lymphocytes, granulocytes and basophilic cells. A cell-suspension rich in macrophages can be obtained, if a phagocytosis inducing agent (liquid paraffin, glyceryl trioletae or proteose-pepton) is injected into the peritoneal cavity of laboratory animals, and the exudate is collected 3 to 6 days later.

2. *Monocytes.* Most of the monocytes are circulating RES cells which are under way from the bone marrow, their site of origin, to the connective tissue or to the site of some pathological lesion.

3. *Microglia.* In the brain tissue, devoid of lymphatics and isolated from circulating cells by the blood-brain barrier, microglia cells fulfill the function of RES.

4. *Sinus cells.* Phagocytosing cells located along the blood and lymphatic sinuses, the most important of them being the Kupffer cells of the liver, and the sinus cells of the bone marrow, spleen, lymph nodes and certain excretory glands.

5. *Reticulum cells.* These are the macrophages of the RES tissue (spleen, lymph nodes, bone marrow, thymus gland). In the lymph nodes and the spleen there are also cells with specific localization which play an important part in the immunological response (cf. Chapter 11). These cells are as follows:

(*a*) free amoeboid macrophages of the sinuses
(*b*) stellate macrophages in between the pulpa
(*c*) dendritic, microglia-like macrophages of the follicles.

The above RES cells are derived from the bone marrow. Experiments using the method of $^3$H-thymidine incorporation have unequivocally shown that the macrophages divide rapidly in the bone marrow but not in the blood and peritoneal cavity [131]. After a labelling period of 8 days all monocytes of the blood are labelled. The dividing cells found in the bone marrow are promonocytes. Half of the monocytes released from the bone marrow into circulation disappear from the blood within 22 h. Emigration commences with adhesion of the monocytes to the endothelium of the vessel wall. The monocytes then intrude themselves through the interspace between the endothelial cells into the interstitium; this is most likely directed by chemotaxis. The turnover of macrophages in the connective tissue is significantly slower [131]. Under special circumstances certain macrophages may have a remarkably long life-span, extending from 60 days to 6 months, for example in a local granuloma [121].

### *Morphological characteristics of macrophages*

Macrophages in preparations made from blood, peritoneal exudate or lymphatic organs may show highly variable shapes both in light- and electron-microscopic examinations. In many instances they cannot be distinguished from cells belonging to the lymphocyte series, while in other cases they show a peculiar and characteristic morphology. Similarly to lymphocytes, macrophages, too, may undergo significant morphological and functional alterations in the course of immunological processes [121]. These cells with variable morphology are classified in the same group on the basis of their common functional characteristics. In fixed preparations these cells may have a diameter of 20 $\mu$m and are thus the largest formed elements of blood. With panoptic staining, their extended cytoplasm has a greyish-blue colour and in most cases contains a fine powder-like azurophilic granulation. Most frequently, the nucleus has the shape of a kidney, although occasionally it may be lobulated and rarely polymorphous. The chromatin of the nucleus forms a loose network, nucleoli are infrequent. When studied in native preparation, the cells have marked extensions and are similar to macrophage monolayer cells.

Under the phase-contrast microscope, the cell membrane of macrophages is thick and crisped, particularly when examined after the cells have been adhered to a slide. The cell membrane has several finger-like projections. The surface of the activated cell may be completely covered with these processes. In the hollow portion of the extensions bright pinocytic vacuoles may be seen. The cytoplasm contains a variable number of dense bodies most likely of lysosomal origin; in addition, there are mitochondria which are thinner than those found in lymphocytes, occasionally phagosomes containing fat droplets. By electron microscope the numerous microvilli covering the surface of the cell can be well observed. The cytoplasm contains micropinocytic vesicles, dense bodies, and a highly developed Golgi apparatus with lamellar and saccular structure. The endoplasmic reticulum assumes a position more distant from the nucleus, usually on the opposite pole of the cell. In the cytoplasm deficient in glycogen the ribosomes and polysomes have a scattered localization. The nucleus contains one or two nucleoli. The above organelles can be detected in the macrophages in variable numbers and sites.

## *Surface properties of macrophages*

The surface of macrophages shows characteristic properties. Electron- and stereoscan electron-microscopic examinations have revealed that the surface of macrophages is covered with microvilli similar to those seen on the surface of lymphocytes [26, 27]. During enhanced activity of the macrophages these processes increase in length and form a dense network. The activity of lysosomes and the quantity of acidic phosphatase increases in the augmented projections. Intercellular links between adjacent macrophages may also be formed by the processes [81]. The formation of cytoplasmic bridges by human macrophages in response to tuberculin antigen has been termed by McLaurin '*macrophage interlinkage reaction*'.

According to our present knowledge, there are two different receptors on the surface of macrophages, which can be demonstrated on 90 per cent of blood and tissue macrophages [63]. One of them is the *IgG receptor* which combines aspecifically with the Fc fragment of IgG molecules. This receptor of human monocytes is able to distinguish between the subclasses of IgG molecules. Erythrocytes coated with specific IgG antibody are attached to the IgG receptors of macrophages by means of the 'outward arranged' Fc fragments of IgG molecules, thereby leading to characteristic 'rosette' formation which can be easily detected even by low-power magnification. This reaction is inhibited by the presence of free, non-specific IgG, indicating a competition between the specific IgG present in the antigen–antibody complex and the non-specific IgG for the macrophage receptors. This receptor can be demonstrated not only on the macrophages and monocytes but also on neutrophil granulocytes [77]. The receptors are not sensitive to trypsin and their function is not influenced by bivalent cations ($Mg^{++}$, $Ca^{++}$).

The other, trypsin-sensitive receptor on the surface of macrophages is specific for the C3 factor of the complement system. Those antigen particles which form complexes with IgM type antibodies can be attached to the surface of macrophages only in the presence of C factors (C1-C4-C2-C3) through the C3 complement receptor. This reaction requires the presence of $Mg^{++}$ ions [64, 65, 77]. Similarly, IgG–antigen–C-complexes can also be attached to the receptor. The above two receptors may have an important part in binding the antigen.

## *Functional characteristics of macrophages*

### *Adherence properties*

Adherence is one of the most characteristic properties of macrophages. In a medium containing neither $Ca^{++}$ nor $Mg^{++}$ ions this ability of macrophages disappears reversibly. This property is utilized when separating macrophages from other cells, by washing the cell suspension through columns of glass-wool or beads. Lymphocytes pass the columns, while adhering cells can be subsequently washed off by fractionated elutions with $Ca^{++}$-free solutions; by this means, neutrophil leukocytes and thrombocytes, etc., can be separated from the macrophages. In cell cultures, macrophages adhere to the wall of the vessel and form there a monolayer, thereby providing another possibility for the separation from other cells. Adherence is significantly reduced on smooth or plastic surfaces.

### *Phagocytosis*

The macrophages are able to ingest foreign particles, e.g. India ink and dye particles, bacteria, etc., as well as liquid substances. Both phagocytosis* and pinocytosis* are temperature and energy-dependent processes, i.e. they occur only in a medium of 37 °C and can be inhibited with actinomycin-D [29]. The substances taken into the cell are subjected to enzymatic degradation, particularly in the phagolysosomes. The following lysosomal enzymes are involved in the process of degradation: acid phosphatase, $\beta$-glucuronidase, cathepsin, esterase. During the process of maturation these enzymes accumulate in growing amounts in the macrophage.

Macrophages exert a bactericidal effect on the phagocytosed Gram-positive bacteria, but they cannot destroy the Gram-negative ones and M. *tuberculosis*, *Listeria* and *Brucella*. The bacteriocidal effect of macrophages as well as their ability to suspend bacterial immunogenicity is significantly weaker than in the case of granulocytes, which might be due to differences in the enzyme constituents of their lysosomes. Lysosome (muramidase) and peroxidase activity is more marked in monocytes than in other cells [124]. The process of degradation is not perfect, for about 10 per cent of the ingested antigen is still to be detected in the macrophages even after a considerable length of time [129]. Proteins are degraded

* The following synonyms have been suggested recently: inchondriosis for phagocytosis, and inchylocytosis for pinocytosis (75).

to and eliminated as amino acids. Macrophages can be isolated and differentiated also on the basis of their phagocytosing function. According to one of the methods the cell suspension containing the macrophages is mixed with powderized iron, and the phagocytosing cells can be then separated with a magnet [30]. Albumin labelled with $^{131}I$ is also suitable for the identification of macrophages; since labelled proteins are also taken up by the macrophages it is easy to recognize them by autoradiography.

An 'uneven' surface, e.g. alveolar endothelium, fibrin network, glass surface, etc., or the presence of opsonins is necessary to induce phagocytosis [139]. Opsonins usually facilitate the foreign particle's coming into contact with the surface of macrophages. Opsonins are mostly specific antibodies which attach the antigen to the surface of the cell through the IgG receptor of the macrophage. To attain 50 per cent phagocytosis it is necessary to coat each erythrocyte with approximately 3,000 IgG molecules. The factors C1-C4-C2-C3 of the C system possess similar opsonizing effect facilitating the attachment of the antigen to the surface of the macrophage by means of the C3 component receptor [64, 69]. Opsonizing property has also been attributed to a compound found in the 5–6S $\beta$-pseudoglobulin fraction. This most probably acts by inhibiting the inactivation of the C3 component [64]. The opsonizing effects of specific IgG and C seem to mutually complement each other, since in the presence of unattached IgG, i.e. after the IgG receptors have been saturated in a non-specific manner, the macrophage is still able to bind antigen by help of C. It is possible that the two main opsonizing processes induce two different types of antigen handling. Antigen–IgM–C complexes tend to persist longer on the surface of macrophages and may facilitate cell interactions, whilst opsonization through IgG receptor leads to quick phagocytosis. The relevance of these data is discussed in Chapter 11.

### *Migration and motility*

Migration and motility are specific properties of macrophages easily detectable also *in vitro* [40]. A chemotactic factor has been found in the serum of normal rabbits, which converted the adirectional movement of macrophages to unidirectional [136]. The chemotactic factors of macrophages and neutrophil granulocytes were found to be different. It has been shown that the antigen–antibody complex promotes the migration of neutrophils while inhibiting the migraton of macrophages. This latter phenomenon is believed to play a part in the regulation of antibody production.

### *Synthesis of macromolecules*

Macrophages have been shown to synthetize macromolecules. DNA and RNA synthesis could be observed in activated macrophage which have already been released from the bone marrow. The presence of endoplasmic reticulum, free ribosomes and polysomes indicate that the macrophages are involved in the synthesis of various proteins. It has been unequivocally demonstrated that macrophages produce interferon, endogenous pyrogenic compounds, $\beta_1$C and $\beta_1$E serum proteins and transferrin [29].

## THE ROLE OF THE MACROPHAGES IN ANTIBODY PRODUCTION

Macrophages play an important part in the process of antibody production, first of all in the presenting of the antigen. In the newborn antibody production is deficient, which has been attributed, at least in part, to insufficient processing of the antigen by the macrophages [3]. If newborn animals are given peritoneal macrophages derived from an adult animal, antibody production becomes normal. This cannot be achieved, however, by the introduction of immunologically competent splenic and lymphoglandular cells. The decrease in antibody production after total body irradiation is also attributed to the radiation injury of the macrophages [47], claiming that the uptake and transfer of information is affected. The induction of antibody production *in vitro* requires the interaction of two or three cells; one of them is the 'adherent macrophage' which processes the antigen [89]. All these data point to macrophages being an important link in the process of antibody production, particularly in the immunological response to thymus-dependent antigens (see earlier, p. 191). Nevertheless, the exact role of macrophages in antibody production is still far from being clear (see Chapter 11).

### *Antigen uptake*

Antigen injected under the skin of the hindlimb appears in the medullary macrophages of the regional lymph node within a few hours. The $^{131}$I-labelled flagellar antigen of *Salmonella adelaidae* enters the cell by two routes: either by direct penetration across the cell membrane, or by pinocytosis. The antigen is then quickly surrounded by protolysosomes derived from the Golgi apparatus which turn into phagolysosomes by confluence after 24 h. The phagolysosomes can contain several antigens at the same time [109]. Certain antigens may be recognized in the phagolysosomes even after 3 weeks [1, 97]. Observations using $^{131}$I-labelled haemocyanin antigen have shown that the majority of antigen is chemically processed by the macrophage within 2 to 5 h [129]. Nevertheless, the antibody production-inducing effect was unimpaired even when the cell had already degraded 90 per cent of the antigen. It may be that only the intact residue of antigen remaining in the macrophage is immunogenic.

Investigations have pointed to the significance of antigens attached to the surface of macrophages in the induction of antibody production [127]. In electron-microscopic autoradiographic studies Nossal et al. [97] found the labelled flagellar antigen to be accumulated mainly extracellularly in the lymph node follicles. The antigen could be detected on the cell surface, attached to the processes of dendritic macrophages, which penetrate tentacle-like among the lymphocytes. It has been demonstrated *in vitro* that the haemocyanin antigen persists on the surface of macrophages for 72 h and does not penetrate the cell [130]. Out of 1,000 antigen molecules, 33 were taken up by a single macrophage, but only one remained on the surface of the cell. Adherence to the surface is most likely effected through C3 receptors [105].

The question arises whether the antigen in the macrophage is bound to some macromolecule that might play a part in the coding of antibody production and protein synthesis. There are numerous data available indicating that there are

RNA fractions present in the macrophages which are capable of inducing antibody production [45, 110]. Two RNA fractions could be isolated from macrophages sensitized *in vitro* with T'2 phage; the one was a low mol. wt. (4 to 7 S) fraction which did not contain antigen fragments and was susceptible to ribonuclease; it induced IgM production when added to lymphocytes. The other fraction having a higher mol. wt. (15 to 30 S) was relatively resistant to ribonuclease and contained antigen which induced IgG synthesis. In this latter case RNA acted as adjuvant, thus the antigen–RNA complex was a *superantigen* [48].

### *Macrophage–lymphocyte interaction*

It is a common observation that, in tissue cultures, macrophages and lymphocytes are clumped together and form clusters. Clustering of the two types of leukocytes in tissue cultures derived from patients with autoimmune diseases has been termed 'rosette' formation or 'peripolesis'. Each macrophage is usually surrounded by several lymphocytes. It could be successfully demonstrated that in the course of peripolesis cytoplasmic bridges were formed between the macrophages and lymphocytes. It has been supposed that these bridges serve for the transfer of immunogenic material into the lymphocytes. The lymphocytes have a special organelle, the so-called uropod, for the establishment of lymphocyte–macrophage link. Nevertheless, it is also possible that the mere purpose of the lymphocyte–macrophage linkage is to maintain a close contact between the antigen located on the surface of the macrophage and the cell surface of the lymphocyte [36]. In the infections the collaboration between T cells and macrophages operates on two levels: T cells attract or arrest blood monocytes, thus promoting their accumulation in foci of infection, and there influence their metabolic state to produce activated macrophages. In several bacterial infections the activation of macrophages is probably of primary importance.

### *Antibody production of macrophages*

The morphology of antibody forming cells involved in natural immunity has been studied by electron-microscopic autoradiography, based on the principle that the antigen is attached to the surface of the antibody forming cells [17]. It has been found that in non-immunized animals about 85 per cent of the cells believed to be antibody forming are monocytes and macrophages and 15 per cent lymphocytes and plasmacytes. In immunized animals, on the other hand, the proportion of antibody forming monocytes and macrophages dropped to 10 per cent. This finding has been seriously challenged on the strength of various methodological objections, for all data concerning the antibody production of macrophages have to be accepted with reservation as long as an exact distinction between lymphocytes and macrophages is impossible.

Other investigators have also presented data indicating that macrophages might possess the ability of producing antibody. Following intrapulmonary immunization, it was possible to find histiocyte antibody producing cells in 20 to 25 per cent in the alveolar exudate [61]. These antibody forming macrophages appeared by electron microscopy as less differentiated cells, the antibody production of which could be blocked with silica and actinomycin-D. Further, Möller [90] reported on peritoneal macrophages which were able to haemolyse erythrocytes in the absence of antibody and C; he claimed that this phenomenon was distinctly different from all processes resulting in haemolysis so far studied. Active participation of the macrophages was necessary for the phenomenon of haemolysis to occur.

## THE ROLE OF MACROPHAGES IN CELL-MEDIATED IMMUNITY

In the efferent side of delayed, tuberculin-type hypersensitivity and in the transplantation immune reaction, macrophages are involved in great number, i.e. in mononuclear cellular infiltration. Isotope studies using $^3$H-thymidine have shown that the majority of cells taking part in the tuberculin-type response are macrophages and monocytes derived from the bone marrow [7, 16]. Further, there are numerous data available pointing to the active participation of macrophages in cell-mediated immune reactions. After selective destruction of mouse macrophages by silica particles smaller than 0.45 $\mu$m; skin allografts showed a significantly prolonged survival [102*a*]. Transfer experiments, on the other hand, have unequivocally demonstrated that immunocytes derived from syngeneic sensitized animals and labelled with $^3$H-thymidine were only involved in insignificant numbers in the allograft reaction of the recipient. The majority of cells in the infiltrate were the recipient's own cells, mainly monocytes [7]. It is a well-known fact that even the non-sensitized animal rejects the graft much more rapidly if lymphocytes derived from a sensitized syngeneic animal are injected into the recipient. Nevertheless, an enhanced rejection of skin allografts occurs also if cells of peritoneal exudate are given to the recipient in doses one-third of the optimum dose of lymphocytes [102*b*].

These findings allow the conclusion that the macrophages play a significant role in the efferent side of the cell-mediated immune reaction. Most likely, the macrophages are involved mainly aspecifically, activated by factors released by the effector lymphocytes (see below).

### *Effect of the migration inhibition factor (MIF) on macrophages*

Sensitized lymphocytes, when encountering the specific antigen, release an agent termed *migration inhibiting factor* (MIF). This factor inhibits the growth and migration of macrophages *in vitro* by promoting the adherence of macrophages to various surfaces [37*b*, 39, 49]. This phenomenon is of considerable significance *in vivo*, too, because at the sites where this factor is released by lymphocytes the circulating macrophages adhere to the capillary endothelium and then migrate into the interstitial space. This factor also enhances the clustering of lymphocytes to macrophages, and presumably also the cytotoxic effect of macrophages [5, 6, 7].

MIF is a cytophilic substance which exerts its effect on the surface of the macrophage. After destroying the cell surface by trypsin MIF fails to exert its effect. Macrophages have presumably a specific receptor to bind MIF [5, 6].

### *Macrophage–lymphocyte interaction*

A direct contact of the two types of cells can also be demonstrated in connection with delayed hypersensitivity reactions. *In vitro* studies have shown [6] that an immediate contact is established between sensitized and normal cells, irrespective of whether it was the macrophages or the lymphocytes that have been derived from sensitized animals. In the course of this reaction, either the lymphocytes surround the macrophages or the other way round. Due to the direct contact, macrophages derived from animals sensitized with the antigen induced a significantly more marked blast transformation than the antigen alone (e.g. PPD, Streptokinase, Streptolysin O, etc.) [59]. Adding tuberculin antigen to a monocyte suspension obtained from tuberculin-positive subjects and mixing this suspension with autologous lymphocytes after appropriate washing, it was possible to induce lymphoblast transformation in 19 of a total of 29 cases even in the absence of the tuberculin antigen due to the monocyte–lymphocyte interaction. The transformation could be induced even if the ratio of sensitized macrophages and lymphocytes was only 1 to 100.

All these data support the concept that the direct interaction of macrophages and lymphocytes plays an important part in the induction of the cell-mediated immunity.

### *Cytotoxic effect of macrophages*

Similarly to lymphocytes, macrophages are also able of a cytotoxic effect on target cells. Sensitized peritoneal exudate cells killed methylcholantrene induced tumour target cells with a five times higher activity than sensitized lymphocytes [103]. Immune macrophages adhere to the target cells in tumour monolayer cultures, causing their lysis within a few hours; however, the macrophages themselves succumb in this process ('allergic death'). The mechanism of the cytotoxic killing by macrophages has not been discovered as yet.

Non-sensitized macrophages also possess the above properties; in this case, cytophilic antibodies, either alone or together with C factors, seem to play an important part by causing adherence of the target cells around the macrophage [7, 41]. Recently it has been shown that lymphocytes shed their cytophilic receptors in the surrounding medium which bind to macrophages, thus rendering the macrophages cytotoxic [77*a*].

### *Macrophage cytophilic antibodies*

Boyden [18] was the first who described a method for the demonstration of macrophage *cytophilic antibodies*. He succeeded in demonstrating antibodies attached to the surface of macrophages derived from guinea pigs following immunization with sheep erythrocytes in Freund's adjuvant. *In vitro*, the 'rosette' formation of sheep erythrocytes around the macrophages, indicated the adherence of cytophilic antibodies to the cell surface. The so-called direct *in vitro* immunocyte-adherence technique is based on the sensitization of macrophages with the antibody-containing serum [18] (cf. below the description of the indirect method).

The macrophage cytophilic antibody can be detected in the $IgG_2$ fraction and it is only loosely attached to the surface of the macrophage. Its significance lies chiefly in opsonization, since the rosette formation occurring at room temperature is immediately followed by phagocytosis at 37 °C. Macrophage cytophilic antibodies are formed not only against erythrocytes but also against other antigens, and can be detected by passive rosette formation after adsorption of the sensitizing antigen to erythrocytes [92].

Macrophage cytophilic antibodies can also be detected using an indirect method [12]. The serum is first incubated with sheep erythrocytes, then these opsonized erythrocytes are allowed to react with the macrophages. This modification considerably enhances the sensitivity of the reaction, however, in contrast to the results obtained with the direct method, no correlation with delayed hypersensitivity is obtained. The test can be performed also with sera obtained from animals immunized i.p. with sheep erythrocytes without adjuvant. With the introduction of the indirect method our knowledge concerning the cytophilic antibodies had to be revised. The assumption that these antibodies have *specific* properties has been seriously challenged based on the fact that the method employed for their detection can be used for the identification of the IgG receptor of the macrophage (see section 'Surface properties of macrophages'). At the time when the IgG receptor of the macrophage was still unknown, it was justified to postulate a cytophilic antibody adhering to the cell, i.e. to the macrophage. Nevertheless, recent investigations are aimed at studying the factors which determine the binding of the IgG–antigen, IgG–antigen–C, and IgM–antigen–C complexes to the macrophage receptors as well as the intensity of this adherence. It is being investigated when this binding results in phagocytosis, in surface antigen retention, or cytotoxic process in case of a cellular antigen.

## THE ROLE OF MACROPHAGES IN THE ANTIBACTERIAL CELLULAR DEFENSE MECHANISMS

The macrophages have a primary role in the defense mechanisms against bacteria like *Salmonellae, M. tuberculosis, Listeria, Brucella,* etc. These pathogens by their continuous multiplication in the body constitute a persistent antigenic stimulus to the macrophages; however, the latter cannot destroy them even after phagocytosis. The macrophages show further maturation, proliferate and produce new lysosomal hydrolases under their influence. This cellular defense mechanism bound to the macrophages is not specific immunologically, since the established defense against some of the bacteria provides protection also against other bacteria growing intracellularly [95].

## REFERENCES


1. Ada, G. L.: In *Immunity, Cancer and Chemotherapy. Basic Relationship on the Cellular Level.* Ed. by Mihich, E. Academic Press, New York 1967, p. 17.

1*a*. Aiuti, F. and Wigzell, H.: *Clin. exp. Immunol.* **13,** 183 (1973).

2. Alm, G. V. and Peterson, R. D. A.: *J. exp. Med.* **129,** 1247 (1969).

3. Argyris, B. F.: *J. exp. Med.* **128,** 459 (1968).

4. Armstrong, W. D. and Diener, M.: *J. exp. Med.* **129,** 371 (1969).
4*a*. Asofsky, R., Cantor, H. and Tigelaar, R. E.: In *Progress on Immunology*. Ed. by Amos, B. D. Academic Press, New York 1971, p. 369.
5. Bartfeld, H. and Atoynatan, T.: *Proc. Soc. exp. Biol. Med. (N.Y.)* **130,** 497 (1969).
6. Bartfeld, H. and Kelly, R.: *J. Immunol.* **100,** 1000 (1968).
7. Benaceraff, B.: *Cancer Res.* **28,** 1392 (1968).
8. Benaceraff, B. and Levin, B. B.: *J. exp. Med.* **115,** 2023 (1962).
9. Benezra, D., Gery, I. and Davies, A. M.: *Clin. exp. Immunol.* **5,** 155 (1969).
10. Bennet, B. and Bloom, B. R.: *Transplantation* **5,** 996 (1967).
11. Berke, G., Ax, W., Ginsburg, H. and Feldman, M.: *Immunology* **16,** 643 (1969).
12. Berken, B. and Benaceraff, B.: *J. exp. Med.* **123,** 119 (1966).
13. Bert, G., Massaro, A. L., Lajolo di Gossano, D. and Maja, M.: *Immunology* **17,** 1 (1969).
14. Biozzi, G., Binaghi, R. A., Stiffel, C. and Mouton, D.: *Immunology* **16,** 349 (1969).
15. Bondevik, H. and Mannick, J. A.: *Proc. Soc. exp. Biol. (N.Y.)* **129,** 264 (1968).
16. Bosman, C. and Feldman, J. D.: *Exp. Hematol.* **16,** 34 (1968).
17. Bosman, C., Feldman, J. D. and Pick, E.: *J. exp. Med.* **129,** 1029 (1969).
18. Boyden, S. V.: *Immunology* **7,** 474 (1964).
19. Börjeson, J., Chessin, L. N. and Landry, M.: *Int. Arch. Allergy* **31,** 184 (1967).
20. Bradfield, J. W. and Born, C. W.: *Nature* **222,** 1183 (1969).
21. Brondz, B. D.: *Folia biol.* **14,** 115 (1968).
22. Brunner, K. T., Manel, J., Cerottini, J. C. and Chapius, B.: *Immunology* **14,** 181 (1968).
23. Buckton, K. E. and Pike, M. C.: *Nature* **202,** 714 (1964).
24. Byfield, P. and Sercarz, E.: *J. exp. Med.* 129, 897 (1969).
25. Campbell, P. A. and Kind, P.: *J. Immunol.* **102,** 1084 (1969).
26. Carr, I.: *J. Path. Bact.* **94,** 323 (1967).
27. Clarke, J. A., Salsburg, A. J. and Rowland, G. F.: *Brit. J. Haematol.* **14,** 533 (1968).
28. Cline, M. J. and Swett, V. C.: *J. exp. Med.* **128,** 1309 (1968).
29. Cohn, Z. A.: *Advanc. Immunol.* **9,** 163 (1969).
29*a*. Cooper, M. G. and Ada, G. L.: *Scand. J. Immunol.* **1,** 247 (1972).
30. Coulson, A. S. and Chalmers, D. G.: *Immunology* **12,** 417 (1967).
31. Craddock, C. G., Winkelstein, A., Matsuyuki, Y. and Lawrence, J. S.: *J. exp. Med.* **125,** 1149 (1967).
32. Crowhter, D., Fairley, G. H. and Sewell, R. L.: *J. exp. Med.* **129,** 849 (1969).
33. Cudkowicz, G., Shearer, C. M. and Priore, R. L.: *J. exp. Med.* **180,** 48 (1969).
34. Cunningham, A. J.: *Immunology* **16,** 621 (1969).
35. Dameshek, W.: *Blood* **21,** 243 (1963).
36. Daniels, J. C., Ritzmann, J. E. and Levin, W. C.: *Texas Rep. Biol. Med.* **26,** 5 (1968).
37*a*. David, J. E.: *Proc. nat. Acad. Sci. (Wash.)* **56,** 72 (1966).
37*b*. id. *Cancer Res.* **28,** 1387 (1968).
37*c*. id., *Fed. Proc.* **30,** 1730 (1971).
38. David, J. R., Al-Askati, S., Lawrence, H. S. and Thomas, L.: *J. Immunology* **93,** 264 (1964).
39. David, J. R., Lawrence, H. S. and Thomas, L.: *J. Immunol.* **93,** 279 (1964).
40. Denham, S., Hall, J. G., Wolf, A. and Alexander, P.: *Transplantation* **7,** 194 (1969).
41. Dumonde, D. C.: *Brit. med. Bull.* **23,** 9, (1968).
42. Dumonde, D. C., Page, D. A., Matthew, M. and Wolstencroft, R. A.: *Clin. Immunol.* **10,** 25 (1972).
43. Ehrlich, P. and Lazarus, A.: *Die Anaemie. I. Abteilung. Normale und pathologische Histologie des Blutes.* Alfred Holder, Vienna 1898.
44. Everett, N. B., Caffrey, R. W. and Ricke, W. O.: *Ann. N. Y. Acad. Sci.* **113,** 887 (1964).
45. Fishman, M. and Adler, F. L., In *Immunity, Cancer and Chemotherapy. Basic Relationship on the Cellular Level.* Ed. by Mihich, E. Academic Press, New York 1967.

46. Fitzgerald, P. H.: *J. theor. Biol.* **6,** 12 (1964).
47. Gallily, R. and Feldman, M.: *Israel J. med. Sci.* **2,** 358 (1966).
48. Garvey, J. and Campbell, D.: *J. exp. Med.* **105,** 361 (1957).
49. George, M. and Vaugham, J.: *Proc. Soc. exp. Biol. (N.Y.)* **111,** 514 (1962).
50. Gery, J., Benezra, D. and Davies, A. M.: *Immunology* **16,** 381 (1969).
51. Good, R. A. and Gabrielson, A. E.: In *Human Transplantation*. Ed. by Rapaport, F. T. and Dausset, J. D. Grune Stratton, New York 1968, p. 526.
52. Gowans, J. L. and Mc Gregor, D. D.: *Progr. Allergy* **9,** 1 (1965).
53. Granger, G. A., Shacks, S. J., Williams, T. W. and Kolb, W. P.: *Nature* **221,** 1155 (1969).
54. Greaves, M. F., Roitt, I. M. and Rose, M. E.: *Nature* **220,** 293 (1968).
55. Greaves, M. F., Roitt, I. M., Zamir, R. and Carnagham, R. S. A.: *Lancet* **ii,** 1317 (1967).
56. Greaves, M. F., Torrigiani, G. and Roitt, I. M.: *Nature* **22,** 885 (1969).
57. Hamashoka, T., Kitagawa, M., Matsuoka, Y. and Yamenura, Y.: *Immunology* **17,** 55 (1969).
58. Hamilton, L. D.: *Nature* **178,** 597 (1956).
59. Hersh, E. M. and Harris, J. E.: *J. Immunol.* **100,** 1184 (1968).
60. Hirschhorn, R., Troll, W., Brittinger, G. and Weismann, G.: *Nature* **222,** 1247 (1969).
61. Holub, M. and Hauser, E. R.: *Immunology* **17,** 207 (1969).
62. Huber, H., Douglas, S. D. and Fudenberg, H. H.: *Immunology* **17,** 7 (1969).
63. Huber, H., Douglas, S. D., Huber, C. and Goldberg, S. L.: *Int. Arch. Allergy* **41,** 262 (1971).
64. Huber, H. and Pastner, D.: *Med. Klin.* **64,** 1183 (1969).
65. Huber, H., Polley, M. J., Linsrott, N. D., Fudenberg, H. H. and Müller-Ebenhardt, H. J.: *Science* **162,** 1281 (1968).
66. Humphrey, J. H. and White, R. G.: *Immunology for Students of Medicine*. 2nd ed. Blackwell, London 1967.
67. Jerne, N. K., Nordin, A. A. and Henry, C., In *Cell-Bound Antibodies*. Ed. by Amos, B., and Koprowski, H. Wistar Inst. Philadelphia 1963, p. 109.
68. Johnson, L. I., LoBue, J., Chau, P. Ch., Monette, C. F., Rubin, A. D., Gordon, A. S. and Dameshek, A. S.: *Proc. Soc. exp. Biol. (N.Y.)* **130,** 675 (1969).
69. Johnston, R. B. and Klemper, M. R.: *J. exp. Med.* **129,** 1275 (1969).
70. Jurezir, R. E., Thor, D. E. and Dray, S.: *J. Immunology* **101,** 823 (1968).
71. Kammermeyer, J. K., Roof, R. K., Stites, D. P., Glade, P. R. and Chassin, L. N.: *Proc. Soc. exp. Biol. (N.Y.)* **129,** 522 (1968).
72. Kelly, R. H., Wolstencroft, R. A., Dumonde, D. C. and Balfour, M. B.: *Clin. exp. Immunol.* **10,** 49 (1972).
73. Klein, J., In *Histocompatibility Testing*. Ed. by Curtoni, E. S., Mattiuz, P. C. and Tosi, R. M. Munksgaard, Copenhagen 1967.
74. Krisch, R. E.: *Nature* **222,** 1295 (1969).
75. LaBella, F. S. and Kross, M. E.: *Nature* **220,** 1141 (1968).
76. Lance, E. M. and Taub, R. N.: *Nature* **221,** 841 (1969).
77. Lay, W. H. and Nussenzweig, V.: *J. exp. Med.* **128,** 991 (1968).
77*a*. Lohmann-Matthes, M. L., Ziegier, F. G. and Fisher, H.: *Eur. J. Immunol.* **3,** 56 (1973).
78. MacFarland, W.: *Science* **163,** 818 (1969).
79. MacFarland, W., Heilman, D. H. and Moorhead, J. F.: *J. exp. Med.* **124,** 851 (1966).
80. Mackaness, G. B.: *J. exp. Med.* **129,** 973 (1969).
81. MacLaurin, B. D.: *Aust. J. exp. Biol. med. Sci.* **47,** 105 (1969).
82. Maini, R. N., Dumonde, D. C., Faux, J. A., Hargreave, F. E. and Pepys, J.: *Clin. exp. Immunol.* **9,** 449 (1971).
83. Marshall, H. W., Valentine, F. T. and Lawrence, H. S.: *J. exp. Med.* **130,** 327 (1969).
84. Marshall, W. H. and Roberts, K. B.: *Quart. J. exp. Physiol.* **50,** 361 (1965).
85. Matsuoka, Y. and Takehaski, M.: *J. Immunol.* **101,** 1111 (1968).
86. Meuwissen, H. J., Kaplan, C. T., Percy, D. Y. and Good, R. A.: *Proc. Soc. exp. Biol. (N.Y.)* **130,** 300 (1969).

87. Micklem, H. S., Ford, C. E., Evans, E. P. and Gray, J.: *Proc. roy. Soc. Biol.* **165,** 78 (1966).
88. Miller, J. F. A. P.: *Brit. J. Haemat.* **16,** 331 (1969).
89. Mosier, D. E. and Coppleson, L. W.: *Proc. nat. Acad. Sci. (Wash.)* **61,** 542 (1968).
90. Möller, E.: *Immunology,* **16,** 609 (1969).
91. Möller, E. and Lapp, W.: *Immunology,* **16,** 561 (1969).
92. Nelson, D. S. and Boyden, S. V.: *Brit. med. Bull.* **23,** 15 (1967).
93*a*. Noltenius, H. and Chakin, M.: *Experientia (Basel)* **25,** 401 (1969).
93*b*. id., *Naturwissenschaften,* **56,** 140 (1969).
94. Noltenius, H., Chakin, M. and Rüppel, V.: *Naturwissenschaften,* **56,** 216 (1969).
95. North, R. J.: *J. exp. Med.* **130,** 299 (1969).
96*a*. Nossal, G. J. V.: In *Human Transplantation.* Ed. by Rapaport, F. T. and Dausset, J. Grune and Stratton, New York 1968, p. 643.
96*b*. id., *Klin. Wschr.* **47,** 568 (1969).
96*c*. id., *Circulation* **39,** 5 (1969).
97. Nossal, G. V. J., Abbot, A. and Mitchell, J.: *J. exp. Med.* **127,** 263 (1968).
98. Nossal, G. V. J., Abbot, A., Mitchell, J. and Immens, Z.: *J. exp. Med.* **127,** 277 (1968).
99. Nossal, G. V. J., Cunningham, F. A., Mitchell, G. F. and Miller, J. F. A. P.: *J. exp. Med.* **128,** 839 (1968).
100. Osoba, D.: *J. exp. Med.* **129,** 141 (1969).
101. Ottesen, J.: *Acta physiol. scand.* **32,** 75 (1954).
102*a*. Pearsall, N. N. and Weiser, R. S.: *Reticuloendothel. Soc.* **5,** 107 (1968).
102*b*. ibid., **5,** 121 (1968).
103. Pearson, G. R., Hodes, R. J. and Friberg, S.: *Clin. exp. Immunol.* **5,** 273 (1969).
104. Perlmann, P., Perlmann, H., Müller-Eberhard, H. J. and Manni, J. A.: *Science* **163,** 937 (1969).
105. Phillips-Quaglieta, J. M., Levin, B. B. and Uhr, J. W.: *Nature* **222,** 1290 (1969).
106. Pierce, C. W.: *J. exp. Med.* **130,** 345 (1969).
107. Raff, M., Nase, S. and Mitchison, N. A.: *Nature* **230,** 50 (1971).
107*a*. Raff, M. C. and Cantor, H.: In *Progress in Immunology.* Ed. by Amos, B. D. Academic Press, New York 1971, p. 83.
108. Rebuck, J. H., Coffman, H. I., Bluhm, G. B. and Barth, C. L.: *Ann. N.Y. Acad. Sci.* **113,** 595 (1964).
109. Rhodes, J. M., Lind, J., Birkch-Andersen, A. and Ravn, H.: *Immunology* **17,** 445 (1969).
110. Roelants, E. G. and Goodman, J. W.: *J. exp. Med.* **130,** 557 (1969).
111. Roitt, I. M., Greaves, M. F., Torrigiani, G., Brostoff, J. J. and Playfair, A. L.: *Lancet* **ii,** 367 (1969).
112. Roseman, J. M. and Leserman, L. D.: *J. Immunol.* **102,** 1002 (1969).
113. Ruddle, N. H. and Waksman, B. V.: *J. exp. Med.* **128,** 1237 (1968).
114. Saunders, G. C.: *J. exp. Med.* **130,** 543 (1969).
115. Sell, S.: *J. exp. Med.* **127,** 1139 (1968).
116. Shearer, G. M. and Cudkowicz, G.: *J. exp. Med.* **129,** 935 (1969).
117. Shelton, E.: *J. cell. Biol.* **12,** 652 (1962).
118. Shortman, K. and Szengberg, A.: *Austr. J. exp. Biol. med. Sci.* **47,** 1 (1969).
119. Singhal, S. K. and Richter, M.: *J. exp. Med.* **128,** 1099 (1968).
120. Skamene, E. and Iványi, J.: *Nature* **221,** 681 (1969).
121. Spector, W. G. and Ryan, G. B.: *Nature* **221,** 860 (1969).
121*a*. Sprent, J. and Miller, J. F. A. P.: *Nature (new Biol.)* **234,** 195 (1971).
122. Steffen, C.: *Allgemeine und experimentelle Immunologie und Immunpathologie.* Thieme, Stuttgart 1968.
123. Stobbe, H.: *Hämatologischer Atlas,* Akademie Verlag, Berlin 1959.
124. Syren, E. and Raeste, A. A.: *Acta haemat.* **45,** 29 (1971).
125. Tannenberg, W. J. K. and Malavya, A. N.: *J. exp. Med.* **128,** 895 (1968).
126. Thor, D. E. and Dray, S. K.: *J. Immunol.* **101,** 469 (1968).
127. Tizard, J. R.: *Int. Arch. Allergy* **36,** 332 (1969).
128*a*. Turk, J. L.: *Transplantation* **5,** 952 (1967)

128*b*. id., In *Immunity, Cancer and Chemotherapy. Basic Relationship on the Cellular Level*. Ed. by Mikich, E. Academic Press, New York 1967, p. 1.
129. Unanue, E. R. and Askonas, B. A.: *J. exp. Med.* **127,** 915 (1968).
130. Unanue, E. R., Cerottini, J. C. and Bedford, M.: *Nature* **222,** 1193 (1969).
131. van Furth, R. and Cohn, Z. A.: *J. exp. Med.* **128,** 415 (1968).
132. Walters, C. S. and Jackson, A. L.: *J. Immunol.* **101,** 541 (1968).
133. Weiss, L.: *J. Immunol.* **101,** 1346 (1968).
134. *WHO Scientific Group:* Clinical Immunology. *Wld Hlth Org. techn. Rep. Ser.* No. 496. WHO, Geneva 1972, p. 19.
134*a*. WHO Scientific Group: Cell-Mediated Immunity and Resistance to Infection. *Wld Hlth Org. techn. Rep. Ser.* No. 519. WHO, Geneva 1972, p. 10.
134*b*. ibid., p. 20.
135. Wigzell, H. and Anderson, B.: *J. exp. Med.* **129,** 23 (1969).
136. Wilkinson, P. C., Borel, J. F., Stecher-Levin, V. J. and Sorkin, E.: *Nature* **222,** 244 (1969).
137. Wilson, D. B.: *Transplantation* **5,** 986 (1967).
138. Wilson, J. D. and Nossal, G. J. V.: *Lancet* **ii,** 1153 (1971).
139. Wood, W. B., Smith, M. R. and Watson, B.: *Science* **104,** 28 (1946).
140. Wortis, H. H., Dresser, D. W. and Anderson, H. R.: *Immunology* **17,** 93 (1969).

CHAPTER 9

# THE THYMUS

by

I. SZERI



## INTRODUCTION

The immunological role of the thymus has been recognized only in the last decade, following Miller's investigations on newborn rodents [94*b*, *c*, *d*]. A new, productive branch of immunology developed from his contribution, the results of which are summarized in numerous reviews [57, 56, 92*k*, 100].

In this section a brief survey of the results which elucidate the immunological role of the thymus will be presented.

## MORPHOLOGY AND DEVELOPMENT OF THE THYMUS

The thymus is an encapsulated, greyish-white, lymphoepithelial organ. It is generally situated in the chest, in the upper part of the anterior mediastinum. In some species (e.g. birds, crocodile, certain marsupials, guinea pig) it is localized in the neck. Species having both a cervical and a mediastinal thymus are also known (e.g. certain marsupials, mole). In most species the substance of the thymus is divided by fibrous septa into lobules. In most species the individual lobules consist of a central medullary substance and a surrounding cortex. The size of the thymus varies between wide limits in different species, however, the size of the individual lobules shows a close similarity. On this basis it was suggested that the thickness of the cortex is restricted in relation to the size of the medulla within certain critical limits [92*l*].

On the phylogenetic scale the thymus first appears in vertebrates. In the earlier round-mouthed types no thymus was found. In the spindle fish, however, a substance resembling a thymus is present, which is called protothymus. From the bony fishes on, all the vertebrate species develop a similar thymus structure. With regard to its origin, it is a branchiogenic organ and usually develops as a diverticulum of the IIIrd and IVth branchial clefts. In species at a low level of development, it originates from the dorsal, while in mammals from the ventral wall of the branchial cleft; an intermediate stage can be found in marsupials.

During embryogenesis the thymus initially appears as an accumulation of epithelial cells, while after several divisions, it is transformed into an epithelial cord and becomes separated from the branchial clefts. It is called epithelial thymus at this stage. In later stages, the distance between the epithelial cells increases, and the cells form a network, the so-called epithelial reticulum. Septa from the surrounding connective tissue subdivide the area. Within these areas a cortical and a medullary substance can be distinguished. The epithelial reticulum of the cortex becomes filled with small, round lymphoid cells. Thus the lymphatic thymus develops. In the fully developed thymus only remnants of the epithelial cells are present in the form of Hassall's corpuscles.

Following sexual maturation, the involution of the thymus begins resulting in a weight loss of the organ. The atrophy first affects the lymphoid substance of the cortex, resulting in a gradual shift of the previously constant cortico-medullary ratio.

Finally, the lymphoid tissue becomes replaced by adipose tissue; giving rise to the so-called adipose thymus.

The ontogenesis of the human thymus has been studied in detail [62]. The epithelial arrangement of the thymus develops from the ventral wall of the IIIrd and IVth branchial clefts at 4–8.5 mm length of the embryo; at approx. 30 mm body length the lymphoid cells appear; while marrow production is initiated at 40 mm length of the embryo. The first Hassall's corpuscle appears at about 50 mm body length. By the end of the second month the organ is situated in the anterior mediastinum, and both of its lobes are developed. The organ keeps growing reaching its maximum weight at adolescence, thereafter its involution starts. In old age only epithelial islands surrounded by connective tissue are usually found.

A close similarity has been discovered between the development and morphology of the thymus and of the dorsal diverticulum-like gland situated close to the cloaca of birds, which is named bursa of Fabricius after its describer Hieronymus Fabricius. On the 12th day of incubation a thickening appears in the cloacal epithelium, which continues to grow. On the 14th day lymphoid cells appear in the epithelial clumps, and by the 18th day the bursa has a true lymphoid structure. Eight to ten days after hatching the cortex and medulla can be distinguished. Involution of the bursa, similarly to the thymus, starts after sexual maturity is reached. The age-related involution among lymphoid organs affects only the thymus and the bursa, not being evident in other lymphoid organs. Birds have both a thymus and a bursa. In mammals the Peyer patches, as well as the lymphoid cells of the intestinal epithelium of the appendix and of the tonsils are considered as being equivalents of the bursa of birds.

In recent years, the origin of the small round lymphoid cells, which fill up the spaces in the cortical epithelial reticulum of the thymus, has been debated. These cells are referred to as thymocytes by a number of investigators. Two theories have been put forward: according to the pseudomorphosis (infiltration) theory the lymphocytes develop from mesenchymal cells migrating into the thymus epithelium during early development; according to the transformation theory, however, the thymus lymphocytes are considered to be derived from the epithelial cells of thymus.

To resolve this problem experiments were devised, in which donor and host lymphoid cells could be easily distinguished by using chromosome markers and isotope techniques. When an irradiated thymus was implanted into an irradiated host, the implanted organ retained its epithelial structure [94*j*]. If, however, an irradiated thymus was transferred to a non-irradiated host, only the host cells took part in lymphoid regeneration [32]. These results support the pseudomorphosis theory, indicating that the lymphoid cells are not derived from the epithelial cells, but from cells leaving circulation.

Furthermore, the identification of the earliest precursors of thymic lymphocytes, which ensure the replacement and the continuity of the system is of considerable interest. Cells with chromosome markers from bone marrow, thymus and lymph node were implanted into lethally irradiated animals. The cells originating from the bone marrow proliferated both in the thymus and the bone marrow, but cells derived from the thymus and the lymph nodes showed proliferation only in the lymph nodes [48]. Small labelled lymphocytes from the thoracic duct, when transferred to a lethally irradiated rat, readily formed colonies in lymphoid organs but not in the thymus [58]. Accordingly, it was concluded that the precursors of the thymic lymphoid cells are derived from the bone marrow, which assumption was also confirmed by more recent findings [29, 99, 102*b*, 105].

The existence of bone marrow stem cells was also indicated by earlier experiments, showing that normal thymic transplants into sublethally irradiated animals grew only poorly compared with transplants into normal or irradiated and bone marrow-transplanted hosts [14]. However, it appears that the age-related involution of the thymus is not due to a lack of stem cells [92*i*].

## THYMIC LYMPHOCYTES

The kinetics of the thymus lymphocyte were studied by morphologic and isotopic techniques, as well as by the measurement of DNS turnover rate. One mg of thymus tissue contains approx. 3 million lymphoid cells [8]. Mitosis is evident in 0.6 per cent of the lymphoid cells. In lymphatic organs of rodents the established mitotic indices show that the mitotic activity of the lymphoid cells is 5–10 times higher in the thymus cortex than in other lymphatic organs. Similar results were obtained by establishing the other index of cell proliferation, i.e. by the measurement of DNS turnover rate [4, 36]. The lymphoid cells in the thymic medulla, in contrast to the cortical lymphocytes, show little mitotic activity [92*g*]. The mitotic activity of the thymic lymphoid cells is greatest in the newborn period, and it begins to diminish with the age-related involution, becoming equivalent to the mitotic activity of lymphoid cells in other lymphatic organs [3, 92*g*]. Isotopic studies [93] show that the entire population of small lymphocytes in the thymic cortex is renewed in 3–4 days. Ninety-five per cent of the small lymphocytes have a short life-span while 5 per cent show a longer one. Of the latter a few may be localized in the medulla. According to calculations, 1 million lymphocytes are produced daily by 1 mg of thymic tissue [100].

Despite the rapid turnover of small lymphocytes, the size of the thymus remains constant for considerable periods. Therefore a control mechanism causing either a continuous cell loss or cell destruction must be present. The outflow of lymphocytes from the thymus has been confirmed and the lymphocyte content of blood draining the thymus has been found to be increased [35]. Isotope studies confirmed the production of colonies in the peripheral lymphatic organs by lymphoid cells originating from the thymus. Colony formation is more frequent in the early years of life than later [108]. Using chromosome markers it was shown that lymphocytes originating from a thymus graft appear in the surrounding lymphatic organs [32, 101]. However, in adult animals significantly fewer lymphocytes flow out from the thymus to form colonies in the peripheral lymphatic organs, than are produced in the thymus. In this respect, experiments performed with multiple thymus grafts are especially convincing. The lymphoid organs of a mouse implanted with 24 thymus grafts showed no significant deviation from the normal in their weight, constitution, and mitotic activity. Moreover, both the peripheral blood and the thymus of the host showed normal morphology and there was no lymphoid infiltration in any other tissues either [92*f*]. The few cells leaving the thymus may be identical with the small lymphocytes having a longer life span [156].

An outflow of cells from the thymus corresponding to the rate of proliferation could not be verified by experiments. Thus only one explanation remains for the constancy of weight of the thymus: a large proportion of the small lymphocytes of the thymus degenerate after 3–4 days of life in the organ itself. Neither the significance of the intensive lymphopoiesis in the thymus, nor the function of the short-lived cells is known. It was proposed that the short-lived lymphocytes functioned as trophocytes, supplying building materials for the growth and differentiation of the other tissue cells [85]. According to another explanation, the intensive thymic lymphopoiesis provides the organism with lymphoid cells reactive with various types of antigens; the degeneration of lymphocytes in the thymus would correspond to a protective mechanism eliminating the continuously produced autoaggressive cells [149]. The trophocytic function of the lymphocytes could not be convincingly proved, moreover experimentally supported considerations make it also improbable that 95 per cent of the thymic lymphocytes are autoaggressive [100]. Thus the function of the short lived thymic lymphocytes remains unknown.

## THE IMMUNOLOGICAL FUNCTION OF THE THYMUS

According to our present knowledge, the thymus plays a basic role in the development of the immune mechanisms of the organism. According to both phylogenetic and ontogenetic data the appearance of thymus and of organized lymphoid tissue coincides with the development of adaptive immunologic responsiveness.

Certainly, in the most primitive bony and cartilaginous fishes definite thymic and lymphoid tissues are already present.

These animals exhibit accordingly a capability for an adaptive immune response, which is characterized by formation of specific immunoglobulins in response to antigenic stimulation and by the development of an immunological memory. The lowest step on the developmental scale is represented by the two main orders of Cyclostomata, which are the most primitive among living vertebrates, i.e. by the more ancient hagfish (Eptatretidae) and the lamprey (Petromyzonidae). Their immunological behaviour shows marked differences. *Eptatretus stoncii* has neither thymic nor lymphoid tissues, and is incapable of adaptive immune responses; *Petromyzon marinus* possessing a rudimentary thymus displays a primitive adaptive immune response [115]. During embryogenesis in the frog [18] and opossum [76], adaptive immune reactions become manifest only when lymphocytes appear in the circulation.

For the last decade research has been mainly concerned with the elucidation of the role of thymus and of the thymus dependent lymphocyte system in immune mechanisms. Valuable observations have been obtained by the analysis of thymic lymphopoiesis, by the study of the effects of thymectomy, and of the methods suitable to overcome its consequences.

## LYMPHOPOIESIS IN THE THYMUS

The reaction of antigen with thymus lymphocytes differs principally from the antigen stimulated lymphocyte response of other lymphatic organs. Antigenic stimulation does not produce a proliferation of thymic lymphocytes, no germinal centres develop in the thymus and there is no evident plasma cell reaction [42, 141]. Neither is a humoral antibody response detectable [96, 141]. The cells of the thymus fail to bring about a graft-versus-host reaction in the rat, even in very large doses [12]. Hence thymic lymphocytes are immunologically not fully competent.

However, quite contradictory results were also published. For example, the introduction of antigen directly into the thymus was successful in producing germinal centres in the organ, in eliciting a plasma cell reaction and the synthesis of immunoglobulins [129]. Thymus implanted into the anterior chamber of the eye was able to produce tetanus antitoxin [131]. A GVH reaction could be elicited by cells derived from the thymus of adult or newborn mice [17]. Based on these results, it was thought that the apparent immunological passivity of the thymus lymphocytes is determined not by their quality, but by their location. It was proposed that a barrier exists between the thymus and circulation [98], which prevents the circulating antigens from reaching the cells of the thymus. The existence of this hypothetical barrier was refuted by investigations demonstrating that injected dyes, colloidal substances, and foreign serum albumin readily enter the thymic tissue and even the thymus cells themselves [15]. Neither can the immunological passivity of the thymus be explained by assuming the lack of phagocytic activity within the organ, as the normal thymus contains large numbers of reticulo-endothelial cells, histiocytes and macrophages, and their effective phagocytic activity could also be verified [61].

Experiments in which immunological reactivity of thymus lymphocytes removed from the organism were investigated were of utmost importance. Thymus lymphoid cells transferred to an irradiated recipient produced an immunological response significantly lower than that elicited by a similar quantity of splenic cells [140]. Following antigen stimulation no haemolysin producing cells could be demonstrated in the spleen of lethally irradiated recipients transplanted with thymic cells [77]. These results unanimously demonstrate that cells originating from the thymus are not, or only slightly sensitive to antigen even outside the thymus. Thus, it is not an inhibitory factor which affects thymus lymphocytes within the organ, but they differ qualitatively from antigen sensitive cells.

According to quantitative and morphological considerations, it seems probable that the few antigen sensitive cells observed among those obtained from the thymus were probably extrathymic, immunologically competent lymphocytes. Small numbers of immunologically competent cells derived from the circulation, especially from the interlobular blood vessels of the thymus, and from the small lymph nodes which are difficult to separate from the organ may become mixed with the cells of the thymus. This theory is also corroborated by experimental evidence. It has been demonstrated with immunofluorescent techniques that plasma cells and medium sized lymphocytes localized in the perivascular connective tissue were responsible for the production of IgG and IgA antibodies within the thymus [50]. In other cases, the tissue destructive effects of the antigens used may have caused the entry of antibody producing cells from circulation into the thymus. Thus, after intravenous injection of the somatic antigen of *Salmonella enteritidis*, antibody producing cells were demonstrable in the thymus, but at the same time, disorganization of the thymus structure was also observed [80]. Contamination by extrathymic immunocompetent cells may also explain the success of GVH reactions elicited by thymus cells [12]. However, many times as much cells were necessary from the thymus than from the spleen or lymph nodes to produce a GVH reaction.

According to some experiments, the usual presence of antigen sensitive cells among thymus cells can be explained assuming that a few cells in the thymus may reach the stage of maturity necessary for reaction to an antigen. Successful GVH reactions were produced using the same amounts of cell suspension from newborn thymus as is necessary from adult thymus. However, a similar dose of newborn splenic cells was not enough to produce a GVH reaction [17]. These results imply that a few cells exist in the thymus which are capable of inducing a GVH reaction but their number does not increase with age.

According to experiments carried out on chicken thymus, the lymphocytes of the thymic medulla, and those of the lymph nodes and spleen, possess similar immunological competence. Contrary to the lymphocytes of the cortex, they will produce an immune response to antigenic stimulation [151], i.e. only the cortical lymphocytes of the thymus lack antigen sensitivity.

The passive transfer of tuberculin sensitivity by thymic lymphocytes [130] has not been satisfactorily proved, as the participation of lymphocytes derived from lymph nodes could not be ruled out.

Thus according to the experimental results, the large majority of the cortical lymphocytes of the thymus, contrary to those localized in the lymph node and spleen, is unable to interact with antigen: there is no cell proliferation and antibody production following antigenic stimulation, they cannot elicit a GVH reaction and transfer tuberculin sensitivity.

The cortical lymphocytes of the thymus differ also in other properties from splenic and lymph node lymphocytes while the lymphocytes of the medulla are similar to the latter in several properties. To stimulation by phytohaemagglutinin, none, or only a few lymphocytes, mainly those derived from the medulla of the thymus, respond with a blastoid transformation [128, 154, 159]. The lymphocytes of the thymic medulla, as well as those of the spleen and lymph nodes contain more mitochondria and a more abundant endoplasmic reticulum together with a better developed nucleus than the lymphocytes of the cortex [106]. The radiosensitivity of the medullary lymphocytes is smaller ($LD_{70} = 180$ r) than that of the cortical lymphocytes ($LD_{70} = 46$ r) [147].

With regard to the origin of the medullary lymphocytes, several hypotheses have been proposed: they develop as the result of recirculation of the peripheral, small lymphocytes with a long life-span; they are more mature forms of their precursors localized in the cortex; or the two types of lymphocytes have different origins. The cortical lymphocytes, contrary to medullary ones, show very high mitotic activity, the lymphopoiesis in the thymic cortex is more intense than in the medulla. This lymphopoiesis in the thymic cortex differs from that occurring in lymph nodes or spleen, because it is independent of antigenic stimulation [100] as shown by several experiments. In the foetus, relatively protected from antigenic stimulation, the number of divisions of lymphoid cells is relatively large in the thymic cortex, and is small, or entirely absent in other lymphoid organs [92*g*]. The mitotic rate of the lymphoid cells in the thymus of both germ-free and conventionally kept mice is similar, while it is considerably lowered in the lymphatic tissue of the germ-free mice, contrary to those kept conventionally [157]. Antigenic stimulation by parenteral injection does not stimulate thymic lymphoid cell divisions [92*e*]. It seems that lymphopoiesis within the thymus is primarily determined not by external factors, but by the thymus itself. External factors which may have certain effect upon thymic lymphopoiesis are of endocrine nature. However, the age-related involution cannot be prevented by any endocrine intervention [30].

According to experiments with thymus grafts, age-related thymic involution is not influenced by the age of the host. The developmental dynamics of thymic grafts implanted into hosts of varying ages was independent of the thymus of the host, but agreed with that found in intact animals of the same group from which the thymus graft had been taken [92*g*]. The growth of the individual thymus graft was not influenced by the presence or absence of the host's thymus, or by the presence of multiple thymus grafts [32, 90, 92*f*, *g*]. On the contrary, using multiple splenic grafts, the mass of the grafts showed such a large decrease that the total weight of the grafted spleens was approximately similar to the weight of the spleen of a normal mouse [92*h*]. The removal of the spleen and lymph nodes did not influence either the growth of the thymic graft, or the proliferation of the thymic lymphoid cells [92*g*]. It appears, therefore, that the growth of the thymus is not influenced by external factors, and the development of the thymus is not subject to factors responsible for endocrine homeostasis [92*h*]. According to experimental evidence, the cytoreticulum of the thymic epithelium itself is responsible for the stimulus resulting in thymic lymphoid cell proliferation, which also determines the age-related involution of the thymus [92*i*, 94*c*]. However, the presence of medullary tissue is necessary in some way for the uninterrupted lymphopoiesis [92*f*]. Morphological analyses showed a close connection between the lymphocytes and epithelial cells of the thymus. It was proposed that in this way information can be transferred from the epithelial cells to lymphocytes [142, 143].

Summing up the above results, it may be proposed that the thymus is built up from several independent sub-units, in which the division of the primitive lymphoid cells gives rise to many small lymphocytes capable of differentiation, whose number is, nevertheless limited. These events are not controlled by some external feed-back mechanism, but by an internal, so far unknown, feed-back mechanism, which determines the size of the sub-units and the degree of differentiation of the lymphocytes [100]. The basic function of the thymus is the intensive lymphopoiesis which appears to be autonomous, and independent of antigenic stimulation. All these characteristics distinguish the thymus as a primary, central lymphatic organ, from the secondary, peripheral lymphatic organs, i.e. the spleen and the lymph nodes.

## THE CONSEQUENCES OF THYMECTOMY

Information concerning the function of the thymus may be obtained by observing the consequences of thymectomy.

### *Changes in lymphopoiesis*

The most significant consequence of thymectomy performed on mice [92*d*, 94*a*], rats [117], and guinea pigs [16, 118] belonging to different age groups was a diminution of the lymphocyte population. Similar results were obtained with chickens [19, 72], dogs [139], and also in man [75]. The small lymphocytes were absent from the blood and from the thoracic duct lymph. The lack of small lymphocytes was most pronounced when thymectomy was performed postnatally, when the lymphocyte depletion appeared early, the number of small lymphocytes remained at the low level observed at birth, in contrast with the increasing values found during growth of the control animals. Thymectomy performed on adult animals produced a gradual decrease in the number of small lymphocytes requiring several months to reach a minimum.

In parallel with the depletion of the small lymphocytes in the blood and the thoracic duct lymph, following thymectomy, characteristic alterations appeared in the histological picture of the secondary lymphatic organs. Well marked lymphocyte depletion was found around the central arterioles of the splenic follicles, and also in the paracortical areas of the lymph nodes [94*d*, 112*a*]. These areas of the peripheral lymphatic organs showing a lymphocyte depletion, as a consequence of thymectomy, were named thymus dependent areas [118].

In rats and mice, following thymectomy, neither a poor development of the germinal centres of the peripheral lymphatic organs nor a decrease in the number of the plasma cells could be observed [118, 150]. It was concluded that the formation of germinal centres, and the function of plasmacytopoiesis are not thymus dependent processes. This suggestion was reinforced by results obtained in birds.

Thymectomy performed during incubation of chickens resulted in a diminution of the number of small lymphocytes in the blood and spleen, but it did not diminish the number of plasma cells in the spleen [152*a*]. However, in freshly hatched chickens, which had undergone bursectomy and irradiation, the follicles and the plasma cells were absent [19]. Thus the concept of bursa dependent lymphoid tissues was put forward. According to this hypothesis, the central, clear, short-lived large lymphoid cells of the germinal centres and the widely distributed plasma cells are primarily dependent upon the bursa. The distinction between the bursa- and thymus dependent lymphoid systems appeared justified from other aspects, too. For example, there is no proof that thymus derived lymphoid cells would be able to transform into plasma cells on the periphery [108].

The latest publications corroborate the earlier proposition of the existence of two types of lymphocyte populations [100]. They proved that during differentiation of stem cells derived from the bone marrow, two independent lymphocyte populations are formed [51]. One population, the so-called T lymphocytes, is dependent upon the presence of the thymus, while the other population, referred to as B lymphocytes (bursa equivalent) is independent of it [124].

The number of lymphocytes in the bone marrow did not vary in rats following thymectomy at different ages [11, 62]. It seems, therefore, that the origin of the bone marrow lymphocytes is independent of the thymus.

Phytohaemagglutinin (PHA) produces the blast transformation predominantly of lymphocytes originating from the thymus. In fact, it was demonstrated using chromosome markers that upon PHA stimulation, cells responding with a blast transformation were all of thymic origin [25]. In rodents thymectomized in the newborn period, the number of circulating lymphocytes responding to PHA stimulation decreased [87]. In newborn chickens following thymectomy but not bursectomy peripheral blood lymphocytes cannot be stimulated with PHA [60]. Thus, the extent of the mitogenic effect of PHA on lymphocytes may be used as an indicator of the origin of the lymphocyte population. Anti-lymphocyte serum has a selective destructive effect upon thymus dependent lymphocytes [83, 88, 138]. On this basis it was established that the so-called 'theta' isoantigen can be regarded as an indicator of lymphocytes derived from the thymus [120, 127].

The experiments have shown that the thymus is responsible for the development of the T lymphocyte population during the early part of life, and for maintaining it on the required level in the blood as well as in the thymus dependent areas of the peripheral lymphatic organs.

Following thymectomy, other histological changes can be demonstrated in lymphatic organs. One can frequently observe, following thymectomy in the newborn period, a generalized hyperplasia of the reticulo-endothelial elements, when reticulum cells, histiocytes and macrophages appear in the cortical substance of lymph nodes which is poor in lymphocytes. Occasionally, extramedullary haemopoiesis is also observed [97]. The thymus does not influence either erythropoiesis, or myelopoiesis. Thymectomy after irradiation hinders lymphoid, but not myelo- and erythropoietic regeneration [7, 52].

## *Changes in immunological reactivity*

Disturbed lymphopoiesis is the immediate consequence of thymectomy and, in turn, leads to changes in immunological reactivity. Experimental results have unanimously proved that thymectomy causes an insufficiency of cell-mediated immune response.

Following neonatal thymectomy homograft acceptance was shown in mice [54, 94*b*, *d*, 98], rats [5], and chickens [72, 152*a*]; acceptance of allogeneic tumour tissue in mice [110, 113] and rats [104]; that of allogeneic lymphoid tissue in mice [89] and rats [2]. Thymectomy in the newborn period weakened the development of a delayed hypersensitivity reaction in rats challenged with tuberculin and bovine serum albumin [5, 70], and in chickens following tuberculin treatment [73, 134]. The development of an allergic encephalomyelitis in rats [5] and chickens was also inhibited [73]. Thymectomy in the newborn period defended mice against lethal meningitis, representing a hypersensitivity reaction following an intracerebral infection with the virus of lymphocytic choriomeningitis [49, 125].

Cells derived from the lymphoid tissue of mice thymectomized in the newborn period [56, 98] were less capable of inducing a graft-versus-host reaction than those derived from normal animals.

A dog at birth already possesses a well developed lymphoid system, and this probably explains the reason why dogs thymectomized neonatally do not tolerate homografts [47]. Mice, in which thymectomy was performed two weeks after birth [56, 94*e*] developed only a partial homograft tolerance.

Thymectomy, when performed on adult animals did not result in homograft tolerance [94*h*]; if, however, thymectomy was combined with total body irradiation, the animals became tolerant to skin homografts [54, 74], tumour homografts [53] and allogeneic lymphoid cells [46]. Adult thymectomy and total body irradiation did not result in homograft tolerance if sensitization against the tissue occurred prior to the irradiation [26]. Lymphoid cells from thymectomized adult mice are capable of eliciting graft-versus-host reaction, but this capacity is limited for many months following thymectomy [94*i*]. In freshly hatched chickens bursectomized on the day of hatching but with an intact thymus, no homograft tolerance was found [116, 153].

Results concerning the effect of thymectomy on the humoral immune response are not unanimous. Adult animals, following neonatal thymectomy, either did not show any significant change as compared to controls [43, 68], or exhibited a diminished rate of primary antibody production against antigens [43, 56, 68, 94*e*, 96, 98, 112*a*]. The existence of the so-called 'thymus dependent' and 'thymus independent' antigens was proposed [124] based on observations showing that following thymectomy in the newborn period, primary antibody formation was diminished only against certain antigens. In neonatally thymectomized mice using sheep erythrocytes as antigen, two to three antigen sensitive cells were found among 1 million circulating lymphocytes as opposed to around sixty found in sham operated controls [102*a*]. The anamnestic response of animals neonatally thymectomized was found to be less affected than the primary responses [66].

Contrasting opinions expressed concerning the immunoglobulin producing capacity of animals thymectomized neonatally [6, 68] may be explained partly by the various nomenclatures used for the designation of the immunoglobulins. Thymectomy in chickens at the time of hatching has no inhibitory effect either upon primary antibody formation or upon immunoglobulin production [152*b*]. However, bursectomy performed at the time of hatching results in a loss of primary antibody formation [19, 69, 119, 153] and also IgG globulin was found to be absent from the serum of bursectomized chickens [69, 111].

Following thymectomy in adult animals no difference was observed in the antibody forming capacity against primary antigenic stimulation as compared with sham operated animals [45]. However, diminished antibody production was observed in these animals when the antigen stimulus followed several months after thymectomy [92*j*]. The capacity for primary immune response was lost in adult animals which had been thymectomized and at the same time exposed to sublethal total body irradiation. It was found to be essential that the antigen should be given only when the control animals receiving only irradiation show complete immunological regeneration [22]. The combined effect of thymectomy and irradiation, however, only influenced the reactivity against those antigens which were applied after irradiation, and not against those given before it [20]. In contrast to the selective depression of antibody formation, an elevation of the blood properdin level was found in thymectomized rats [37].

The consequences of thymectomy performed in several species at various ages of life, primarily affect the cell-mediated immune responses. The damage is more serious following thymectomy in the newborn period than if it is performed at a later age of life. Bursectomy performed at the time of hatching results in the loss of primary antibody formation and has no influence upon cell-mediated immunity. The different effects of thymectomy and bursectomy on the immune response show that thymus dependent and thymus independent (i.e. the bursa equivalent) lymphocyte populations, can be functionally well differentiated [100]. It has been demonstrated that the T lymphocyte population is responsible for cell-mediated immune responses, while the actual antibody synthesis is performed by effector cells of B lymphocytic origin [109]. It is also well established that for the undisturbed production of antibody against the so-called thymus dependent antigens, the collaboration of T lymphocytes in a so far unclarified manner is required [124]. Experimental observations have shown that co-operation between the two lymphocyte systems occurs in the course of antibody formation [103, 121].

The existence of the T and B lymphocyte populations and their functional separation is supported also by some human diseases. Thus the di George syndrome and the Bruton-type agammaglobulinaemia are characterized by pathological changes resulting from the selective absence of the T and B lymphocyte populations, respectively (see Chapter 77 in Volume 2). According to our present knowledge, the cells derived from the thymus dependent, antigen sensitive small lymphocyte population are responsible both for antigen stimulated cell-mediated responses and for the immunological memory. Furthermore, in the case of certain antigens, they take part in the humoral immune responses by stimulating the B lymphocytes.

However, the specific immune response is only one possible way of reaction to antigenic stimulation. Under certain conditions a specific immunological tolerance may also occur (see Chapter 5). The possibility to produce specific immunological tolerance to antigenic stimulation following thymectomy in adult animals shows that the presence of the thymus is not necessary for this reaction. The presence of mature, immunocompetent cells is sufficient. A certain time after antigenic stimulation has been finished, the artificially created immunological tolerance ceases, and the immunological responsiveness against the used antigen returns [86]. It can be assumed that of the continuously formed immunologically competent cells those are responsible for the reaction, which were produced following the withdrawal of the antigen causing the tolerance.

It has been proved that the cessation of tolerance is caused by a thymus dependent mechanism [162]. Specific immunological tolerance artificially produced in adult animals showed to be irreversible if the animals were thymectomized [139]. The state of specific immunological tolerance becomes irreversible with removal of the thymus, hence the return of an immunological reactivity is related to the thymus. These experiments demonstrate in addition that the thymus plays a role in the immune mechanisms also in adults.

### *Consequences of diminished immunological reactivity*

Neonatally thymectomized animals are much more susceptible to infection with viruses [33], bacteria [9, 123] and fungi [126] than sham-thymectomized controls. The susceptibility to infections can be adequately interpreted as the consequence of the diminished immunological reactivity of thymectomized animals. Also, a basic role is attributed to infections in the pathomechanism of autoimmune diseases seen more frequently than usual in the absence or incorrect function of the thymus dependent immune system [100].

Previously, other explanations were proposed concerning the role of the abnormal function or absence of the thymus in the development of autoimmune diseases. It was suggested that either the production of so-called 'forbidden clones' by the thymus, or the lack of their elimination may cause autoimmune diseases [13]. These assumptions could not be verified by experiments, no evidence supporting the persistence of forbidden clones within the thymus in autoimmune diseases has been found [149, 153].

If the production of forbidden clones by the thymus would be responsible for the development of autoimmune diseases, it could be prevented by neonatal thymectomy. Also the implantation of normal thymus would be effective if autoimmune diseases were caused by diminished elimination of forbidden clones. On the contrary, thymectomy in the newborn period did not prevent, in fact it enhanced, the manifestations of the disease in a mouse strain suffering from autoimmune disease [67]. Implantation of normal thymus into such mice were not succesful in preventing the manifestation of autoimmune disease.

Much evidence argues in favour of an increased susceptibility of neonatally thymectomized experimental animals towards oncogenic viruses [27, 81*a*, 148] and chemicals [59]. The tumours caused by oncogenic viruses and chemical carcinogens contain new cellular antigens which are foreign to the organism and therefore give rise to a homograft-type reaction in case of an intact immune system [64, 110]. The lack of a thymus dependent immune system following neonatal thymectomy results not only in homograft tolerance, but also enhances the growth of the tumour possessing a new, foreign antigen.

The enhanced susceptibility of an animal to infections, autoimmune diseases and neoplasm following neonatal thymectomy can be explained by the reduced immunological reactivity consequent upon the absence of a thymus dependent immune system.

## *The wasting syndrome*

Miller, in his first publications on the consequences of neonatal thymectomy described, besides the lymphoid atrophy and disturbances of immune mechanisms, other effects, too [94*b*, *c*, *d*]. He found that the mice which had been neonatally thymectomized developed normally for a time, but after weaning, at the age of 6–8 weeks, signs of a peculiar atrophy, the so-called wasting syndrome, appeared. The animals lag behind in development, their fur becomes ruffled, dermatitis develops, the animals assume a characteristic hunched posture, periorbital oedema appears, they become lethargic, develop diarrhoea and finally die within two or three weeks. Autopsy reveals macroscopically that the whole lymphatic apparatus is atrophied, the spleen and lymph nodes show no follicles, and proliferation of reticulo-endothelial elements is observable [97]. In 50 per cent of the wasted mice necrotic foci were found in the liver, together with accumulations of polynuclear granulocytes, macrophages and giant cells [33]. The hepatic lesions are explained by the presence of hepatotrophic virus [33]. In wasted mice the subcutaneous adipose tissue disappears, the skin and intestinal wall becomes thin and anaemia develops [94*e*, 98]. In mice suffering from the wasting syndrome, following neonatal thymectomy serious skeletal lesions were found [10]. Atrophy of endocrine organs has also been reported in this condition [82, 107].

The earlier the age at which thymectomy had been performed, the greater was the percentage of animals in which the wasting syndrome developed [94*g*].

The time at which wasting develops may vary depending upon the mouse strain. The disease may appear in certain inbred strains at the age of 4 weeks, while in hybrids and non-inbred strains it may occur even after the fourth month [94*g*]. Thymectomy performed in young, adult animals only slightly interferes with the increase of body weight [41, 100], the state of the lymphatic organs [39], and with the function of the endocrine organs [41] during the weeks following the operation.

The pathogenesis of the wasting syndrome is a much debated topic. It was previously assumed that the wasting results from the loss of the trephocyte function of the lymphocytes [85]. This possibility has not been verified. The symptoms of the wasting syndrome were found similar to those of runt disease developing as a consequence of a graft-versus-host reaction [97, 98]. On the basis of the similarity it was suggested that autoimmune processes may play a role also in the pathogenesis of the wasting syndrome [97].

However, results obtained in mice contained in a germ-free environment point to a difference in the pathogenesis of the two types of wasted state. Thymectomized newborn germ-free mice did not develop a wasting syndrome [91, 158]. However, following transfer to conventional environment wasting appeared in 4 to 8 weeks [158]. Non-thymectomized mice maintained in a germ-free environment show a low number of lymphocytes; however, these mice do not accept foreign skin grafts, and they are capable of a normal immune response. On the other hand, neonatally germ-free thymectomized mice display homograft tolerance and a generalized depression of the immune state without the symptoms of wasting [91]. Acceptance of the foreign skin graft shows that the lack of immune reactivity is directly due to the absence of the thymus and is not a secondary effect of wasting syndrome. The transfer of lymphoid cells from germ-free mice into other germ-free mice results in the development of runt disease [91], which is a type of wasting syndrome consequent to a graft-versus-host reaction. Thus the wasting secondary to a graft-versus-host reaction will also occur in germ-free animals.

These results were interpreted to mean that the pathogenesis of the two states of atrophy is different. The introduced immunocompetent cells are themselves responsible for the atrophy following a graft-versus-host reaction, while in the development of the wasting syndrome secondary to neonatal thymectomy bacteria seem to have some pathogenic role. Later observations supported this possibility. The wasting syndrome in newborn thymectomized mice develops more quickly and more frequently after treatment with the endotoxin of *Salmonella typhi* [126], or after intracerebral infection with LCM virus [137]. Antibiotic treatment diminishes the frequency of the wasting syndrome in newborn thymectomized rats [9]. Other results also point to the role of antigens in the pathogenesis of the atrophic state. A fatal cachexia with signs similar to the wasting syndrome can be induced by neonatal glucocorticoid treatment in mice [122], rats [23, 38, 133], and dogs [40]. Atrophy developing as a result of this treatment may be diminished by antibiotic treatment [31], or by keeping the animals in germ-free environment [122]. Similarly to conventionally kept animals, the atrophy will appear in germ-free mice following oral monocontamination with *Escherichia coli* [122]. In other cases, the administration of streptococcal and staphylococcal antigens to mice in the state of neonatal immunological depression resulted in the appearance of atrophy resembling the wasting syndrome [34]. LCM virus infection enhances the appearance of the post-graft-versus-host reaction atrophic syndrome [79].

Based on the experimental results, the following generalization appears permissible: in various states of immunological depression (neonatal period, neonatal thymectomy, glucocorticoid treatment, graft-versus-host reaction), the most varied antigens (normal flora, *E. coli*, LCM virus, strepto- and staphylococcal antigen) will produce the same non-specific disease, the atrophic syndrome [137]. In the pathogenesis of the wasting syndrome a prominent role is attributed to the infecting agent, or one or more of its products, against which sensitivity is displayed only in a state of immunological depression. It is assumed that the bacteria, or the released cell fragment following cell destruction caused by their products, may initiate autoimmune reactions, although an autoimmune process cannot be demonstrated directly, and cannot be passively transferred [91].

Mice afflicted with the wasting syndrome following neonatal thymectomy show, besides the disturbance in the adaptive immune reactivity, other disturbances of adaptation. Their responses to stress differ from that of normal animals. They respond with a marked sensitivity and a diminished lymphopenic reaction to cold stress [136]. It is, therefore, assumed that apart from the immunological adaptive function of the thymus, it also plays a part in other adaptive processes. It is suggested moreover that the generalized disorder of adaptation plays a basic role in the pathogenesis of the wasting syndrome [136].

## PROTECTION AGAINST THE EFFECTS OF THYMECTOMY

Protection against the consequences of thymectomy performed in newborn and adult animals has been tried by several methods including the injection of lymphoid cells, the use of thymus grafts and thymus extracts.

### *Lymphoid cells*

With the injection of at least 5 million splenic cells into mice thymectomized neonatally, the development of the wasting syndrome was prevented and the immune mechanism was restored [24, 144]. The immunological restoration of thymectomized and irradiated mice was only successful with splenic cells derived from normal mice. The splenic cells from neonatally thymectomized mice were ineffective [21].

The injection of cells from the lymph nodes into neonatally thymectomized mice prevented the development of the wasting syndrome in 60 to 80 per cent of the cases and restored the immunological reactivity against skin homografts [94*f*]. The protective effect of 5 million lymph node cells per mouse given a week after neonatal thymectomy was still evident [24, 94*g*]. Also, following thymectomy and irradation in adult mice, the administration of cells from the lymph nodes restored immunological reactivity [54]. The immunological reactivity of neonatally thymectomized rats was also successfully restored with lymph node cells [71]. However, it appears that splenic and lymph node cells are not able to prevent entirely and irreversibly the consequences of neonatal thymectomy. Twenty per cent of the neonatally thymectomized mice treated with splenic or lymph node cells died at three to seven months of age, showing the characteristic signs of weight loss and a marked decrease in the number of circulating lymphocytes [144].

Thymus cells derived from newborn and adult mice are able to restore immunological reactivity, and to protect against the wasting syndrome only when used in very large doses: 100–300 million cells per mouse, and only if injected several weeks before the appearance of the wasting syndrome [161], or rather before the application of the antigenic stimulus. These data suggest that the maturation of thymus lymphocytes into immunologically competent cells may occur outside the thymus, but some time is necessary for this. Large quantities of bone marrow cells, in doses of 40 million cells per mouse, were not able to restore immunological reactivity in thymectomized and irradiated mice [21]. This was also the case when foetal liver cells were used [21].

Following thymectomy both in newborn [24, 94*b*, *g*, 95], and also adult mice—in the latter combined with irradiation [32]—the correction of immunological reactivity was successful with thymus grafts implanted subcutaneously or under the renal capsule. The correction was equally successful when normal irradiated isogeneic or allogeneic thymus grafts were used. The correction of immunological reactivity was successful even if the neonatally thymectomized recipient carried the isogenic graft for one week [95].

When allogeneic thymus grafts were used, a specific immunological tolerance towards the skin type of the thymus donor [24] could be observed. In other cases immunological tolerance did not appear, and the implanted allogeneic thymus restored the immunological reactivity of thymectomized and irradiated recipients in such a way that they were capable of an immune reaction against tumour grafts of the donor's type [44]. Following immunological restoration with rat thymus 60 to 70 per cent of the neonatally thymectomized mice successfully rejected skin grafts of the type of the thymus donor [81*b*]. The correction of the immunological reactivity of neonatally thymectomized hosts failed when thymus irradiated with a dose of 2000 r was used, while restoration was successful following irradiation with only 500 r [95].

In a thymus graft devoid of lymphocytes due to *in vitro* irradiation small, 'lymphocyte-like' cells appeared between the 4th and 8th days after implantation. They were first observed in the capillaries; later their number increased and they could be seen throughout the entire thymus. The 'lymphocyte-like' small cells had a dense chromatin structure, and relatively little cytoplasm besides the nucleus [32]. These cells must have originated from the host, as no such cells were found when the host was lethally irradiated and not treated with bone marrow [94*j*]. The analysis of the splenic cells of mice thymectomized neonatally and subsequently grafted with an allogeneic thymus showed that the cells of the host are primarily responsible for the immunological reactivity [24]. Using chromosome markers it was found that in the lymphoid tissue of a host thymectomized neonatally and subsequently implanted with a thymus graft, both the host and donor cells were dividing, but the majority of the dividing cells were of the host type [101].

The results show that the correction of immunological reactivity in mice thymectomized neonatally is possible using thymus grafts, but the cells capable of an immune response are generally derived from the host. The host cells receive some kind of stimulus from the cytoreticulum of the thymus which triggers their differentiation into immunologically competent cells. A further question is whether the stimulus is conveyed by a direct cellular transfer on host cells which have migrated into the thymus, or whether it has distant effects on lymphocyte precursors. The latter possibility is supported by experiments using thymus grafts enclosed in diffusion chambers. The immunological reactivity of neonatally thymectomized mice [84, 114] and of mice thymectomized and irradiated in adult age [9] was successfully restored with embryonic, neonatal or adult thymus grafts placed into the peritoneal cavity enclosed in a millipore chamber preventing cellular transfer across its wall. Similar results were obtained in rats [1], and rabbits [146]. It appears that the restoration of lymphopoiesis depends upon the pore size of the millipore chamber. Normalization of the blood lymphocytes was observed using a chamber with pores of 0.45 $\mu$ in diameter [112*a*], but not when the diameter was decreased to 0.1 $\mu$ [160]. The correction of the immunological reactivity was equally effective with allogeneic and isogeneic thymus grafts enclosed in a diffusion chamber. Other lymphatic organs, however, such as the spleen and the lymph nodes, were ineffective [112*a*].

The results of the diffusion chamber experiments indicate that the thymus produces a humoral substance which is believed to trigger the differentiation and maturation of immunologically competent cells from the lymphoid precursor cells of neonatally thymectomized mice [112*a*, 114]. Thymus epithelial reticulum enclosed in a diffusion chamber and containing no lymphocytes was able to restore immunological reactivity [160]. Histological examination of implanted thymus tissue, enclosed in a diffusion chamber, revealed that the thymus lymphocytes degenerate and disappear within two weeks, while many epithelial cells survive [155]. This implies that the thymus epithelial cells are responsible for the production of the humoral substance initiating the differentiation of the lymphoid precursor cells into immunologically competent cells.

The return of immunological reactivity during pregnancy and delivery in neonatally thymectomized female mice provides further evidence for the existence of such a humoral factor [112*b*]. Hormonally produced pseudopregnancy had no such effect. Using chromosome markers it was not possible to demonstrate either the transfer of foetal lymphoid cells to the pregnant mouse, or the presence of maternal cells in the thymus of the newborn animals. These facts suggest that a foetal, thymus-produced humoral factor is transferred to the mother, which brings about the correction of the immune mechanisms in the mother [100]. Immunological reactivity in bursectomized chickens may be corrected by isogeneic or allogeneic bursal grafts [69], implanted either free or enclosed in a diffusion chamber [132], indicating that the bursa of Fabricius, too, has some humoral influence upon the differentiation of the precursor cells of the host into antibody forming cells.

### *Thymus extracts*

The existence of a humoral factor produced by the thymus and affecting lymphopoiesis would be supported by direct evidence if lymphopoiesis and immunological reactivity could be corrected by thymus extracts in neonatally thymectomized animals. The results obtained are, however, contradictory. Thymus extracts generally do not correct the immune mechanisms in neonatally thymectomized mice. A growth promoting substance purified from the thymus [135] did not prevent the onset of the wasting syndrome, nor did it correct the immunological reactivity of neonatally thymectomized mice [24]. The repeated injection of a protein fraction derived from calf thymus, restored the immune mechanisms of adult, thymectomized and irradiated mice [145].

Many attempts were made to induce lymphopoiesis with thymus extracts. According to previous experiences lymphocytosis in the peripheral blood of mice could be produced by the injection of the plasma of patients suffering from chronic lymphoid leukaemia, lymphosarcoma, and myelofibrosis [92*a*]. No such effect was produced by normal human plasma. Thymus extracts from patients suffering from the above diseases had also a lymphocyte stimulating effect. However, the same effect was also elicited by emulsions of a normal human or mouse thymus [92*b*]. An increased incorporation of tritiated thymidine into DNA was observed in the lymph nodes of mice treated with thymus extracts [78]. Similar effects were reported following the use of purified protein from calf thymus both *in vitro* and *in vivo* [55].

The lymphocytosis produced in the peripheral blood by thymus extracts demonstrates the presence of a humoral 'lymphocytosis stimulating factor' (LSF) in the thymus [92*c*]. This factor stimulates the differentiation and proliferation of lymphoid precursor cells which are not sensitive to the antigen. Similar effect has been attributed to a so-called 'competence inducing factor' (CIF), which was postulated on the basis of experiments with diffusion chambers [94*h*]. It is assumed that LSF and CIF are identical. As its effect is analogous to that of erythropoietin it could be called lymphopoietin [100]. It is assumed that thymus lymphoid cells insensitive to antigen are converted into antigen sensitive cells by lymphopoietin. In the course of differentiation, the cells lose their sensitivity to lymphopoietin [100]. The assumed, thymus derived, humoral factor controlling lymphoid proliferation has not yet been isolated in a biologically active form.

In the cytoplasm of thymic lymphocytes and epithelial cells of various germ-free and normally kept mouse strains, typical virus particles were demonstrated. Their presence could not be correlated with any disease. It might be that these virus-like particles, transferred together with the cell-free extracts of the thymus, are responsible for the lymphocytosis stimulating effect [28].

## CONCLUSIONS

Present knowledge concerning the function of the thymus in immune mechanisms may be summarized as follows:

1. The. thymus plays a basic role in lymphopoiesis. Antigen insensitive, bone marrow derived, lymphoid precursor cells differentiate into antigen sensitive, immunocompetent cells in the thymus. The differentiation is triggered by a so far unidentified factor derived from the epithelial cytoreticulum. This process ensures in the course of ontogenesis, the appearance and the continuous supply of a thymus dependent, antigen sensitive, small lymphocyte population on the periphery.
2. Cells derived from the thymus dependent, antigen sensitive, small lymphocyte population play a significant role in the immunological responses of the organism: they are responsible for cell-mediated immune responses and for immunological memory; they contribute, in cooperation with the thymus independent, antigen sensitive small lymphocytes, to the humoral responses, too.

Thus the function of the thymus is the initiation of differentiation processes, which starting from the perinatal period, continuously proceed through the later stages of life. In essence, the mechanism of differentiation occurring in an adult organism, cannot be distinguished from that involved in embryogenesis. Therefore, a more detailed knowledge of embryonic differentiation would support the understanding of extra-uterine differentiation, and *vice versa*. In addition, a better understanding of differentiation would help the elucidation of many unanswered questions concerning the function of the thymus.

## REFERENCES


1. Aisenberg, A. C. and Wilkes, B.: *Nature* **205,** 716 (1965).
2. Aisenberg, A. C., Wilkes, B. and Waksman, B. H.: *J. exp. Med.* **117,** 759 (1962).
3. Andreasen, E. and Christensen, S.: *Anat. Rec.* **103,** 401 (1949).
4. Andreasen, E. and Ottesen, J.: *Acta physiol. scand.* **10,** 258 (1945).
5. Arnason, B. G., Jankovic, B. D., Waksman, B. H. and Wennersten, C.: *J. exp. Med.* **116,** 177 (1962).
6. Arnason, B. G., de Vaux St. Cyr., C. and Grabar, P.: *Nature* **199,** 1199 (1963).
7. Auerbach, R.: *Science* **139,** 1061 (1963).
8. Axelrad, A. A. and Van der Gaag, H. C.: *J. nat. Cancer Inst.* **28,** 1065 (1962).
9. Azar, H. A.: *Proc. Soc. exp. Biol. (N.Y.)* **116,** 817 (1964).
10. Berek, L., Bános, Zs., Szeri, I., Anderlik, P. and Aszódi, K.: *Experientia (Basel)* **24,** 721 (1968).
11. Bierring, F.: *Acta anat.* **55,** 9 (1963).
12. Billingham, R. E., Defendi, V., Silvers, W. K. and Steinmuller, D.: *J. nat. Cancer Inst.* **28,** 365 (1962).
13. Burnet, F. M.: *Austr. Ann. Med.* **11,** 79 (1962).
14. Carnes, W. H., Kaplan, H. S., Brown, M. B. and Hirsch, B. B.: *Cancer Res.* **16,** 429 (1956).
15. Clark, S. L., jr.: In *The Thymus.* Ed. by Defendi, V. and Metcalf, D. Wistar Inst. Press, Philadelphia 1964, p. 9.
16. Clark, W. G. B., Williams, C. B. and Yoffey, J. M.: *J. Lab. clin. Med.* **67,** 439 (1966).
17. Cohen, M. W., Thorbecke, G. J., Hochwald, G. M. and Jacobson, E. B.: *Proc. Soc. exp. Biol. (N.Y.)* **114,** 242 (1963).
18. Cooper, E. L. and Hildemann, W. H.: *Ann. N. Y. Acad. Sci.* **126,** 661 (1965).
19. Cooper, M. D., Peterson, R. D. A., South, M. A. and Good, R. A.: *J. exp. Med.* **123,** 75 (1966).
20. Cross, A. M., Leuchars, E. and Davies, A. J. S.: *Nature* **203,** 1042 (1964).
21. Cross, A. M., Leuchars, E. and Miller, J. F. A. P.: *J. exp. Med.* **119,** 837 (1964).
22. Csaba, G., Dunay, C. and Fischer, J.: *Experientia (Basel)* **22,** 253 (1966).
23. Csaba, G. and Fischer, J.: *Acta biol. Acad. Sci. hung.* **17,** 75 (1966).
24. Dalmasso, A. P., Martinez, C., Sjodin, K. and Good, R. A.: *J. exp. Med.* **118,** 1089 (1963).
25. Davies, A. S. J., Festenstein, H., Leuchars, E., Wallis, V. J. and Doenhoff, M. J.: *Lancet* **i,** 183 (1968).
26. Davies, E. W., jr., Tyan, M. L. and Cole, L. J.: *Science* **145,** 394 (1964).
27. Defendi, V. and Roosa, R. A.: *Cancer Res.* **25,** 300 (1965).
28. De Harven, E.: *J. exp. Med.* **119,** 177 (1964).
29. Doria, G. and Agarossi, G.: *Nature* **221,** 871 (1969).
30. Dougherty, T. F.: *Physiol. Rev.* **32,** 379 (1952).
31. Duhig, J. T.: *Nature* **207,** 651 (1965).
32. Dukor, P., Miller, J. F. A. P., House, W. and Allman, V.: *Transplantation* **3,** 639 (1965).
33. East, J., Parrott, D. M. V., Chesterman, F. C. and Pomerance, A.: *J. exp. Med.* **118,** 106g (1963).
34. Ekstedt, R. D. and Nishimura, E. T.: *Exp. Med.* **120,** 795 (1964).
35. Ernström, U., Gyllensten, L. and Larssön, B.: *Nature* **207,** 540 (1965).

36. Everett, N. B., Rieke, W. O., Reinhardt, W. O. and Yoffey, J. M.: In *Ciba Found. Symp. Haemopoiesis: Cell Production and its Regulation.* Ed. by Wolstenholme, G. E. W. and O'Connor, M. Churchill, London 1960, p. 43.
37. Fachet, J. and Cseh, G.: *Med. exp.* **39,** 10 (1964).
38. Fachet, J., Palkovits, M., Vallent, K. and Stark, E.: *Acta endocrin. (Kbh.)* **51,** 71 (1966).
39. Fachet, J., Stark, E., Palkovits, M. and Mihály, K.: *Acta med. Acad. Sci. hung.* **21,** 297 (1965).
40. Fachet, J., Stark, E., Palkovits, M. and Vallent, K.: *Gen. and Comp. Endocrin.* **9,** 449 (1967).
41. Fachet, J., Stark, E., Vallent, K. and Palkovits, M.: *Acta med. Acad. Sci. hung.* **15,** 461 (1962).
42. Fagraeus, A. and Gormsen, H.: *Acta path. microbiol. scand.* **33,** 421 (1953).
43. Fahey, J. L., Barth, W. F. and Law, L. W.: *J. nat. Cancer Inst.* **35,** 663 (1965).
44. Feldman, M. and Globerson, A.: *Ann. N. Y. Acad. Sci.* **120,** 182 (1964).
45. Fichtelius, K. E., Laurell, G. and Phillipssön, L.: *Acta path. microbiol. scand.* **51,** 81 (1961).
46. Field, E. O. and Gibbs, J. F.: *Transplantation* **3,** 634 (1965).
47. Fisher, B., Fisher, E. R., Lee, S. and Sakay, A.: *Transplantation* **3,** 49 (1965).
48. Ford, C. E. and Micklem, H. S.: *Lancet* **i,** 359 (1963).
49. Földes, P., Szeri, I., Bános, S., Anderlik, P. and Balázs, M.: *Acta microbiol. Acad. Sci. hung.* **11,** 227 (1964–65).
50. Furth, R. Van, Schuit, H. R. E. and Hijmans, W.: *Immunology* **11,** 19 (1966).
51. Gabrielsen, A. E., Cooper, M. D., Peterson, R. D. A. and Good, R. A.: In *The Textbook of Immunopathology.* Ed. by Miescher, P. A. and Müller-Eberhard, H. J. Grune and Stratton, New York 1969, Vol. I, p. 385.
52. Globerson, A. and Feldman, M.: *Transplantation* **2,** 212 (1964).
53. Globerson, A., Fiore-Donati, L. and Feldman, M.: *Exp. Cell Res.* **28,** 455 (1962).
54. Goedbloed, J. F. and Vos, O.: *Transplantation* **3,** 368 (1965).
55. Goldstein, A. L., Slater, F. D. and White, A.: *Proc. nat. Acad. Sci. (Wash.)* **56,** 1010 (1966).
56. Good, R. A., Dalmasso, A. P., Martinez, C., Archer, O. K., Pierce, J. C. and Papermaster, B. W.: *J. exp. Med.* **116,** 773 (1962).
57. Good, R. A. and Gabrielsen, A. E.: *The Thymus in Immunbiology.* Harper and Row, New York 1964.
58. Gowans, J. L. and Knight, E. J.: *Proc. roy. Soc. (Lond.) Ser. B.* **159,** 257 (1964).
59. Grant, G. A., Roe, F. J. C. and Pike, M. C.: *Nature* **210,** 603 (1966).
60. Greaves, M. F., Roitt, I. M. and Rose, M. E.: *Nature* **220,** 293 (1968).
61. Green, I. and Block, K.: *Nature* **200,** 1099 (1964).
62. Hammar, J. A.: *Endocrinology* **5,** 543 (1921).
63. Harris, C.: *Blood* **18,** 691 (1961).
64. Hellström, K. E. and Möllner, G.: *Progr. Allergy* **9,** 158 (1965).
65. Hess, M. W.: *Experimental Thymectomy.* Springer, Berlin 1968.
66. Hess, M. W. and Stoner, R. D.: *Int. Arch. Allergy* **30,** 37 (1966).
67. Howie, J. B. and Helyer, B. J.: In *Ciba Found. Symp. Thymus: Experimental and Clinical Studies.* Ed. by Porter, R. and Wolstenholme, G. E. W. Churchill London 1966, p. 360.
68. Humphrey, J. H., Parrott, D. M. V. and East, J.: *Immunology* **7,** 419 (1964).
69. Isakovic, K., Jankovic, B. D., Popeskovic, L. and Milosevic, D.: *Nature* **200,** 273 (1963).
70. Isakovic, K. and Waksman, B. H.: *Proc. Soc. exp. Biol. (N.Y.)* **119,** 676 (1965).
71. Isakovic, K., Waksman, B. H. and Wennersten, C.: *J. Immunol.* **95,** 602 (1965).
72. Jankovic, B. D. and Isakovic, K.: *Int. Arch. Allergy* **24,** 278 (1964).
73. Jankovic, B. D., Isvaneski, M., Milosevic, D. and Popeskovic, L.: *Nature* **198,** 298 (1963).
74. Jeejeebhoy, H. F.: *Immunology* **9,** 417 (1965).
75. Joske, F. A.: *Med. J. Austr.* **45,** 859 (1958).
76. Kalmutz, S. E.: *Nature* **193,** 851 (1962).
77. Kennedy, J. C., Siminovitch, L., Till, J. E. and McCulloch, A. E.: *Proc. Soc. exp. Biol. (N.Y.)* **120,** 868 (1965).

78. Klein, J. J., Goldstein, A. L. and White, A.: *Ann. N. Y. Acad. Sci.* **135,** 485 (1966).
79. Koltay, M., Virág, I., Bános, S., Anderlik, P. and Szeri, I.: *Experientia (Basel)* **24,** 63 (1968).
80. Landy, M., Sanderson, R.P., Bernstein, M. T. and Lerner, E. M.: *Science* **147,** 1591 (1965).
81*a*. Law, L. W.: *Cancer Res.* **26,** 551 (1966).
81*b*. id., *Nature* **210,** 1118 (1966).
82. Law, L. W., Dunn, T. B., Trainin, N. and Levey, R. H.: In *The Thymus*. Ed. by Defendi, V. and Metcalf, D. Wistar Inst. Monogr. No. 2. Wistar Inst. Press, Philadelphia 1964, p. 105.
83. Levey, R. H. and Medawar, P. B.: *Ann. N. Y. Acad. Sci.* **129,** 164 (1966).
84. Levey, R. H., Trainin, N., Law, L. W. and Black, P. H.: *Science* **143,** 1049 (1963).
85. Loutit, J. F.: *Lancet* **ii,** 1106 (1962).
86. Makela, O. and Nossal, G. J. V.: *J. Immunology* **88,** 613 (1962).
87. Martial-Lasfargues, C., Liacopolous-Briot, M. and Halpern, B.-N.: *C. R. Soc. Biol. (Paris)* **160,** 2013 (1966).
88. Martin, W. J. and Miller, J. F. A. P.: *Lancet* **ii,** 1285 (1967).
89. Martinez, C., Dalmasso, A. P., Blaese, M. and Good, R. A.: *Proc. Soc. exp. Biol. (N.Y.)* **111,** 404 (1962).
90. Matsuyama, M., Wiadrowski, M. N. and Metcalf, D.: *J. exp. Med.* **123,** 559 (1966).
91. McIntire, K. R., Sell, S. and Miller, J. F. A. P.: *Nature* **204,** 151 (1964).
92*a*. Metcalf, D.: *Brit. J. Cancer* **10,** 431 (1956).
92*b*. ibid., **10,** 442 (1956).
92*c*. id., *Ann. N. Y. Acad. Sci.* **73,** 113 (1958).
92*d*. id., *Brit. J. Haematol.* **6,** 324 (1960).
92*e*. id., *Brit. J. Cancer* **15,** 769 (1961).
92*f*. id., *Austr. J. exp. Biol. med. Sci.* **41,** 437 (1963).
92*g*. id., In Good, R. A. and Gabrielsen, A. E.: *The Thymus in Immunobiology*. Harper and Row, New York 1964, p. 150.
92*h*. id., *Transplantation* **2,** 387 (1964).
92*i*. id., *Nature* **208,** 87 (1965).
92*j*. ibid., **208,** 1336 (1965).
92*k*. id., *The Thymus*. Springer, Berlin 1966.
92*l*. ibid., p. 1.
93. Metcalf, D. and Wiadrowski, M.: *Cancer Res.* **26,** 483 (1966).
94*a*. Miller, J. F. A. P.: *Brit. J. Cancer* **14,** 244 (1960).
94*b*. id., *Lancet* **ii,** 748 (1961).
94*c*. id., *Nature* **191,** 248 (1961).
94*d*. id., In *Ciba Found. Symp. Transplantation*. Ed. by Wolstenholme, G. E. W. and Cameron, M. P. Churchill, London 1962, p. 384.
94*e*. id., *Proc. roy. Soc. (Lond.) Ser. B.* **156,** 415 (1962).
94*f*. id., *Lancet* **i,** 43 (1963).
94*g*. id., in, Good, R. A. and Gabrielsen, A. E.: *The Thymus in Immunbiology*. Harper and Row, New York, 1964, p. 436.
94*h*. id., *Brit. med. Bull.* **21,** 111 (1965).
94*i*. id. *Nature* **208,** 1337 (1965).
94*j*. id., In *Ciba Found. Symp. Thymus: Experimental and Clinical Studies*. Ed. by Porter, P. and Wolstenholme, G. E. W. Churchill, London 1966, p. 153.
95. Miller, J. F. A. P., De Burgh, P. M., Dukor, P., Grant, G., Allman, V. and House, W.: *Clin. exp. Immunol.* **1,** 61 (1966).
96. Miller, J. F. A. P., De Burgh, P. M. and Grant, G. A.: *Nature* **208,** 1332 (1965).
97. Miller, J. F. A. P. and Howard, J. G.: *J. Reticuloend. Soc.* **1,** 369 (1964).
98. Miller, J. F. A. P., Marshall, A. H. E. and White, R. G.: *Advanc. Immunol.* **2,** 111 (1962).
99. Miller, J. F. A. P. and Mitchell, G. F.: *Transplantation Rev.* **1,** 3 (1969).
100. Miller, J. F. A. P. and Osoba, D.: *Physiol. Rev.* **47,** 437 (1967).
101. Miller, J. F. A. P., Osoba, D. and Dukor, P.: *Ann. N. Y. Acad. Sci.* **124,** 95 (1965)
102*a*. Mitchell, G. F. and Miller, J. F. A. P.: *Nature* **214,** 992 (1967).

102*b*. id., *J. exp. Med.* **128,** 821 (1968).
103. Mitchison, N. A.: In *Immunological Tolerance.* Ed. by Landy, M. and Braun, W. Academic Press, New York 1969, p. 115.
104. Money, W. L., Typond, P. and Rawson, R. W.: *Cancer Res.* **25,** 423 (1965).
105. Moore, M. A. S. and Metcalf, D.: *Brit. J. Haemat.* **18,** 279 (1970).
106. Murray, R. G., Murray, A. and Pizzo, A.: *Anat. Rec.* **151,** 17 (1965).
107. Nishizuka, Y. and Sakakura, T.: *Science* **166,** 753 (1969).
108. Nossal, G. J. V.: *Ann. N. Y. Acad. Sci.* **120,** 171 (1964).
109. Nossal, G. J. V., Cunningham, A., Mitchell, G. F. and Miller, J. F. A. P.: *J. exp. Med.* **128,** 839 (1968).
110. Old, L. J. and Boyse, E. A.: *Ann. Rev. Med.* **15,** 167 (1964).
111. Ortega, L. G. and Der, B. K.: *Fed. Proc.* **23,** 546 (1964).
112*a*. Osoba, D.: *J. exp. Med.* **122,** 633 (1965).
112*b*. id., *Science* **147,** 298 (1965).
113. Osoba, D. and Auersperg, N.: *J. nat. Cancer Inst.* **36,** 523 (1966).
114. Osoba, D. and Miller, J. F. A. P.: *Nature* **199,** 653 (1963).
115. Papermaster, B. W., Condie, R. M., Finstad, J. and Good, R. A.: *J. exp. Med.* **119,** 105 (1964).
116. Papermaster, B. W. and Good, R. A.: *Nature* **196,** 838 (1962).
117. Pappenheimer, A. M.: *J. exp. Med.* **19,** 319 (1914).
118. Parrott, D. M. V., Sousa, M. A. B. and East, J.: *J. exp. Med.* **123,** 191 (1966).
119. Pierce, A. E., Chubb, R. C. and Long, P. L.: *Immunology* **10,** 321 (1966).
120. Raff, M. C.: *Nature* **224,** 378 (1969).
121. Rajewsky, K., Schirrmacher, V., Nase, J. and Jerne, N. K.: *J. exp. Med.* **129,** 1131 (1969).
122. Reed, N. D. and Jutila, J. W.: *Science* **150,** 356 (1965).
123. Rees, R. J. W.: *Nature* **211,** 657 (1966).
124. Roitt, I. M., Greaves, M. F., Torrigiani, G., Brostoff, J. and Playfair, J. H. L.: *Lancet* **ii,** 367 (1969).
125. Rowe, W. P., Black, P. H., and Levey, R. H.: *Proc. Soc. exp. Biol. (N.Y.)* **114,** 248 (1963).
126. Salvin, S. B., Peterson, R. D. A. and Good, R. A.: *J. Lab. clin. Med.* **65,** 1004 (1965).
127. Schlesinger, M. and Yron, I.: *Science* **164,** 1412 (1969).
128. Schwarz, M. R. and Rieke, W. O.: *Anat. Record.* **155,** 493 (1966).
129. Sherman, J. D., Adner, M. M. and Dameshek, W.: *Proc. Soc. exp. Biol. (N.Y.)* **115,** 866 (1964).
130. Skog, E.: *Acta derm.-venerol.* **35,** 253 (1955).
131. Stoner, R. D. and Hale, W. M.: *J. Immunol.* **75,** 203 (1955).
132. St. Pierre, R. L. and Ackerman, G. A.: *Science* **147,** 1307 (1965).
133. Szeberényi, Sz.: *J. Endocrinol.* **35,** 323 (1966).
134. Szenberg, A. and Warner, N. L.: *Brit. med. Bull.* **23,** 30 (1967).
135. Szent-Györgyi, A., Hegyeli, A. and McLaughlin, J. A.: *Proc. nat. Acad. Sci. (Wash.)* **48,** 1439 (1962).
136. Szeri, I., Anderlik, P. and Bános, S.: *Acta microbiol. Acad. Sci. hung.* **15,** 1 (1968).
137. Szeri, I., Bános, Zs., Anderlik, P., Balázs, M. and Földes, P.: *Acta microbiol. Acad. Sci. hung.* **13,** 255 (1966).
138. Taub, R. M. and Lance, E. M.: *Immunology* **15,** 633 (1968).
139. Taylor, R. B.: *Immunology* **7,** 595 (1964).
140. Thorbecke, G. J. and Cohen, M. W.: In *The Thymus.* Ed. by Defendi, V. and Metcalf, D. Wistar Inst. Press, Philadelphia, 1964, p. 33.
141. Thorbecke, G. J. and Keuning, F. J.: *J. Immunol.* **70,** 129 (1953).
142. Törő, I. and Oláh, I.: *Acta morph. Acad. Sci. hung.* **14,** 275 (1966).
143. Törő, I., Pályi, I., Csapó, I. and Gazsó, L.: *Acta morph. Acad. Sci. hung.* **13,** 51 (1964).
144. Trainin, N., Law, L. W. and Levey, R. H.: *Proc. Soc. exp. Biol. (N.Y.)* **118,** 79 (1965).
145. Trainin, N. and Linker-Israeli, M.: *Cancer Res.* **27,** 309 (1967).
146. Trench, C. A. H., Watson, J. W., Walker, F. C., Gardner, P. S. and Green, C. A.: *Immunology* **10,** 187 (1966).

147. Trowell, O. A.: *Int. J. Radiation Biol.* **4,** 163 (1961).
148. Vandeputte, M., Denys, J., Leyton, R. and De Somer, P.: *Life Sci.* **7,** 475 (1963).
149. Vries, M. J. De and Hijmans, W.: *J. Path. Bact.* **91,** 487 (1966).
150. Waksman, B. H., Arnason, B. G. and Jankovic, B. D.: *J. exp. Med.* **116,** 187 (1962).
151. Warner, N. L.: *Austr. J. exp. Biol. med. Sci.* **42,** 401 (1964).
152*a*. Warner, N. L. and Szenberg, A.: *Nature* **196,** 784 (1962).
152*b*. id., In Good, R. A. and Gabrielsen, A. E.: *The Thymus in Immunbiology*. Harper and Row, New York, 1964, p. 395.
153. Warner, N. L., Szenberg, A. and Burnet, F. M.: *Austr. J. exp. Biol. med. Sci* **40,** 373 (1962).
154. Weber, W. T.: *J. cell. comp. Physiol.* **68,** 117 (1966).
155. Weiss, L. and Miller, J. F. A. P.: *Fed. Proc.* **25,** 613 (1966).
156. Weissman, I.: *J. exp. Med.* **126,** 291 (1967).
157. Wilson, R., Bealmear, M. and Sobonya, R.: *Proc. Soc. exp. Biol. (N.Y.)* **118,** 97 (1965).
158. Wilson, R., Sjodin, K. and Bealmear, M.: *Proc. Soc. exp. Biol. (N.Y.)* **117,** 237 (1964).
159. Winkelstein, A. and Craddock, C. G.: *Blood* **26,** 876 (1965).
160. Wong, F. M., Taub, R. N., Sherman, J. D. and Dameshek, W.: *Blood* **28,** 40 (1966).
161. Yunis, E. J., Hilgard, H., Sjodin, K., Martinez, C. and Good, R. A.: *Nature* **201,** 784 (1964).
162. Zaalberg, O. B. and Van Der Meul, V. A.: *Transplantation* **4,** 274 (1966).

CHAPTER 10

# ANTIBODIES

by

Z. CSIZÉR



## TERMINOLOGY [26]

Substances (*i*) which introduced into the body by infection or by other means are recognized as foreign and induce a specific immune response, or (*ii*) substances involved in specific immunological reactions *in vivo* or *in vitro* are termed antigens. However, these two properties are often dissociated. For this reason, it is convenient to use the term immunogen for substances which are able to elicit antibody formation (humoral immune response) or sensitization (cell-mediated response) *de novo*, and the term hapten for chemical molecules or groups of small size which in themselves do not elicit antibody formation but can unite in natural or artificial conditions with proteins to form compounds having specific antigenic properties; haptens, on the other hand, are capable of interacting with the specific antibodies. The site or area of an antigen molecule which is responsible for its specific interaction with antibody molecules evoked by the same or a similar antigen is called antigenic determinant or epitope. Chemical groups (haptens) conjugated artificially to a protein can elicit specific antibody formation which is often directed against the hapten, that is, against an antigenic determinant of the molecule. Various substances, e.g. nucleic acids or purified polysaccharides, which evoke specific immune responses in a preimmunized animal and can react with preformed antibody but do not elicit specific immune response *de novo*, are also called haptens. In both cases the carrier molecules of haptens are proteins also referred to as 'schleppers'.

Antibodies are proteins formed in plasma cells (and secreted into the blood serum and tissue fluids) as a result of a specific response to the introduction of antigen. These antibodies are the so-called humoral or secreted antibodies. On the other hand, antigens can induce specific sensitization of cells. Under physiological conditions the characteristic property of both antibodies and sensitized cells is to combine specifically with the antigen in response to which they were formed.

The term sensitized cell has two distinct meanings. (*i*) it covers cells, especially macrophages, which are bearing antibodies (cytophilic antibodies) on their surface; (*ii*) it is also used for specifically sensitized lymphocytes taking part in cell-mediated immunity, which have the property to react with the specific antigen by antibody-like macromolecules or, perhaps, antibodies.

Antibodies which are attached to tissues firmly enough to resist washing are called sessile antibodies. Homocytotropic antibodies sensitize the cells of the same or closely related species, and heterocytotropic ones are special examples of cytophilic antibodies which attach to the cells of unrelated species.

According to recent data, the macrophages carrying cytophilic antibodies, the thymus-derived lymphocytes (T lymphocytes or antigen-reactive cells) bearing receptors which are possibly antibodies partly buried by the cell membrane and the bone-marrow-derived lymphocytes (B lymphocytes or precursors of antibody-forming cells) also bearing receptors, which are possibly class-specific immunoglobulins, seem to be the cells which cooperate in developing both humoral and cell-mediated immune responses. Chemically, antibodies are of globulin nature.

Immunoglobulin as a general term is used for all proteins which have antibody activity and those proteins without known antibody activity which possess a common antigenic specificity with them and are produced by similar cells. The latter group includes myeloma proteins, Bence–Jones proteins, Waldenström macroglobulin and subunits of antibodies.

## HUMORAL ANTIBODIES [24]

The antibody activity of serum is due to immunoglobulins which have distinct physical, chemical, and biological properties. The extreme heterogeneity of immunoglobulin classes with respect to structure, molecular weight, sedimentation coefficient, and electrophoretic mobility (Fig. 10-1) is reviewed in Chapter 13. Furthermore, each class of immunoglobulins to which antibodies belong differs from most other plasma proteins in consisting of heterogenous proteins with overlapping physical and chemical properties. The currently used nomenclature of immunoglobulins was accepted by the WHO in 1964 [12].

Our present purpose is to highlight very briefly some of the essential features of the function and biological properties of humoral antibodies (Table 10-I).

Both the humoral and cellular mechanisms of the specific immune response first appear in the most primitive true vertebrates. The investigations in this respect are based on experiments on two species of cyclostomes. The more primitive one, the hagfish (*Eptatretus stoutii*), neither forms humoral antibodies nor develops delayed hypersensitivity yet, but it rejects homografts. The hagfish has no thymus and no lymph nodes, but possesses a primitive spleen. Its tissues do not contain plasma cells and lymphocytes, but contain primitive granulocytes. The higher cyclostome which has been studied, the lamprey (*Petromyzon marinus*), is able to produce antibodies against certain antigens, can develop delayed hyper-

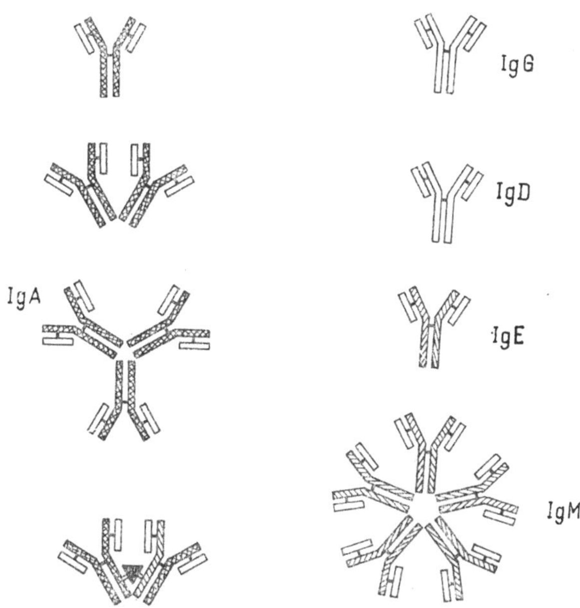


Fig. 10-1. Primary forms of humoral immunoglobulins. IgG, IgD and IgE exist as single tetramers, IgM as aggregate of five tetramers, and IgA is variable. The black triangle represents the transport piece in the secretory IgA molecule (lower right) [24]

sensitivity to tuberculin and rejects skin homografts. The lamprey has thymus, and foci of lymphocytes in the bone marrow and spleen, but does not possess plasma cells. In the course of the phylogenetic development of the immune response the structure of immunoglobulins differentiates, different classes of heavy and light chains are developed from a single class of heavy chain, lymphocytes and germinal centres, as well as the phenomenon of immunological memory appear [26]. (For detailed information on the antibody formation and the connected theories see Chapter 11).

The most important function of antibodies is their ability to combine specifically with the corresponding determinant group(s). Most natural antigens, e. g. bacteria, are very complex and may contain a mosaic of hundreds of unrelated antigenic determinants. Sera obtained after immunization with such antigens will contam various antibodies against the different antigenic determinants. The analysis of these sera is very complicated. More exact information can be obtained if animals are immunized with proteins to which some sort of hapten has been linked artificially. From such studies it appears that IgG antibodies have two combining sites with identical specificity. Hybrid molecules of IgG capable of combining with two different antigenic determinants can be produced *in vitro,* but have never been found naturally.

The antigenic determinant groups of certain polysaccharide antigens usually

TABLE 10-I

*Biological properties of immunoglobulins*

| Properties | IgG | IgA | IgM | IgD | IgE |
|---|---|---|---|---|---|
| Antibody activity | Major antibacterial and antiviral activity in serum | Major antibody of external secretions | Initial antibody formed to new antigens; anti-polysaccharide | Antinuclear activity | Reaginic antibody |
| Complement fixation | + (except IgG4) | − | + | − | − |
| Placental transfer | + | − | − | − | − |
| Presence in milk | + | + | − (or trace) | − | − |
| Skin fixation | − | − | − | − | + |
| Seromucous secretions | + (no selective secretion) | + | − | − | − |
| Passive cutaneous anaphylaxis | + (except IgG1) | − | − | − | − |

contain three to six monosaccharide residues, those of protein antigens contain 8 to 12 amino acid residues. In consequence of this, it is possible that the size of the antibody combining site is similar to that of the antigenic determinant, i.e. about 10 to 20 amino acids are involved in it. The combination between antigen and antibody molecules is reversible and does not involve stable chemical bonds. The complex formation is mainly due to ionic bindings and van der Waals forces, but hydrogen bonds may occur, too. The strength of such forces in holding the complex together will depend upon fitness and nearness of the opposite surfaces of components. The forces are the strongest at physiological conditions of pH and ionic strength. At pH values below 3 or above 10.5 the forces are so weak that the complex may dissociate. Antibodies, even those against a given antigenic determinant formed in a single animal, can vary significantly in the strength with which they combine, or in their affinity, depending on minor differences in fitness. The specific term avidity is used for the expression of the affinity of the antibody. Such variation can be estimated by the Law of Mass Action according to the equation

$$Ko = \frac{[AbH]}{[Ab]\,[H]}$$

where $Ko$ = equilibrium constant expressed in units of litres per mol,
$[Ab]$ = antibody concentration in mols per litre at equilibrium,
$[H]$ = hapten concentration in mols per litre at equilibrium,
$[AbH]$ = concentration of antibody–hapten complex in mols per litre at equilibrium.

Experimentally values for $Ko$, i.e. avidity may vary from $10^5$ to $10^{12}$ even for antibodies against a single hapten group. It is usually observed that the earliest antibodies obtained soon after the beginning of immunization are of low avidity and highly specific, but after prolonged immunization the antibodies become more avid and less specific. Since the antibody molecules are produced by individual antibody-forming cells, the functional and structural differences observed within a population of antibody molecules reflect the degree of diversity among the cells capable of responding to a given antigen. The variability of the avidity of antibody molecules are thought to be due to an antigen-mediated cell selection process in which cells capable of synthesizing antibody of high or low avidity are stimulated to different degrees depending on the dose of antigen [2*a*]. On the other hand, at the beginning of immunization there is hardly any cross-reaction even with closely related antigens, but later on cross-reactions with similar or related antigens may be found. It is possible that the early antibodies are directed against few distinct antigenic determinants and there is little chance for the same determinants to occur on other, even related, antigens [53].

A variety of factors may influence the class of the antibody produced [45]. One of them is the chemical structure of antigen, which can influence the proportion of IgM and IgG produced. Protein antigens, viruses, bacteriophages, and simple haptens have usually been found to stimulate mainly the IgG antibody formation after an early IgM response [4, 5, 7, 23, 34]. Lipopolysaccharide somatic antigens of Gram-negative bacteria elicit predominantly IgM antibodies [5]. Particle size may be another factor, since polymer forms of flagellin stimulate greater amounts of IgM antibody than monomer forms [1]. The dosage of antigen, the intensity of antigenic stimulation, the presence or absence of adjuvant, the time schedule of immunization and the route of antigen administration may also play an important role. Little amounts of bacterial lipopolysaccharide antigen elicit only IgM, whereas larger amounts of the same antigens injected over longer periods of time can stimulate IgG antibodies [47]. The fact that polysaccharide antigens are good immunogens in guinea pig but not in man and rabbit shows the role of species [9]. In an *in vitro* system it was found that the optimal concentration of antigen was the same for the formation of IgG, IgM and IgE antibodies. Furthermore, the optimal concentration of antigen and the distribution of anti-hapten antibodies between IgG and IgM classes were decided by the population of hapten-specific memory cells rather than carrier-specific helper cells [349].

### *IgM*

IgM comprises about 7 per cent of the immunoglobulins and has a half-life of 5.1 days. It circulates mainly within the vascular space, presumably because of its large size, which hinders crossing the capillary wall in the absence of local inflammation. It does not pass the placental barrier and is not present in significant amounts in milk or seromucous secretions. Despite its large molecular weight (about 900,000), IgM has a basically similar structure in several species to that of other immunoglobulins. Existing as a polymer of five tetramers each IgM antibody molecule should have ten antibody combining sites. There is no doubt that each molecule is multivalent, some of them having ten, but others only five, effective sites. The structure of IgM appears to be adapted for protective activity against microbes and other large antigens which have some repeating pattern of antigenic determinants close together on their surfaces. For example, the cell wall O-antigen of Gram-negative bacteria, the pneumococcal capsules, bacterial flagella or viruses have such a pattern of determinants. Since each combining site is of relatively low avidity, i.e. has a relatively small association constant, the combined action of multiple sites increases the avidity of the whole antibody molecule, in other words, the site avidity of IgM antibody is low but its effective avidity specific for such kinds of antigens may be very high [3]. The IgM molecules are probably distorted by combination with such particulate antigens and therefore a single IgM antibody molecule can fix and activate complement. On the other hand, for soluble antigens like ordinary proteins, being not associated with an organized structure and having a variety of different antigenic determinants, the IgM antibody has no special advantage. Its multiple combining sites, having low avidity each, cannot attach to the same antigenic determinant and therefore they readily dissociate.

The foetus synthesizes some IgM during the third trimester, but increased serum levels of IgM in the newborn indicate intrauterine infection. IgM antibody tends to be formed very early in the typical primary immune response. It is suggested on phylogenetic and ontogenetic basis that the IgM response is more primitive than the responses resulting in increasing levels of other classes of immunoglobulin. This conception seems to be connected with the fact that most, if not all, natural antibodies formed against different antigens have been found to belong to this class. The initial increased IgM antibody level is present rather transiently, usually declines or disappears completely in a few weeks if the antigen is soluble, but it may persist over much longer periods of time in response to, at least some, particulate antigens. Nevertheless, IgM antibodies are most active in agglutination and lytic reactions and less efficient in precipitation and complement fixation. They have virus-neutralizing capacity, but fail to neutralize bacterial exotoxins and enzymes.

When IgG and IgM antibodies against the cell wall O-antigen of Gram-negative bacteria were comparatively studied on the weight basis, the IgM antibodies were found to be more than 20 times as active in agglutinating, more than 100 times as effective in complement-dependent killing, and about 1,000 times as potent for opsonization. On the other hand, in neutralizing of diphtheria toxin or a small virus as poliovirus, IgM was found less efficient than IgG.

Recently, it has been shown that B lymphocytes could be stimulated by pokeweed mitogen. The B lymphocyte response to the non-specific effect of pokeweed mitogen was polyclonal and the secreted IgM was heterogeneous [42].

### *IgG*

IgG constitutes about 75 per cent of the total immunoglobulins in the serum of adults. It is exchanged readily between blood and extravascular fluid, 45 per cent occurring intravascularly, and has a relatively long half-life of 23 days. IgG seems to be unique among the immunoglobulins in that the fractional catabolic rate (per cent of intravascular pool per day) increases with the concentration of IgG in the blood. In the case of other immunoglobulins the fraction catabolized daily is constant, irrespective of their concentration in the blood. As a consequence, the significantly raised IgG levels in IgG myelomas or chronic malaria are accompanied by a shortened half-life of all the IgG. If a patient suffering from one of these diseases continues to produce a given antibody only at the normal rate, its absolute blood level will drop. This phenomenon may partly explain the occurrence of antibody deficiency syndromes in these diseases. The control of fractional catabolic rate has been found to depend upon the Fc portion of the IgG heavy chain. Passively administered specific 7S antibody can inhibit both the IgM and IgG responses to antigen. In initiation of humoral immune responses to heterologous erythrocytes three types of cells (T and B lymphocytes and macrophages) are involved. Recent findings suggest that previous association of the Fc portion of specific 7S antibody with the surface of macrophages alters the subsequent macrophage–antigen interaction in such a way that the antigen is not presented to the lymphoid cells in an immunogenic form [1*a*].

In all mammalian species IgG crosses the placenta and is present in the milk. It is present in variable amounts in seromucous secretions but no selective mechanisms are involved. The exact biological significance of the four sub-classes of IgG is not known, although there are some differences between them. All of the sub-classes except IgG1 elicit reversed passive cutaneous anaphylaxis in the guinea pig and all of them except IgG4 fix complement. IgG antibodies can directly neutralize bacterial exotoxins, enzymes and small viruses, and are highly effective precipitins. They account for the major portion of the complement fixing activity of the serum, and in this way the complement fixation of antigen–antibody complexes followed by the complement chain reaction is the mechanism which significantly promotes the biological effectiveness of IgG antibodies in phagocytosis and killing of microbes. These properties endow IgG with extra significance for the overall protection of the organism against infections.

IgG antibody response replaces the declining primary IgM response and persists for long periods of time. Secondary stimulus and hyperimmunization elicit great amounts of IgG. Although this pattern of sequential appearance seems to be a general one, there are variations depending on the kind of antigen and adjuvant, the dosage, the route of immunization, and the species. In naturally occurring infections or experimentally infected volunteers IgG agglutinins were not found until about 2 weeks after the infection [38, 46, 49]. According to recent findings, however, simultaneous appearance of IgM and IgG antibodies have been detected by means of radioimmuno-electrophoresis [20, 41]. If the methods used for measuring antibody activity favour the detection of IgM (e.g. agglutination), it is obvious that IgM appears to predominate in early sera.

### *IgA*

The third principal immunoglobulin designated IgA was described only in 1959 [25]. Although IgA constitutes about 15 per cent of serum immunoglobulins, it was confused with IgG for a long time. The half-life of human IgA is 5.8 days, much shorter than that of IgG. This means that, although the serum concentration is about one quarter, the amount of IgA synthesized daily is nearly the same as that of IgG. Synthesis of IgA begins a few days after birth and achieves adult levels by the age of 5 to 10 years. IgA antibodies do not activate complement, but can neutralize bacterial exotoxins and viruses. They do not kill Gram-negative bacteria *in vitro* in the presence of complement, but exert an anti-bacterial antibody activity in the presence of lysozyme [2]. Certain IgA antibodies do not precipitate, others do so. IgA is the most abundant immunoglobulin in human colostrum, and predominance and selective concentrating of IgA was shown in various other external secretions, such as, parotid saliva, tears, nasal mucus and tracheobronchial washings [60]. A large fraction of antibodies in the urethral exudates and in the middle ear fluid is secretory IgA [25*a*, 32*a*]. Furthermore, there is some evidence of selective passage of IgA into the small intestine lumen. It is probable that the bactericidal activity of the IgA-lysozyme system is of great biological importance, since IgA and lysozyme coexist in several secreted fluids [2]. IgA occurs intravascularly in 42 per cent. Some difference has been described between the IgA isolated from serum and external secretions. The IgA isolated from colostrum and parotid saliva sediments more rapidly (sedimentation coefficient, 11S) than its 7S serum counterpart. This 11S IgA, called secretory IgA, has a unique polypeptide component termed secretory or transport piece which is covalently linked to the heavy chains of the antibody molecule [59]. The function of the secretory piece is unknown. This component is probably synthesized in the epithelial cells of IgA-secreting glands and attached to IgA during the process of secretion. The IgA itself may be synthesized locally by plasma cells or arrive there via the circulation. There is no convincing evidence, however, about the transport function of the secretory piece in the secretion process of IgA [61]. The secretory IgA has been shown to have an increased resistance to digestion by proteolytic enzymes, suggesting that the secretory piece is involved, in some way, in this relative resistance [58].

Secretory IgA possesses yet another polypeptide chain, called J-chain. The J-chain is present also on the polymeric forms of serum IgA and IgM. Its role has been suggested to consist in joining several monomeric immunoglobulin molecules during polymerization [23*a*, 36*a*]. The demonstration of selective concentration of IgA in certain secretions suggests that the secretory IgA system may be of considerable importance in the defense mechanism preventing the microbial invasion of mucous surfaces. The increased resistance of the secreted form of IgA to the proteolytic enzymes of the gut gives great importance to this type of immunoglobulins appearing as copro-antibodies. The intestinal secretions from the jejunum, terminal ileum, and proximal colon have been found to contain qualitatively the same immunoglobulins as the serum and colostrum. Secretory IgA is present in the intestinal walls, intestinal contents, and faecal extracts at a significantly higher level than in the serum. It has been established that IgA can be synthesized by cells in the lamina propria of the intestine, and that cells producing IgA predominate over those forming other classes of antibody [13]. Since IgA does not fix or activate complement, a direct action against Gram-negative bacteria seems to be unlikely, in spite of the fact that IgA in the presence of lysozyme may have such a direct effect [2]. It has been demonstrated, however, that IgA has a powerful opsonic effect to promote the phagocytic activity of mononuclear and other phagocytic cells present on the epithelial surface of the intestine [63]. Although local antigen administration stimulates the formation of far greater numbers of IgA-producing cells than of IgG- or IgM-producing cells, there are appreciable amounts of IgM and IgG in the intestinal juices. The available data are insufficient to justify the supposition that copro-antibodies and IgA are identical.

In the light of these new findings it is interesting to mention that Besredka suggested the existence of local immunity distinct from serum antibody more than fifty years ago [8]. A great number of outstanding studies dealing with the protective role of local antibody in man have utilized local and systemic immunization with respiratory viruses. These studies have shown that exposure of the nasal and bronchial mucosa to virus results in the formation of predominantly IgA antibody to the virus in the local secretion [32]. On the other hand, local immunization does not elicit serum antibody. Nevertheless, the level of local antibody is correlated even in the absence of serum antibody with the resistance to infection. Similarly, copro-antibodies are produced by oral, but not parenteral, immunization [40]. In certain cases there seems to be no difference between local and systemic immunization. Immunization with aerosols the particles of which can reach the alveoli may act as systemic immunization.

### *IgD*

The existence of this class of human immunoglobulin was recognized on the basis of its precipitation by an antibody to a very rare form of myeloma protein that lacked determinants for the other classes of human immunoglobulins [51]. Subsequently, the presence of IgD has been shown in the plasma of normal persons. It has been demonstrated to occur predominantly in the vascular space (75 per cent) and to have a very short half-life, 2.8 days. IgD does not cross the placenta and was not detected in cord sera. Since the original description of IgD no specific antibody activity has been recognized to be associated with this class. According to recent findings, however, different antibody activities of IgD have been described. Anti-nuclear, anti-thyroid [31], anti-insulin [16], and anti-penicilloyl [22] antibodies were demonstrated. Moreover, a definite elevation of mean IgD concentration was found in the serum of pregnant women, and it seems that oral contraceptives may produce a rise in serum IgD. Three alternative hypotheses may be considered to explain this finding: (*i*) the rising IgD level reflects an antibody response to the foeto-maternal relationship, (*ii*) in pregnancy the usual IgD metabolism is altered, and (*iii*) the IgD level is regulated by sex steroids [35]. Approximately 18 per cent of all circulating lymphocytes with demonstrable surface immunoglobulin can be shown to have membrane-associated IgD. It has been suggested that cell-associated IgD may have an important biological role [9*a*].

### *IgE* [54*b*]

The biological and physicochemical properties of reagins were already known around 1940 based principally on the Prausnitz–Küstner reaction. These are, briefly, binding to isologous and closely related heterologous tissues, heat lability (destroyed by 56 °C in 1 h), activity in the absence of complement, failing to cross the placenta, moving in the fast $\gamma$ region on electrophoresis, and an approximately 8S sedimentation coefficient. Further evidence that reagins were probably a unique class of human immunoglobulin was obtained by a series of brilliant experiments in Ishizaka's laboratory [27*a*, *b*, 28]. They fractionated active preparations of sera from patients showing marked hypersensitivity to ragweed pollen, developed the very sensitive radioimmuno-diffusion techniques for the measuring of reagin, produced anti-reagin antisera which were rendered specific by absorption with the major classes of human immunoglobulins, and used radioimmunoelectrophoresis to show the complex formation of radiolabelled ragweed allergen (E) and reagin. They suggested that a unique immunoglobulin, termed IgE, was responsible for the reagin activity. The existence of IgE was confirmed by the isolation of an atypical myeloma protein which lacked the characteristic antigenic determinants of IgG, IgM, IgA and IgD [29, 30]. IgE has the shortest half-life, 2.3 days, as compared to other immunoglobulins and 51 per cent of it is distributed intravascularly. Inhibition test with the Fc portion of myeloma IgE protein has led to the conclusion that the IgE antibodies can attach firmly to certain tissue cells, mainly mast cells, of the same species (homocytotropic antibodies) by their Fc portion. The combination of this type of sensitized cells with specific allergen is shown in Fig. 10-2. Increased amounts of IgE have been found in the serum of patients suffering from some forms of immediate hypersensitivity. There seems to be, however, no quantitative relationship between the size of skin test reactions and the level of specific circulating reaginic antibody [28*a*]. It is suggested that in the classical allergen-reagin-mediated reaction of certain tissue cells conformational changes of attached IgE molecules may lead to the formation of tissue-activation sites which are distinct from the tissue-binding sites of IgE [54*a*]. As a consequence of these conformational changes, cross-linking of the Fab portions of IgE antibody molecules may occur eliciting the tissue activation sites and triggering the release of pharmacologically active mediators, e.g. of histamine (Fig. 10-3). This cross-linking of IgE molecules may be realized within their Fc portions, too. For example, protein A of *Staphylo-*

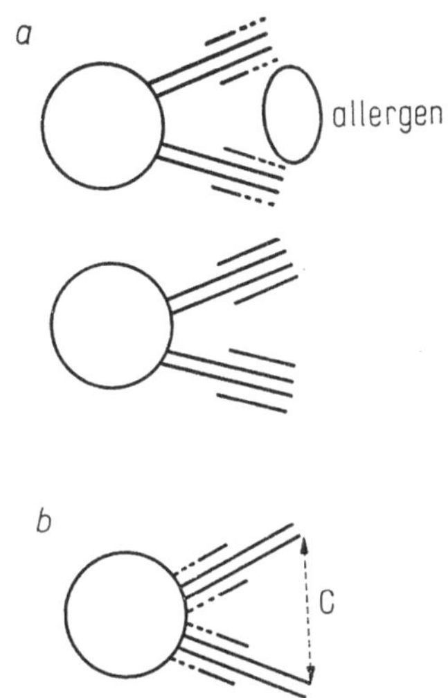


Fig. 10-2. *a)* Diagrammatic comparison of the properties of antibody and myeloma IgE molecules, showing the mode of attachment to target cells by means of sites in the Fc regions. *b)* Mode of interaction of IgG type cytolytic antibody molecules with target cells, showing subsequent interaction of complement with sites located in the Fc regions [54*b*]

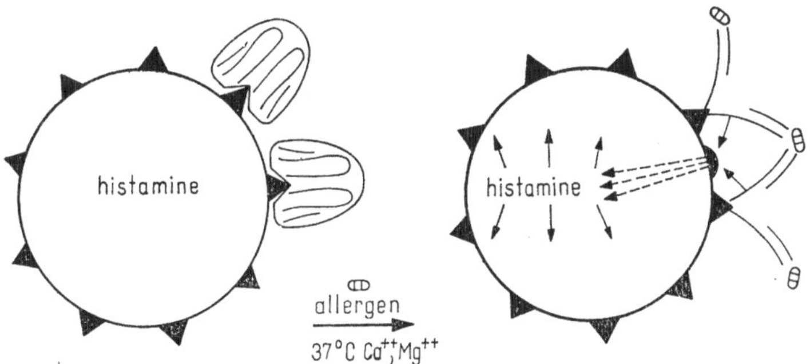


Fig. 10-3. Postulated mode of interaction between cell-fixed IgE antibodies and allergen leading to the triggering of release of vaso-active amines [54*b*]

*coccus aureus,* which possesses an unusual capacity for combination with the Fc regions of immunoglobulins [19, 55], may play an important role in these reactions (Fig. 10-4).

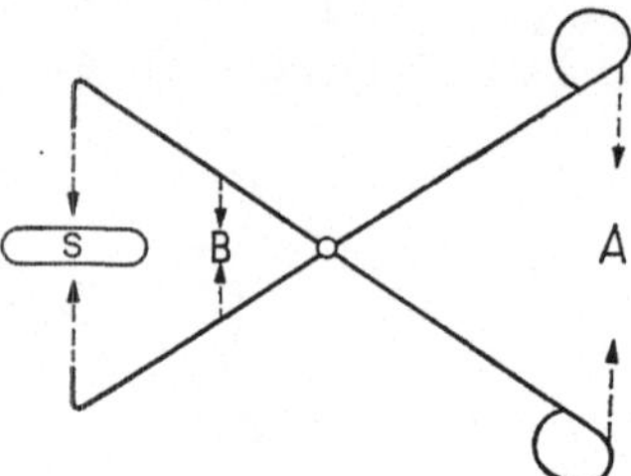


Fig. 10-4. Model illustrating various methods of inducing an allosteric transformation within cell-fixed IgE antibody molecules. Application of a force at position A would be more effective than at position B to form the activation site at position S. Position A corresponds to the sites in the Fab regions, and position B corresponds to the sites in the Fc regions [54*b*]

In certain circumstances, however, IgE antibodies are not deleterious, even may fulfill a protective role. Studies made on rat, infected with *Nippostrongylus brasiliensis,* have brought some evidence of association between a marked rise in the number of intestinal mast cells, an alteration of mucosal permeability and the expulsion of the nematode by a so-called self-cure mechanism [37].

## NATURAL OR NORMAL ANTIBODIES [64]

Antitoxins and natural antibodies play an important role in the defense mechanisms of the host. These specific antibodies have been produced in response to natural infection or to artificial immunization. An adequate survey of the blood of any subject living under natural conditions who has never suffered from a particular disease or has never been immunized artificially may show circulating antibodies which react *in vivo* and *in vitro* in the same way as specifically induced antibodies. The frequency of any particular antibody found in the non-immune sera may vary widely from one species to another, from group to group within the same species in accordance with age, and with some environmental conditions. These antibodies may possess a variety of biological activities as antitoxins, agglutinins, precipitins, bactericidal antibodies, and so on. It is possible that they arise in both passive and active ways. The newborn animal of an immune mother is endowed with a congenital passive immunity (naturally acquired congenital immunity) by prenatal or postnatal acquisition. The prenatal acquisition of maternal antibodies may be due to transplancental transmission from the maternal blood to the foetus. Since humoral antibodies can pass into the lumen of the uterus in the rat and guinea pig, it is another possibility that the foetus acquires these antibodies through the gut via the amnion. As a third possibility in the rat, rabbit and guinea pig the antibody passes to the yolk sac and is absorbed into the foetal circulation from here. The postnatal acquisition of maternal antibodies is due to early transference to the newborn animal via colostrum, and, later in smaller amounts, via milk. The acquired congenital immunity is, however, of relatively short duration. On the other hand, it is supposed that these so-called natural antibodies may arise in an active way as a result of true immune response to unrecognized antigenic stimulus. The synthesis of immunoglobulins begins a few days after birth. In the early years of life the immunoglobulin levels increase and parallelly natural antibodies appear in the serum. This true immune response may be due to an unrecognized infection. The presence of diphtheria and scarlet fever antitoxins, e.g. in the serum of persons who have never suffered from clinical diphtheria or scarlet fever can be explained on the basis of unrecognized contact with *Corynebacterium diphtheriae* and *Streptococcus pyogenes*, respectively. But it is unlikely that the wide variety of normal antibodies present in the serum are due to latent disease or carrier state. It was shown that the sera of young animals contain antibodies against most of the ubiquitous and exotic microbes. The antigens of dead bacterial cells pass from the intestines into the tissues, stimulating antibody formation. Many members of the normal intestinal bacterial flora contain antigens in common with related, and even unrelated, organisms. In so-called germ-free animals (deprived of living bacteria in their food and environment), although immunoglobulins are at relatively low levels, certain natural antibodies are present which may be attributed to stimuli by dead bacteria on the immune apparatus. In these cases chemical similarity of antigens has been suggested. Furthermore, similarity was described not only between the antigens of different species of bacteria, but even between bacterial antigens and antigens of plant or animal tissues. The idea that such antibodies arise rather by heterologous than by homologous stimulation widens the classical definition and meaning of specificity. Specificity is thus not absolutely connected and correlated with biological classifications but may rather be explained in terms of chemical constitution.

The specificity of natural antibodies is disputable. According to some investigations they are less specific than would be expected of antibodies resulting from an immune response. On the other hand, recent data obtained by studies on different bactericidal reactions have shown that in the case of Gram-negative bacteria, being the most susceptible to the combined action of antibody and complement system, there is a high specificity of natural antibodies against the *Bordetella* species [48*a*, *b*]. These natural antibodies seem to be anti-endotoxin in nature [14, 36]. Some authors suggest that all natural antibodies are anti-endotoxins, and therefore the normal intestinal Gram-negative bacterial flora has a great biological importance in the defense mechanisms stimulating the immune apparatus throughout life. It is possible that most of the natural antibodies belong to the IgM class. The IgM antibodies are more sensitive to heat inactivation than IgG antibodies. Perhaps, partly this is the reason why natural antibodies are more sensitive to heat inactivation than antibodies obtained by hyperimmunization.

## CYTOPHILIC ANTIBODIES [10*a*, 39*b*]

After antigen administration, the host is likely to produce humoral antibody of various types, including cytophilic antibody. The term cytophilic has been used to describe a special property of immunoglobulins for attachment to the surface of certain cells in virtue not of their antibody combining sites but of the cytophilic property of the Fc portion of the molecule [6, 11]. This antibody can be bound by homologous and heterologous cells and its affinity for cells seems to be limited mainly to macrophages. Cells bearing cytophilic antibodies on their surface are capable of specifically adsorbing antigen.

After recent findings this definition seems to be too narrow. Cytophilic antibodies may be present in the sera of non-immunized animals as well. Such antibodies may arise by unrecognized contact of a particular antigen or rather heterologous than homologous stimulation supported by some chemically similar antigen. The above-mentioned definition is narrow from another point of view, too. Some cytophilic antibodies may be better characterized by virtue of their conferring on cells a reactivity with antigen than by uptake of antigen. For example, reaginic antibodies responsible for some form of anaphylaxis may also be considered as cytophilic antibodies. Some of these bind to mast cells, and when the sensitized mast cells react with the specific antigen, degranulation occurs with a release of vasoactive amines. After all, it is prospected that the definition of cytophilic antibody will become wider in the future years in consequence of new experimental tools to be utilized in detecting and measuring this particular type of antibodies.

There are several methods for the detection of cytophilic antibodies in the serum and on the cell surface. The most useful one depends on visualization of the attachment of particulate antigens to the cells, which can be seen in wet preparations by phase-contrast microscopy. The most convenient form of this technique is the rosette test. In this test sheep erythrocytes are mainly used as indicators. The steps in the rosette test are as follows: (*i*) formation of a monolayer of cultured macrophages, (*ii*) incubation of washed monolayer with dilutions of serum containing cytophilic antibody, (*iii*) washing to remove free serum from the monolayer, (*iv*) incubation with a particulate antigen (for example, sheep erythrocytes), (*v*) washing to remove unattached particles, and (*vi*) microscopic examination. Sheep red cells can be used not only as antigens but also as carriers of antigens since soluble antigens can be coupled to them by means of bis-diazotized benzidine. The above method has been defined as the direct technique [10*b*]. In the indirect technique the antigen-coated erythrocytes as indicator cells and the antibody are made to react first [6]. These immune complexes are then mixed with untreated macrophages.

The indirect technique of rosette formation can also be used for visual identification of antibody producing cells. Rosette forming cells increase in number rapidly after the inoculation of antigen, indicating an active secretion of antibodies. Analysis of doubly immunized animals shows that lymphocytes and plasma cells are nearly all single producers, i. e. stimulated only by one of the antigens, indicating that passive sensitization of cytophilic antibodies can only be effective in a small proportion of them. The proportion of double producers is much higher amongst the peritoneal macrophages, but single reactors are in majority even there, suggesting that these cells are mainly modified immunocytes derived from lymphoid cells. From these findings it seems to be questionable that the cytophilic antibodies play an essential role in any major immunological phenomenon, but there is no wholly acceptable disproof of their importance. However, the cytophilic antibodies may, hypothetically, play some part in the non-specific stimulation of immunocytes. With the local liberation of antibody, some cytophilic antibodies may attach to immunocytes of unrelated immune pattern, which will then be stimulated non-specifically to antibody production.

The factors affecting the production of cytophilic antibodies in experimental animals have not been studied in detail [6, 10*b*]. In the majority of the respective experiments sheep erythrocytes were used. Both the route of immunization and the type of adjuvant (Freund's complete or incomplete adjuvant) are important. The ratio of cytophilic antibody to total antibody in the sera of immunized animals may vary greatly. The cytophilic antibodies may be 7S $\gamma_2$-globulins, 19S (IgM) globulins, and $\alpha_1$-globulins in the sera of mice and slow 7S $\gamma_2$-globulins in the sera of guinea pigs.

Factors affecting the attachment of cytophilic antibodies to macrophages have been examined recently. Chemical modification of lysine or tryptophan groups of rabbit IgG antibody by carbamylation or amidination of lysine and benzylation of tryptophan residues can effectively suppress cytophilic activity [57]. Such techniques lead to loss of complement fixing ability but have no significant effect on the primary union of antibody with antigen. These results suggest that only the Fc portion alters and the Fab combining site remains intact, and the properties of cytophilic binding and complement fixation can reside on the same antibody molecule. There seems to exist no functional relationship between cytophilic binding and complement fixation in the Fc portion since cytophilic binding can occur in the absence of complement. According to our present knowledge, the sensitization of macrophages is mainly an immunological, but not energy dependent, active process. The receptors on mouse and guinea pig macrophages for 7S $\gamma_2$-globulin are resistant to treatment with proteolytic enzymes and are of phospholipid nature. The alveolar macrophages can take up more cytophilic antibodies than the peritoneal ones, probably because the alveolar macrophages possess more binding sites or are more reactive. Besides macrophages, other types of cells as neutrophils, lymphocytes, mast cells may carry cytophilic antibodies [43, 62].

Cytophilic antibodies may play some role in the attachment phase of the phagocytic process [6, 62]. Attachment can occur if the particle has been treated with either cytophilic or non-cytophilic specific antibody and if the macrophage has been sensitized with cytophilic antibody. Consequently, the indirect technique of rosette formation is a more sensitive method than the direct one. It is not yet clear whether the immune complexes attach to the same receptors as do antibodies which are cytophilic *per se* or complex formation in the indirect procedure leads to conformational changes of the Fc portion which facilitate the attachment of non-cytophilic antibodies to macrophages. The attachment of complexes can be promoted by adding complement. It is possible that in this case the receptor may be similar to or identical with the immune adherence receptor. Opsonization may occur to promote the engulfment of particles, the second step of phagocytosis [6, 62]. Natural or immune cytophilic antibodies take part as opsonins in this process. The ability of mouse macrophages to take up red cells of various species has been examined and it has been found that there are marked differences depending on the presence of natural cytophilic antibodies. In mice, a cytophilic form of IgM antibody against *Salmonella typhimurium* has been described which attaches to the macrophages and significantly increases their capacity to ingest and kill the virulent organisms.

According to numerous experimental data, cytophilic antibodies may play some role in delayed hypersensitivity. Delayed-type allergic reactions cannot be shown to relate to humoral antibody, but seem to be specific allergic cell-mediated processes. The peritoneal macrophage disappearance reaction, based on a characteristic *in vivo* activity of macrophages, is used for investigating delayed hypersensitivity [39*a*]. In guinea pigs with delayed hypersensitivity the injection of the specific antigen by any route, but especially intraperitoneally, is followed promptly by a striking fall in the number of free-floating macrophages. It is very convenient to use for such experiments BCG-vaccinated guinea pigs and the purified protein derivative of tuberculin (PPD). It was found that local passive transfer of the macrophage disappearance reaction was effected by (*i*) cells but not by serum, (*ii*) cells from sensitized donors only if the donors had been exposed to the antigen, and (*iii*) normal cells treated with serum of sensitized animals. From these experiments cytophilic antibody appears to be an immunological mediator of reactivity. It seems possible that the local passive transfer of the macrophage disappearance reaction may be conferred by macrophages carrying cytophilic antibodies and the effect on recipient macrophages can be due to a pharmacological mediator. Macrophage disappearance reaction can also be produced by injection of bacterial endotoxins. It is possible that this effect of endotoxins depends on the existence of natural delayed hypersensitivity. On the other hand, cytophilic antibodies seem not to play any role in the migration inhibition reaction. These findings suggest that the reaction of antigen with lymphocytes from sensitized guinea pigs results in the release of the migration inhibition factor, which inhibits the migration of macrophages and the affected macrophages do not react directly with the antigen [15]. In spite of these findings, it is also possible that large amounts of cytophilic antibodies on guinea pig macrophages, reacting with specific antigen, inhibit the migration.

Some other data about the role of macrophage cytophilic antibodies in delayed hypersensitivity are listed in the following. In mice, there is a correlation between the existence of delayed hypersensitivity and the actual cytophilic antibody content of the serum. The injection of suitable antigens, e.g. brain in complete Freund's adjuvant, produces in the guinea pig a significant elevation of $\gamma_2$-antibody, an increased level of cytophilic antibody and delayed hypersensitivity, leading to an allergic encephalomyelitis in this particular case. In the guinea pig, however, there is no correlation between the intensity of delayed skin reaction and the cytophilic antibody titres. It has also been shown in guinea pigs that the local passive transfer of delayed skin reactivity to sheep erythrocytes can be carried out by means of normal peritoneal cells sensitized with cytophilic antibodies *in vitro*. Normal guinea pigs injected with serum containing cytophilic antibodies of 7S $\gamma_2$-globulin do not develop delayed hypersensitivity. On the other hand, the migration inhibition reaction can be reduced by treatment with trypsin, suggesting that $\alpha_1$-globulin (which is not a conventional immunoglobulin) and

19S globulin cytophilic antibodies on mouse macrophages, and cytophilic factors other than 7S $\gamma_2$-globulins on guinea pig macrophages may also play some role in this *in vitro* delayed hypersensitivity.

Although, due to new findings, our knowledge about cytophilic antibodies is expanding, we cannot give any general explanation of their role and importance [56]. It is possible that they enhance antibody formation through more effective capture and retention of antigen, but, on the other hand, they may be involved in the feedback control mechanism of antibody formation by preventing the antigen from reaching antibody forming cells. We may say that examination of this special type of antibody is promising for the understanding of the whole immunological function.

## SPECIFICALLY SENSITIZED CELLS INVOLVED IN CELL-MEDIATED IMMUNITY [17, 44]

The development of specific cell-mediated immunity (homograft rejection, delayed hypersensitivity) is based on the formation of specifically sensitized T lymphocytes which can be stimulated by contact between specific antigen (which may be macrophage-processed) and specific antibody or antibody-like macromolecules or receptors on their surfaces *in vivo* and *in vitro* [21]. It is to be noted that T cells can be stimulated also non-specifically *in vitro* by mitogens, such as phytohaemagglutinin. These stimulated T lymphocytes which do not contain intracellular immunoglobulin may exert two main functions besides taking part in cell-mediated immunity. (*i*) They may divide further to form an expanded population of primed antigen-sensitive cells, which play an important role in immunological memory because of their long life-span and (*ii*) they may co-operate during the immune response to certain antigens by stimulating B lymphocytes to produce humoral antibodies. For further information about antibody formation see Chapter 11.

T cells have two further characteristics forming the basis of the phenomena of specific cell-mediated immunity. They may be killer cells (aggressor cells), i. e. cytotoxic for graft target cells, thus causing graft rejection. On the other hand, on contact with the specific antigen they release different soluble substances possessing several biological activities. It is one of the unanswered questions whether lymphocytes produce a large number of distinct soluble mediators or only a limited number of factors with multiple biological activities. The different biological activities attributed to soluble substances released by T lymphocytes are as follows. A group of them affects macrophages: they inhibit the migration of macrophages of various origins in suspension or as an outgrowth from solid tissue explants; they are chemotactic for macrophages *in vitro*: induce aggregation of macrophages in suspension; promote phagocytosis by macrophages of non-immune animals; cause different morphological changes in the individual cells; inhibit macrophage spreading; activate normal macrophages and cause the release of biologically active mediators from them. Further biological activities include their being chemotactic for polymorphonuclear leukocytes and eosinophils *in vivo* and *in vitro* as well as cytotoxicity towards tumour cells *in vivo* and different kinds of cells in tissue cultures. There is an inflammatory reaction of lymphocyte products in the skin of normal animals, including local increase in vascular permeability. Mitogenic activity means the stimulation of DNA synthesis which causes non-sensitized lymphocytes to divide. Other mediators stimulate acid production by cells in tissue culture, cause release of histamine and other vasoactive amines from platelets, cause histological changes upon injection into lymph nodes [33], and possess interferon-like properties. Activities related to the presence of complement components have also been described.

These various biological mediators found in lymphocyte culture supernatants make it possible that a few specifically sensitized T lymphocytes in the host reacting with the specific antigen can affect a large number of immunologically non-specific effector cells [52].

The properties of different soluble lymphocyte products have been studied recently. The most detailed knowledge has been obtained about the chemical nature of the migration inhibition factor (MIF). MIF is a glycoprotein, sialic acid being necessary for its biological activity. It has an approximate mol. wt. of 35,000 to 50,000. These results were obtained by enzymatic treatment and isopycnic centrifugation in a CsCl density gradient [50]. Application of such a method is promising in characterizing other lymphocyte mediators, too [18].

Up to now there is only suggestive evidence that soluble lymphocyte products studied under *in vitro* conditions are the actual mediators of cellular immune reactions *in vivo*. According to preliminary studies there is a good correlation between a state of delayed hypersensitivity in the intact animal and the ability of its lymphocytes to release soluble factors *in vitro*. The soluble lymphocytic mediators may cause macrophage activation, and in such a way enhance non-specific microbicidal activity. The skin-reactive factor (SRF) formed *in vitro* can cause an inflammatory reaction in the skin resembling the delayed skin test in actively immunized animals. It is possible that further results in the chemical characterization of the soluble lymphocytic products and their modes of action will clarify the cell-mediated immune processes as deeply, as the characterization of the immunoglobulins has clarified the humoral immune reactions.

## REFERENCES


1. Ada, G. L., Nossal, G. V. J. and Austin, C. M.: In *Molecular and Cellular Basis of Antibody Formation*. Ed. by Sterzl, J. Czechoslovak Academy of Sciences, Prague 1965, p. 31.

1*a*. Abrahams, S., Phillips, R. A. and Miller, R. G.: *J. exp. Med.* **137,** 870 (1973).

2. Adinolfi, M., Glynn, A. A., Lindsay, M. and Milne, C. M.: *Immunology* **10,** 517 (1966).

2*a*. Ahlstedt, S., Holmgren, J. and Hanson, J. A.: *Immunology* **24,** 191 (1973).

3. Baker, P. J., Prescott, B., Stashak, P. W. and Amsbaugh, D. F.: *J. Immunol.* **107,** 719 (1971).

4. Bauer, D. C.: *J. Immunol.* **91,** 323 (1963).

5. Bauer, D. C., Mathies, M. J. and Stavitsky, A. B.: *J. exp. Med.* **117,** 889 (1963).

6. Berken, A. and Benacerraf, B.: *J. exp. Med.* **123,** 119 (1966).

7. Berlin, B. S.: *Proc. Soc. exp. Biol. (N.Y.)* **113,** 1013 (1963).

8. Besredka, A.: *Ann. Inst. Pasteur* **33,** 882 (1919).

9. Bloch, K. J., Koursilsky, F. M., Ovary, Z. and Benacerraf, B.: *Proc. Soc. exp. Biol. (N.Y.)* **114,** 52 (1963).

9*a*. Boxel, J. A. van Paul, W. E., Terry, W. D. and Green, I.: *J. Immunol.* **109,** 648 (1972).

10*a*. Boyden, S. V.: In *Cell-bound Antibodies*. Ed. by Amos, B. and Korowski, H Wistar Institute Press, Philadelphia 1963, p. 7.
10*b*. id., *Immunology* **7,** 474 (1964).
11. Boyden, S. V. and Sorkin, E.: *Immunology* **3,** 272 (1960).
12. Ceppellini, R., Dray, S., Edelman, G., Fahey, J., Franek, F., Franklin, H., Goodman, H. C., Grabar, P., Currick, A. N., Heremans, J. F., Isliker, H., Karush, F., Presse, N. and Truka, Z.: *Bull. Wld Hlth Org.* **30,** 447 (1964).
13. Crabbe, P. A., Nash, D. R., Bazin, H., Eyssen, H. and Heremans, J. F.: *J. exp. Med.* **130,** 723 (1969).
14. Daguillard, F. and Edsall, G.: *J. Immunol.* **100,** 1112 (1968).
15. David, J. R., Al-Askari, S., Lawrence, H. S. and Thomas, L.: *J. Immunol.* **93,** 264 (1964).
16. Devey, M., Sanderson, D. J., Carter, D. and Coombs, R. R. A.: *Lancet* **ii,** 1281 (1970).
17. Dumonde, D. C. and Maini, R. N.: *Clin. Allergy* **1,** 123 (1971).
18. Dumonde, D. C., Page, D. A., Matthew, M. and Wolstencroft, R. A.: *Clin. exp. Immunol.* **10,** 25 (1972).
19. Forsgren, A. and Sjöquist, J.: *J. Immunol.* **97,** 822 (1966).
20. Freeman, M. J. and Stavitsky, A. B.: *J. Immunol.* **95,** 981 (1965).
21. Fudenberg, H. H., Good, R. A., Goodman, H. C., Hitzig, W., Kunkel, H. G., Roitt, I. M., Rosen, F. S., Rowe, D. S., Seligmann, M. and Soothill, J. R.: *Bull. Wld Hlth Org.* **45,** 125 (1971).
22. Gleich, G. E., Bieger, R. C. and Stankievic, R.: *Science* **165,** 606 (1969)
23. Grey, H. M.: *Immunology* **7,** 82 (1964).
23*a*. Halpern, M. S. and Koshland, M. E.: *Nature (Lond.)* **228,** 1276 (1970).
24. Harkness, D. R.: *Postgrad. Med.* **48,** 64 (1970).
25. Heremans, J. F., Heremans, M.-Th. and Schultze, H. E.: *Clin. chim. Acta* **4,** 96 (1959).
25*a*. Howie, V. M., Ploussard, J. H., Sloyer, J. L. and Johnston, R. B.: *Inf. Immunol.* **7,** 589 (1973).
26. Humphrey, J. H. and White, R. G.: *Immunology for Students of Medicine*. 3rd ed. Blackwell, Oxford 1970.
27*a*. Ishizaka, K. and Ishizaka, T.: *J. Allergy* **42,** 330 (1968).
27*b*. id., *J. Immunol.* **100,** 554 (1968).
28. Ishizaka, K., Ishizaka, T. and Hornbrook, M. M.: *J. Immunol.* **97,** 35 (1966).
28*a*. Jarrett, E. E. E. and Stewart, D. C.: *Immunology* **24,** 37 (1973).
29. Johansson, S. G. O. and Bennich, H.: *Immunology* **13,** 381 (1967).
30. Johansson, S. G. O., Bennich, H. and Wide, L.: *Immunology* **14,** 265 (1968).
31. Kantor, G. L., Van Herle, A. J. and Barnett, E. V.: *Clin. exp. Immunol.* **6,** 951 (1970).
32. Kasel, J. A., Rossen, R. D., Fulk, R. V., Fedson, D. S., Couch, R. B. and Brown, P.: *Ann. intern. Med.* **71,** 369 (1969).
32*a*. Kearus, D. H., O'Reilly, R. J., Lee, L. and Welch, B. G.: *J. inf. Dis.* **127,** 99 (1973).
33. Kelly, R. H., Wolstencroft, R. A., Dumonde, D. C. and Balfour, B. M.: *Clin. exp. Immunol.* **10,** 49 (1972).
34. Kim, Y. B., Bradley, S. G. and Watson, D. W.: *J. Immunol.* **93,** 798 (1964).
34*a*. Kishimoto, T. and Ishizaka, K.: *J. Immunol.* **109,** 612 (1972).
35. Klapper, D. G. and Mendenhall, H. W.: *J. Immunol.* **107,** 912 (1971).
36. Mergenhagen, S. E., Gewurz, H., Bladen, H. A., Nowotny, A., Kasai, N. and Lüderitz, O.: *J. Immunol.* **100,** 227 (1968).
36*a*. Mestecky, J., Kulhavy, R. and Kraus, F. W.: *J. Immunol.* **108,** 738 (1972).
37. Miller, H. R. P. and Jarrett, W. F. H.: *Immunology* **20,** 277 (1971).
38. Murray, E. S., O'Connor, J. M. and Gaon, J. A.: *J. Immunol.* **94,** 734 (1965).
39*a*. Nelson, D. S. and Boyden, S. V.: *Med. Res.* **1,** 20 (1961).
39*b*. id., *Brit. med. Bull.* **23,** 15 (1967).
40. Ogra, P. L. and Karzon, D. T.: *J. Immunol.* **102,** 1423 (1969).
41. Osler, A. G., Mulligan, J. J. and Rodriguez, E.: *J. Immunol.* **96,** 334 (1966).
42. Parkhouse, R. M. E., Jánossy, G. and Greaves, M. F.: *Nature (Lond.)* **235,** 21 (1972).
43. Phillips-Quagliata, J. M., Levine, B. B. and Uhr, J. W.: *Nature (Lond.)* **222,** 1296 (1969).

44. Pick, E. and Turk, J. L.: *Clin. exp. Immunol.* **10,** 1 (1972).
45. Pike, R. M.: *Bact. Rev.* **31,** 157 (1967).
46. Pike, R. M., McBrayer, H. L., Schulze, M. L. and Chandler, C. H.: *Proc. Soc. exp. Biol. (N.Y.)* **120,** 786 (1965).
47. Pike, R. M., Schulze, M. L. and Chandler, C. H.: *J. Bact.* **92,** 880 (1966).
48*a*. Pusztai, Zs., Csizér, Z. and Joó, I.: *Z. Immun.-Forsch.* **141,** 1 (1971).
48*b*. ibid., **141,** 129 (1971).
49. Reddin, J. L., Anderson, R. K., Jenness, R. and Spink, W. W.: *New Engl. J. Med.* **272,** 1263 (1965).
50. Remold, H. G. and David, J. R.: *J. Immunol.* **107,** 1090 (1971).
51. Rowe, D. S. and Fahey, J. L.: *J. exp. Med.* **121,** 171 (1965).
52. Salvin, S. B., Sell, S. and Nishio, J.: *J. Immunol.* **107,** 655 (1971).
53. Siskind, G. W. and Benacerraf, B.: *Advanc. Immunol.* **10,** 1 (1969).
54*a*. Stanworth, D. R.: *Clin. exp. Immunol.* **6,** 1 (1970).
54*b*. id., *Nature (Lond.)* **233,** 310 (1971).
55. Stanworth, D. R., Matthews, N. and Sjöquist, J. (in preparation).
56. Sulitzeanu, D.: *Bact. Rev.* **32,** 404 (1968).
57. Thrasher, S. G. and Cohen, S.: *J. Immunol.* **107,** 672 (1971).
58. Tomasi, T. and Calvanico, N.: *Fed. Proc.* **27,** 617 (1968).
59. Tomasi, T. B., Tan, E. M. and Solomon, A.: *J. exp. Med.* **121,** 101, (1965).
60. Tomasi, T. B. and Zigelbaum, S.: *J. clin. Invest.* **42,** 1552 (1963).
61. Tourville, D. R., Adler, R. H. and Bienenstock, J.: *J. exp. Med.* **129,** 411 (1969).
62. Uhr, J. W.: *Proc. nat. Acad. Sci. (Wash.)* **54,** 1599 (1965).
63. Wernet, P., Breu, H., Knop, J. and Rowley, D.: *J. inf. Dis.* **124,** 223 (1971).
64. Wilson, G. S. and Miles, A. A.: *Topley and Wilson's Principles of Bacteriology and Immunity.* 5th ed. Arnold, London 1964, p. 1315.

CHAPTER 11

# ANTIBODY PRODUCTION AND ITS THEORIES

by

G. JÁNOSSY and G. GY. PETRÁNYI



## INTRODUCTION

Jerne [76*b*] classified theoretical immunologists into two categories, namely, 'trans-immunologists' who, starting from the chemical structure of antibodies, investigate the process of antibody production backwards and 'cis-immunologists' who examine the sequence of the events immediately following the antigen stimulus. The present chapter will be concerned with problems belonging to the realm of cis-immunology. In the light of the results of recent years' research, however, we may expect that the two camps of immunologists will soon meet somewhere at the 'middle' of the immune process and in this way numerous important questions will be put in a new, *common*, light. Besides the highly developed immunological techniques applied by trans-immunologists, other newly developed methods, such as transfer experiments on inbred animals, use of chemically well-defined antigens, exact cytokinetic studies and the wide-spread use of *in vitro* culture technique, have substantially contributed to the rapid development of immunology in recent years. It appears that immunology has gone a long way towards the solution of the riddle of the 'three-cell interaction', which is expected to throw light on the basic question of differentiation.

To make the large experimental material easier to survey, we have divided this chapter into three parts. In the first part, the basic phenomena of humoral immunity are briefly summarized. In the second part, the cellular events occurring in the course of the basic phenomena are described, together with theoretical considerations concerning the steps of immune response. At last, the third part reviews the selective and instructive theories of antibody production.

## BASIC PHENOMENA OF ANTIBODY PRODUCTION

### DEFINITION OF PRIMARY AND SECONDARY HUMORAL IMMUNE RESPONSES

Antibody production may be defined as *de novo* synthesis of $\gamma$-globulins stereospecific for a given antigen. These $\gamma$-globulins are formed by immunocytes committed to produce a given antibody. Such specific immunocytes arise in the course of the immune response. A foreign substance (antigen) when entering the body for the first time induces a *primary immune response* in the course of which serum antibodies appear after a relatively long interval and their level rises slowly up to a relatively low peak. The height of the peak depends on the dose of the antigen. After the second introduction of the antigen, the pre-existing antibody level shows a sudden drop due to the neutralizing effect of the antigen. Soon thereafter, however, the antibody level will rise steeply and may exceed the level reached during the primary response even 10–30-fold (*secondary immune response*). Further repeated stimuli by not too large doses of the antigen administered at not too short intervals induce ever higher peaks of serum antibody level. The animal sensitized by repeated stimuli may be considered *hyperimmunized*.

### PHASES OF PRIMARY IMMUNE RESPONSE

The immune response as investigated by serological methods is characterized by the following successive stages (Fig. 11-1): latency; exponential rise in antibody production; plateau; decline of antibody production. The latency is due to several factors. Handling of the antigen and the cell interactions necessary for the initiation of antibody formation take time but not more than several minutes or, at most, several hours. In fact, however, latency has usually been found longer because of the insufficient sensitivity of the serological tests.

The exponential phase usually lasts (in the mouse) from the 2nd to the 4th day after the introduction of the antigen. During this period, owing to the rapid

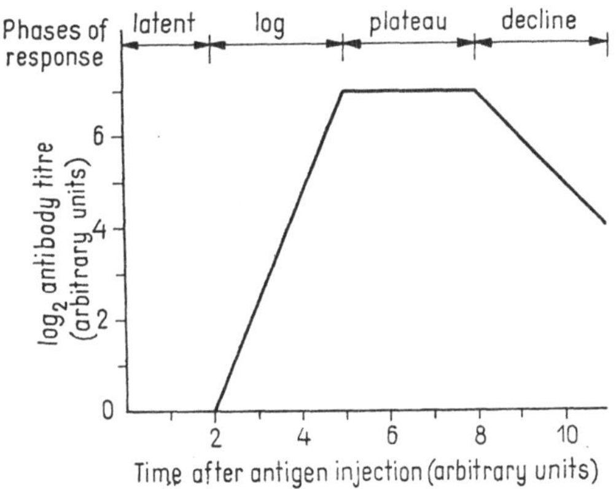


Fig. 11-1. Phases of antibody response (see text)

production of antibody, concentration in the serum is doubled every 8 h. In this way, the amount of the antibody in the serum grows ~1,000-fold. In immunized animals, the lymph nodes and the spleen substantially grow in size, especially in the early period of the exponential phase, which is characterized histologically by plasma cell formation in the medullary areas and hyperplasy of the germinal centres. In the exponential phase, the rise in the antibody level is due to an increase in the number of antibody forming cells.

The plateau and the decline in antibody production are both phases very variable in length because the production during these periods of the individual classes of immunoglobulins are each regulated by different mechanisms to be outlined below. The regulation impacts, if highly intensive, may stop the production of the antibodies belonging to some of the immunoglobulin classes. In this case, the antibody level falls without any plateau, at a rate corresponding to the half-life in the serum of similar immunoglobulin molecules introduced passively. In other cases, there is a well-defined plateau and the antibody production declines slowly, in a protracted manner.

## RULES OF THE PRODUCTION OF ANTIBODIES OF DIFFERENT CLASSES

The most striking property of immunoglobulins is their extraordinary heterogeneity. Besides having specific combining sites for different antigens, they are also heterogeneous, due to their class variability, in size, form, composition and biological function. The different immunoglobulin classes being governed by different regulation mechanisms, the same antigen may induce immune responses of several types, i.e. different mechanisms of B cell triggering may occur simultaneously or successively; the produced antibodies show different class specificities. The events follow one another according to a time table which, apart from a few exceptions, is subjected to general rules.

Twenty hours after the injection of a particulate antigen antibodies of the

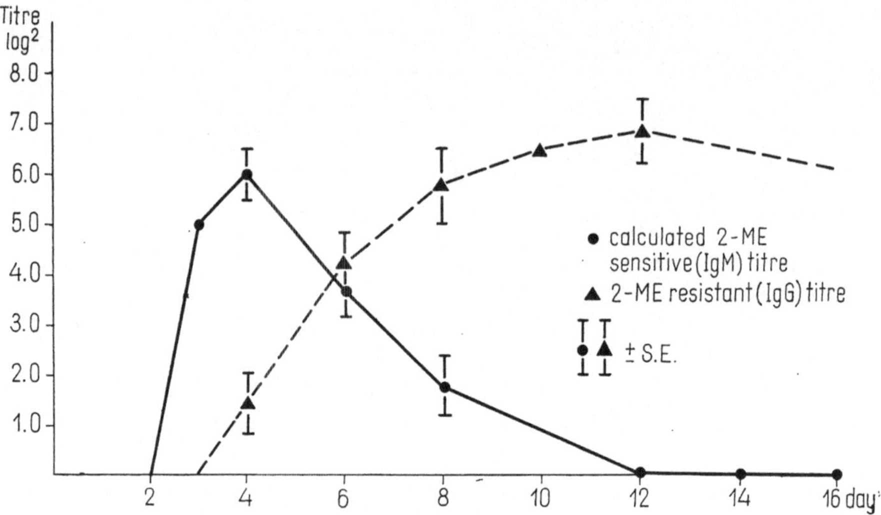


Fig. 11-2. IgM and IgG antibody production in mice after a single intraperitoneal injection of $2 \times 10^6$ sheep red blood cells

macroglobulin type (IgM)* can be demonstrated in the serum of the recipient mouse. The length of latency thus defined depends on the sensitivity of the method of detection. It is to be added that the first small amounts of antibody secreted into serum may be bound by the introduced antigen itself. From the first day on, IgM antibodies are continuously produced yielding an exponential curve. The peak of the IgM response is usually reached on the 3rd to 5th day (Fig. 11-2). On days 6–10, the titre of the IgM antibodies is rapidly declining while the half-life of these antibodies is approximately equal to that of the IgM molecules passively administered to normal animals (approx. 24 h). This phenomenon points to an intensive (almost complete) inhibition of the IgM synthesis. The dynamics of the IgM synthesis as outlined above proved to be nearly the same when heterologous erythrocytes [38, 126], influenza virus [9], or $F_2$ bacteriophage [3] was administered as antigen to mice, when flagellar antigen [109] was administered to rats or $\Phi$x phage to guinea pigs [163*a*] etc. The cells producing IgM antibodies show characteristic morphological changes while the production proceeds. In the spleen of rats immunized three days earlier with heterologous erythrocytes, the IgM haemolysins were found to be produced in 84 per cent by lymphoblasts and plasmablasts while the contribution of immunocytes showing transient maturity and of mature plasma cells was 11 per cent and 5 per cent, respectively [126]. On the 5th day, on the other hand, this distribution showed a shift in favour of

* Owing to lack of space, the description of methods had to be omitted. In this chapter, the immunoglobulins which are detectable by the direct haemolysin plaque method [38, 151*a*] and/or proved to be sensitive to 2-mercapto-ethanol (2-ME) in the course of serological titration [163*a*] are called IgM globulins. Most of these belong to the 19S class. The antibodies defined by the indirect plaque method and the 2-ME resistant antibodies are called IgG (7S) globulins.

mature plasma cells: immature forms (plasmablasts) were demonstrated at a rate as low as 23 per cent. After the 5th day, early signs of degeneration, suggestive of the half of IgM antibody production, appeared in immature plasma cells [88].

Antibodies of the IgG type appear in the serum three to four days after the administration of a particulate antigen. However, the latency may be more variable in length and is highly dependent on the antigen dose. It is almost a rule that in the course of the primary response IgG antibodies never appear before the IgM globulins. In the mouse, globulins of the $IgG_1$ sub-class can be demonstrated earliest, almost simultaneously with the IgM macroglobulins. These globulins attain a peak on the 4th or 5th day [171]. The peak for the $IgG_2$ antibodies, which make up the bulk of the IgG globulins, appears between the 6th and 14th days (Fig. 11-2) and is followed by a long plateau and a slow decline. $IgG_2$ antibodies may be demonstrable in the serum even several months after the primary antigen stimulus [163*a*]. The dynamics of the IgG-type antibodies have been found to follow this pattern, irrespective of the quality of the antigen [3, 109, 163*a*].

In the beginning (on the 4th day), the cells producing IgG antibodies in the spleen are mainly plasma- and lymphoblasts; in a later phase, plasma cells gradually take over this activity. These cells may also enter circulation [88, 126].

If the dose of antigen exceeds the optimal dose by two or three orders of magnitude, IgA antibodies are also produced from the 4th–6th day on. Maximum production of these antibodies is to be observed between the 8th and 14th days after the antigen has been introduced.

The pattern of antibody production is somewhat different if the antigen is soluble, i.e. not particulate. Initial investigations suggested [163*b*] that the latency period of the production of IgM antibody to soluble antigens was more protracted, lasting from several days to several weeks. Subsequently, it was shown with more sensitive methods that even in case of soluble antigens, the IgM production starts early, but substantially less IgM antibody is produced [109, 162]. IgG antibody production, on the other hand, is independent of the physical properties of the antigen [109, 162].

In larger animals (e.g. rabbit), as well as in man, the kinetics of antibody production are similar: after an initial IgM production, IgG production gradually becomes predominant. In man, experimental primary immune response is usually induced with the haemocyanin of the sea-snail (*Megathura crenulata*) [32, 154] because spontaneous immunization with this antigen never occurs. Experimental data indicate that in man the peak of the IgM antibody production occurs on the 14th day, whereas the IgG response reaches its maximum between the 45th and 56th days.

## PHASES OF THE SECONDARY IMMUNE RESPONSE

If several weeks after the induction of primary response the same antigen is administered again, the secondary response will exceed the primary one in intensity [163*b*]. As a result of the primary response, IgG antibodies may persist in the serum, which are immediately bound by the antigen. The latency period is much shorter than in the case of the primary response. Latency is followed by the exponential phase of IgG antibody production, which lasts till the 5th–7th day following the administration of the antigen. Microplaque experiments have shown that these IgG antibodies are exclusively produced by plasma cells in the spleen after an extraordinarily rapid maturation process [75]. Although the sequence of the phases of secondary response may be modified by previous immunological events (see Chapter 8, section on immunological memory), the amounts of IgM antibody produced are generally below the sensitivity threshold of the serological tests and can be demonstrated only by ultracentrifugation. During the exponential phase of the secondary response the antibody doubling time is 5 to 7 h. The exponential phase is relatively short. Subsequently, antibody production continues at a slower rate for several weeks. The characteristics of the secondary response are less influenced by the quality of the antigen than those of the primary response [153, 163*b*].

## CELLULAR EVENTS OCCURRING DURING ANTIBODY PRODUCTION

### METHODS FOR FOLLOWING THE CELLULAR EVENTS OF ANTIBODY FORMATION

During the phases of fast antibody production, the dynamics of the process are reliably reflected by the increase in antibody concentration [163*b*]. From the end of the proliferation phase, however, serum titre gives no suitable information on the kinetics of antibody production because the titres are substantially influenced by the decomposition of antibodies and their distribution in the organism [88, 163*b*]. For this reason, the introduction of the haemolytic plaque test by Jerne et al. [77] for the detection of antibody forming cells has been of great importance. Lymphoid cells from animals immunized against sheep erythrocytes are mixed with sheep erythrocytes in a medium containing agar. Subsequently, complement (C) is added. Antibody (haemolysin) production is indicated by a haemolytic zone appearing around antibody forming cells (direct IgM plaque). The number of the plaques gives information about the cytokinetics of the antibody response. This ingenious method has proved to be very sensitive. Even a single antibody producing cell is demonstrable. The method was soon modified and thus made suitable for the detection of cells producing haemagglutinins of the IgG type. These antibodies do not fix C until they have been incubated with anti-IgG. After such a treatment a haemolytic zone appears also around the cells producing IgG antibodies (indirect IgG plaque) [38, 151*a*].

The plaque method has become a classical example of the use of functional-morphological tests in immunology, for the immunocyte in the centre of each plaque can be examined microscopically and also electron microscopically (direct and indirect microplaque method) [142] and because antigens other than erythrocytes can be detected by coating the erythrocytes with the antigen [83, 166].

Investigation of the cellular events of humoral immunity are made difficult by the fact that the antibody production depends on several interdependent factors:

1. The number of progenitor cell (PC) or, according to the modern terminology, antigen sensitive units (ASU);

2. The effective antigen dose (AD);

3. The number and producing capacity of the antibody forming cells (AFC) developing from an ASU, the number of the developing memory cells (MC) and the rate of the repeated involvement of MCs in the immune response;

4. The volume (V) in which AFCs develop and proliferate;

5. Other regulation factors (R).

Antibody production being dependent on all the above factors, the role of the individual factors cannot be studied in the living animal; for instance, the number of ASUs cannot be varied without influencing V and R and, through these factors, AD [88]. To overcome these difficulties, the use of inbred mouse strains became necessary, for immunocyte pools consisting of known numbers of immunocytes can be established by transferring isologous cells (transfer method). For transfer experiments, the immune response of the host organism must be eliminated either by irradiating the recipient with a sublethal dose or by rendering it tolerant to the given antigen in the neonatal age (*in vivo* culture method) [24, 121]. Otherwise, the precise kinetical investigations would be disturbed by undesirable reactions taking place in the recipient, such as the reaction of the host against the antigen or suboptimal proliferation of transferred competent cells.

However, even the *in vivo* culture has its limitations. In an open system like this the appearance of a given cell type or a decrease in the number of such cells may be attributed to cell migration. Besides, the cell population under study is hardly accessible for cytological investigation. To eliminate these difficulties, the '*in vivo* diffusion chamber' has been developed [88], which is a chamber containing antigen and a known number of immunocytes; it is sealed with a membrane having pores 0.1–0.4 $\mu$m diam. and implanted in the irradiated recipient. The membrane is permeable to metabolites, but impermeable to cells. The course of the immune response can be followed by examining the cells present in the chamber [16, 108] or by titrating the homologous antibody in the recipient's serum [108].

One of the greatest achievements in the immunological methodology has been the development of the method of *in vitro* primary antibody response [49*a*, 90, 99]. This method seems to be simple today and is employed with success in studying antibody production not only to heterologous erythrocytes, but also to chemically defined antigens. However, the elaboration of the special conditions for culturing and the standardization of the variable factors (species and strain differences, the cell types developing antigen sensitive units in different cell suspensions, etc.) have been a difficult task.

The use of antigens consisting of chemically defined haptens plus carrier molecules has been a further achievement of modern methodology. Special anti-thymocyte [131] and anti-macrophage [68] sera, antisera of high (mouse-) strain specificity (anti-CBA, anti-$C_{57}$Bl, etc.) and anti-allotype antisera [61, 98], in combination with transfer experiments, have enabled an accurate analysis of the contribution of different cells. Chromosome markers [31, 33] and cell-separation methods have also been developed [62, 170].

When dealing with the cellular kinetics of antibody production preference was given to data obtained with the simplest experimental methods. Consequently, the results of the *in vitro* studies are preferentially discussed below.

## CELLULAR EVENTS OF THE LATENT PHASE OF ANTIBODY PRODUCTION

The process of differentiation which follows the antigen's entry into the organism and precedes antibody production is difficult to investigate. No specific antibodies which would direct attention to the differentiating cells are produced in this phase as yet. On the other hand, the immunogenic fraction of the entering antigen cannot be distinguished from the foreign material to be decomposed non-specifically on the basis of the histological localization of the former until the course of the immune response has been recognized.

### *Frequency of antigen sensitive units (ASU) in the lymphoid population*

In the following the frequency of occurrence of antigen sensitive cells in lymphoid populations originating from animals which have not been in previous contact with the antigen will be discussed. According to a calculation based on the plaque number in the spleen and the kinetics of the immune response, among $10^6$ nucleated spleen cells there was only a single precursor cell from which proliferation of antibody forming cells started [77]. In transfer experiments, $2.5 \times 10^5$ to $1 \times 10^6$ lymphoid cells in the inoculum give rise to a haemolytic focus in the recipient's spleen after immunization with heterologous erythrocytes [88, 115, 151*b*]. An average of $10^6$ cells are needed to form a haemolytic area also in *in vitro* tests [90, 139, 143*a*].

The spleen of a young adult mouse contains about $1.5 \times 10^8$ lymphoid cells, which means that one-third of the whole lymphoid cell population ($5 \times 10^8$ cells) is to be found in the spleen [88]. Accordingly, the spleen of a mouse contains about 150, the whole animal possesses approx. 500 antigen sensitive cells against sheep erythrocytes. Obviously, it is difficult to demonstrate antigen sensitive cells, and it is not surprising that precursor function had been attributed in the past to almost all cell types of the lymphoid and vascular system.

The frequency of precursor cells is influenced by several factors. Firstly, cells giving rise to haemolysis have been detected even in the spleen of animals which had received no antigen stimulus at all (background plaques) [65*b*, 77]. It would be plausible to assume that these cells are precursors that begin functioning as a result of immunization. In fact, however, it is not so, and the role in the immune response of cells forming background plaques is doubtful [65*b*].

Secondly, there are substantial strain differences in the number of precursor cells. As a result, e.g. spleen cells from $C_{57}B1$ mice fail to give an *in vitro* immune response to sheep erythrocytes [62]. On this basis, it was assumed that primary *in vitro* haemolysin production by cells from other strains was, in fact, a secondary response due to a cross-reaction with an antigenic determinant of the animal's own bacterium flora or any other antigen. Since, however, *in vitro* primary immune response can be induced not only to complex antigens (e.g. heterologous erythrocytes) but also to chemically defined synthetic ones [45], the above values for the numbers of precursor cells of primary immune response may be accepted as real.

Claman et al. [23] inoculated irradiated mice with $5 \times 10^7$ thymocytes. Subsequently, only 12 per cent of the spleen fragments of the animals showed haemolytic activity. Mice treated with $10^7$ bone marrow cells showed still lower activity (1.3 per cent). If, however, the animals received $5 \times 10^7$ thymocytes and $10^7$ bone marrow cells simultaneously, the response was 54 per cent instead of the expected 13.3 per cent. This finding has pointed to a possible interaction between thymic and bone marrow cells which may result in promoting the normal course of immune response. This was also supported by the finding that the immune response to differently diluted spleen cell suspensions did not result in a linear curve, which would have been expected if the antibody production had arisen from precursors of a single cell type. Reduction of cell dose resulted in a greater decrease in the number of plaque forming cells than expected, suggesting that, in fact, the probability of the interaction between more than one type of cells was reduced.

Thus, it has been supposed that immune response needs an interaction between two cells to start. In this sense, therefore, it is better to interpret the above data as referring to the frequency of *antigen sensitive units* (ASU) instead of antigen sensitive cells, supposing that it is informative of the probability of interactions between the different cells composing the functional unit.

### *Characteristics of the cell types forming the antigen sensitive unit (ASU)*

Extensive studies with the aim of recognizing the cell types taking part in initiating antibody production have been commenced. The antibody production of irradiated animals could be restituted with thymic and bone marrow cells given together, but neither with thymic cells nor with bone marrow cells alone [49*b*, 100, 143*b*]. The chromosome marker of the transplanted bone marrow cells made it possible to establish that cells deriving from the bone marrow are the precursors (P-AFC) of the antibody forming cells and that the antigen reactive cells (ARC) are thymocytes. This view is supported by the fact that ARC is not contained by the thymocytes of antigen-tolerant animals [98].*

* Accordingly, two major populations of lymphocytes take part in the process of antibody formation. These are called differently by various authors. In Chapter 8 of the present book, the thymus dependent lymphocytes (category I) are called T lymphocytes as suggested by Roitt et al. [134]. These cells are responsible for cell-mediated immunity recognizable by their blastogenic response to phytohaemagglutinin and to histoincompatible lymphocytes (mixed lymphocyte reaction) [168]. The cells mentioned by Mitchell and Miller [100] as 'antigen sensitive cells' and by Cudkovitz et al. [30] as 'antigen reactive cells' belong to this population. To category II belong the thymus-independent (B) lymphocytes, precursors of plasma cells which are responsible for the secretion of humoral antibody [168]. These cells mature in birds under the influence of the bursa of Fabricius (a 'bursa equivalent' which has also been postulated in mammals). These cells are termed variably 'precursors of antibody forming cells' (P-AFC) [100], 'precursors of plaque forming cells' [30] or 'marrow derived cells'. In the present paper the designations T cell and B cell (lymphocyte) will be used. Further research may show the existence of various subpopulations within these types [168].

*In vitro* studies have shown that a further cell type is also necessary to the immune response. When the cell adhering to the wall of the culture flask were removed from a spleen cell suspension, the non-adherent population, although containing both thymus derived and bone marrow derived cells, gave no antibody response [11, 156]. The adherent cells have been found to correspond to macrophages both morphologically and functionally. Their role was not discovered in *in vivo* transfer experiments because this sub-population of macrophages is relatively resistant to radiation, retaining their function for one or two days after having been irradiated [62, 156]. The cells of the population of macrophage character when mixed *in vitro* with cells of thymus and bone marrow origin tend to give rise to clustered cell groups [62, 102*b*]. Such a tendency of cluster formation was not demonstrated in homogeneous suspensions of any of the three cell types.

Apparently, the micro-milieu determined by the three cell types is a prerequisite of the differentiation process initiated by the antigen. Cells separated from clusters mechanically form clusters again. However, cluster formation was prevented by the presence of antibodies homologous to the given antigen [102*b*].

Of the three interacting cell types, macrophage is supposed to be the first to be active in the initiation of antibody production. This is supported by experiments [104] in the course of which adhering monolayers of macrophages were incubated with heterologous erythrocytes and subsequently washed. Erythrocytes were fixed by a small antigen sensitive sub-population (1–10 in 10,000), and yet induction of antibody production could be observed. This has only been demonstrated for the *in vitro* primary IgM response, but not for other types of interaction. Macrophages are regarded as non-specific participants of the interaction [11], their involvement being due to cytophilic (mainly of IgM type) antibodies produced previously [66, 69]. Peritoneal macrophages from immunized animals showed a more intensive effect on the induction of adaptive immune response than cells from normal animals, and mild heating resulted in the separation of an antigen-specific extract—presumably cytophilic antibody—which stimulated the immune response [81]. Consequently, the adhering cells of the spleen are not the only cells capable of inducing primary response *in vitro*: they can be substituted by cells of the peritoneal exudate [69]. Haemolysin production induced *in vitro* by $10^7$ spleen cells was substantially stimulated by $2 \times 10^5$ exudate cells and intensively inhibited by a tenfold dose. This phenomenon might be explained by assuming a competition between the scavenger (phagocytosing) and immune-response-inducing functions of the macrophages; predominance of the scavenger function results in a decreased immune response. This phenomenon has been induced in various ways, e.g. with large macrophage doses [69, 120], incubation of the antigen with IgG antibodies (see section dealing with the regulatory role of antibodies, p. 267) or by stimulation of peritoneal macrophages with phytohaemagglutinin *in vivo* [43, 126].

We have already mentioned that within the ASU, thymus derived cells (ARC, T cell) are able to recognize the foreign antigen. In B cell excess the animals had to be inoculated with $10^7$ thymocytes to establish at least one ASU per animal [143*b*]. Taking into consideration that the spleen of an irradiated animal is reached by 10 per cent of the inoculated cells, i.e. by $10^6$ thymocytes in the experiment cited, the number of the ASUs in these experiments is likely to be limited by the low number of ARCs in the T cell pool. A single antigen reactive T cell (ARC) that had reached the spleen was able to participate in more than one ASU producing antibodies of both IgM and IgG types, whence it can be concluded that T cells fail to determine the antibody class, i.e. the type of the B cells committed to produce immunoglobulin [143*b*]. T cells (ARCs) bear the theta ($\theta$) antigen on their surface. These long lived cells recirculate in the organism and do not adhere to glass surface.

Considering that thymus dependent cells do not secrete demonstrable quantities of antibodies [33], it has been questionable from the beginning whether they bear antigen sensitive receptors of immunoglobulin nature on their surface [39]. However, the antigen recognition by T cells could be inhibited by anti-Fab and anti-light-chain antibodies [22, 53*a*, 55]. The receptor carried by T cell could be a result of passive fixation of cytophilic antibodies on the cell surface, or the receptor is a constituent of the cell membrane [53*a*]. Presumably, the receptor contains no free light-chain molecule, it is of $F(ab')_2$ character [54]. A still unknown heavy chain, however, may be a constituent of the receptor if its constant part is buried in, and covered by, the cell membrane. Thus, the receptor of the T cell may be of immunoglobulin character. It is tentatively termed IgX [134]. The presence of immunoglobulin on the surface of T lymphocytes has been proved by the very sensitive method of opsonic adherence, too. However, high concentrations of anti-Fab serum were needed for the opsonization, suggesting that the T cell surface is poor in receptors [53*a*]. This might be the reason why the fixation to T lymphocytes of fluorescein-labelled anti-Fab serum fails to give a positive result [132]. It is characteristic of T cells that, in spite of the paucity of receptors on their surface, they are readily activated by antigen and relatively low antigen concentrations may induce their lymphoblastic transformation and clonal division [80].

The third cell type taking part in the interaction is the protagonist of antibody production. As shown both by strain-specific serum and the chromosome-marker method, the precursors of the antibody-forming (plaque-forming) cells (P-AFC, B cells) derive from these cells, which originate in the bone marrow and mature in the 'bursa equivalent' lymphoid organs [111]. Mice irradiated, and subsequently inoculated with excess thymus cells, required about $5 \times 10^4$–$10^5$ bone marrow cells to develop one or two ASUs in the spleen [30]. The resulting plaques mainly contained antibodies of the IgM type. Plaques of the IgG type required 6 to 15 times larger doses of bone marrow cells [30]. Accordingly, the B cells in the bone marrow would be committed to produce antibodies of a given immunoglobulin class and the proportion of the different types of B cells in the bone marrow would be predetermined [30, 58]. However, in the light of recent experiments, these views should be reconsidered (see below).

B lymphocytes have a fast turnover rate and a short life-span. Having not passed through the thymus, these cells do not bear the theta ($\theta$) antigen. Their rate of recirculation in the organism is slow and they tend to adhere to glass surface, but less intensively than macrophages. Their surface is rich in receptors as shown by the positive opsonic adherence test with low-concentration anti-Fab sera [53*a*]. Fixation of fluorescent anti-Fab antibody on their surface is well demonstrable [132]. Despite their richness in receptors, these cells cannot be stimulated to lymphoblastic transformation by antigen and their clonal division needs special conditions of culture [40].

The antigen sensitive receptors of B lymphocytes, like those of the T lymphocytes, are supposed to be formed by a membrane-fixed $F(ab')_2$ structure. On the stimulating effect of the antigen (e.g. heterologous erythrocytes), a fragment of the Fc part of the heavy chain becomes demonstrable on the recently activated antigen sensitive B lymphocytes (cells forming rosette with erythrocytes, RFC). In accordance with this, rosette formation can be inhibited by specially selected anti-heavy-chain antisera [53*a*].

Experiments on the development of primary antibody response *in vitro* have shown that all the three cell types necessary for ASU formation are present in the spleen. Therefore *in vitro* antibody production can be brought about with spleen cells. There are both T and B lymphocytes in the thoracic duct [98, 100]. In adult animals, ARCs are more frequent among lymphocytes in the thoracic duct than among those in the thymus [98].

### *Co-operation of carrier-specific and hapten-specific cells in the initiation of antibody formation*

Recent investigations have yielded important data on the role and functional significance of the co-operation between T and B cells. It is well known that antibodies are produced to haptens, i.e. to the determinant groups of conjugated antigens, yet, immune response cannot be induced by isolated haptens, for these are too small to be immunogenic. Besides, during the humoral immune response, phenomena can be observed suggesting that even the molecules carrying the hapten give rise to immunologically specific events (carrier effect) while the antibodies to the carried hapten are formed. The above statements are based on the following experimental observations [101*a*]:

1. The binding of hapten to serum antibodies is influenced by changes in the hapten structure to a greater degree than by those in the carrier molecule. The opposite is valid for the lymphoblastic transformation inducible with the antigen.
2. In animals tolerant to the carrier molecule, anti-hapten antibodies cannot be induced with a conjugate containing the same carrier, whereas anti-hapten antibody production does occur after immunization with the same hapten molecule bound to another carrier protein. It may be concluded that hapten-specific receptors are present in the animals, but fail to be stimulated if the carrier proteins are processed in the organism in a manner different from the normal immunological events [64, 118, 132].
3. Cells sensitized to a conjugate of hapten and type A carrier protein (H–A) were mixed with cells pre-immunized with type B carrier protein. The resulting antibody production was very intensive if the mixed cell suspension was stimulated with the conjugate of the hapten and type B carrier molecule (H–B) (Table 11-I).
4. The immunogenic zone of the carrier molecule is not located in the immediate neighbourhood of the hapten [5, 6].

To interpret the above data, one should assume that an interaction between cells plays some part in the immune response. Some cells bear the receptor reacting

TABLE 11-I

*Effect of anti-θ serum on co-operative secondary anti-hapten immune response of spleen cells immunized with hapten (hapten + A carrier) and carrier (B carrier) in transfer experiment (based on data of Raff) [131]*

| Cells immunized with hapten + carrier A | *In vitro* treatment before transfer | Cells immunized with B carrier | *In vitro* treatment before transfer | Secondary challenge by hapten + B carrier | Anti-hapten immune response* |
|---|---|---|---|---|---|
| + | 0 | + | 0 | 0 | 0.12 |
| + | 0 | 0 | 0 | + | 1.9 |
| + | 0 | + | 0 | + | 10.0 |
| + | 0 | + | anti-θ serum + C | + | 0.54 |
| + | anti-θ serum + C | + | 0 | + | 9.8 |

* Antigen binding capacity in $\times$ $10^{-8}$ M

with the hapten, others bear that reacting with the carrier molecule [169c]. The two kinds of cells might support each other in the induction of hapten-specific antibodies [101a]. It is reasonable to suppose that the receptors sensitive to the hapten may be carried by B lymphocytes, i.e. by the cell giving rise to the anti-hapten antibody producing clone. In this case, T lymphocytes would bear the carrier-specific receptor. The increase in the immune response induced by carrier-specific cells is in direct relation to the number of thymus derived AR cells [101b]. Table 11-I shows the effect on the cell co-operation of the anti-theta (θ) serum, i.e. an antiserum which destroys the cells of thymus origin in the presence of C. The cells sensitive to the B carrier could be destroyed by the antiserum, suggesting that the T lymphocytes contained this population. On the other hand, the intensity of the immune response was not influenced by treatment of the hapten-specific cell population (population immunized by hapten) with the anti-θ serum, indicating that the hapten receptor is carried on the surface of B lymphocytes [131].

Owing to methodological reasons, the role of macrophages in cell co-operations was not investigated on the transfer experiments referred to above. If the function of macrophages in the co-operation is relatively resistant to radiation, the macrophages of the irradiated recipient may contribute to the induction of antibody production [62]. On the other hand, pre-existing antibodies (like those which substantially influence the participation of macrophages in the secondary response under normal circumstances) are not present under conditions of transfer experiments. This has been shown by recent findings. The non-specific macrophage may become an active and specific member of the cell co-operation by binding the specific cytophilic antibody on its surface. Although the antibody production against an antigen is in general inhibited by passively administered homologous antibody, the phenomenon below was mostly observed in case of heterogeneous antigens. The suppression of the antibody production to the strongly immunogenic fraction of $\gamma_2$-globulin was associated with an increase in the antibody production to the *other* part of the same molecule after antibody administration [128]. Similar results were obtained in chickens where the immunogenicity of the blood-group isoantigens inherited on different loci is variable. The isoantigens directed by the complex locus B induce high-titre haemagglutinin production, whereas, among others, those directed by locus A fail to induce detectable haemagglutinin production even after several inoculations (especially in young recipients). Surprisingly, the recipient who is unable to start an anti-A immune response will be capable of high-titre response to both A and B antigens after immunization with erythrocytes bearing both antigens [140].

McBride [94], using the above experimental system, succeeded in producing in chickens an extremely intensive immune response to the weak A antigen by administering erythrocytes bearing A and B isoantigens covered by anti-B antibodies. In this case, it is reasonable to suppose that the carrier-specific cells were not T lymphocytes; it is more likely that the antibody turned hapten B into a carrier molecule by fixing the antigen on the macrophage surface.

### *Sequence of events of the latent phase of antibody production*

There are different opinions about the length of the latency in antibody production. Methods of low sensitivity have shown latencies lasting for several days whereas chicken erythrocytes injected into non-sensitized guinea pigs could already be detected in the lymph nodes within 10 sec and the lysis of these erythrocytes started within 7 min. In sensitized guinea pigs, the lysis started within 30 sec [86]. These data suggest that the lymphoid system of immunologically reactive animals is capable of starting an immune response without any cell proliferation, but the manifestation of this capability requires cell interactions.

This view is supported by *in vitro* findings. The sensitivity of the applied tests and, consequently, the measured periods are variable [102*b*, 139], yet, on the whole, the following data are acceptable. In the course of an immune response brought about *in vitro* with spleen cells, ASUs developed very early and 10 haemolysin producing foci per $10^7$ spleen cells appeared within 4 h (Fig. 11-3). The plaque number significantly exceeds the background plaque number. Subsequently, the plaque forming cells show no significant change in number up to the 19th h of culturing. If, however, the spleen cell suspension is stirred at 19 h and spread over an erythrocyte layer in another vessel, the number of plaque forming cells will be doubled [139].

According to the experiments cited above, the latency phase of antibody production should be subdivided into three main periods. The first includes the handling of the antigen. The length of this period highly depends on the quality of the antigen, and the site of its injection. In the second period, specific cell associations (ASU) come into existence and the interaction among the cells of the ASU starts. Soon after the end of this period, the lysis of cells surrounding the ASUs becomes apparent. The *in vitro* course of the second period takes about 4 h, with a wide variation in different experiments [102*b*, 103, 139]. The third period of the latency phase is a preparation for the proliferation phase.

Plaque formation is not inhibited by 5-fluoro-2-deoxyuridine, indicating that the start of antibody production requires neither cell division nor *de novo* DNA or RNA synthesis [139]. It may be assumed that B lymphocytes are uniformly in phase $G_1$ (see p. 264) at the time of the induction, for the cell division starts in various ASUs synchronously, around the 19th hour of culturing.

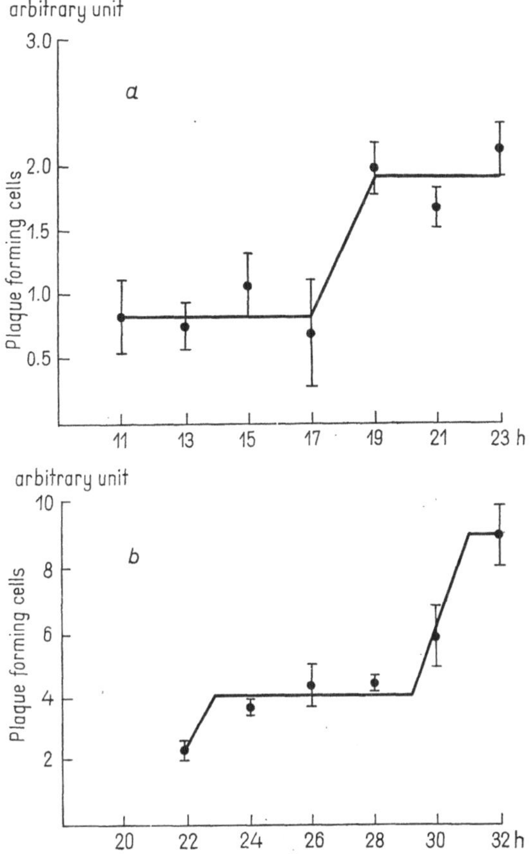


Fig. 11-3. The proliferation of haemolytic plaque forming (antibody producing) cells during the primary immune response *in vitro* (Saunders) [139]. Murine spleen cells ($10^7$) were sensitized on a layer of sheep red blood cells (SRBC) and the original number of haemolytic precursor cells in the early culture (4–10 h) has been determined. When the number of plaques after different periods of culturing have been compared with the original number of precursor cells, synchronous cell doublings were observed with a generation time of 7–8 h. Results are expressed as ratio of PFC/precursor cells. *a)* Interval from 11–23 h after initiation of culture; *b)* interval from 22–32 h

There is no precise information available on the exact nature of the cell interaction within the ASU. Adler et al. [1] succeeded in inducing production of specific IgM antibodies by an RNA (messenger RNA) prepared from macrophages of immunized animals. Further experiments were suggestive of an information transfer concerning the light-chain synthesis among the cells taking part in the interaction [4, 26]. Other investigators failed to reproduce the latter experiment and the supposed role of macrophage RNA has also been disproved experimentally. Consequently, the essence of cell co-operations should not be sought in the field of information transfer.

Anyhow, numerous cell co-operations of various types must be involved in the stimulation process occurring during the period of cell interactions, indicating that B lymphocytes can be activated in different ways (Fig. 11-4). There are numerous antigens (e.g. haemocyanin, equine ferritin, pneumococcus polysaccharide, *E. coli* endotoxin) which do not require the co-operation of cells of thymus origin in the initiation of antibody production [44, 71, 105*b*]. It is common in the structure of these thymus independent antigens that some antigenic determinant occurs in the same molecule repeatedly, i.e. the thymus independent antigens are multivalent (Fig. 11-4, *a*). Fixation of a single molecule on the surface of a B lymphocyte may stimulate more than one receptor simultaneously. Heterologous erythrocytes, on the other hand, if applied in small doses, may be considered thymus dependent antigens, but their large doses tend to induce haemolysin production without co-operation of thymocytes [147, 159].

The importance of the interaction between T and B cells has been pointed out in the previous section. According to indirect evidence, the most important function of T lymphocytes seems to be due to its ability to accumulate the antigen on its surface in a form that makes the hapten accessible for B lymphocytes (helper theory). On the surface of a T cell, the antigen may reach a cumulation corresponding to 100-fold of its average concentration in the organism [101*b*]. T and B lymphocytes may be linked together by several antigen bridges [158] which assure the simultaneous stimulation of several surface receptors of the B cell and the effective contact of the cells (Fig. 11-4, *b*).

B lymphocytes may be linked by multivalent bridges also with a macrophage covered by specific antibodies (Fig. 11-4, *c*). In the case, as already mentioned, the antibody-covered hapten turns into a functional carrier, and a B cell, specific for some uncovered hapten, is activated.

The rules dealt with in this section have been discovered only recently. The individual processes of the interaction have not yet been outlined and the relative importance of the interactions in immune reactions of different types (primary, secondary, IgM, IgG) has not yet been recognized. Until more precise data will become available, we may suppose that an optimal response (e.g. satisfactory detection of haemolysin production during primary antibody formation *in vitro*) needs the presence of three types of cells, namely macrophage and the T and B lymphocytes (Fig. 11-4, *d*). The macrophage binds the B cell on its surface, and it may be supported in this function by the T cell, which presumably secretes little amounts of cytophilic antibody undetectable by any method except by the demonstration of its role in the interaction. Multiple bridges are formed between T and B lymphocytes as well as between macrophages and B cells; consequently, the hapten presented in an immunogenic form on the surface of B cells attains a concentration high enough to stimulate plasma cell clone formation from B cells. B lymphocytes undergo blast transformation and, as a result of successive cell divisions, the plasmablasts turn into plasma cells. As is known from *in vitro* stimulation experiments, the antigen starts the transformation and clonal division of T lymphocytes as well.

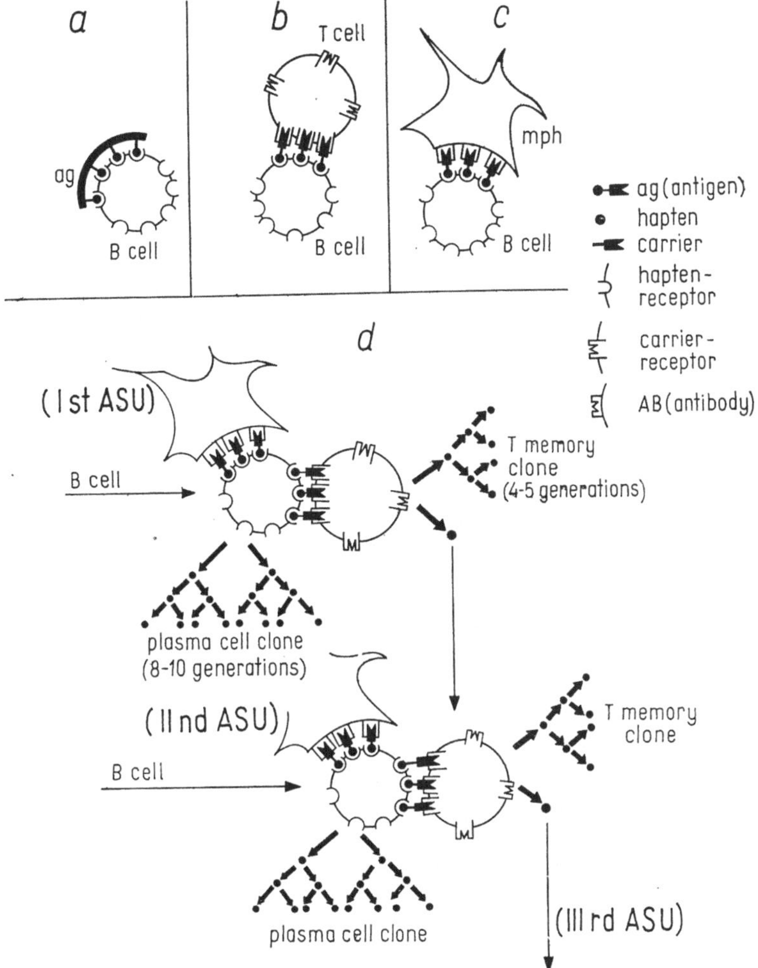


**Fig. 11-4.** Cell interactions in the activation of P-AFC (precursor of antibody forming cells = B lymphocytes). *a)* Activation of B cell by thymus independent (multivalent) antigen. *b)* Interaction of ARC (antigen reactive = T cell) and P-AFC (B lymphocyte). Antigen (carrier-hapten complex) forms a cell-cell contact between carrier-specific (T) and hapten-specific (B) cells ('antigen bridge'). *c)* Interaction of macrophage and B cell. The interaction is facilitated by cytophilic antibody attached to the macrophage surface. *d)* Induction of proliferation of B cells in antigen sensitive units (ASU). The clonal proliferation of plasma cell clones (deriving from B cell) as well as the proliferation of T-memory cell clones (deriving from T cell) are schematically depicted. The phenomenon called 'recruitment' can be explained if members of the T-memory clone successively participate in more than one ASU as described in text. Abbreviations: ag, antigen; mph, macrophage; ASU, antigen sensitive unit

## CELLULAR EVENTS OF THE EXPONENTIAL PHASE OF ANTIBODY PRODUCTION

To characterize the cellular dynamics of the exponential phase of antibody production, one should explain the 1,000-fold increase in the number of the antibody forming cells and the 100-fold increase in the number of antibody sensitive memory cells which occur within a short time [19, 88, 165]. Firstly, we must return to Saunders' [139] *in vitro* experiments (see Fig. 11-3). Beginning from the 17th h of the incubation of a spleen cell suspension with antigen, the doubling time for the haemolysin forming cells was approximately 8 h.

Accordingly, the antibody forming cells develop from proliferating B cells. For the generation time* of these cells, different authors have published variable values ranging, in general, from 8 to 13 h [88, 122, 136, 157]. The cells produce antibodies over 8–9 generations continuously. Towards the end of the exponential phase, the cells appear as plasma cells and lymphocytes with widened cytoplasm. The life-span of these cells is short, usually 2 days.

The data in Fig. 11-3 leave no doubt that the antibody forming cells proliferate. It is demonstrable even in *in vivo* systems that all antibody forming cells are descendants of cells having undergone a proliferative process [122, 155, 157]. This must be pointed out because in *in vivo* systems more antibody forming cells developed than expected on the basis of the proliferation process calculated from the generation time. According to Tannenberg and Malaviya [157], the generation time of the cells dividing in the course of a haemolysin response ranges about 13 h, whereas the doubling time of plaque forming cells in the spleen is 6–7 h. Perkins et al. [122] determined the number of haemolysin producing plaques of spleens from 10 mice in every hour 2–96 h following an injection of heterologous erythrocytes. The increase in the plaque number was step-wise during the response. There was no increase for 8–9 h. Then sudden increase occurred. This is in accord with the observation that the proliferating antibody forming cells undergo a synchronous division every 8th to 9th hour. However, the steps were greater than would correspond to mere doubling. Therefore, the doubling time was as short as 6 hours.

The phenomenon that the rate of increase of the antibody forming cell number exceeds the rate of proliferation is termed *recruitment*. The extent and the significance of recruitment are being disputed in the literature. Nevertheless, data have been published which may be helpful in approaching this problem. The changes occurring in the number of T cells in the course of the immune response suggest that T lymphocytes undergo proliferation [19, 23, 34, 106]. Although these cells are called memory cells** in the next chapter, it is reasonable to assume that some

* Generation time should be distinguished from doubling time. The former means the rate of division and can be determined by isotope methods on the basis of the DNA metabolism of cells. It consists of phases $G_1$, S, $G_2$ and M. It is reasonable to accept as a rule that the generation time for continuously dividing lymphoid cells of mammals (man, mouse and rat) ranges from 8 to 10 h [78, 91, 157]. Doubling time means the period during which a group of cells in a given population (or serum antibody titre) is doubled. This value, being influenced by cell division, cell death, emigration and immigration and regulation mechanisms, may be very variable.

** In this chapter memory cells are not dealt with in detail, therefore the phenomenon of B lymphocyte populations also being able to develop memory cells is not discussed here.

cells of the ever increasing antigen reactive T cell population immediately contribute to the strengthening of the immune response. This assumption is in agreement with the observation that in the spleen of animals irradiated and subsequently restituted with bone marrow cells, a thymus cell dose containing only one T cell gives rise to more than one haemolysin-producing clones. There were several animals in whose spleen as many as three B cells (three foci) were activated [143*b*].

It would be perhaps a simplification to assume as a cellular basis of recruitment that one T cell is able to activate numerous B cells successively. It is more plausible to suppose that, in addition to the antibody producing clone developing by proliferation from activated B cells, T cells may also undergo blast transformation and mitosis under antigenic effect (see Fig. 11-4*d*) and thus give rise to a clone of developing memory cells. Another member of the same memory clone may interact with the antigen present on the surface of macrophages, thus forming an ASU in which a further B cell may be activated. Accordingly, the sub-clones developing from the secondary ASU also result from proliferation. Supposing that the rate of division for the sub-clones is the same as that for the primary clones, it is not surprising that the stepwise course described by Perkins et al. [122] is not disturbed by recruitment; instead, the latter may increase the height of the individual steps (see above).

The question whether the approximately 1,000-fold increase in the number of antibody forming cells and the 100-fold increase in the number of memory cells is explainable by the cellular phenomena occurring during the exponential phase, may be answered based on Fig. 11-4*d* as follows. We may assume that a B lymphocyte in an ASU gives rise to 512 plasma cells as a result of 9 successive divisions, while the T cell divides into two cells. One of these joins a second ASU, the other undergoes 4 or 5 division cycles resulting in a clone consisting of 16–32 memory cells. The second ASU, too, is supposed to produce 512 plasma cells and 16–32 memory cells, and one of the memory cells may stimulate a third ASU. Assuming that four activations occur, we may calculate the number of plasma cells to be $4 \times 500$, and that of the memory cells $4 \times (16–32)$. About a half of the plasma cells die within two days. Such an oversimplified calculation might explain the production of 1,000 plasma cells and 64–128 memory cells.*

The phenomena of the lymphoblastic transformation have been followed by microcinematography. In the lymphocyte population obtained from a sensitized subject, the antigen induced clonal division in the course of which a single T cell gave rise to 4 or 5 successive generations [91]. The phenomenon as described above might explain the explosive dynamics of the primary immune response.

* In fact, the T lymphocyte is not the only source of memory cells.

## REGULATORY ROLE OF ANTIGENS AND ANTIBODIES IN THE STIMULATION AND INHIBITION OF THE IMMUNE RESPONSE

### *Stimulation of immune response by antibodies*

In exceptional cases, antigen–antibody complexes may be found to be more immunogenic than the antigen itself [8, 160]. This phenomenon cannot be reproduced with sera containing both IgM and IgG, except when little amounts of such sera are applied [119, 135]. Henry and Jerne [66] have shown that the stimulation is primarily due to specific IgM antibodies. If the preparation is contaminated with IgG antibodies, the immunosuppressive effect of the latter becomes predominant. An increase in the dose of pure IgM is followed by increased stimulation (Fig. 11-5).

We return here to the data which indicate that an antigen molecule may be highly immunogenic if one of its two different hapten groups is covered with antibodies (see Fig. 11-4, *c*). The antibody-covered haptens thus obtain a carrier

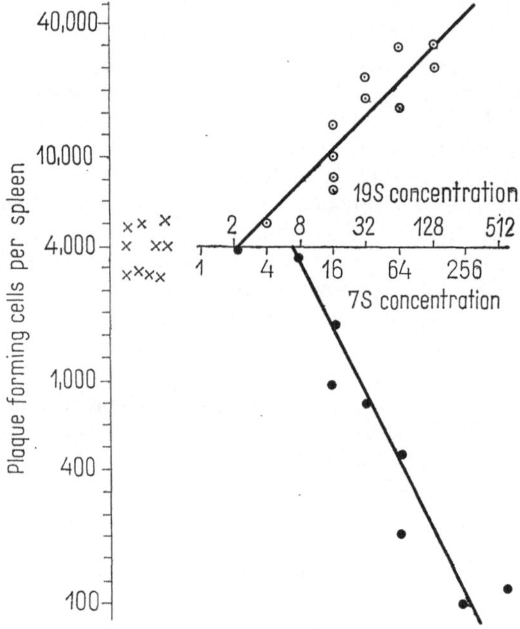


Fig. 11-5. Elevation by specific IgM antibody, and depression by specific IgG antibody, of the primary immune response of mice to a single intravenous injection of $4 \times 10^5$ sheep red blood cells as measured by the number of plaque forming cells per total spleen 6 days later. The antibody was injected 1–2 h before the SRBC. The open symbols represent the responses of mice that received IgM antibody, the solid circles represent the responses of mice that received IgG (Henry and Jerne) [66]

character and will contribute to the immunogenicity of the hapten of the other type [94]. The antibody playing role in this phenomenon is probably of IgM nature, for the IgM molecule, being polyvalent, is capable of a more intensive stimulation than the bivalent IgG molecules. The phenomenon may serve to explain the plateau of the curve representing the dynamics of the antibody level in the immunized organism. It should be noted that the fixation of IgM antibodies on the surface of the macrophage is mediated by complement, and this type of fixation does not stimulate the phagocytosis of the antigen–antibody complex [84].

### *Suppression of immune response by antibodies*

By the end of the exponential phase, we may calculate with a 1,000-fold increase in the number of antibody forming cells and with a 100-fold increase in the number of AR cells. However, the factors regulating the immunological events have remained unclear. A further exponential increase in the immune response would be undesirable because relative overproduction of antibodies in relation to the antigen is already apparent during the exponential phase [163*b*].

To throw light on the regulation mechanism of the antibody production, sera from immunized animals were deprived of antibodies by an immune adsorbent and the resulting sera were retransfused to the animals. The antibody production started again at an exponential rate after one or two days' delay [52]. Other investigators [105*a*] transplanted spleen cells from animals immunized with sheep erythrocytes into irradiated isologous animals. An extraordinarily intensive immune response was observed in the recipient. By the 7th day, the number of plaque forming cells in the spleen approximated or exceeded $10^7$ and the serum titre had reached values ranging between $2^{15}$ and $2^{25}$ [105*a*]. These experiments point to the regulatory role of the antibodies appearing in the serum in the course of the immune response. Without this regulation, exponential-type antibody production would persist until the exhaustion of the immune apparatus (Fig. 11-5).

The regulatory role of antibodies has its peculiar rules. Antibodies added to the culture medium during immune response *in vitro* prevents cluster formation [102*b*]. This inhibition is antigen specific [102*b*]. It has been proved by using chemically defined antigens that the antigen specificity of inhibiting antibody is limited to the hapten, i.e. it does not involve the whole molecule [13, 29, 135]. Suppression shows a linear correlation with antigen concentration in the culture medium and the suppressive effect of IgG antibody can be prevented to some extent by adding excess antigen to the medium. Incubation of adherent macrophage-type cells with IgG antibody, either before the antigen is added or subsequently, results in a suppressive effect [127].

The following conclusions can be drawn from these *in vitro* experiments:

1. Cells of the macrophage type play part in the suppressive effect of antibodies. A possible mode of the action of the passive antibody is that, fixed on the surface of the macrophage-type cell, it alters the character of antigen processing and covers the antigenic determinants fixed on the same cell.

2. In the *in vitro* system the suppressive effects are competitive in two ways. Firstly, there is a competition between the passively induced antibodies and the B cell receptors for the antigenic determinants fixed on the macrophage. Secondly, the determinants of the free antigen molecules compete for the antibodies with those of the antigen molecules fixed on macrophages.

*In vivo* investigations have pointed to two further important phenomena concerning the suppressive effect of antibodies. The *in vivo* suppression by passive antibodies of the antibody production always shows a delay of about 48 h, during which period the antibody production proceeds undisturbed. The delay is independent of the dose of the antibody. The 48 h delay is in accordance with the fact that the maturation of the plasma cell clone lasts 48 h; meanwhile, due to the cell proliferation, the newly-produced cells provide an ample supplementation for the decaying cells. Furthermore, antibody production was easily suppressed in the early stages of the immune response, whereas only large doses of hyperimmune sera of high affinity were effective later on [169*b*].

Further experimental data may be taken into account in the analysis of the mechanism of action of passively administered antibody. In *in vitro* experiments macrophages and heterologous erythrocytes were incubated in the presence of passive antiserum (opsonization). Haemolysis occurred, and the macrophages showed an intensive phagocytosis [2]. Subsequently, these macrophages were injected into isologous animals, where they induced only a slight immune response, despite the intensive phagocytosis [70].

These experiments suggest that passively introduced antibodies exert their suppressive effect at the level of the recognition of antigen. Supposedly, the same is valid for the autologous antibodies produced in the course of immune response. The suppressive effect of antibodies is a complex process. It should be taken into account that the immunogenic antigenic determinants are covered with antibodies. (This has been evidenced by *in vitro* experiments.) Furthermore, the opsonized antigen is phagocytosed at an increased rate [70], which is unfavourable for the immune response. Finally, the recognizing capacity of macrophages remains specifically impaired by antisera for a long time [137].

A further aspect of the suppressive effect of antibodies has not yet been clarified. On the 4th or 5th day, due to the appearance of IgG antibodies in the serum [138, 169*b*], IgM antibodies suddenly stop being produced and give place to IgG antibodies. The cause of this phenomenon is unknown. One might say that the IgM memory cells are much more sensitive to the suppressive effect of antibodies than the memory cells of the IgG type. However, we wish to avoid this explanation for reasons to be discussed below. A clarification of this question would be difficult because full primary response of the IgG type has never been induced *in vitro*. The rapid and effective blocking of IgM antibody production is suggestive of a mechanism limited to the surface of B cells. There is so far a single experimental finding available [45] suggesting that, in addition to the 'peripheral' inhibition resulting from the elimination of the antigen from the surface of macrophages, a 'central' inhibition on the B cell surface might also occur. Normal spleen cells were incubated with a mixture of antigen and IgG antibody *in vitro*. The cells were then washed and treated for the second time with antigen alone. These cells failed to induce antibody production, whereas cells of the same origin having been incubated with the antibody without antigen after washing gave a normal response to antigen. The kinetics of the immunosuppression induced by the antibody–antigen complex proved to be similar to the kinetics of the tolerance induced in the same system. The suppression required both the antigen and the homologous antibody covering the antigen on the B cell surface. The mechanism of this inhibition is still unknown. Another difficulty is that this hypothetic immunosuppressive system (see Fig. 11-4c) has been proposed, on the basis of *in vivo* experiments, to be a prototype of cell co-operations leading to antibody production. The contradiction may be merely apparent, for a process which inhibits the primary IgM antibody response might at the same time stimulate another response, e.g. an IgG response which, due to methodical reasons, may not develop fully *in vitro*. We shall return to this question later in this chapter.

## THE MEMORY IN THE HUMORAL IMMUNE RESPONSE AND THE CELLULAR BASIS OF THE SECONDARY HUMORAL IMMUNE RESPONSE

In this field of contemporary immunology acceptance of a uniform view would probably be the most difficult. This is reflected by the great differences found in the theories of immunological memory [12, 17, 40, 89, 152]. The question is obviously complex because, as a result of proliferation and recruitment, memory cells are produced in highly variable numbers and the function of the memory cells is influenced by the extremely variable quantity of the antigen persisting on the surface of macrophages at the time of the secondary stimulus.

Elimination of the suppressive effect of antibodies in transfer experiments leads to a continuous exponential increase and an enormous extension of the immune response [105*a*]. The secondary stimulus, on the other hand, sometimes results in hardly any titre rise [163*b*] because the pre-existing antibodies may fix a substantial proportion of the antigen and thus modify the course of antigen processing. There is an optimum time when a secondary response can be most effectively elicited (in the mouse the 8th and 9th week after a primary stimulus). At that time memory cells are still present in a declining, yet satisfactory number and the amount of circulating antibodies has already fallen to a level which allows the secondary response to proceed. The secondary stimulus applied at the time results in a response which is preceded by a time interval shorter than the latency phase of the primary response and may give rise to antibody titres even ten times as high as the peak reached during the primary response [79, 163*b*].

In the proliferating clones, the generation time is equal to that experienced during the primary response (8–9 h), whereas the doubling time is shortened (5–7 h) [65*a*, 157, 163*b*] because of the more intensive recruitment. Possibly, an increased transformation tendency of memory cells contributes to the shortening of the latency [18]. If the interval between the two stimuli is longer than the optimum, the memory cells are gradually decreasing in number, but never diminish to the pre-immunization level [51, 144, 169*a*].

All our information concerning the memory cells became questionable as soon as the importance of co-operation between carrier- and hapten-specific cells was recognized. In the light of this discovery, the secondary response cannot be explained by the activity of a single type of memory cell. We can only speak of an increased probability of cell interaction due to the more intensive proliferation of some or both of the interacting cell types.

In the process of antibody production, contribution of two kinds of memory cells may be assumed. These are T memory cells deriving from ARCs, and B memory cells deriving from P-AFCs. The existence of T memory cells has been proved. Roitt et al. [134] pointed out that the descendants of T cells develop a memory cell population having a long life-span [50] (see Fig. 11-4D). Following the injection of heterologous erythrocytes, a wave of cell divisions [33, 34] is running through the population of the cells of thymus origin located in the lymph nodes and in the spleen. At the same time, in transfer experiments the precursors increase in number [19]. *In vitro,* such a population of memory cells responds to antigenic stimulus by blast transformation [40, 48, 91, 145].

Like the T lymphocyte, the T memory cell fails to determine the immunoglobulin class of the antibodies produced due to its interaction with B cells. In the course of adoptive secondary immune response, pronounced early IgM antibody production can be experienced even if the spleen cells have been taken from donors having reached the IgG phase of antibody production [58, 60, 82, 169*b*]. In these experiments, production of IgG antibodies starts only after the IgM phase.

The existence and development of B memory cells supposedly deriving from B cells as well as their importance is disputable*. Firstly, the function of T memory cells may, in general, be sufficient to explain the cell kinetics of recruitment and of the secondary response. Secondly, it is unclear whether it is justified to assume a simultaneous development of a plasma cell clone and a B memory cell clone at the time of activation of B lymphocytes. An unequal division [12, 152] in the first generation has not been proved and the various suggestions are not convincing. Thirdly, accepting the existence of B memory cell, we ought to suppose that these, like B lymphocytes in general, have a short life-span. Consequently, the existence of long-lived B memory cell needs further experimental evidence.

The antibodies produced during the secondary response against a chemically defined hapten showed much higher affinity to the hapten than the antibodies induced by the same dose at the corresponding stage of the primary response [117, 149]. Even the antibodies produced in the earliest phase of the secondary response showed high affinity and the capacity of fast production of antibodies of high affinity was demonstrable in rabbits for at least two years after the primary stimulus [149]. The persistence of the memory of hapten receptors formed in a previous immune response is therefore possible. If so, the B memory cell population should be considered, in our present knowledge, to be of long life-span.

Evidence pointing to the existence of memory cell populations committed to produce antibodies of the IgA, IgG1, IgG2a or IgG2b sub-classes would strongly support the existence of a B memory. On the basis of physical separation of memory cells *in vitro,* it seems probable that IgG1 and IgG2 memories are mediated by different cell populations in transfer experiments [73]. Observation of the physical properties of these cell populations have also suggested that in the

* The existence of B memory has since been unequivocally proven (cf. Miller, J. F. A. P. and Sprent, J.: *J. exp. Med.* **134,** 66 1971). The cellular events during its development are still unknown.

spleen the appearance of IgG1 memory cells precedes that of the IgG2a cells [58, 170]. The experiments to be described also provided some information in this respect. Spleen cells from donors immunized with heterologous erythrocytes were passed through a column of plastic beads covered with the antigen. The memory cells were fixed by the column. In the subsequent experiment, the spleen cells were incubated with anti-IgG1 (or anti-IgG2) serum before being passed through the column covering IgG1 (or IgG2) receptors on the cells, thus preventing one (or the other) type in attaching to the column-bound antigen. The cell suspension recovered from the column was injected into animals. The recipients developed anti-erythrocyte antibodies of IgG1 (or IgG2) class, but not of IgG2 (or IgG1) class. These experiments suggest that there exist cell populations committed to produce IgG1 or IgG2 antibodies, and these are supplied with IgG1 and IgG2 surface receptors, respectively.

The results of these experiments may be utilized with relation to the memory cells if we accept the receptor theory (see below), i.e. the principle that antibody forming cells bear on their surface the receptor which is synthesized by them in the form of antibody. The correctness of the receptor theory is supported by numerous experiments [101*b*]. In this respect, the study of rosette forming cells (RFC)* is of interest [54]. Five to 7 days after administration of heterologous erythrocytes, a substantial proportion of the RFCs (presumably the population of non-secreting B memory cells) lost their antigen-fixing capacity if they had been incubated with any kind of anti-heavy-chain antiserum (the degree of inhibition of rosette formation with the individual antisera is as follows: anti-IgA, 33 per cent; anti-IgG1, 48 per cent; anti-IgG2a, 47 per cent; anti-IgG2b, 41 per cent; anti-IgM, 76 per cent. Anti-IgM serum inhibits T rosettes as well). If serum containing antibodies specific for two different immunoglobulin classes were added to the incubation mixture, no or very little summation occurred [10, 54, 95]. According to control experiments, the phenomenon cannot be simply attributed to cross-reactions or cell-fixed cytophilic antibodies [54]. These results imply that, in contrast to the antigen forming plasma cells, recently activated rosette forming (memory) cells show an incomplete restriction in relation to the immunoglobulin classes [10, 54, 141]. However later, on the 15th day following the antigenic stimulus, the B-type RFCs only carried IgG-type surface receptors [53*b*], i.e. in this late phase of the immune response, B memory cells lost their IgM receptors and thus became completely restricted to the production of a given IgG. Supposedly, these late B memory cells are those which proved to be separable by IgG sub-class on the plastic-bead column (see above).

* Rosette forming cells (RFC) are formed while a lymphoid population capable of an immune response to heterologous red blood cells (HRBC) are incubated with HRBC *in vitro*. HRBCs adhere to the cells bearing receptors recognizing the HRBC antigen (rosette formation). The RFC population is heterogeneous. In non-immunized animals, 40–50 per cent are of thymus origin, i.e. T lymphocytes. The rest are B lymphocytes. The cell receptors are formed by the $F(ab)_2$ part of Ig and the corresponding heavy chain (Fc) is covered by the cell membrane [54]. Following immunization with HRBC, part of the Fc fragment will become demonstrable on the multiplying RFCs, by anti-heavy-chain serum. A new type of RFC — ASC (antibody secreting cell) — appears which binds HRBCs in several layers. ASC is an early form of antibody forming cell, a member of the plasma cell population. On the 5th day following immunization, the percentage distribution of RFCs is as follows: ASC, 30 per cent; non-secreting B lymphocyte, 34 per cent; T lymphocyte, 36 per cent.

## CELLULAR PHENOMENA DETERMINING THE QUALITATIVE CHARACTERISTICS OF ANTIBODIES

As a result of the successive cellular events occurring during the immune response, the contribution to the production of antibodies of different qualities is continuously changing in favour of antibodies produced to sterically small determinants. Besides, late antibodies show an increased affinity to these determinants. The class distribution of the antibodies is shifted towards the IgG class. This section deals with the cellular events resulting in these complex phenomena. There is increasing evidence indicating that the individual cells within a clone committed to antibody production produce antibodies of given antigen specificity, of the same affinity, and belonging to a single immunoglobulin class. Therefore, we should reconsider some theoretical aspects in order to provide appropriate explanation for facts apparently irreconcilable with the clone theory (see section 'Theories of Antibody Formation').

### *Antigen specificity of the process of antibody production*

Antibodies are specific for antigenic determinants (haptens) (see Chapter 7). The antigen specificity of antibody production raises two questions, namely (*i*) to how many antigenic determinants does a single cell produce antibody? (*ii*) what is the role of the structure of the carrier molecule in the specific immune response (carrier specificity)?

(*i*) As regards the first question, opinions appear to be consistent. The only inconsistent observation has been published by Hiramoto and Hamlin [67], who found cells producing mixed antibodies in 45 per cent, presumably due to having worked with cross-reactive reagents [56]. Other investigators using very sensitive methods have unequivocally proved that all the antibody produced by the same cell is directed to the same antigen [21, 57, 114]. The restricted commitment of immunocytes is considered by these authors as a basic evidence for the clone theory. None of 16,000 cells from animals simultaneously hyperimmunized by two phages showed antibody production to both phages [92*b*]. In another experimental series, following simultaneous immunization, 5,675 cells showed antibody production to one of the antigens, 6,990 to the other antigen and as few as 21 cells showed double production. Such a rare occurrence of double-producing cells falls within the limit of error of the method applied [124].

The high-degree of commitment is valid for the receptors of the lymphocytes as well [92*a*, 116]. According to Cross and Mäkelä [29], the cells responsible for IgG antibody production show a relatively high sensitivity to the inhibiting action of antibodies. This is in accord with the relatively high specificity shown by IgG antibodies in binding haptens. The immunosuppressive effect of passive antibodies has proved in many cases that antibodies are specific for a given determinant and not for the whole of the antigen molecule. The hapten-specific antibody production was not inhibited by antibodies produced to a hapten of different character, conjugated to the same carrier [13, 125].

(*ii*) The effective stimulation of antibody forming cells needs the participation of the antigen reactive cell (ARC) bearing carrier-specific surface receptors. Using the same chemically defined hapten conjugated with different carriers, it has been proved that the intensity of the immune response is determined by the quality of the carrier molecule. In mice, the most intensive immune response to dinitrophenol (DNP) hapten was induced if the highly immunogenic haemocyanin was used as carrier. The immune response was less intensive to DNP conjugated with human IgG, and murine IgG as carrier often caused specific tolerance to DNP [64]. This shows that it is difficult to induce a humoral response to antigens consisting of a hapten and of such a carrier which is unable to induce delayed hypersensitivity. The process of specific antibody production to haptens starts on the basis of the carrier-specific delayed hypersensitivity reaction, an immune process based on T lymphocyte function. The specificity of T lymphocytes in immune responses is dealt with in Chapter 8. An appropriate co-operation of cells sensitive to the antigenic determinant (hapten) with those sensitive to the carrier molecule is important primarily from the aspect of the induction of antibody production; therefore, this has been discussed in the section dealing with the events of the latency period.

### *The affinity of antibodies produced by a clone*

Cells of different affinity produce antibodies of different affinity even after immunization with a single hapten [92*a*]. The antibodies produced early in the course of the primary immune response show low affinity, those produced in the late phase show high affinity. In general, IgM antibodies are of lower affinity than IgG antibodies. It is not known whether these changes in affinity occur within a given clone or whether the phenomenon is due to a shift in the relative contribution of cells belonging to different clones. On columns of antigen-covered particles, cells with receptors of different affinities can be separated from one another. The cells thus separated retained their affinities after having been re-introduced into the animals [170].

It is another question whether precursors of cells committed to produce highly specific late antibodies to a given antigen already exist before immunization. This question will be dealt with later on.

### *Production of antibodies of different immunoglobulin classes*

Antibodies directed against the same antigen, but belonging to different immunoglobulin classes may be simultaneously present in the serum. It is not quite clear whether the same clone (or even the same cell) may produce all these antibodies. Considering that investigators usually failed to demonstrate immunoglobulins containing different heavy chains within the same plasma cell [20, 169*c*], it was initially supposed that simultaneous production of two different heavy chains does not occur in cells of the same clone except in the short period of time when the production of IgM globulins is stopped and the cell begins producing IgG globulins (Nossal switch) [113]. Although plasmocytomas simultaneously synthesizing immunoglobulins of two different heavy chains have rarely been demonstrated [28, 167], evidence obtained in recent years favours the view that, from the induction of antibody production on, the cells of a given plasma cell clone form antibodies of a given class specificity throughout [21, 30, 169*c*].

It is a further question whether B cells are multipotent or not. The data presented in the chapter discussing immunological memory suggest that the B memory cells produced during the early phase of primary antibody production may be multipotent i.e. the type of cell interaction and the quality of the antigen determine the class of antibodies to be produced by a given B cell. In the late phase of the primary response, and supposedly during the secondary response, on the other hand, the B memory cells are committed to produce IgG antibodies of a given sub-class [54] (see section 'Theories of Antibody Formation').

The following experiment fails to answer the question of the multipotency of B cells, but proves that antigens are able to stimulate preferentially the B cell surface receptors to which they have an increased affinity. This shows that the ratio of plasma cell clones producing IgM antibodies to those producing IgG antibodies may be influenced by the type of the antigen. Nitroiodophenyl (NIP) hapten molecules were conjugated with ovalbumin (OA) carrier molecules to produce monovalent $NIP_{0.5}$ OA and multivalent $NIP_8$ OA antigens, and animals were immunized with the two conjugates. Doses which resulted in production of approximately equal amounts of IgG-type anti-NIP antibodies induced significantly different IgM responses. The IgM response to the polyvalent antigen conjugate was four times that induced by the monovalent conjugate as measured by the antigen-binding capacity of antibodies [93]. Considering that to $NIP_{0.5}$BSA and other monovalent conjugates IgM antibodies show substantially lower affinity than IgG antibodies [14], the experiment is suggestive of the existence of cell surface receptors resembling multivalent (IgM) or bivalent (IgG) antibodies. These receptors, in accordance with the receptor theory, may be helpful in the selection of the appropriate receptors in the course of the restriction of multipotent precursors.

It has been mentioned earlier in this chapter that soluble proteins, as compared to particulate ones, induce in general a very weak, hardly detectable, IgM antibody response, whereas approximately equal quantities of IgG antibodies are produced to soluble and particulate antigens. It may be supposed that soluble antigens are less capable of stimulating IgM receptors than particulate proteins.

## THEORIES OF ANTIBODY FORMATION

The exactly co-ordinated variable system of nature, which has governed antibody production for millions of years seems to be so extremely specific and precise that there is no hope in the near future to elaborate any 'human-made' theory that gives an approximate explanation for its perfection. The theory must meet the highest requirements and explain the following facts [72]:

1. The high-degree specificity of antigen–antibody reaction despite the very large number of antigenic groups potentially able to induce specific antibodies.
2. The difference in course between primary and secondary immune responses.
3. The fact that an antigen molecule may induce the production of 100,000 or more antibody molecules.

4. The individual being able to distinguish between its own antigens and foreign antigens (self or not-self).
5. The phenomenon of immunological tolerance.

There are two main possibilities to approach these apparently insoluble problems. The literature refers to the corresponding two theories, different in their basic principles, as selective and directive (instructive) theories.

## BASIC CHARACTERISTICS OF THE SELECTIVE AND DIRECTIVE (INSTRUCTIVE) THEORIES

Ehrlich (1900) was the first to propose a selective theory [42]. He assumed the existence on the cell surface of haptophore groups, i.e. chemically defined receptors which are able to recognize nutrient metabolites and foreign proteins and to combine with them. According to the theory, the nutrient metabolite would be taken up by the cell, whereas the haptophore group in combination with a foreign substance would be thrown off from the cell surface. The separation of the haptophore group would stimulate the organism to produce, and even overproduce, the same haptophore group, the appearance of which in the serum as specific antibody was considered by Ehrlich a special kind of overproduction. The essence of the selective theories is therefore a selection by the antigen of a pre-existing receptor. In this way, a type of cell is selected which starts antibody formation. To this theory, an objection was immediately raised, namely that the existence of such an extraordinarily large number of predetermined cell receptors is hard to imagine.

Haurowitz [63] developed an early version of the directive (instructive) theory in the early 1930s. He supposed that antigen enters an originally multipotent cell and directs the metabolism of the cell in such a way that the antigen may serve as a template for antibody formation. According to this theory, therefore, the antigen gives the cell an instruction to start specific antibody production. However, this theory was unable to face an objection which was immediately raised. It is unlikely that the ability to produce antibodies to any of the potential antigens of the organism is continuously blocked in all cells which are potentially capable of producing antibodies. Without such a blocking, the organism would produce auto-antibodies.

Both the selective and the instructive theories have been developed in accordance with the advance of the related fields. Nevertheless, recent data appear to favour the selective theory. This does not mean that the instructive theory is less ingenious. In the 1930s, there was no sign suggesting that DNA strands, and not stable proteins, serve as templates in the living organism. Considering that the selective theories are in better agreement with the concept of a DNA-directed genetic control of antibody production, they appear to involve a greater part of truth than the instructive theories.

The first modern selective theory, the 'natural selection theory', was proposed by Jerne in 1955 [76a]. He assumed that, of the continuously synthesized $\gamma$-globulin molecules, those showing a sufficient specificity form a complex with antigen particles. The complex is phagocytosed by macrophages, and this step is the signal for the specific antibody production to get started. According to this theory, the role of the antigen consists in selecting from the globulin pool, and introducing into the macrophage, the globulin which is to be synthesized during the antibody response. Burnet's [15] 'clonal selection theory' is only one step further, but this step is very important. Burnet was puzzled by the phenomenon described by Simonsen [146] that mature chicken leukocytes inoculated into chick embryos caused proliferative lesions in the spleen and in the thymus. On this basis, Burnet supposed that a contact with antigenic determinants exerts its effect not on the immunoglobulins, but on sensitive cells, strictly speaking, on the receptors of sensitive cells. The cells thus affected will proliferate showing a clonal character. Burnet attributed the main role in immune reactions to small lymphocytes, and this assumption has proved to be correct. Furthermore, Burnet suggested that if antigen is fixed to any of the surface receptors of immunocytes before the full maturation of the immune apparatus, the corresponding clone will not proliferate, but will be suppressed. Thus, Burnet was the first to explain why the organism does not start an immune response to its own constituents. Starting from Burnet's conception, Medawar [96] inoculated newborn mice with cells deriving from a different mouse strain. The mice, having grown up, did not reject the grafts deriving from the same donor strain, i.e. developed specific tolerance.

The next step was taken by Nossal and Lederberg [112], who had shown that the clonal selection theory was basically correct by examining the antibody production of lymph-node cells. It became also evident that immunoparalysis is the specific deficiency of reactive cells [129]. Perhaps the strongest evidence in favour of the clonal selection theory has been furnished by immunochemical observations in human myelomatosis. These results have definitely demonstrated (*i*) the uniformity, i.e. monoclonal character, of the immunoglobulins formed in the same immunocyte; (*ii*) the exact way of somatic inheritance of, and the restriction in, the phenotype of plasmocytomas; and (*iii*) the randomness of the mutations giving rise to $\gamma$-globulins varying substantially in structure. In this manner, nearly all the characteristics of the supposed clonal selection have been demonstrated in the myelomatosis system.

Based on the selective theories, the development of the immune response is supposed to consist of five large steps: (*i*) randomization, in the course of which a wide range of reactive units develop which are capable of directing the production of specific antibodies to different antigens; (*ii*) a mechanism which prevents the immune reaction to self antigen and recognizes foreign antigenic determinants; (*iii*) the activation of antibody synthesis; (*iv*) intensification of the immune response; (*v*) as a last step the antibodies protect the organism at several levels against an undesirable overproduction of antibodies.

## STEPS OF THE IMMUNE RESPONSE IN ACCORDANCE WITH THE CLONAL SELECTION THEORY

(*i*) The conformation of the combining sites of the immunoglobulin molecule is determined by the amino acid sequence of the variable regions ($V_L$ and $V_H$) of the N-terminal part of the light and heavy chains. The variability of the amino acids extends to half of the 106–108 amino acids constituting the $V_L$ and $V_H$

regions. Supposing that the combining sites of the antibody molecules are not larger than the antigen determinants, and are determined by 5 or 6 amino acids, the number of variable penta- or hexa-peptides might be estimated between $3 \times 10^6$ and $60 \times 10^6$. In fact, the number of possibilities must be lower ($\sim 10^6$) because, due to steric reasons, certain amino acids must be excluded [35]. However, in the same peptide chain several (2–3) sites may be capable of recognizing hapten, thus increasing the number of variations. We do not know whether all the possible variations are, in fact, realized during randomization, but the clonal theory cannot be disproved on genetical basis, for the existence of approximately $10^6$ distinct precursors is in accordance with the above data.

The central lymphoid organs have special roles, namely the thymus in the production of T lymphocytes and the bursa-equivalent lymphatic organ in the production of B lymphocytes. Considering the origin of the B cells, it may be of interest to examine the randomization process in the light of the recent theories concerning the bursa. In the chick embryo, the first cells containing $\mu$ heavy chain appear in the bursa on the 14th day of incubation [27], i.e. one day after the inflow of stem cells into the bursa. Cells containing IgG are first detectable a week later. To decide whether IgM and IgG are synthesized during different phases of the development of a single cell line or whether they are synthesized by different populations appearing in different phases of ontogenesis, 13-day embryos were treated with antiserum to the heavy chain of IgM (anti-$\mu$ serum). After hatching, the chickens produced very little IgM antibody but their IgG synthesis was still more impaired, indicating that the IgM → IgG switch occurs in the cells having differentiated in the bursa, within a single cell line. According to the hypothesis of Cooper et al. [27], the heterogeneity of the combining sites of antibodies develops in the micro-environment of the bursa in the phase of the initiation of IgM synthesis. The descendants of these cells are responsible for the IgM → IgG switch, and in mammals also for the later IgG → IgA switch. B lymphocytes belonging to the same cell line may leave the bursa in different phases of their differentiation and thus appear in the periphery as IgM, IgG or IgA precursors.

(*ii*) At present, the somatic mutation of the few gene loci ('generator of diversity') appears to be the most probable explanation for the development of about $10^6$ distinct precursor cells. This mutation occurs in the V (variable) genes of the immunoglobulins at a hypernormal mutation rate. The theories concerning the function of the generator of diversity are discussed in literary reviews [41, 85, 93, 148]. From among the resulting cells those possessing recognizing sites to self antigens are eliminated. It was shown that of the cells brought about in the thymus more than 99 per cent are eliminated [97]. The immunocytes having no recognizing site to self antigens migrate from the central lymphatic organ to the periphery.

Lymphocytes that have undergone randomization are responsible for the recognition of foreign antigens. According to the modern minimum clone theory, antigens are recognized by receptors located on the surface of cells. The essence of the minimum theory is as follows [101*a*]. We may suppose that the antigen is recognized by an antibody. If so, it may also be supposed that the receptor itself that recognizes the antigen is an antibody, which is already present on the cell surface before the cell meets the antigen; it is formed by the precursor, due to a genetic information that was acquired during randomization, and retained by the cell thereafter. The descendants of the precursor cell are supposed to produce the antibody on the same information after a successful stimulation of the clone. According to the minimum theory, therefore, the relation of the end product to the receptor appears to be simple: a given plasma cell synthesizes a single immunoglobulin pattern and the same pattern is shared by the receptor of the progenitor lymphocyte.

The receptor is a structure consisting of several chains. The presence of more than one chain in it increases the variability of the recognizing site, which is determined by the sequence of several amino acids [101*b*]. Antibodies consisting of more than one chain developed in an early phase of phylogenesis. The receptor must resemble the F(ab')$_2$ fragment of the antibody, for the Fc of the heavy chain is enclosed in, or covered by the cell membrane [54].

(*iii*) While since the last decade numerous data have contributed to our knowledge on the specific and non-specific stimulation of T lymphocytes [44, 117, 133], much less is known about the activation of B lymphocytes. While T lymphocytes are readily stimulated by antigens, the stimulation of B lymphocytes *in vitro* meets difficulties, though, they are rich in receptors. In the case of thymus independent and thymus dependent antigens, they require help from macrophages [107] and T lymphocytes, respectively. During stimulation of a T lymphocyte population, numerous substances are released (mitogenic factor, chemotactic factor, MIF, etc., see Chapter 8). Some of these may be capable of activating B lymphocytes, and antigen bridges between the two different types of cells may secure the high efficacy of the mediator. Furthermore, B lymphocytes are cells very liable to injury, which appear to require the presence of feeder cells *in vivo* as well as *in vitro*.

As regards the difference in antigen sensitivity between T and B lymphocytes, it seems to be important that the antigen doses rendering T and B lymphocytes tolerant are also different. Both 'low-dose' and 'high-dose' tolerance can be induced [37]. These are due to the specific paralysis of T-type memory cells and B cells, respectively.

(*iv*) Several simultaneous processes are responsible for the intensification of the immune response. The view disregarding the contribution of other processes in addition to the clonal division of plasma cells should be considered obsolete. There is no doubt that 500 to 1,000 plasma cells can develop from a single B cell. However, these cells represent the final, decaying forms of the maturation process. The clonal division of plasma cells may be compared to the bunch of grapes at the tip of a wine. In the depth of the intensification of the immune response, there is the explosion-like process which increases the probability of the cell interactions exponentially until the concentration of the stimulating antigen falls below a given concentration. This process is fed by several sources. Firstly, a T-memory clone (helper cells) develops from a T cell and may directly contribute to intensifying the immune response. Secondly, macrophages may turn into carrier-specific cells due to the effect of cytophilic antibodies. Thirdly, B lymphocytes, showing high turnover, are rapidly supplemented from the central lymphatic organ and from stem cells circulating on the periphery (see section on immunological memory in Chapter 8). In addition, development of B memory cells of long life-span committed to IgG synthesis may be supposed.

(*v*) The regulating role of antibodies has its most important manifestation in initiating the production of antibodies of high affinity and in preventing an over-production of antibodies. The two processes are closely related. As the immune response proceeds, antibodies greatly increase in affinity, reaching even a thousand-fold increase [169*b*]. A small dose of the antigen induces antibodies of high affinity [149]. The higher the dose, the larger proportion of the antibodies will show low affinity. The phenomenon is explicable by the clonal selection theory, indicating that cells of variable affinity compete for the antigen and, if the antigen dose is small, the stimulus is accessible only for clones of high affinity. IgG antibodies produced late in the course of the immune response proved to be more effective in inhibiting the immune response than the early IgG antibodies, suggesting that there is a competition between antibodies and receptors and that the antigen covered by antibodies is unable to stimulate receptors. Thus, as the immune response proceeds, the antigen, diminishing in amount, is only accessible for cells supplied with receptors of the highest affinity. Finally, in the latest phase of the immune response when the antigen has been phagocytosed and decomposed, only a few plasma cells of long life-span keep producing antibodies [169*b*]. These cells, which are constantly decreasing in number, do not require the presence of the stimulating antigen for a continuous antibody production. The memory of a previous immune response is retained for years in small lymphocytes developing from long lived memory cells.

## AN ATTEMPT AT THE RECONCILIATION OF IMMUNOLOGICAL THEORIES

In the foregoing, we have attempted to outline the clonal selection theory. Here, Sterzl's [152] conception concerning the course of immune reaction is reviewed in comparison with the clonal theory. Sterzl has proposed to designate the course of the immune response by the transformation X → Y → Z as a final abstraction (Fig. 11-6). X is the precursor cell which is potentially able to respond to an antigenic stimulus, but has not yet met the given antigen. This theory does not say to how many different antigens a precursor cell may react, but implies the multi- or omnipotency of the X cell. The Y cell, which is the central participant of the immune response, develops from the X cell due to antigenic stimulus. Proliferation of Y cells results in generations $Y_1$, $Y_2$, $Y_3$, $Y_4 \ldots Y_n$, which are responsible for immunological memory. Due to further antigenic stimuli, Y cells are transformed into antibody producing Z cells, i.e. plasma cells. Sterzl has attempted to explain the heterogeneity of the antibodies formed in the course of the immune response on the basis of the successive Y generations. Accordingly, Y → Z transformation may occur in any of the generations during proliferation. It may occur, e.g. that a $Y_{10}$ cell is transformed into a $Z_{10}$ cell. The antibodies produced by $Z_{10}$ cells are of much higher affinity than those produced, e.g. by $Z_4$ cells which are the products of the transformation of $Y_4$ memory cells. The dose and administration schedule of the antigen primarily determine which of the Y generations will turn into Z cells. Sterzl [150] has outlined the responses to different immunization schemes (Fig. 11-6*a*) and analysed the successive steps of antibody formation. Sterzl's conception is substantially different from the clonal theory. The latter is based on the principle that the antigen-specificity,

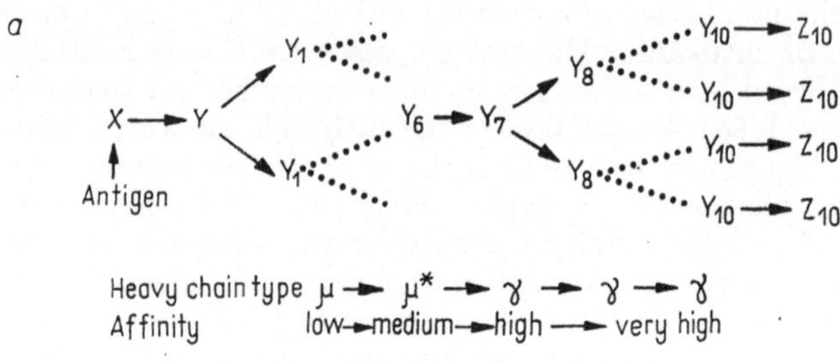


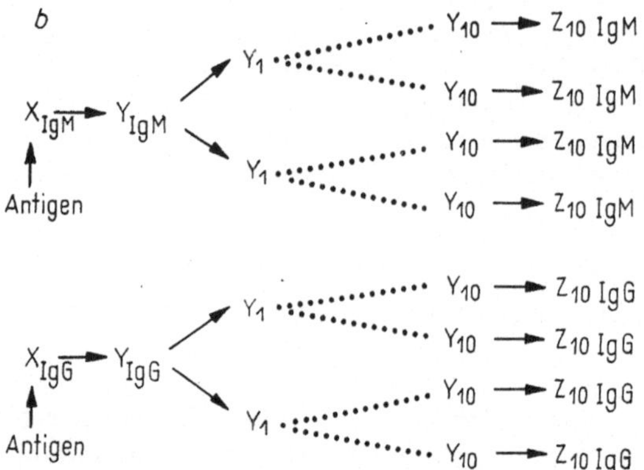


Fig. 11-6. Two possible schemes for immunocyte maturation. *a)* The 'X-Y-Z' scheme by Sterzl [150] postulates that the characteristics of immunoglobulins produced by successive generations of cells in the clone are modified during the 'maturation' of the immune response. *b)* The classical clonal theory postulates numerous precursors and emphasizes that the immunoglobulin molecules assembled by the cells of a given clone are identical

affinity and immunoglobulin class of the antibody to be produced is *predetermined* in the precursor before the precursor meets the antigen (Fig. 11-6*b*).

Antibody forming cells show an extremely high specialization. The individual must be prepared against tens of thousands of potential antigens and the affinity of the antibodies produced in the course of the immune response increases 1,000-fold. The antibodies belong to immunoglobulin groups of about 20 different class-allotype combinations and, in the course of an immune response, antibodies belonging to practically all of these classes are produced in larger or smaller quantities. Of course, the clonal theory cannot explain such a high degree of specialization, in case we ought to suppose that even the precursors of cells producing antibodies of high affinity and belonging to various sub-classes in the *latest* phase of the immune response exist *before* the cell meets the antigen. Considering that the plasma cell is committed to produce a given antibody from the moment of the activation of the plasma cell clone, the solution of the question should be sought in the course of the development of precursor cells. It appears reasonable to discuss the restriction of precursor cells in the light of the immunoglobulin class and in that of affinity.

According to Mäkelä [93], who dealt with the problem of high-affinity precursors developing in the course of the immune response, the antibodies reacting with the antigen in the early phase of antibody production are supposedly of low affinity. Antibodies with an affinity of $K_0 = 10^5/\text{M}$ appear as late as one month after immunization. In the mouse, at least $10^6$ immunocytes are dividing during this month. Considering that the generator of diversity functions not only in the central lymphatic organ but also on the periphery, we may expect a relatively high mutation rate ($10^4$ per cistron per division) during the replication of the gene directing $V_L$ and $V_H$. Accordingly, about 100 different mutants of the $V_L + V_H$ gene may develop and some of these may highly increase the affinity of the cells. Due to the antigenic stimulus, the descendants of the mutant cell may outgrow the population of low affinity. We do not know, however, how many cell divisions occur in the B memory population deriving from B cells during the month following immunization. According to Dresser [36], the increase in the number of spleen cells in the hyperimmunized spleen ranges about $40 \times 10^6$, and only 3 per cent of these cells form antibodies. Thus the number of divisions of B memory cells even might exceed $10^6$. A maturation of the immune response by mutations is therefore theoretically possible, but our knowledge of the population-kinetic events proceeding in the background of antibody production are extremely poor.

On the other hand, the restriction of the immunoglobulin class is a more easily approachable problem. The data of Cooper et al. [27] mentioned in the foregoing have substantially modified our view. We may suppose, accordingly, that precursors develop antigen specificity at the level of the cells committed to produce IgM antibodies, and that the cell line deriving from such a precursor may reach a maturation phase when the cells begin to produce IgG or IgA antibodies. If so, it is not necessary to assume 20 kinds of precursors within a single antigen-specificity. We must, however, raise the question whether the possibility of an IgM $\rightarrow$ IgG switch is acceptable from the immunochemical point of view. In other words, is a linked synthesis of the variable regions in the light and heavy chains ($V_L$ and $V_H$) possible, independent of the synthesis of the constant region $C_H$. Some literary data [87] suggest that, indeed, the $V_H$ and $C_H$ regions are controlled by different genes. In the rabbit, immunoglobulin allotypes Aa1, Aa2 and Aa3 are alleles of the same locus 'a'. Probably, the determinants of these allotypes are located in the $V_H$ region of the globulin molecule [80, 123]. The same Aa determinant is demonstrable in each of the different heavy chains ($\mu$, $\gamma$, $\alpha$) of the same rabbit [159, 161] (Fig. 11-7). If it could be proved that the amino acid sequences in the Aa2 determinants of chains $\mu$ and $\gamma$ are identical (not only similar), this would be strong evidence indicating that two genes co-operate in heavy-chain synthesis [93].

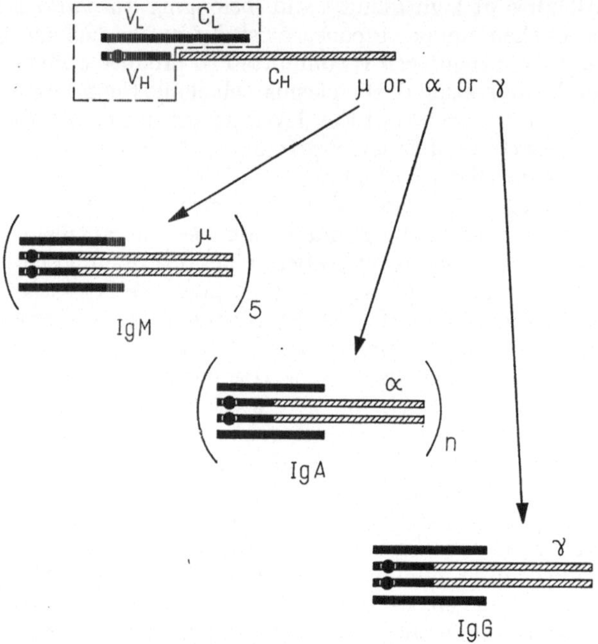


Fig. 11-7. Gene map of IgM, IgA and IgG according to the 'two-gene-cooperation' hypothesis. During the synthesis of heavy chains one of the co-operating genes controls the variable region ($V_H$) and the other controls the constant region ($C_H$). During the development of a B lymphocyte the $V_H$ gene may attach to a $C_H$ gene of $\mu$ or $\alpha$ or $\gamma$ type. As the gene responsible for the synthesis of $C_H$ is determined at a later stage of differentiation than the genes responsible for the synthesis of $V_H$ (and $V_L + C_L$, the light chain), different cells with identical antigen binding sites ($V_H + V_L$) may produce immunoglobulins of different (IgM or IgA or IgG) classes. The hypothesis is based on the fact that the same allotypic determinant of the $V_H$ region (Aa1 or Aa2 or Aa3, depicted in the Figure as solid circle) can be demonstrated in each of the different heavy chains ($\mu$, $\alpha$, $\gamma$) of the same rabbit

Accordingly, the IgM → IgG switch might be imagined immunochemically as follows. The whole light chain and the variable part of the heavy chain $[(C_L + V_L) + V_H]$ are synthesized in harmony, thus developing the recognition site, i.e. the cell receptor, or combining site of the antibody (Fig. 11-7). The gene complex controlling the $[(C_L + V_L) + V_H]$ unit may, depending on the commitment of the cell, be switched from gene $C_H$ controlling the constant region of the heavy chain to another $C_H$ gene. The $C_H$ genes are probably located on the same chromosome in the order $\mu, \alpha_1, \alpha_2, \gamma_4, \gamma_2, \gamma_3, \gamma_1, \delta, \varepsilon$.

If it is accepted that an IgM → IgG switch may occur at a certain point along a cell line, the micro-environment in which the switch actually takes place will be determined by the degree of maturation of the precursor cells. There are three possibilities: (*i*) switch may occur in the central lymphatic organ (bursa). In this case, IgM, IgG and IgA precursors will be found on the periphery (Cooper); (*ii*) it may occur in the course of the cell interaction ensuing upon the encounter with antigen. In this case the character of the interaction will determine the cistron to be activated and, consequently, the corresponding heavy chain; (*iii*) finally, an IgM → IgG switch may occur after the induction of antibody production in the course of the development of the plasma cell clone (Nossal switch). Experimental evidence supports possibilities (*i*) and (*ii*), but does not support (*iii*). An advantage of the second possibility is that it is compatible with a feedback mechanism through which the sub-class of the antibodies to be produced might be regulated by the quality and quantity of the antigen, as well as by the type, cytophilia and quantity of antibodies produced by other cells. In the section on immunological memory of Chapter 8 we have mentioned that according to recent literary data the restriction of a population of rosette forming cells was found to be incomplete 5–7 days after immunization with heterologous erythrocytes, because cells were bearing surface receptors of different classes at the same time [10, 54]. With the progress of the immune response, however, a population committed to produce IgG antibodies developed. It appears to be possible that some B cells may undergo a maturation process *during* the immune response.

In the following, we try to summarize the development of the process of antibody production. Due to the many factors of uncertainty, there is hardly any doubt that the summary is incorrect from some point of view. Nevertheless, we believe that this brief summary may serve for clinicians as a guide for systemization of new, supporting or refuting, data. In Fig. 11-8, the types of cell interaction are not indicated because it is not quite clear how the different interactions (see Fig. 11-4) relate to the clone-activation process outlined in Fig. 11-8. A more detailed illustration of the interrelations is impossible because we know almost nothing about the processes leading to B cell activation. For the same reason, it might be postulated that an antigen–B cell interaction which fails to initiate a plasma cell clone [45], might start a dissimilar differentiation of the B cell, e.g. a development of short lived precursors into long lived (IgG) memory cells and division of the latter.

An interaction between B cell and antigen may have at least four different consequences: (*i*) tolerant (paralysed) B cell may develop; (*ii*) an activation resembling the division of stem cells may result in a progeny showing characteristics identical with those of the mother cell; (*iii*) restriction from some aspect of a multipotent cell and development of a unipotent clone, e.g. of an IgG memory clone from multipotent precursors; (*iv*) induction of a plasma cell clone from a B cell. Following the entry of the antigen, antigen sensitive B cells are activated in cell interactions (see Fig. 11-4). This cell population of bursa-equivalent origin probably varies in degree of the maturity of the member cells, indicating that although B cells are committed to produce antibodies of a given affinity to a given antigen, their restriction as regards commitment to immunoglobulin class is variable. In such a cell population, B cells committed to produce IgG antibodies may occur, making up at most one-seventh of the B cell population [30]. The bulk of the B cells is made up by forms which are able to respond to antigenic stimulus by developing an IgM-producing plasma cell clone. Such an antigen

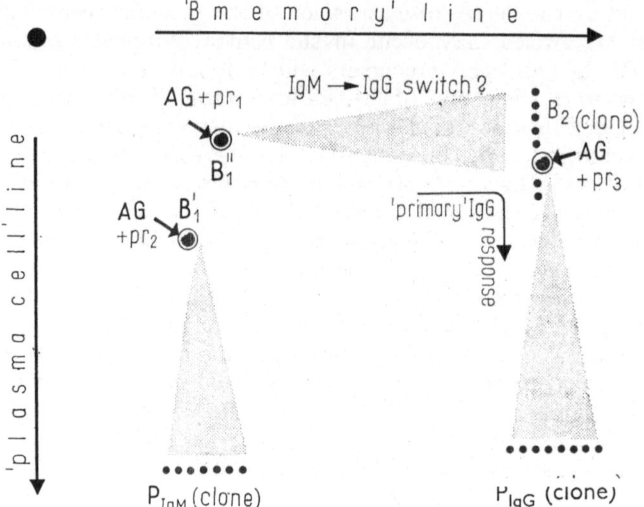


Fig. 11-8. Production of 'plasma cell' and 'B-memory cell' clones. Certain B cells (e.g. $B_1'$ cells) are stimulated and give rise to IgM producing plasma cells ($P_{IgM}$ clone). The development of IgG response is probably more complex. At the early stage of the immune response only relatively few cells are triggered successfully to produce large amounts of IgG, whilst in late stages IgG plasma cells are numerous and B cell memory (predominantly IgG) also develops. For this, it is postulated that certain B cells (e.g. $B_1''$) are also stimulated by antigen and proliferate but do not produce excessive amounts of Ig as plasma cells do. They rather develop into sensitized cells of lymphoid character ($B_2$ cells, which without further stimulus may become B memory cells). If the stimulus is protracted or repeated, even within the frame of the primary response (see text), they rapidly form IgG plasma cell clones ($P_{IgG}$). $B_1'$ and $B_1''$ could be cells of different maturity and/or the presentation of antigen ($pr_1$, $pr_2$, $pr_3$) by macrophages and T lymphocytes can influence which way B cells develop. IgG response is more dependent upon the collaboration of T cells and more sensitive to different immunosuppressive treatments than the IgM response

stimulation *in vitro* requires, in the case of most of the antigens, the presence of helper cells, i.e. carrier-specific T lymphocytes and macrophages ('T-dependent' antigens, e.g. heterologous red blood cells). Other antigens ('T-independent' antigens, e.g. polysaccharides) do not require the participation of T cells in the ASUs. However, as a general rule, IgM antibody synthesis is considered *relatively* T cell independent *in vivo*. Some antigens, e.g. soluble proteins [109, 162] and conjugates carrying monovalent hapten [92], may undergo such an activation with difficulty. The IgM antibody production to these antigens is poor.

Some additional antigen reactive cells within the B cell population may be theoretically capable of producing IgG, but only after a maturation process involving activation of B cells different from the activation described above (Fig. 11-8). The circumstances of this type of activation have not been studied, because these proliferating B cells do not produce large quantities of immunoglobulin; they can be detected by rosette formation (after immunization with red blood cells). IgG receptors appear on their surface in growing numbers and, parallel to this, the cells lose their IgM-producing capacity. In a late stage of their maturation (about the 15th day), and subsequently, they carry only IgG-subclass (IgG1 or IgG2a or IgG2b) receptors, and are committed to produce antibodies of the sub-class determined by their receptor (class restriction). This type of activation is T cell dependent.

To explain the shutting off of IgM formation at the start of IgG formation, two assumptions appear to be reasonable, firstly a competition may be assumed between the two kinds of stimulation of B cells and, due to the start of the maturation of B cells in the direction of IgG production, IgM precursors may be exhausted. The start in the IgG direction may be supported by a facettation of antigens persisting in the organism, due to their combination with early IgM antibodies. Facetted antigens do not stop being immunogenic, only the number of adjacent free determinants will be reduced. The other alternative is more probable. Accordingly, the distribution and mode of processing of the antigen changes in parallel with the appearance of early antibodies. Antigen–antibody complexes tend to accumulate in germinal centres [60] and, presumably, the number of IgM-type B cells as compared with those of the IgG-type ones is low just at this site (see below).

It is reasonable to suppose that mature, committed IgG precursors give rise to plasma cell clones only as a result of a repeated stimulus. If such cells meet an antigen repeatedly, they start producing and secreting IgG. If mature IgG precursors do not repeatedly meet an antigen during the primary immune response, they turn into B memory cells and in the secondary response these cells will immediately start producing IgG antibodies.

According to experimental data [159], initiation of IgG production and secondary response is much more dependent on helper (T) cells than the successful induction of primary IgM response. It may be supposed that, due to the close proximity of T and B cells in cell interactions ('antigen bridge' see Fig. 11-4), T cells may influence the metabolism of B precursors significantly; IgM $\rightarrow$ IgG switch may also be the result of such an effect.

Although discussion of the anatomical sites of antibody production is outside the scope of the present chapter, the following data should be mentioned. The proliferation of T lymphocytes, which appears to be the prelude of antibody production, occurs in the paracortical areas of the spleen and of the lymph nodes [33]. In these regions, it is associated with the division of IgM-producing B lymphocytes [19, 33]. The germinal centres in the cortical area develop with a delay of one or two days. These centres are the centres of the IgG antibody production and secondary response [33, 74]. The appearance of germinal centres seems to be preceded by migration of cells from the paracortical region into the cortical area. This flux of cells whirls into the cortical area newly-produced T lymphocyte progeny and B cells that have started maturing into IgG precursors. In addition, the antigen–antibody complexes that have been removed from the blood stream accumulate on the surface of dendritic macrophages in the germinal centres [59]. It is reasonable to suppose that in the germinal centres two kinds of clonal division are proceeding, namely, the maturation of IgG precursors may be completed (development of B memory) and, on repeated stimulus, the latter cells evolve the IgG-producing plasma cell clones. It is of interest that no further clonal division of T cells occurs in the germinal centres [33].

Administration of suboptimal doses of antigen [110, 164], appropriately timed treatment with cortisone [7] or passive antibodies [51], irradiation of animals [125, 163*b*], and intraperitoneal phytohaemagglutinin pretreatment [47, 75] each induce the same alteration in antibody production. As a consequence, IgG antibodies are not produced, germinal centres are not formed and, consequently, IgM is produced persistently. In such animals, the secondary response may be mainly of the IgM type. The alteration in the immune response cannot be attributed to an inhibition of the development of plasma cell clones, for the latter process has been proved to be drug- and radiation-resistant in the course of the therapeutic treatment of the secondary response. The maturation of B cells into IgG precursors is probably inhibited by the above interventions. It seems probable that the affected process is a proliferation associated with a drug-sensitive differentiation (Fig. 11-8).

Evidence showing the existence of B memory cells having a long life-span would substantially contribute to the importance of the interaction between T and B lymphocytes. It might be supposed that such an interaction may provide a mutagenic environment for B lymphocytes. The suggestion of Mäkelä and Cross [93] that the generator of diversity functions even at the division of peripheral lymphatic cells may be consistent with such an interaction. Favourable mutants are stimulated by the antigen more intensely, whence antibodies of greater affinity may come about. If it is so, we must not suppose the pre-existence of precursors supplied with receptors of high affinity; they may develop during the immune response.

If, after all, we compare Sterzl's theory with the classical clonal theory (Fig. 11-6), we may state that the two theories are reconcilable. However, we cannot state that the ideas presented in this chapter are necessarily correct. Numerous authors have pointed out, e.g. the possibility of an intercellular information transfer [4, 25, 26, 46*a*, *b*]. If the existence of such a transfer could be proved, the above outlined theories would need a profound reconsideration. As regards the details, all the cited data need supplementation, or may be interpreted differently. We only wanted to emphasize that the tremendously growing knowledge in the field of immunology tends to create a solid basis for a uniform synthetic view as regards the mechanisms involved in antibody formation.

## REFERENCES


1. Adler, F. L., Fishman, M. and Dray, S.: *J. Immunol.* **95,** 583 (1965).
2. Argyris, B. F.: *J. Reticuloend. Soc.* **6,** 498 (1969).
3. Basch, R.: cited by 163*b*.
4. Bell, C. and Dray, S.: *J. Immunol.* **103,** 1196 (1969).
5. Benacerraf, B., Green, I. and Paul, W. E.: *Cold Spring Harb. Symp. quant. Biol.* **32,** 569 (1967).

6. Benacerraf, B. and Levine, B. B.: *J. exp. Med.* **115,** 1023 (1962).
7. Benczur, M., Petrányi, Gy. and Alföldy, P.: *Orv. Hetil.* **112,** 183 (1971).
8. Berdardini, A., Imporato, S. and Plescia, O. U.: *Immunology* **18,** 187 (1970).
9. Berlin, B. S.: *J. exp. Med.* **113,** 1013 (1963).
10. Biozzi, G., Bianghi, R. A., Stittel, C. and Monton, D.: *Immunology* **16,** 349 (1969).
11. Boak, J. L., Kolsch, E. and Mitchison, N. A.: *Antibiot. et Chemother. (Basel)* **15,** 98 (1969).
12. Bosman, C. and Feldman, J. D.: *J. exp. Med.* **128,** 293 (1968).
13. Brody, N. I., Walker, J. G. and Siskind, G. W.: *J. exp. Med.* **126,** 81 (1967).
14. Browstone, A., Mitchison, N. A. and Pitt-Rivers, R.: *Immunology* **10,** 481 (1966).
15. Burnet, F. M.: *Cold Spring Harb. Symp. quant. Biol.* **32,** 1 (1967).
16. Bursard, A. E. and Andersson, S. G.: *Immunology* **11,** 67 (1966).
17. Byers, V. S. and Sercarz, E.: *J. exp. Med.* **128,** 715 (1968).
18. Byfield, P. and Sercarz, E.: *J. exp. Med.* **129,** 897 (1969).
19. Campbell, P. A. and Kind, P.: *J. Immunol.* **102,** 1084 (1969).
20. Cebra, J. J., Colberg, J. E. and Dray, S.: *J. exp. Med.* **123,** 547 (1966).
21. Celada, F. and Wigzell, H.: *Immunology* **11,** 453 (1966).
22. Chon, C. T., Cinader, B. and Dubiski, S.: *Cold Spring Harb. Symp. quant. Biol.* **32,** 317 (1967).
23. Claman, H. N., Chaperon, E. A. and Triplett, R. F.: *J. Immunol.* **97,** 828 (1966).
24. Cochrane, C. G. and Dixon, F. J.: *Adv. Immunol.* **2,** 205 (1962).
25. Cohen, E. P.: *Nature* **213,** 462 (1967).
26. Cohen, E. P. and Raska, K.: *Cold Spring Harb. Symp. quant. Biol.* **32,** 349 (1967).
27. Cooper, M. D., Kincade, P. W. and Lawton, A. R.: In *Immunologic Incompetence.* Ed. by Kagan, B. M. and Stiehm, E. R. Year Book Medical Publishers, Chicago 1971, p. 85.
28. Costea, N., Yakulis, U. J., Libnoch, J. A., Pilz, C. G. and Heller, P.: *Amer. J. Med.* **42,** 630 (1967).
29. Cross, A. M. and Mäkelä, O.: *Immunology* **15,** 389 (1968).
30. Cudkovitz, G., Shearer, G. M. and Priore, R. L.: *J. exp. Med.* **130,** 481 (1969).
31. Cunningham, A. J.: *Immunology* **17,** 933 (1969).
32. Curtis, J. E., Hersh, E. M., Harris, J. E., McBridge, C. and Freireich, E. J.: *Clin. exp. Immunol.* **6,** 473 (1970).
33. Davies, A. J. S., Carter, R. L., Lechars, E., Wallis, V. and Koller, P. C.: *Immunology* **16,** 57 (1969).
34. Davies, A. J. S., Lenechars, E., Wallis, V. and Koller, P. G.: *Transplantation* **4,** 438 (1966).
35. Doolittle, R. F. and Singer, S. J.: *Proc. nat. Acad. Sci. (Wash.)* **54,** 1773 (1965).
36. Dresser, D. W.: In *Proc. 4th Int. Cong. Pharmacol.* Springer, Berlin–Heidelberg 1969, p. 45.
37. Dresser, D. W. and Mitchison, N. A.: *Advanc. Immunol.* **10,** 350 (1968).
38. Dresser, D. W. and Wortis, H. H.: *Nature* **208,** 859 (1965).
39. Dubiski, S.: *Cold Spring Harb. Symp. quant. Biol.* **32,** 311 (1967).
40. Dutton, R. W.: *Advanc. Immunol.* **6,** 253 (1967).
41. Edelman, G. M. and Gall, W. E.: *Ann. Rev. Biochem.* **38,** 415 (1969).
42. Ehrlich, P.: cited by 119.
43. Elves, M. W.: *Int. Arch. Allergy* **37,** 353 (1968).
44. Fahey, J. L., Barth, W. F. and Law, L. W.: *J. nat. Cancer Inst.* **35,** 663 (1965).
45. Feldmann, M. and Diener, E.: *J. exp. Med.* **131,** 247 (1970).
46*a*. Fishman, M. and Adler, F. L.: *J. exp. Med.* **117,** 595 (1963).
46*b*. id., *Cold Spring Harb. Symp. quant. Biol.* **32,** 343 (1967).
47. Gengozian, N. and Hubner, K. F.: *J. Immunol.* **99,** 184 (1967).
48. Gery, I., Benezra, D. and Davies, A. M.: *Immunology* **16,** 381 (1969).
49*a*. Globersson, A. and Auerbach, R.: *J. exp. Med.* **124,** 1001 (1966).
49*b*. ibid., **126,** 223 (1967).
50. Gowans, J. L. and McGregor, D. D.: *Progr. Allergy* **9,** 1 (1965).
51. Gowans, J. L. and Uhr, J. W.: *J. exp. Med.* **124,** 1017 (1966).
52. Graf, M. W. and Uhr, J. W.: *J. exp. Med.* **130,** 1175 (1969).
53*a*. Greaves, M. F.: *Transplant. Rev.* **5,** 45 (1970).

53*b*. id., *Europ. J. Immunol.* **1,** 195 (1971).
54. Greaves, M. F. and Hogg, N. M.: In *Third Sigrid Jaselius Foundation Symposium on Cell Interactions in the Immune Response*. Ed. by Cross, A. Academic Press, New York 1970, p. 145.
55. Greaves, M. F., Torrigiani, G. and Roitt, I. M.: *Nature* **222,** 885 (1969).
56. Green, I., Vassalli, P., Nussenzweig, V. and Benacerraf, B.: *J. exp. Med.* **125,** 511 (1967).
57. Guillien, P., Avrameas, S. and Burtin, P.: *Immunology* **18,** 483 (1970).
58. Hamaoka, T., Kitagawa, M., Matsuoka, Y. and Yamamura, Y.: *Immunology* **17,** 55 (1969).
59. Hanna, M. G., Francis, M. W. and Peters, L. C.: *Immunology* **15,** 75 (1968).
60. Hanna, M. G., Nettesheim, P. and Francis, M. W.: *J. exp. Med.* **129,** 953 (1969).
61. Harris, G.: *Immunology* **17,** 911 (1969).
62. Haskill, J. S., Byrt, P. and Marbrook, J.: *J. exp. Med.* **131,** 57 (1970).
63. Haurowitz, F.: *Cold Spring Harb. Symp. quant. Biol.* **32,** 559 (1967).
64. Havas, H. F.: *Immunology* **17,** 819 (1969).
65*a*. Hege, J. S. and Cole, L. J.: *J. Immunol.* **96,** 559 (1966).
65*b*. ibid., **99,** 61 (1967).
66. Henry, C. and Jerne, N. K.: *J. exp. Med.* **128,** 133 (1968).
67. Hiramoto, R. N. and Hamlin, H.: *J. Immunol.* **95,** 214 (1965).
68. Hirsch, M. S., Gary, G. W. and Murphy, F. A.: *J. Immunol.* **102,** 656 (1969).
69. Hoffmann, M.: *Immunology* **18,** 791 (1970).
70. Huber, H., Douglas, S. D. and Fudenberg, H. H.: *Immunology* **17,** 7 (1969).
71. Humphrey, J. H., Parrott, D. M. V. and June, E.: *Immunology* **7,** 419 (1964).
72. Humphrey, J. H. and White, R. G.: *Immunology for Students of Medicine*. Blackwell, Oxford 1966. p. 163.
73. Jacobson, E. B., L'age-Stehr, J. and Herzenberg, L. A.: *J. exp. Med.* **131,** 1109 (1970).
74. Jacobson, E. B. and Thorbecke, G. J.: *Lab. Invest.* **19,** 635 (1968).
75. Jánossy, Gy., Petrányi, Gy. and Alföldy, P.: *Folia biol. (Prague)* **15,** 453 (1969).
76*a*. Jerne, N. K.: *Proc. nat. Acad. Sci. (Wash.)* **41,** 849 (1955).
76*b*. id., *Cold Spring Harb. Symp. quant. Biol.* **32,** 591 (1967).
77. Jerne, N. K., Nordin, A. A. and Henry, C.: In *Cell Bound Antibodies*. Ed. by Amos, B. D. and Koprowski, H. Wistar Inst. Press, Philadelphia 1963, p. 109.
78. Johnson, L. I., Sullivan, P. A., Siegel, C. D. and Chan, P.: *Brit. J. Haemat.* **13,** 168 (1967).
79. Jókay, I. and Karcag, E.: *Orvostud. (Budapest)* **19,** 221 (1968).
80. Kelus, A. S. and Gell, P. G. H.: *Progr. Allergy* **11,** 141 (1967).
81. Kennedy, J. C., Treadwell, P. E. and Lennox, E. S.: *J. exp. Med.* **132,** 353 (1970).
82. Kontiainen, S. and Mäkelä, O.: *Int. Arch. Allergy* **34,** 417 (1968).
83. Landy, M., Sanderson, R. P. and Jackson, A. L.: *J. exp. Med.* **122,** 483 (1965).
84. Lay, W. H. and Nussenzweig, V.: *J. exp. Med.* **128,** 991 (1968).
85. Lennox, E. and Cohn, M.: *Ann. Rev. Biochem.* **36,** 365 (1967).
86. Litt, M.: *Cold Spring Harb. Symp. quant. Biol.* **32,** 477 (1967).
87. Mage, R. G., Young, G. O. and Reisfeld, R. A.: *J. Immunol.* **101,** 617 (1968).
88. Makinodan, T. and Albright, J. F.: *Progr. Allergy* **10,** 1 (1967).
89. Makinodan, T. and Peterson, W. J.: *Develop. Biol.* **14,** 112 (1966).
90. Marbrook, J.: *Clin. exp. Immunol.* **3,** 367 (1968).
91. Marshall, W. H., Valentine, F. T. and Lawrence, H. S.: *J. exp. Med.* **130,** 327 (1969).
92*a*. Mäkelä, O.: *J. exp. Med.* **126,** 159 (1967).
92*b*. id., *Cold Spring Harb. Symp. quant. Biol.* **32,** 423 (1967).
93. Mäkelä, O. and Cross, A. M.: *Progr. Allergy* **14,** 145 (1970).
94. McBride, R. A. and Schierman, L. W.: *J. exp. Med.* **131,** 377 (1970).
95. McConell, I., Munroe, A., Gurner, B. N. and Coombs, R. R. A.: *Int. Arch. Allergy* **35,** 209 (1969).
96. Medawar, P. B.: *Proc. roy. Soc. Edinb.* '*B*' **148,** 145 (1958).
97. Metcalf, D.: *The Thymus*. Springer Berlin–Heidelberg 1966. p. 29.
98. Miller, J. F. A. P. and Mitchell, G. F.: *J. exp. Med.* **128,** 801 (1968).
99. Mishell, R. I. and Dutton, R. W.: *J. exp. Med.* **126,** 423 (1967).

100. Mitchell, G. F. and Miller, J. F. A. P.: *J. exp. Med.* **128,** 821 (1968).
101*a*. Mitchison, N. A.: *Cold Spring Harb. Symp. quant. Biol.* **32,** 431 (1967).
101*b*. id., In *Transptantation Today*. Ed. by Balner, H., van Bektum, B. W. and Rapaport, F. T. Grune-Stratton, New York 1971, p. 953.
102*a*. Mosier, D. E.: *Science* **158,** 1573 (1967).
102*b*. id., *J. exp. Med.* **129,** 351 (1969).
103. Mosier, D. E. and Cohen, E. P.: *Nature* **219,** 969 (1968).
104. Mosier, D. E. and Coppleson, L. W.: *Proc. nat. Acad. Sci. (Wash.)* **61,** 542 (1968).
105*a*. Möller, G.· *J. exp. Med.* **127,** 291 (1968).
105*b*. id. EMBO Int. Training Course. Stockholm 1970.
106. Möller, G. and Greaves, M. F.: *Cell. Immunol.* **1,** 372 (1970).
107. Munroe, A. and Hunter, P.: *Immunology* **23,** 69 (1972).
108. Nettesheim, P. and Makinodan, T.: *J. Immunol.* **94,** 868 (1965).
109. Nossal, G. J. V., Ada, G. L. and Austin, C. M.: *Austr. J. exp. Biol. Med. Sci.* **42,** 283 (1964).
110. Nossal, G. J. V., Austin, C. M. and Ada, G. L.: *Immunology* **9,** 333 (1965).
111. Nossal, G. J. V., Cunningham, A., Mitchell, G. F. and Miller, J. F. A. P.: *J. exp. Med.* **128,** 839 (1968).
112. Nossal, G. J. V. and Lederberg, J.: *Nature* **181,** 1419 (1958).
113. Nossal, G. J. V., Szenberg, A., Ada, G. L. and Austin, C. M.: *J. exp. Med.* **119,** 485 (1964).
114. Osoba, D.: *J. exp. Med.* **129,** 141 (1969).
115. Papermaster, B. W.: *Cold Spring Harb. Symp. quant. Biol.* **32,** 453 (1967).
116. Paul, W. E. and Siskind, G. W.: *Immunology* **18,** 921 (1970).
117. Paul, W. E., Siskind, G. W. and Benacerraf, B.: *Immunology* **13,** 147 (1967).
118. Paul, W. E., Thorbecke, J., Siskind, G. W. and Benacerraf, B.: *Immunology* **17,** 85 (1969).
119. Pearlman, D. S.: *J. exp. Med.* **126,** 127 (1967).
120. Perkins, E. H. and Makinodan, T.: *J. Immunol.* **94,** 765 (1965).
121. Perkins, E. H., Robinson, N. A. and Makinodan, T.: *J. Immunol.* **86,** 533 (1961).
122. Perkins, E. H., Sado, T. and Makinodan, T.: *J. Immunol.* **103,** 668 (1969).
123. Pernis, B., Torrigiani, G., Amante, L. Kelus, A. S. and Gebra, J. J.: *Immunology* **14,** 445 (1968).
124. Peterson, B. W. and Ingraham, J. S.: *Immunochem.* **6,** 479 (1969).
125. Petrányi, Gy.: Effects of cytostatics and irradiation on humoral and cellular immunity. Thesis. Budapest 1969.
126. Petrányi, Gy., Jánossy, Gy. and Alföldy, P.: *Nature* **221,** 77 (1969).
127. Pierce, C. W.: *J. exp. Med.* **130,** 365 (1969).
128. Pincus, C. S. and Nussenzweig, V.: *Nature* **222,** 594 (1969).
129. Putman, F. W., Titani, K., Winkler, M. and Shinoda, T.: *Cold Spring Harb. Symp. quant. Biol.* **32,** 9 (1967).
130. Radovich, J., Hemmingsen, H. and Talmage, D. W.: *J. Immunol.* **100,** 756 (1968).
131. Raff, M. C.: *Nature* **226,** 1257 (1970).
132. Raff, M. C., Sternberg, M. and Taylor, R. B.: *Nature* **225,** 553 (1970).
133. Rajewsky, K., Rosslander, E., Pelke, G. and Muller, B.: *J. exp. Med.* **126,** 581 (1967).
134. Roitt, I. M., Greaves, M. F., Torrigiani, G. and Playfair, J. H. L.: *Lancet* **ii,** 367 (1969).
135. Rowley, D. A. and Fitch, F. W.: *J. exp. Med.* **120,** 987 (1964).
136. Rowley, D. A., Fitch, F. W., Mosier, D. E., Solliday, S., Cappleson, L. W. and Brown, B. W.: *J. exp. Med.* **127,** 983 (1968).
137. Ryder, R. J. W. and Schwartz, R. S.: *J. Immunol.* **103,** 970 (1969).
138. Sahiar, K. and Schwarz, R. W.: *Science* **145,** 395 (1964).
139. Saunders, G. C.: *J. exp. Med.* **130,** 543 (1969).
140. Schierman, L. W. and McBride, R. A.: *Science* **156,** 658 (1967).
141. Sell, S.: *J. exp. Med.* **127,** 1139 (1968).
142. Sell, S. and Asofsky, R.: *Progr. Allergy* **12,** 86 (1968).
143*a*. Shearer, G. M., Cudkowitz, G. and Priore, R. L.: *J. exp. Med.* **129,** 185 (1969).
143*b*. ibid., **130,** 467 (1969).

144. Sercarz, E. and Byers, V. S.: *J. Immunol.* **98,** 836 (1967).
145. Simons, M. J. and Fitzgerald, M. G.: *Clin. Exp. Immunol.* **4,** 55 (1969).
146. Simonsen, M.: *Progr. Allergy* **6,** 349 (1962).
147. Sinclair, N. R. St. C. and Elliot, E. V.: *Immunology* **15,** 325 (1968).
148. Smithies, O.: *Cold Spring Harb. Symp. quant. Biol.* **32,** 161 (1967).
149. Steiner, L. A. and Eisen, H. N.: *J. exp. Med.* **126,** 1185 (1967).
150. Sterzl, J.: *Cold Spring Harbor Symp. quant. Biol.* **32,** 493 (1967).
151*a*. Sterzl, J. and Riha, I.: *Nature* **208,** 858 (1965).
151*b*. id., *Folia microbiol. (Prague)* **9,** 173 (1965).
152. Sterzl, J. and Silverstein, A. M.: *Adv. Immunol.* **6,** 337 (1967).
153. Svehag, S. E. and Mandel, B.: *J. exp. Med.* **119,** 21 (1964).
154. Swanson, M. A. and Schwartz, R. S.: *New Engl. J. Med.* **277,** 163 (1967).
155. Szenberg, A. and Cunningham, A. J.: *Nature* **217,** 747 (1968).
156. Talmage, D. W., Radovich, J. and Hemmingsen, H.: *J. Allergy* **43,** 323 (1969).
157. Tannenberg, W. J. K. and Malaviya, A. N.: *J. exp. Med.* **128,** 895 (1968).
158. Taylor, R. B.: *Transplant. Rev.* **1,** 114 (1969).
159. Taylor, R. B. and Wortis, H. H.: *Nature* **220,** 927 (1968).
160. Terres, G. and Wolins, H.: *Proc. Soc. exp. Biol. (N.Y.)* **102,** 632 (1959).
161. Todd, G. W. and Inman, F. P.: *Immunochemistry* **4,** 407 (1967).
162. Torrigiani, G. and Roitt, I. M.: *J. exp. Med.* **122,** 181 (1965).
163*a*. Uhr, J. W. and Finkelstein, M. S.: *J. exp. med.* **117,** 457 (1963).
163*b*. id., *Progr. Allergy* **10,** 37 (1967).
164. Valentova, V., Cerny, J. and Ivanyi, J.: *Folia biol. (Prague)* **13,** 100 (1967).
165. Vazquez, J. J. and Makinodan, T.: *Fed. Proc.* **25,** 1727 (1966).
166. Walsh, P., Maurer, P. and Egan, M.: *J. Immunol.* **98,** 344 (1967).
167. Wang, A. C., Wang, I. Y. F., McCormick, J. N. and Fudenberg, H. H.: *Immunochemistry* **6,** 451 (1969).
168. WHO Scientific Group: *Clinical Immunology. Wld Hlth Org. techn. Rep. Ser.* No. 496. WHO. Geneva 1972.
169*a*. Wigzell, H.: *Ann. Med. Exp. Fenn.* **44,** 208 (1966).
169*b*. id., *Cold Spring Harb. Symp. quant. Biol.* **32,** 507 (1967).
169*c*. id., *Quart. Rev. Biophys.* **1,** 347 (1969).
170. Wigzell, H. and Andersson, B.: *J. exp. Med.* **129,** 23 (1969).
171. Wortis, H. H., Dresser, D. W. and Andersson, H. R.: *Immunology* **17,** 93 (1969).

CHAPTER 12

# HUMAN SERUM PROTEINS

by

G. SÁNDOR



## INTRODUCTION

Modern immunochemistry has been started, we may say, in the Pasteur Institute of Paris as a result of Oudin and Grabar's work. The need for immunochemical methods arose when individual blood serum proteins had to be identified and for the study of components obtained through purification processes. The immunoelectrophoretic analyses made by Grabar and Williams showed that a very great number of various proteins is present in blood serum. In the following we shall discuss individually those proteins which have so far been fairly accurately defined. It would be very difficult to present an overall picture, for instance, with the help of an immunoelectrophoretogram. Indeed many components are present only in trace amounts and so they are not represented in blood serum immunoelectrophoresis.

To avoid repetitions we must underline that except for serum albumin (and perhaps retinol binding globulin), all serum proteins do contain carbohydrates which are composed in most cases, or possibly invariably, only of N-acetylneuraminic acid, N-acetylglucosamine, galactose, mannose and fucose. Carbohydrates are bound chemically to the polypeptide chain and the link is established, except for some IgA-paraproteins, always between the $\beta$-carboxylic acid of an asparagine residue and the pseudo-aldehydic function of a glucosamine residue.

In agreement with Oudin, we will speak about allotypes only when immunochemical differences were well established between genetically determined protein sub-classes. Therefore, we cannot speak for the time being about allotypes in the case of haptoglobins, tranferrins and albumins. This distinction is more or less arbitrary since in every case in which physicochemical differences were observed, sooner or later immunochemical ones were also discovered. A good example is that of anomalous haemoglobins; though they differ only in the nature of one amino acid residue, immunochemical differences were eventually discovered.

## SERUM ALBUMIN

Serum albumin is, from the quantitative point of view, by far the most important component. Its concentration cannot be precisely assessed with the help of the conventional techniques [48a]; immunochemistry only is able to do this. The latter provides us with two evaluations, the results of which are as follows:

| No. of cases | Mean values | Limits in 5% approximation | References |
|---|---|---|---|
| 42 | 4.30% | 3.80–4.90% | [45] |
| 98 | 4.06% | 3.38–4.74% | [22] |

The mean value is somewhat higher in the male, than in the female [22], but the statistical significance of this difference has not been firmly established. The most important physicochemical properties are the following: 15.7–16.1 per cent N; $E^{1}_{280\,m\mu}$, 1 cm $= 5.3–6.6$; $s^{20,W}_{C\to 0} = 4.1–5.5$; $D = 6.1 \cdot 10^{-7}$ cm$^2$/sec; $V = 0.73–0.74$; mol. wt.: (*i*) Svedberg's equation, 64–66,000; (*ii*) sedimentation equilibrium, 67–71,000; osmotic pressure, 68–71,000; light scattering, 70–77,000. The data are given within the limits of the technical errors.

All experimental results show that an albumin molecule is composed of only one polypeptide chain. The latter has in all known cases N-terminal aspartic acid. The nature of the C-terminal amino acid depends upon the animal species and we have leucine in the case of man. It does not contain fat, however, one or two molecules of fatty acids are *in vivo* firmly bound to it and contribute notably to its properties.

In a neutral aqueous medium the albumin molecule has probably a nearly spherical shape, but the latter is modified in acid and in alkaline medium. At present, we might accept the hypothesis of Harrington and Foster maintaining that the albumin molecule consists of little spherical parts linked together by flexible chains; the latter become straight in alkaline, as well as in acid medium This hypothesis has been proved by electron-microscopic evidence [58].

Probably as a consequence of this plastic mechanical character, albumin shows conspicuous and diversified affinities to various organic as well as mineral substances. It has a real chemical affinity to strong mineral anions, a peculiar fact for macromolecular anions. Among other mineral substances, we must mention zinc and copper ion as well as molecular iodine. Serum albumin combines readily with neutral and acid organic substances yielding a great number of various compounds. Its reaction with organic dyes are used for albumin determinations. However, here we will report primarily on combinations in which albumin is present in the native state and 40 per cent of the free fatty acids, the totality of bilirubin, about 50 per cent of sex hormones (among them the natural oestrogen, oestradiol 17 B) are linked to it. The affinity of serum albumin to the ferri-heme complexes is also conspicuous whereby methaemoglobin is linked to it. It reacts also with thyroxine and the indol residue; the affinity for the latter allows it to bind tryptophan. Penicillin and sulphonamides are drugs which are linked to albumin in the blood.

Mostly, covalent linkages do not seem to be responsible for the association of these compounds, the nature of the interaction being more complex. However, one or two great-affinity binding sites are present in many cases:

| | $Zn^{++}$ | $Cu^{++}$ | $Cl^-$ | Thyroxine | Indol | Progesterone | Fatty acids |
|---|---|---|---|---|---|---|---|
| No. of binding sites | 2 | 1 | 1–2 | 1 | 1 | 2 | 2 |

In the case of $Cu^{++}$ the site is almost certainly the N-terminal tripeptide: Asp-Thr-His [38]. Iodine is covalently bound as mono- and diiodothyrosine [61] and I-albumin is also present in the thyroid gland [53].

Presumably, these products play, at least in some cases, a physiological role. I-albumin probably takes part in iodine transport [41] and the fatty acid linking in fat metabolism.

Hereditary albumin sub-classes were first described by Knedel, Nennstiel and Becht in 1957. This is due to a very rare anomalous gene which is a co-dominant allele at the albumin locus. This is seen mostly in heterozygotes when two albumin bands appear in the electrophoretogram. However, two individuals homozygous with respect to the anomalous gene were also reported. This abnormality has no pathological consequences. Five varieties were characterized according to the electrophoretic mobility ($A_1$ . . . $A_5$ with increasing speed). A chemical analysis of the anomalous albumin was performed only in one case showing that the difference between the anomalous and the normal albumin concerns only one or two amino acids.

## ANALBUMINAEMIA

The almost total absence of serum albumin is most probably a hereditary abnormality. This very rare syndrome was first described by Bennhold in 1954, who called it analbuminaemia. The cases described by Bennhold were those of two brothers. Other cases have also been described since. Undoubtedly the pathological trait is recessively inherited; however, the albumin content remains normal for the family members who do not carry the anomalous trait. This is rather difficult to understand if we have a co-dominant anomalous gene.

Serum albumin is, in fact, not lacking entirely. Ott found in one of Bennhold's cases 18 mg per litre; others found 3–8 per cent of the normal value [31]. The lack of albumin is partly compensated by an increase of the globulin level. Ott found a total protein level of 5 per cent with a prevailing hyperalphaglobulinaemia. A thorough immunochemical study was made by Montgomery et al. with the following pathological to normal value ratios:

| Tf | $\alpha_2$M | $\beta$-lipoprot. | IgM | IgG |
|---|---|---|---|---|
| 2–3 | 3 | 3 | 3 | 1.6 |

As we see, globulin values were in most cases considerably increased. This abnormality shows that serum albumin is not absolutely necessary for life.

## LIPOPROTEINS

Quantitatively total lipoprotein comes immediately after serum albumin in importance. One litre of human serum contains 10–12 g lipoproteins [48*c*]. The great importance of lipoproteins as constituents of the living cell is well known. Though Hoppe-Seyler had supposed their existence, his hypothesis was chemically substantiated by Macheboeuf's work carried out on blood serum. In 1927 he obtained from horse serum a protein containing in defined proportions polypeptide, phosphatides and cholesterol esters. The definitive confirmation was furnished by Cohn et al. only 20 years later. By alcoholic fractionation they isolated two lipoproteins from human blood serum; one contained about 80 per cent lipids; migrating with $\beta$-globulins, it was called $\beta$-lipoprotein; the other had a lipid level of about 50 per cent and $\alpha$-globulin mobility; it was called $\alpha$-lipoprotein. Though fractionation through alcohol does not allow to obtain native lipoproteins, the fundamental facts were well established: there are low density $\beta$-lipoproteins and high density $\alpha$-lipoproteins.

A more effective purification technique was first applied by Pedersen making use of the ultracentrifuge; this was called flotation. The molecular density of lipid-free proteins equals 1.33, whereas the greatest part of blood serum lipoproteins have a molecular density less than 1.21; when the density of the solvent is at least 1.21, during ultracentrifugation lipoproteins move to the surface of the solution and other proteins descend. This flotation process, when carried out in an analytical ultracentrifuge, allows to determine the number and proportion of the individual components in a lipoprotein mixture. This latter technique was first applied to blood serum by Lewis and Page, however, the fundamental work was carried out by Goffman and his co-workers. They demonstrated the existence of low density and high density lipoproteins. The first group seems to be an extremely heterogeneous one and it is not possible to define sub-classes by the means of analytical ultracentrifugation, although this would be necessary from the physiological and pathological points of view. However, in the case of high density lipoproteins analytical ultracentrifugation revealed readily distinguishable sub-classes.

The presence in blood serum of lipoproteins with a density higher than 1.21 has been debated for a long time. According to Phillips and his co-workers such lipoproteins are present in blood serum in exceedingly small amounts and contain only glycerides and phosphatides bound to polypeptides.

## LOW DENSITY LIPOPROTEINS

When the molecular density is lower than 1.04, we speak about low density lipoproteins. They have 3 sub-classes: (*i*) low density lipoproteins proper (LDL); (*ii*) very low density lipoproteins (VLDL); (*iii*) chylomicrons.

At first it is necessary to comment on the meaning of the flotation coefficient of Goffman. Flotation is opposite in sign to the usual direction of sedimentation, and $s_F$ is the speed expressed in Svedberg units, with which the lipoprotein molecule moves during ultracentrifugation if the density of the solution is adjusted to 1.063. This coefficient, therefore, characterizes only low density lipoproteins. The peculiar relationship of an increasing mol. wt. and decreasing density with increasing $s_F$ values has been demonstrated.

The sub-group LDL itself is extremely heterogeneous. It contains a great number of substances with various fat levels, fat compositions and molecular weights. In a more or less conventional fashion, we may say that lipoproteins having molecular densities between 1.006 and 1.04 and $s_F$ values ranging between 0 and 20 belong to the LDL sub-group. Most probably they have the following mean composition:

| Poly-peptides | Cholesterol | Phospho-lipids | Glycerides | $\frac{\text{Free cholesterol}}{\text{Total cholesterol}}$ |
|---|---|---|---|---|
| 20% | 46.5% | 23% | 10.5% | 0.2 |

The lipoproteins defined in that manner make out at least 90 per cent of the fasting subjects' low density lipoproteins; therefore they determine predominantly the flotation diagram of blood serum at a density of 1.063. However, the composition and also the flotation diagram of LDL show individual variations depending perhaps upon hereditary factors [30]. The LDL concentration is not constant either; e.g. it is relatively high for man having group A blood. Individual hereditary factors are even more decisive. It is well known that there are families the blood sera of whose members show high LDL levels; in these families atheroma is frequent. Another most probably hereditary character is a high glyceride level in LDL; atheroma in relatively young subjects is frequent also in this case.

LDL is highly resistant to protease action. Pepsin has no detectable effect and papain and chymotrypsin are effective only until about 20 per cent of the polypeptide chain has been distroyed without, however, any fats being liberated. Whereas after the extraction of the native lipoproteins with organic solvents the remaining polypeptide part could not be dissolved in water, when the same extraction is carried out after protease action, a water-soluble polypeptide part is left [47] whose physicochemical properties can be readily studied. In the presence of sodium dodecylsulphate the peptide part having a high molecular weight yields homogeneous 15–20,000 mol. wt. fragments [47]. At least one glutamic acid can be detected in N-terminal position and one serine residue in C-terminal position. Sugar content is as follows: 3.2 per cent hexose; 1.2 per cent hexosamine; 0.3 per cent neuraminic acid. However, it is certain today that LDL is heterogeneous from the chemical point of view. It seems to contain, in low concentrations, the peptide with C-terminal alanine which is present in a high proportion in the VLDL-apoprotein, as well as the peptide with C-terminal threonine, chief component of HDL.

As far as immunochemical properties are concerned, we must underline the fact that they do not depend at all upon the lipid components; this is a common law for serum lipoproteins. Therefore *a priori* it was possible that all LDL subgroups may have the same immunological specificity though their fat content and composition are very different. However, today the chemical and immunological heterogeneity of LDL is generally accepted. The present idea is that all serum lipoproteins contain the same apoproteins the number of which is at least 3 and their individual levels vary from one lipoprotein group to the other. Apo-A is the chief component of HDL, apo-B that of LDL, and apo-C is present in all groups in smaller amounts. It must be recalled that the latter is the main component of an anomalous lipoprotein, which is present in great amounts in patients suffering from obstructive jaundice; it has a high phosphatide level and its apoprotein contains also serum albumin.

The blood serum level of the second low density lipoprotein group (VLDL) is very low; they can be evidenced only in certain hyperlipaemias. Normally three lipoprotein bands of the human serum appear during paper electrophoresis; two of these are always present: (*i*) LDL moving with $\beta$-globulins; and (*ii*) HDL moving with $\alpha$-globulins. The third lipoprotein band remains as a rule at the site of the serum depot (0-band) and appears here only in those hyperlipaemias in which the glyceride level is very high. In such cases there may be an increase in the VLDL and chylomicron levels.

However, when electrophoresis is carried out in the presence of a solution containing 1 per cent serum albumin, the greatest part of VLDL reaches the zone between $\beta$- and $\alpha$-globulins (pre-$\beta$-lipoprotein), but the chylomicrons remain at the depot site [25]. It is generally accepted [17*a*, *b*] that the molecular density of VLDL remains between 0.93 and 1.006, whereas its $s_F$ value ranges between 20 and 400 [13]. Mean composition is as follows:

| Protein | Triglycerides | Cholesterol free | Cholesterol ester | Phosphatides | Sugars |
|---|---|---|---|---|---|
| 10% | 50–70% | 10% | 5% | 15–20% | < 1% |

Ninety per cent of the apoprotein of VLDL is constitued by 4 different polypeptides, about 40 per cent of which are LDL-apoprotein (B-apo). A small amount of the HDL-apoprotein (A-apo) is also present.

Great quantities of chylomicrons appear in the chyle after a meal rich in fats giving the milky appearance of the chyle. Only a very small amount reaches the blood in healthy subjects; nevertheless high levels appear in certain pathological conditions, mostly giant molecules having $s_F$ values above 400 S. The mean values of several determinations are as follows:

| Protein | Triglycerides | Cholesterol free | Cholesterol ester | Phosphatides |
|---|---|---|---|---|
| 1–2% | 80–95% | 1–5% | 2–4% | 3–8% |

The exact nature of the chylomicron-apoprotein is not yet known. Chylomicrons adsorb vigorously albumin and $\gamma$-globulins, but this is most probably due to secondary physical processes. It is almost sure that LDL-apoprotein (B-apo) is one of their components; indeed in the hereditary disease called a-$\beta$-lipoproteinaemia, in which this apoprotein is lacking, chylomicrons cannot be synthesized.

A number of purely conventional physicochemical statements have been made in the preceeding paragraphs. Some of the LDL have undoubtedly $s_F$ values above 20 S and no sharp distinction can be made between VLDL and chylomicrons. However, these 3 lipoproteins can mostly be well distinguished by physiological or pathological considerations. LDLs are especially rich in cholesterol; their increased level, which is often a hereditary trait, is responsible for hypercholesterolaemia and atheromatous disease. In typical cases increased VLDL and chylomicron levels produce two different hyperglyceridaemic syndromes. Ahrens and his co-workers were the first to differentiate between the two, i.e. between endogenous and exogenous hyperglyceridaemias; the first one is elicited by a diet rich in carbohydrates in some acquired or hereditary pathologic states, whereas the second type is caused, under the same conditions, by fatty diet. Glycerides are joined to VLDLs in endogenous hyperlipaemias and to chylomicrons in the exogenous form of the disease [13, 28].

This supposition is undoubtedly valid in its general outlines. In 1956 Gilliers et al. studied the fatty acid composition of the different kinds of LDL. They showed that the arachidonic and linoleic acid levels are relatively high in the 0–20 S sub-group, whereas oleic acid is the chief component of the unsaturated fatty acids in the case of the 20–400 S sub-group. This is also true for the depot-fat of the body, therefore the 20–400 S sub-group might be of endogenous origin [13]. On the contrary, the fatty acid composition of chylomicrons is the same as that of alimentary fat. However, atypical hyperglyceridaemias occur frequently, and it is, therefore, not always easy to distinguish between VLDL and chylomicrons on the one hand, and endogenous and exogenous hyperlipaemias, on the other. It must be added that not only chylomicrons but also VLDLs are synthesized in the small bowel making their participation in exogenous fatty acid transport probable.

## HIGH DENSITY LIPOPROTEINS

Of the three HDLs characterized by Goffman only two could be isolated and studied. The least dense one ($HDL_1$) has a molecular density of only 1.05, therefore it remains for the most part with LDL during fractionation processes. The other two HDLs are $HDL_2$ and $HDL_3$, the latter being the densest. They have the following chemical properties:

| | Total fat | Composition of lipids | | | Free cholesterol / Total cholesterol |
|---|---|---|---|---|---|
| | | phosphatides | cholesterol | glycerides | |
| $HDL_2$ | 67% | 43.3% | 44.6% | 11.9% | 0.3 |
| $HDL_3$ | 41% | 48.8% | 36.6% | 14.6% | 0.13 |

Some of the glycerides are free fatty acids comprising, according to Lindgren and his co-workers, 6 per cent of the total fatty substances of the HDL. Highly purified HDLs have the following physicochemical properties according to two independent studies:

| | $HDL_2$ | | $HDL_3$ | |
|---|---|---|---|---|
| | I | II | I | II |
| Molecular density | 1.099 | 1.106 | 1.149 | 1.153 |
| Sedimentation coefficient | 5.5 S | 5.44 S | 5 S | 4.64 S |
| Molecular weight | | | | |
| Stoke's law | 365,000 | — | 165,000 | — |
| sedimentation equilibrium | 435,000 | 400,000 | 145,000 | 174,000 |

I = determination made by Shore; II = determination made by Hazelwood

Both HDLs have the same amino acid composition and the chief terminal amino acids are also identical (N-terminal aspartic acid and C-terminal threonine) [57*a, b*]; therefore, their apoproteins must be identical. It was supposed that $HDL_3$ is only an artifact resulting at ultracentrifugation.

HDL-apoprotein is relatively easy to obtain in a water soluble state. Its aqueous solution shows heterodispersity with a chief component of 2.3–2.6 S [57*a, b*]. However, in the presence of dodecylsulphate only one ultracentrifugal component appears having a molecular weight of 20–30,000 [46, 57*a, b*]. A chemical heterogeneity nevertheless remains, since two different polypeptide chains correspond to the one ultracentrifugal component. It is possible that the structure of the HDL-apoprotein is even more complex. By gel filtration on Sephadex G 200 three chief components can be evidenced; further a very small part of the apoprotein (3–5 per cent) seems to be a polypeptide mixture comprising also VLDL-apoproteins.

All HDL-apoproteins have the following properties: 16.2 per cent N; 0.85 per cent hexose; 0.6 per cent fucose; 0.48 per cent neuraminic acid; $E^{1\%, 1cm}_{289 m\mu} = 10.8$. It binds strongly various lipids. When a phosphatide emulsion is added in excess to its aqueous solution, a compound with constant composition is obtained [51] (about 33 per cent phosphatides; $s = 3.6$ S; mol. wt., 94,000). This affinity is not altered by denaturation and other chemical influences.

There is no immunological difference between $HDL_2$ and $HDL_3$. We have reported above that according to Alaupovic and others all serum proteins contain the same apoproteins varying only in their relative proportions. It must, however, be recalled that up to now we could not detect any immunological relation between HDL and LDL.

## LIPOPROTEIN LEVEL IN THE BLOOD SERUM OF HEALTHY PEOPLE

It is not easy to evaluate the normal lipoprotein content of blood serum owing to differences in the way of life and hereditary factors as well as to technical difficulties. Using the analytical ultracentrifuge the same research group obtained the following two sets of results; in g per litre (11 years elapsed between the two determinations):

| LDL | | | $HDL_2$ | $HDL_3$ | LDL / Total LP | Total |
|---|---|---|---|---|---|---|
| 400 S | 12–400 S | 0–12 S | | | | |
| 0.07 | 1.11 | 3.36 | 1.13 | 2.43 | 0.56 | 8.1 |
| — | 2.6 | 3.64 | 0.61 | 1.78 | 0.72 | 8.63 |

Considering that mean values are quoted, the differences are rather great.

TABLE 12-I

*Human blood serum lipoprotein levels*

| Age (years) | Sex | LDL 0–12 S | LDL 12–400 S | HDL | Total LP | LDL / Total LP |
|---|---|---|---|---|---|---|
| 20–39 | M | 2.57 | 2.21 | 2.55 | 7.33 | 0.65 |
| | F | 2.98 | 1.36 | 3.21 | 7.55 | 0.58 |
| 40–65 | M | 3.81 | 2.35 | 2.59 | 8.75 | 0.7 |
| | F | 3.57 | 2.03 | 3.23 | 8.83 | 0.63 |

| Sex | (1) LDL 400 S | 100—400 S | 20—100 S | 12–20 S | 0–12 S |
|---|---|---|---|---|---|
| M | 0.11 | 0.36 | 0.89 | 0.40 | 3.69 |
| F | 0.03 | 0.06 | 0.30 | 0.20 | 3.03 |

| Sex | (2) HDL $HDL_2$ | $HDL_3$ | total HDL | LDL / Total LP | Total LP |
|---|---|---|---|---|---|
| M | 0.53 | 2.22 | 2.75 | 0.67 | 8.14 |
| F | 1.72 | 2.64 | 4.37 | 0.45 | 7.99 |

*Note.* Levels are expressed in g per litre

Serum lipoprotein concentration varies with sex (Table 12-I). The two series of mean values in the Table are noticeably different, however a higher HDL value in females is characteristic throughout. Cohn's alcohol fractionation method, too, yields higher $\alpha$-lipoprotein values for women. Further the following values were obtained by Barr and his co-workers in 1951 with the help of preparative flotation:

| Age (years) | Sex | HDL | LDL | LDL / Total LP |
|---|---|---|---|---|
| 30–39 | male | 3.46 | 4.78 | 0.58 |
| | female | 4.35 | 4.70 | 0.52 |

Table 12-I shows that especially $HDL_2$ shows an increased level in female serum; according to some authors [4] the $HDL_2$ level increases during the first two weeks of the menstrual cycle. No differences as regards the LDL level can be established between men and women. Nevertheless, in 1958 Burstein using the specific dextran sulphate precipitation technique, obtained notably higher LDL values for young men than for young women.

It seems that the LDL level increases with age. The results in Table 12-I show significant differences between men older and younger than 40 years; comparable results were obtained also by other workers [13]. According to Burstein LDL changes with age as follows (in g per litre):

| Mean age (years) | 25 | 35 | 45 | 55 |
|---|---|---|---|---|
| Men | 3.85 | 4.20 | 4.65 | 5 |
| Women | 3.1 | 3.4 | 4.25 | 4.65 |

On the contrary, the HDL level does not seem to vary with age.

## SERUM LIPID LEVEL AND COMPOSITION

Serum lipids are in general bound to proteins. From a critical evaluation of the rather contradictory literature, the following most probable lipid composition can be deduced (in g per litre) [48*b*]:

| | Total cholesterol | Phosphatides | Total lipids | Difference | Free cholesterol / Total cholesterol |
|---|---|---|---|---|---|
| Mean | 2.1 | 3.3 | 7.3–7.9 | 2.25 | 0.27 |
| S.D. | 1 | 0.3 | — | — | 0.014 |

'Difference' is that between total lipids, on the one hand, and the sum of total cholesterol and cholesterol esters, as well as phosphatides, on the other. The value found: 2.25 g per litre, is much higher than the glyceride concentration, which is about 0.8 g per litre in young subjects, and 1.2 g per litre in the aged. Our knowledge of serum lipid composition is at present rather scanty; paraffines are most probably present, but only in small amounts.

The glyceride level increases with age; therefore the concentration of lipoproteins with $s_F$ values greater than 20 S would also increase with age, since only this group of lipoproteins carries noticeable amounts of glycerides. However, data obtained by analytical ultracentrifugation do not confirm this supposition. We notice also a slight increase of the serum cholesterol level with age together with an increasee in the LDL level. It must be added that at birth, umbilical cord serum contains only small quantities of lipids (0.8 g cholesterol, 1.2 g phosphatides, 0.34 g glycerides per litre). Women's blood serum shows a slightly lower level of glycerides than that of men; however, no difference in the cholesterol level has been demonstrated.

## LIPOPROTEIN ALLOTYPES

It is interesting to recall that the Australia hepatitis antigen was first taken for an allotype of human serum lipoproteins. Real allotypes were, however, discovered in the LDL group; they pertain to two groups: (*i*) the Ag system has been demonstrated by isoimmunization—we know today four allotypes of this kind; (*ii*) the Lp system has been detected by heteroimmunization. Two genetic loci are supposed to exist: Lp(a) and Lp(x) and of the possible allotypes three have been recognized: Lp($a^+x^+$), Lp($a^+x^-$) anf Lp($a^-x^+$). The trait is most probably autosomal and dominant. It must be added that no relationship could be detected between the Ag and the Lp systems. Lipoprotein allotypes have been described also in rabbits.

### *Abetalipoproteinaemia (acanthocytosis)*

A considerable decrease or total lack of LPL appears as a rare hereditary trait causing a well-defined clinical syndrome, which was first recognized by Bassen and Kornzweig in 1950 in the case of two brothers. The basic symptoms were detected on a third case one year later by Singer.

Today this syndrome is mostly known as abetalipoproteinaemia, but the term acanthocytosis, originally proposed by Druez, is also used. The latter expression is connected with the sea-urchin-like appearance of erythrocytes, a chief characteristic of this condition. However, abetalipoproteinaemia is a more correct term, since acanthocytosis may occur in other pathological conditions, too.

Acanthocytosis in abetalipoproteinaemia appears with a diarrhoea resembling sprue in the first days after birth; later atypical retinitis pigmentosa makes its appearance, physical and mental development is retarded, and a nervous disease somewhat similar to Friedreich's ataxia is observed. The life span of erythrocytes is greatly reduced and fatty infiltration in the intestinal mucosa and hepatocytes is also characteristic. The sprue syndrome is quickly improved by a restriction of dietary fat.

No $\beta$-lipoproteins appear in the electrophoretograms, but data obtained by more sensitive immunochemical methods are contradictory. Trace amounts were detected by Salt et al. (about 1/1000th of the normal value); Levi et al. [27] reported the absence of all $\beta$-lipoproteins, although they studied members of 6 affected families. Flotation yields a small amount of low density lipoprotein, which, however, shows HDL-specificity and must therefore, contain HDL-apoprotein [27]. HDL level also diminishes, but only that of $HDL_3$ [23]. We quote from the work of Fredrickson et al. [13] the following ranges of lipid levels (in g per litre):

| Cholesterol | Phosphatides | Glycerides |
|---|---|---|
| 0.2–0.9 | 0.35–0.95 | 0.1–0.2 |

As we see, lipids of all classes show decreased levels. Also qualitative changes in blood serum and in the erythrocytes can be observed: the levels of lecithin and plasmalogen decrease while that of sphingomyelin increases. These biochemical symptoms are not to be found in other disturbances of intestinal absorption. A decrease in the level of the indispensable poly-unsaturated fatty acids may also be observed, but this is common to all intestinal absorption deficiencies. The level of nervonic acid, a component of cerebrosides, is also increased. It must be underlined that abetalipoproteinaemic serum gave in all observed cases a precipitate with normal human LDL.

A fundamental defect of the glyceride transport is evidenced by the fatty infiltration of intestinal mucosa and of hepatocytes. Neither endogenous, nor exogenous hyperglyceridaemia can be produced in the affected subjects [27]; however, even a very abundant and protracted blood serum transfusion failed to improve intestinal fat absorption, although the $\beta$-lipoprotein level became normal. On the other hand, acanthocytosis ceases when certain surface active substances are added to the blood.

The syndrome is caused by LDL deficiency. Incomplete intestinal absorption, fatty infiltration of cells and the very low level of glycerides in the serum show that LDLs play a prevailing role in glyceride transport. In fact, this is a task of LDL-apoprotein and not of LDL. It has already been said that LDL-apoprotein is an important component of VLDL, and therefore, it is easy to understand why it is not possible to produce endogenous hyperglyceridaemia in abetalipoproteinaemia. The same fact with exogenous hyperglyceridaemia proves that LDL-apoprotein contributes also to chylomicron synthesis. We can explain also the inefficacy of exogenous LDL given with the aim of improving fat absorption. As far as our present knowledge goes, LDL originates from VLDL through the loss of the glyceride content of the latter; but once produced, LDL cannot undergo any metabolic change which would be necessary for glyceride transport.

The red cell symptom, retinitis, as well as the involvement of the nervous system can be explained by a slow loss of an indispensable cellular lipoprotein whereas the body fluids do not contain LDL [62]. A similar hypothesis was put forward by Dodge et al. in 1967 claiming that acanthocytosis is due to vitamin E deficiency; in 1968 McBridge and Jacob postulated that an increase in the cholesterol content of the cells might be involved.

It may be that abetalipoproteinaemia is not always governed by the same genetic law. In the case of the family studied by Salt et al. many apparently healthy subjects had about the half of the normal LDL level, while in the affected family reported by Ways and his co-workers all healthy subjects had normal LDL concentration. Therefore, the genetic trait seems to be truly dominant and only apparently recessive in Salt's case, whereas in the family observed by Ways a real recessive hereditary character prevailed.

About 20 cases were reported up to now; some atypical hypobetaglobulinaemia cases were also quoted, in which the LDL level was only partially reduced, but the clinical symptoms were the same.

### *Tangier disease*

In rare cases a decrease in serum HDL occurs as a hereditary trait. The syndrome was first observed in two brothers from the island of Tangier; therefore the disease was called Tangier disease. The expression is not correct, since the abnormality was detected later in two other families with no relations with Tangier [26].

The clinical symptoms are discoloured tonsils often associated with spleno- and hepatomegaly, as well as with enlarged lymph nodes. These symptoms are due to the cholesterol surcharge of macrophages.

In homozygotes the serum HDL level is very low, whereas it is moderately decreased in heterozygotes. Further, the small amount of HDL present in the blood serum of homozygotes has anomalous immunochemical characters ('Tangier α-lipoprotein') [26]. In heterozygotes no pathological symptoms can be observed.

When the carbohydrate content of the food is not restricted, patients have a slightly elevated serum glyceride level, but the cholesterol and phosphatide levels are decreased. Fredrickson et al. [13] reported the following values (in g per litre):

| | Cholesterol | Phosphatides | Glycerides |
|---|---|---|---|
| Mean | 0.7 | 1 | — |
| Range | 0.5–1.3 | 0.7–1.4 | 1.2–1.8 |

Glyceride level can be rapidly decreased with carbohydrate restriction and, in turn, hyperglyceridaemia is easily produced with a diet rich in carbohydrates. In this kind of endogenous hyperglyceridaemia VLDL does not appear and the glycerides are linked to LDL, the density of which will thus decrease. On the other hand, chylomicrons are produced by a diet rich in fat, only their cholesterol content is low [13, 27, 28]. This seems to prove that HDL-apoprotein is needed for VLDL synthesis, whereas chylomicrons can be synthesized even without HDL-apoproteins being present.

The genetic trait is autosomal and dominant. According to the simplest explanation there would be two alleles: $G^A$ and $G^a$, at the G locus controlling HDL-apoprotein. HDL level is normal in AA homozygotes, half of the normal level in Aa heterozygotes and there is a total lack of HDL in aa homozygotes.

### *Deficiency of cholesterol-lecithin acyltransferase*

The lack of the serum cholesterol-lecithin-acyltransferase was only observed in three sisters up to now. The clinical symptoms included proteinuria, anaemia, lipid deposition in the tissues and a practically total absence of esterified cholesterol from the serum. Therefore, this disease also supports the earlier hypothesis on the origin of serum esterified cholesterol according to which cholesterol is esterified in the circulating blood at the expense of the fatty acid in $\beta$-position on the lecithin molecule and the reaction is catalyzed by cholesterol-lecithin acyltransferase. High lecithin levels and decreased lyso-lecithin levels were also found in these patients. The small amount of esterified cholesterol present in their serum must have come from the intestines since the fatty acids it contained had the composition of alimentary fat.

## $\alpha_2$M-GLOBULIN

$\alpha_2$M-globulin is present in blood serum in relatively great amounts. It was obtained in a pure state by Brown and his co-workers and by Schultze and Biehl in 1954 at about the same time. Its phys cochemical properties are as follows: $s^{20,w}_{c\to 0} = 19.6$ S; $D = 2.4\times 10^{-7}$ cm²/sec; $\bar{V} = 0.735$; mol. wt., 900,000; isoelectric point, pH 5.4; 14–14.8 per cent N; 5.3 per cent hexose; 3.8 per cent hexosamine; $E^{1\%\ 1cm}_{280\ m\mu} = 12.8$. Reducing substances do not change its molecular weight; the molecule is, however, divided into two parts in concentrated urea solution, the molecular weights of which are 600,000 and 300,000 respectively. The pattern seen at electron-microscopic examination is best explained by presuming that the molecule is composed of five linear monomers.

The serum level of $\alpha_2$M-globulin is mostly determined immunochemically, but it can be determined also indirectly by measuring its peculiar anti-trypsin effect (see later). The levels obtained vary notably, showing, however, a strong correlation with age. According to Ganrot and Schersten [14], its level is high in cord serum, increases further after birth reaching its highest value between 1 and 3 years; thereafter it decreases continuously remaining, however, higher for females than for males above 17 years; the results of these authors were not statistically analysed. Our own results were submitted to a statistical control. We confirmed the continuous decrease with age, but the sex difference could not be established with certainty. A slightly higher value for females than for males was observed only between 20 and 30 years but the significance remained at the limit of the 5 per cent approximation [50].

| Age and sex | <15 years | 15–20 years | 20–30 years men | 20–30 years women | >30 years |
|---|---|---|---|---|---|
| Mean | 3.62 | 3.31 | 2.85 | 3.04 | 2.50 |
| S.D. | 0.54 | 0.31 | 0.22 | 0.36 | 0.32 |

It must be added that above 30 years the level remained constant. The different determinations in adults gave most often concentrations between 2 and 3 g per litre.

$\alpha_2$M-globulin inhibits the action on proteins of several proteases (plasmin, trypsin, chymotrypsin, thrombin), but does not interfere with their effect on esters. It is responsible for about half of the serum anti-thrombin effect [59] and it disappears almost entirely from circulating blood during intra-circulatory fibrinolysis probably through being bound to the activated plasminogen [35].

The age dependence of $\alpha_2$M-globulin level is even more conspicuous in the case of the rat: it entirely disappears from the blood of the adult animal. However, it appears during pregnancy and in cancer-bearing animals.

In human serum two allotypes have been demonstrated [5] and such allotypes have been found in the rabbit and chimpanzee serum as well.

As regards its physiological role, it must have an effect on tissue proliferation, since its level decreases strongly during the growth period. However, according to our own experience, it is not involved in malignant cell proliferation at least not in humans. Physiological and pathological data show that it most probably acts primarily on the lympho-plasma cell system.

## TRANSFERRIN

The entire amount of serum iron is bound to a protein which was first obtained by Koechlin in 1952, who called it siderophilin; the name transferrin, which is generally accepted today, makes reference to its role in iron transport.

According to chemical determinations, blood serum contains 2–2.5 g per litre of transferrin. A precise immunochemical determination has been carried out by Goodman et al. They found a mean value of 2.82 g per litre, and a range of 2.29 to 3.6 g per litre. Its iron binding capacity is saturated only to 1/3 in normal serum. Cord serum contains more iron than adult serum and less transferrin, while pregnant women's blood serum is rich in the latter and poor in iron.

Its physicochemical properties are as follows: mol. wt., 85,000; $s = 5.1\,S$; $D = 5.5 \times 10^{-7}$ cm²/sec; isoelectric point: (*i*) apotransferrin, pH 5.5; (*ii*) iron saturated transferrin, pH 5.1; $E^{1\%\ 1\mathrm{cm}}_{280\mathrm{m}\mu} = 14.1$; 14.7 per cent N; iron content in the iron saturated state: 1.25 mg per g. The $Fe^{+++}$ containing protein is red in colour; its highest light absorption is in the visible at 470 m$\mu$ and the corresponding extinction coefficient is 60. Most probably it contains only one polypeptide chain with an N-terminal valine residue.

Two iron atoms are bound by one molecule transferrin; in a neutral medium this is the strongest iron link known up to now; however, during denaturation the affinity disappears. As regards the iron binding site, it is usually accepted since Vallée and Ulmer's work [60] that the phenolic groups of three tyrosine residues take part in the linking; further 2 or 3 histidine residues add their effect and the protein must bind one molecule $CO_2$.

According to Jamieson [21*a*, *b*], each transferrin molecule contains two identical oligosaccharides, which are bound by different amino acid patterns. The polypeptide is linked to the oligosaccharide by an asparagin residue in both cases, but it is followed by lysine in one of them and by serine in the other. Hen blood transferrin contains two similar oligosaccharides and differs from conalbumin only in the composition of the latter; however, in the rabbit, the same polysaccharide part is found in the transferrin present in blood serum and in that in milk.

Owing to their different electrophoretic mobilities in starch gel, genetically determined transferrin sub-classes could be detected for various species (man, monkey, ox, sheep, rat). Three sub-classes were demonstrated in man by Smithies; he called them in the order of their decreasing migration velocities: $Tf_B$, $Tf_C$, $Tf_D$. In white individuals $Tf_C$ is found mostly in itself, whereas in black people and Australian aborigines often $Tf_C$ and $Tf_D$ are present simultaneously. The three sub-classes are determined by three alleles, but each sub-class has many varieties; 12 different transferrins are known today. Up to now the reason for the differences in electrophoretic mobility is unknown; most probably they are due to differences in amino acid composition, since they do not disappear after neuraminidase treatment.

## $\beta_1$C-GLOBULIN AND THE COMPLEMENT

In the following we shall only discuss the physicochemical properties of proteins having a part in the complement reaction without discussing their role in it. $\beta_1$C-globulin is a quantitatively important protein fairly well known with a generally accepted role in C3 activity. It is characterized by a very limited water solubility and is a typical 'euglobulin'. Oncley et al. postulated its existence more than 20 years ago, however, it was obtained in a pure form only in 1965 [36]. It occurs in fresh blood serum as a slowly moving $\beta_1$-globulin having a 9.5 S sedimentation coefficient; it is very instable, it may undergo modifications of two kinds [33]: (*i*) during immune haemolysis its electrophoretic mobility increases and it becomes a faster moving $\beta_1$-globulin without, however, a change in its molecular weight; Mueller-Eberhard called this modification $\beta_1$-C-globulin; (*ii*) another kind of modification may be due to: (1) the presence of an antigen–antibody complex, (2) blood conservation; (3) some peculiar carbohydrates (zymosan etc.). The molecule dissociates into several fragments the greatest of which is a fast moving $\beta_1$-globulin ($\beta_1$A-globulin) with a sedimentation coefficient of 7 S. Two of the smaller fragments known today are $\alpha_2$-globulin (West et al. 1966; $\alpha_2$D) and a $\beta_2$-globulin. It must be underlined that similar or even identical fragments are also produced by the serum protease, plasmin. The speed of the spontaneous transformation increases with the temperature: at 1 °C it takes 14 days, whereas at 20 °C only a few days. Since the largest fragment,

$\beta_1$A-globulin, preserves most of its immunological properties, when the transformation is not yet complete a characteristic double curved precipitation line appears on the immunoelectrophoretograms one curvature corresponding to the original $\beta_1$C-globulin in the slow $\beta_1$ zone and the other to $\beta_1$A-globulin in the fast $\beta_1$ zone.

The $\beta_1$C-globulin level of human serum has been determined several times by immunochemical methods. Though the results are rather diverse, the most probable mean value is 1.4–1.5 g per litre. A statistically significant decrease in the serum level can be detected above 30 years of age.

It is strange to find such a high level for a complement component. However, several facts point to its participation in C activity. Physicochemical alterations of the $\beta_1$C-globulin cause a disappearance of complement activity; $\beta_1$C-globulin and C disappear together under the effect of cobra venom. There is no close correlation between the $\beta_1$C-globulin value and C activity, however $\beta_1$C-globulin is mostly present when there is a C activity and in opsonization its concentration is limiting as $\beta_1$C-globulin concentration is closely linked to this activity.

$\beta_1$C-globulin has several genetic sub-classes, which can be distinguished thanks to their different electrophoretic mobilities in agarose [2*a*, *b*]. The two most important varieties are the S (slow) and the F (fast) sub-classes, but we know five less frequent varieties with intermediate electrophoretic mobilities. Seven co-dominant alleles correspond to a single locus. The S sub-class occurs in the serum of about 75 per cent of the white population and the F sub-class in the remaining 25 per cent; the latter is somewhat rarer in black man and Asiatic aborigines. The serum of heterozygotes contains both sub-classes in equal amounts.

Several proteins take part in C1 activity; the first of them was isolated by Brumfield and his co-workers (1959, 1961). It is a fast moving $\gamma$-globulin with a $s$ of 11 S ($C1_q$). Its molecular weight is 390,000 and its serum level about 0.1 g per litre; it can be readily dissociated by urea to monomers of mol. wt. of 40–60,000. Two other C1 components are $C1_r$ and $C1_s$; the latter is a proesterase which is activated during C activity. Naff and his co-workers (1964) postulated that the three components are linked together in native blood serum to constitute a single component containing also $Ca^{++}$, but according to Namura and Nelson (1967) no such component exists. Nagaki and his co-workers (1969, 1970) found that activated $C1_s$ is an $\alpha_1$-globulin with a molecular wight of 110,000; its level in human serum would be 33 mg per litre.

C2 of human serum is a $\beta_2$-globulin first isolated by Polley and Mueller-Eberhard [40] ($s = 5.2$ S; $D = 4 \times 10^{-7}$ cm²/sec; mol. wt., 117,000). Its level in human blood serum is $10 \pm 2$ mg per litre.

What was originally defined as C3 activity depends, in fact, not only upon $\beta_1$C-globulin. Of the four other globulins also contributing to it, two were obtained in a pure form [36]. Since the symbol C3 has been preserved for $\beta_1$C-globulin, the new globulins were called C5 and C6. C5 is a $\beta_1$-globulin having a $s$ of 8.7 S; its mean level in human blood serum is 76 mg per litre. C6 has a $\beta_2$-globulin mobility, a $s$ of 5 S and its level in human serum is 24 mg per litre.

C4 of human serum was first isolated by Mueller-Eberhard and Biro [32]; it is a $\beta_1$-'pseudoglobulin' with a $s$ of 10 S. It has a high level in human serum (0.44 $\pm$0.12 g per litre).

Human C8 has been identified by Mann and his co-workers in 1969; it is a $\gamma_1$-

globulin on agarose and an $\alpha_2$-globulin on agar agar; its molecular weight is 50,000 and its serum level 14 mg per litre.

Pillemer's properdin known to destroy C3 in the presence of certain carbohydrates was considered by some authors a complement component. It was thought to be a mixture of heterogeneous substances and even perhaps of antibodies. However, later Pensky et al. [37] isolated properdin in a pure form having the following properties: $s^{1\%}_{20,W} = 5\text{–}5.3$ S; $D = 2.15 \times 10^{-7}$ cm$^2$/sec; mol.wt., 216–230,000. It moves more slowly than $\gamma$-globulins in acrylamide gel or on cellulose acetate; it remains in the $\beta$-globulin zone during immunoelectrophoresis.

Partial or total lack of complement activity was first observed in guinea-pigs as a typical recessive hereditary trait. In certain inbred mouse strains the lack of an immunologically well-defined $\alpha_2$-globulin involves the disappearance of complement activity; it seems to be C5 and the deficiency is transmitted as a dominant hereditary trait. C6 deficiency has been detected in a rabbit strain. Defective C2 in humans has been observed in four families as an autosomal and most probably dominant trait. Instead of the normal mean value of 10 mg per litre, 3–6 mg have been found in heterozygotes and only 0.5–4 per cent of the normal mean in homozygotes.

The lack of complement activity has no pathologic consequences either in man or in animals. However, another hereditary trait which only modifies the complement activity is responsible for the condition called familiary angioneurotic oedema. A deficiency of serum C1 esterase inhibitor activity can be observed in all the cases, but this can result from two different kinds of serum protein disturbances, namely (*i*) lack of the C1 esterase inhibitor [11], or (*ii*) the presence of the inhibitor protein in an inactive form [44]. Forty-four affected families were observed by Alper and his co-workers (1970). In 38 of them the serum of the diseased subjects contained only trace amounts of the inhibitor protein; in the other six families the protein showed normal concentration, but abnormal electrophoretic properties. The inhibitor protein seems to be a well-defined $\alpha_2$-globulin, probably identical with neuramino-glycoprotein (see later). Though the immediate C1 substrate, C2, is often diminished in the patients' serum and disappears entirely during attacks, a decrease in the C4 level is the most characteristic symptom. This, sometimes very severe, condition could in some cases be considerably improved by an artificial C1 inhibitor [trans-4-(aminomethyl)-cyclohexane carboxylic acid].

## COERULOPLASMIN

In 1948 a new serum protein was discovered by Holmberg and Laurell. They called it coeruloplasmin because of its deep blue colour. Coeruloplasmin was found to contain copper.

According to the most precise determinations, its physicochemical properties are as follows: $s^{20,w}_{c\to 0} = 7.11$ S; mol. wt., 143,000$\pm$2,900; copper content 3.1–3.4 mg per g; isoelectric point, pH 4.4. It has a peculiar spectrum in the visible with an absorption maximum at 6,050 Å and the relation of the common protein absorption maximum at 2,800 Å to the latter gives a good measure of its grade of purity. For the pure coeruloplasmin this ratio would be 21.9 according to Deutsch and his co-workers and 22.7 according to Hirsch and his collaborators.

It is probable that coeruloplasmin contains several polypeptides which are not held together by co-valent bonds. Poillon and Bearn [39] observed that the molecule dissociates into two fragments during succinylation and, above pH 12, it was further subdivided into eight parts of equal mol. wt. 17,200, acrylamide gel electrophoresis of which gives two bands of equal intensity. It might be presumed that the coeruloplasmin molecule is composed of eight monomers of two different kinds ($4\alpha$, $4\beta$); investigation of the copper content has shown that each molecule contains precisely eight copper atoms. The incipient trypsin effect is also best explained by the presence of similar monomers, since coeruloplasmin is divided into fractions having *s* values of 3 S and retaining the original deep blue colour. The properties of the carbohydrate part are also in good agreement with the supposition of each molecule being made up of 8 to 10 monomers, since precisely 8 to 10 oligosaccharides are to be found in each molecule. Except for their fucose content, all oligosaccharides seem to have the same composition: 1 N-acetylneuraminic acid, 1 N-acetylglucosamine, 2 galactoses, 2 mannoses [20]. Normal serum coeruloplasmin mean value is 0.3 g per litre, and physiological values remain between 0.2 and 0.4 g per litre. There is no sex difference in adults, however, the coeruloplasmin level is elevated in pubescent girls and in women taking contraceptive drugs.

Blood serum contains about 1 mg copper per litre, 95 per cent of which is firmly bound by coeruloplasmin, and 5 per cent is loosely linked to albumin.

Of the eight copper atoms, four are monovalent and four bivalent. The latter are responsible for a moderate oxydase activity having the specificity of polyphenol oxydases of the laccase type. But the indoxylphenol residue as well as serotonin are also substrates for coeruloplasmin, further coeruloplasmin acts on catecholamines and on vitamin C. Its oxydase activity might, therefore, be of physiological importance. This is shown further by the fact that in the presence of mitochondria coeruloplasmin is reduced by physiological substrates (cytochrome C, diphosphopyridine nucleotide, succinic acid). Owing to its oxydase activity coeruloplasmin is also able to transform $Fe^{++}$ into $Fe^{+++}$ and therefore it was called feroxydase; the reduced copper is spontaneously oxidized again by molecular oxygen.

Copper is bound very strongly in a neutral medium, but it is made free by acids as well as by bases. Cyanide, ethylenediamine tetraacetic acid and urea act similarly in concentrated solutions. There is no chemical equilibrium between the copper and the apoprotein; the latter does not bind $Cu^{++}$ in the blood serum; the reaction can, however, take place in a slightly acid aqueous solution (pH 5.4) when cystein is also present.

Human coeruloplasmin may have sub-classes, too. Buyze and Visser (1966) described two varieties they observed with hydroxyapatite column chromatography; the ratio of the two proteins was constant in all the studied cases except for cord serum and in Wilson's disease.

## WILSON'S DISEASE AND THE PHYSIOLOGICAL ROLE OF COERULOPLASMIN

Wilson's disease is due to an autosomal recessive hereditary trait and is almost always characterized by considerable decrease on the coeruloplasmin level. Markowitz and his co-workers e.g. found in the 14 cases studied by them coeruloplasmin levels between 0.02 and 0.19 g per litre. On the other hand, the 'free' copper loosely bound to albumin is in excess, e.g. in the already quoted 14 cases it ranged between 0.11 and 0.5 mg per litre, as opposed to the normal mean value of 0.05 mg. However, in rare cases the coeruloplasmin level remains in the affected subjects at the lower limit of the normal range [52]. A lower ceruloplasmin level can often be detected in healthy members of affected families [52]. It is, therefore, possible that the true hereditary trait is, in fact, dominant.

Copper metabolism is profoundly disturbed. Exogenous copper appears in the free state in the circulating blood of both normal subjects and those suffering from Wilson's disease. However, after 24 h it is bound to coeruloplasmin in the blood of the former, whereas it remains in the free state in that of the latter.

Coeruloplasmin perfusion does not improve the symptoms; oestrogens, too, are without effect, although they slightly increase coeruloplasmin level. However, penicillamine improves the symptoms because it exhausts the organism's copper depots. In normal subjects it does not act upon the serum coeruloplasmin level, but in Wilson's disease it strongly decreases it.

The pathogenesis of Wilson's disease and the physiological role of coeruloplasmin are related problems. It can be presumed that coeruloplasmin has to detoxify copper ion in the circulating blood. Indeed, at first in most patients most of the copper remains in the body fluids in a free state for several years, and further many symptoms of the disease (Kayser–Fleischer ring, aminoaciduria, inflammatory changes of the parenchymatous organs) are similar to those usually observed in chronic metal poisoning. However, there is no direct relation between the coeruloplasmin level and the time of onset of the disease, as well as its severity. In order to eliminate this contradiction, it must be supposed that an originally low coeruloplasmin level increases in the course of the disease [52], because in most cases when the coeruloplasmin level is relatively high, an advanced liver disease is also present. The latter could have an indirect effect on the coeruloplasmin level, since oestrogen metabolism is inhibited in liver diseases and, as we have already said, oestrogens increase the coeruloplasmin level also in Wilson's disease. Further it might be supposed that the disease is not due to the actually prevailing coeruloplasmin level, but to a disturbance of the homeostasis of coeruloplasmin concentration [19]. The importance of such a disturbance is shown also by the effect of the penicillamine, which causes a strong decrease in the coeruloplasmin level only in patients with Wilson's disease.

There are other hypotheses trying to explain the physiological role of coeruloplasmin. Some authors think that it has a part in oestrogen metabolism owing to its oxydase activity. Undoubtedly, oestrogen effect and coeruloplasmin level are interrelated. Osaki and his co-workers (1966) were the first to postulate that coeruloplasmin changes the iron absorbed in the ferrous state into $Fe^{+++}$; indeed only $Fe^{+++}$ is bound by transferrin. Lee and his co-workers (1970) reported that in the pig in alimentary copper deficiency the blood coeruloplasmin and iron levels decrease simultaneously, whereas a $Fe^{+++}$ injection increases the iron level.

## PLASMINOGEN

At the beginning of the 20th century Delezenne and Pozerski demonstrated that the stirring with chloroform of fresh blood plasma results in a protease activity. The protease detected in this way was first called fibrinolysin and the zymogen, present in native serum, was called profibrinolysin. However, it has no specific action on fibrinogen; it is, in fact, a typical serin-protease acting in slightly alkaline medium. Therefore, today, we prefer the expression plasmin, the zymogen being called plasminogen.

Plasmin is the blood's strongest protease present in the greatest amount. At least in man and of some animal species its zymogen is selectively activated by a protein produced by haemolytic streptococci and called streptokinase. Thus the pathogenic cocci can invade the body by freeing themselves from coagulated blood in which they have been confined. Plasminogen was obtained in a pure form and the streptokinase effect elucidated [42*a*, *b*, 43].

The zymogen is a $\beta_2$-globulin with the following properties: $s = 4.1$ S; mol. wt., 89,000. Neither the molecular weight, nor the amino acid composition change during activation, but the electrophoretic migration velocity increases. Zymogen possesses only one N-terminal lysine residue and one C-terminal asparagine residue; on the activated molecule, however, two terminal residues are to be found on each ends: valine and lysine in N-terminal position and asparagine and arginine at the C-end. The activated molecule is divided into two parts by the breaking of a single S—S bridge. We can suppose, therefore, that only one peptide bond is hydrolysed under the streptokinase effect at an asparaginyl-valine sequence of the polypeptide chain, but the resulting two polypeptide chains are nked together by a S—S bridge.

## PREALBUMIN

Only those proteins might be called prealbumins which during free electrophoresis in a slightly alkaline medium appear before the albumin band. The term cannot be applied to proteins appearing before albumin in other types of electrophoretic separation. Most of these substances are anomalous, or even artificial. Artificial prealbumins are produced, e.g. when in hyperlipaemias, or during the conservation of blood serum, free fatty acids are bound to lipoproteins increasing their anionic character. Only one true prealbumin has been obtained, which has a very low serum level and cannot be demonstrated by conventional electrophoresis in the native serum. Schultze and his co-workers (1955), who first obtained it in a pure form, called it 'tryptophan-rich prealbumin'. Its physicochemical properties are as follows: $u=9\times10^{-5}$/Volt sec at pH 8.6; $s=4.2$ S; mol. wt., 61,000; hexose 0.6 per cent; hexosamine, 0.1 per cent; neuraminic and uronic acids, as well as fucose, 0; P, 0.1 per cent. This very low P level excludes the presence of lipids in noticeable amounts, however its refraction index increment has a very low value (0.1824; 4,360 Å); such values were observed only in the case of lipoproteins. It has a relatively high typtophan content (2.6 per cent) and in this it differs from serum albumin the tryptophan content of which is very low; further it has well defined immunological properties.

The presence of a tyrosine binding prealbumin in human serum was detected by several authors independently from Schultze's work, but today we know that tyrosine binding and tryptophan-rich prealbumins are identical [3]. According to the thyroxine saturation we obtain a level of 0.3–0.31 g per litre for man, whereas the direct immunochemical determination gives a value of 0.27 g per litre.

## RETINOL BINDING GLOBULIN

Retinol binding globulin has to be mentioned in connection with the tryptophan-rich prealbumin. Indeed Alvsaker and his co-workers (1967) first thought that vitamin A alcohol is bound by prealbumin in blood serum, however, Kanai and his co-workers (1968) demonstrated that retinol is bound to another well-defined protein which is bound by prealbumin in the native state. Its precise level determined by Smith and his co-workers (1970) is: 0.48$\pm$0.016 g per litre in males and 0.42$\pm$0.02 g per litre in females. It was obtained in pure form by Peterson as well as Smith and his co-workers (1971) and was found to have the following properties: $\alpha_2$-globulin; $s = 2.3$ S; mol. wt., 21,000; $E_{280\ \mathrm{m}\mu}^{1\%, 1\mathrm{cm}} = 18.7$ (the high extinction coefficient is a consequence of its high tryptophan and tyrosine content); carbohydrates, 0. As we see, this seems to be another serum protein which, similarly to albumin, contains no carbohydrates. Each molecule binds one molecule of retinol. Its bond with prealbumin is broken in media of low ionic strength.

## C-REACTIVE PROTEIN

Though it is probable that C-reactive protein is present in trace amounts in normal human serum, it was unequivocally detected only in various pathological conditions in considerably increased amounts. It was characterized by Tillett in 1930 by its peculiar property to give a precipitate with the somatic C-polysaccharide of pneumococci; he discovered it in febrile human patients as well as in infected rabbits. Only the C-reactive protein of human serum precipitates all C-polysaccharides of pneumococci; that of the rabbit serum is active only in the case of a certain R-pneumococcus; it was also called C-x-reactive protein.

C-reactive protein has no antibody activity; indeed it appears in the blood serum in various diseases (infection, accidental or surgical trauma, coronary thrombosis, neoplastic diseases, etc.). The level of some other serum proteins increases at the same time (haptoglobin, orosomucoid), that is why C-reactive protein as well as the latter were called 'acute phase proteins'. However, since only C-reactive protein is absent from the normal blood serum, its presence is a diagnostic sign in itself. In 1942 McLeod and Avery prepared a specific anti-C-reactive-protein immune serum.

Human serum C-reactive protein has the following physicochemical properties: $s = 7.2$–$7.4$ S; 14.1 per cent N; P, 0; isoelectric point pH 4.82. Its quaternary structure is very complicated. It probably contains 6 polypeptide chains of the same molecular weight (20,000) but without covalent bonds [16]. Its electrophoretic mobility depends upon the supporting medium; during free electrophoresis it appears as a $\beta$-globulin, while it moves with $\gamma$-globulins on paper, in starch gel and agar agar.

The C-reactive protein of blood serum precipitates at low ionic strength in the presence of $Ca^{++}$, probably because it is linked to $\beta$-lipoproteins in the native state. Indeed, precipitation ceases after lipid extraction. $Ca^{++}$ is also necessary for the precipitation of the C-polysaccharide by C-reactive protein, but this reaction is not modified by the extraction of lipids.

It must be underlined that of the animal species studied it was only the rat which did not produce C-reactive protein after injury; however, a considerable increase in the level of a peculiar $\alpha_1$-globulin has been reported.

## SEROMUCOIDS AND HAPTOGLOBINS

These are low molecular weight serum proteins rich in carbohydrates. Therefore, they are more or less soluble in trichloroacetic and sulphosalicylic acid or not precipitated by the latter at all, and relatively resistant to heat. But these are only quantitative characters and besides typical seromucoids many atypical varieties are to be found.

### $\alpha_1$-ANTITRYPSIN

Three different trypsin inhibitors can be detected by appropriate staining methods on the electrophoretogram of human blood serum; one of them is the already mentioned $\alpha_2$M-globulin; the second one appears between $\alpha_1$- and $\alpha_2$-globulins (inter-$\alpha$-inhibitor, see later) and at present we shall deal with the third one which has an $\alpha_1$-globulin mobility and is called $\alpha_1$-antitrypsin. Of all seromucoids this one appears to have the highest concentration. It was first obtained by Schultze in 1955, who called it $\alpha_1$-3,5 S-glycoprotein, as its sedimentation coefficient was 3.5 S. Bundy and Mehl showed that it was identical with the former indirectly characterized $\alpha_1$-trypsin inhibitor. Sometimes it is called $\alpha_1$A-globulin because of its site of appearance on the immuno-electrophoretogram. Its molecular weight is 54,000 and its neuraminic acid level 3.3 per cent. Besides trypsin, it also inhibits elastase, thrombin and plasmin. It is responsible for the 'very quickly acting' antitrypsin effect of serum.

According to the immunochemical study of Augener (1964), its mean level is 2.35 g per litre (S.D. 0.33). This value may seem too high, since the total $\alpha_1$-globulin level of human serum is only 2.3–2.5 g per litre. Notwithstanding, its concentration must be very high.

$\alpha_1$-antitrypsin has various genetic sub-groups showing different electrophoretic mobilities. Seven sub-groups have been described controlled by seven alleles on the same genetic locus.

An important decrease of the $\alpha_1$-antitrypsin level appears as a rare hereditary trait. $\alpha_1$-antitrypsin may disappear entirely in homozygotes, whereas its diminution is only partial in heterozygotes. This serum protein abnormality has no pathological consequences [24].

## HAPTOGLOBINS

Haptoglobins are $\alpha_2$-globulins partly soluble in trichloroacetic and perchloric acids as a consequence of their great carbohydrate content.

In 1939 Polonovski and Jayle demonstrated that human blood serum contains a protein which is able to bind haemoglobin, thereby strongly increasing its peroxydase activity. This haemoglobin binding protein was called haptoglobin by them. Several haptoglobin bands appear on the starch gel electrophoretogram showing individual variations corresponding to three genetically defined subgroups. Two co-dominant alleles: $Hp_1$ and $Hp_2$, control the haptoglobin synthesis. Thus three chief hereditary varieties, Hp(1–1), Hp(2–2) and Hp(1–2), may be defined, of which the first two appear in homozygotes and the third one in heterozygotes.

Haptoglobin level depends on the haptoglobin type and on sex. In Table 12-II the respective results of Nyman (1959) are shown. Differences according to haptoglobin type and sex are statistically significant. The sex effect is best explained by postulating that the haptoglobin level increases under androgen effect and decreases under that of oestrogens.

Smithies et al. [8] demonstrated that the haptoglobin molecule is composed of several polypeptide chains linked by S—S bridges. There are two different polypeptide chains, called $\alpha$ and $\beta$, and monomeric form of haptoglobin corresponds to $2\alpha + 2\beta$. The $\beta$ chain remains the same in all haptoglobin varieties, whereas the $\alpha$ chains vary according to genetic sub-classes; $\alpha 1$ corresponds to $Hp_1$ and

TABLE 12-II

*Haptoglobin levels in human blood serum (g per litre)*
*Male and female*

| | *Male and female* | | | |
|---|---|---|---|---|
| No. of subjects | 277 | 59 | 130 | |
| Type | 1—1+1—2+2—2 | 1—1 | 2—1 | |
| Mean | 1.1 | 1.36 | 1.08 | |
| S. D. | 0.41 | 0.3 | 0.37 | |
| Range* | 0.28–1.92 | 0.77–1.94 | 0.15–1.49 | |
| | *Male* | | | |
| No. of subjects | 144 | 22 | 68 | 54 |
| Type | 1—1+1—2+2—2 | 1—1 | 2—1 | 2—2 |
| Mean | 1.13 | 1.44 | 1.16 | 0.88 |
| S. D. | 0.43 | | | |
| Range | 0.27–1.97 | | | |
| | *Female* | | | |
| No. of subjects | 84 | 24 | 29 | 31 |
| Type | 1—1+1—2+2—2 | 1—1 | 2—1 | 2—2 |
| Mean | 0.94 | 1.15 | 0.95 | 0.79 |
| S. D. | 0.3 | | | |
| Range | 0.34–1.54 | | | |

* The range is given witb 5 per cent approximation.

$\alpha 2$ to $Hp_2$. The molecular weight of the $\alpha$ chain is 18,000, that of the $\beta$ chain is 36,000. The various starch gel electrophoretic bands represent various polymeric forms. The S—S bridges between the basic polypeptide chains have been disputed, since according to Wachs and Alfsen (1968) in strongly diluted solutions haptoglobins may reversibly dissociate. The smallest unit thus produced would have a mol. wt. of 40,000. All haptoglobin types have two N-terminal residues: valine and isoleucine.

In addition to the above-described genotypes a number of varieties have been described, such as those containing two kinds of $\alpha 1$ chains, a fast variety: $\alpha$-1F, and a slow one: $\alpha$-1S. The corresponding genotypes are Hp (1F–1F); Hp (1S–1S); Hp (1S–1F); Hp (2–1F); Hp (2–1S).

As to the amino acid composition, Schultze et al. reported differences between the various haptoglobin types in the relative proportion of glycine, leucine, phenylalanine and tyrosine [55], only the total amount of which would be constant. The primary structure for all three $\alpha$-chains: $\alpha 2$, $\alpha 1$F, $\alpha 1$S, was described by Black and Dixon in 1968. $\alpha 2$ contains 142 amino acid residues, mol. wt. 16,000; $\alpha 1$ chains contain 83 residues, mol. wt. 9,100. $\alpha 1$F differs from $\alpha 1$S only by one amino acid residue; at the 54 position there is glutamic acid in the former and lysine in the latter and, therefore, $\alpha 1$F is formed from $\alpha 1$S by simple point mutation. $Hp_1$ differs from $Hp_2$ only by one tryptic peptide which contains the half cystine residue binding the $\alpha$ chain to the $\beta$ chain. These facts are in good agreement with Smithie's genetic hypothesis: the $\alpha 2$ gene results from an unequal crossing over of two $\alpha 1$ genes and the deletion involves the N-end of one of them and the C-end of the other. Since there is only a very slight difference between $Hp_1$ and $Hp_2$, this crossing over must have taken place only relatively recently during phylogenesis; in fact, in primates only Hp(1–1) is to be found.

All haptoglobin types contain the same amount of a carbohydrate with an identical composition. Schultze and his co-workers (1963) found the following composition for the three chief types: hexosamine: 5.3–6 per cent; hexose: 7.8–7.9 per cent; neuraminic acid: 4.8–5.3 per cent; fucose 0.2 per cent. Analysis of the glycopeptides remaining after advanced protease action shows that only one kind of oligosaccharide is present in all cases; sometimes, however, fucose is lacking. With this restriction, it has the following composition: 2 neuraminic acids, 4 galactoses, 2 mannoses, 4 glucosamines. The carbohydrate content of haptoglobin amounts to about 19 per cent, and, therefore, the monomeric form would bind 10 oligosaccharide residues; however, the peptide environments are not similar.

It has not been firmly established whether there are any immunochemical differences between the various haptoglobin types. Further, haptoglobins having no haemoglobin binding capacity are known [34].

One molecule of haemoglobin is irreversibly bound to one molecule of haptoglobin involving the $\alpha$ chain of the globin. It seems, however, that the binding sites are mostly latent in the tetrameric haemoglobin and become accessible only in the symmetrical dimeric form [6]. Strongly diluted solutions contain this dimeric form, e.g. the circulating blood, the free haemoglobin content of which is always very low. Most probably it is the task of haptoglobin to bind haemoglobin in the circulating blood thus preventing its renal excretion. Heparin and protamin inhibit the binding of haemoglobin by haptoglobin. Haptoglobin inhibits viral haemagglutination.

## OROSOMUCOID

Orosomucoid is the most typical of the quantitatively important seromucoids. It was first characterized indirectly by Winzler and his co-workers by electrophoresis in acid medium, when they called it $MP_1$. Later, in 1950, they obtained it in pure form. The name orosomucoid was proposed many years later by Winzler. Schmid called it $\alpha_1$-acid glycoprotein; the incorrect expression: $\alpha_1$-seromucoid is sometimes to be found in the literature.

Its sedimention coefficient varies between 2.9 and 3.5 S; $V = 0.67$–$0.69$; $D = 5.27 \times 10^{-7}$ cm²/sec; mol. wt., 40–45,000. Its carbohydrate content reaches 40 per cent with 10 per cent neuraminic acid; isoelectric point, pH 2.7. It is not coagulated in a bath of boiling water and remains soluble even in concentrated trichloroacetic acid. However, this solubility is retained even after neuraminidase action.

Its immunochemical properties are accurately known allowing its measurement by immunochemical methods. Normal mean value and S.D. are $0.9 \pm 0.15$ g per litre. The serum level does not depend upon age or sex. The carbohydrate part is composed of several oligosaccharides, but their composition is not yet fully known. Orosomucoid level increases greatly during injury [49]; which makes it typical 'acute phase protein'.

Most probably, orosomucoid has several genetically defined varieties. Two orosomucoid bands appear after neuraminidase action on starch gel electrophoretograms and their electrophoretic mobility is subject to individual variations probably according to three hereditary phenotypes.

## $\beta_1$-SEROMUCOID OR $\beta_1$B-GLOBULIN OR HAEMOPEXIN

Haemopexin was the name given by Grabar and his co-workers to a protein also called $\beta_1$B-globulin after its site of appearance on immunoelectrophoretograms. The former expression refers to its great affinity for heme (hematin) with which it produces equimolecular compounds. But it also binds haemoglobin, myoglobin and cytochrome C.

It was obtained in a pure form by Biserte and his co-workers and Schultze and his co-workers. Its properties are as follows: $s = 4.8$ S; mol. wt., 80,000; it contains about 25 per cent carbohydrates of which 5.8 per cent is neuraminic acid; its tryptophan content is very high (4.7 per cent).

In the literature two immunochemical levels are mentioned: according to Augener (1964) its mean value is 0.86 g per litre, S.D. 0.12; according to Hannstein and Mueller-Eberhard the mean value and the physiological range are: 0.75 g per litre and 0.66–1.0 g per litre, respectively. Starting with a mean value of only 0.18 g per litre at birth, its level increases during childhood.

## VARIOUS SEROMUCOIDS

Ba-$\alpha_2$-glycoprotein, or $\alpha_2$-HS-mucoid, has still a relatively high serum level (0.96 g per litre according to Poortmans). It has the following properties: $s = 3.6$ S; carbohydrate content: 14 per cent; neuraminic acid content: 4.1 per cent.

Another $\alpha_2$-globulin is of importance from the genetic point of view. It was first detected by immunoelectrophoretic analysis and called Gc (group-specific component) by Hirschfeld. Indeed, its precipitation line on immunoelectrophoretograms shows individual variations following certain genetic laws. Hirschfeld demonstrated the existence of three types controlled by two co-dominant alleles: $Gc^1$ and $Gc^2$. The homozygote $Gc_{1-1}$ has a precipitation line with a single curvature in the slow $\alpha_2$-globulin zone; the precipitation line remains in the fast $\alpha_2$-globulin zone for the homozygote $Gc_{2-2}$ having also a single curvature; a very long precipitation line extending over the entire $\alpha_2$-globulin zone is characteristic of the heterozygote $Gc_{2-1}$, but this precipitation line has two curvatures, one in the slow and the other in the fast $\alpha_2$-globulin zone. All three varieties have been obtained separately in pure form by Bearn and Bowman (1963, 1964, 1965, 1969). In soluble starch as well as in acrylamid gel electrophoresis two bands appear for both homozygote types and all the four corresponding bands appear in the heterozygote's serum. Up to now immunochemical differences could not be evidenced between the two homozygote types. Chemically they differ in the nature of the C-terminal tripeptide (valinyl-serinyl-leucine in the case of $Gc_{1-1}$ and alanilyl-asparaginyl-isoleucine in that of $Gc_{2-2}$). No other chemical difference could be detected between the genotypes. It must be added that most probably the Gc molecule contains two polypeptides linked by a S—S bridge. Bowman (1969) modified the hypothesis of Hirschfeld concerning the mode of inheritance. According to him, Gc synthesis is under the control of three genetic loci: $\alpha$, $\beta$ and $\gamma$; further, the $\alpha$ locus may be occupied by two alleles: $\alpha_1$ and $\alpha_2$. Two kinds of molecules are present in the case of both homozygotes; $\alpha_1$, $\beta$, and $\alpha_1$, $\gamma$, in the case of $Gc_{1-1}$ and $\alpha_2$, $\beta$, and $\alpha_2$, $\gamma$, in that of $Gc_{2-2}$. Since the individual polypeptide chains have very similar chemical compositions, it might be supposed that the three genes originate from a single ancestral gene through duplication.

We will only briefly comment on proteins which are present in blood serum in very small amounts and have no apparent physiological roles. The low-molecular-weight $\alpha_2$-globulin characterized by Schmid has the following properties: $s = 2.6$ S; isoelectric point, pH 3.8–3.9; 7 per cent neuraminic acid; serum level, 0.39 g per litre. Schmid and his co-workers as well as Winzler and his collaborators obtained independently a tryptophan-rich $\alpha_2$-glycoprotein each; but as the following data prove, the two products are strikingly similar:

| | $s_{20,w}^{c\to 0}$ (S) | Tryptophan (%) | Tyrosine (%) | Hexose (%) | Hexose-amine (%) | Neuraminic acid (%) | Fucose (%) |
|---|---|---|---|---|---|---|---|
| Winzler | 3.7 | 5.4 | 6.5 | 6 | 3.8 | 5 | 0.5 |
| Schmid | 3.2 | 4.7 | 5.9 | 7 | 4 | 7 | 0.2 |

Therefore, it may be supposed that the two proteins are identical. We can add the following data: $V = 0.706$; mol. wt., 41,000; isoelectric point, pH 3.7–3.8 (Schmid). The $\alpha_1$-X-glycoprotein first obtained by Schultze and his co-workers has, according to Heimburger and Haupt [18], the following properties: $s^{1\%}$: 3.9 S; 11 per cent hexose; 8 per cent glucosamine; 7 per cent neuraminic acid; 0.8 per cent fucose; mol. wt., 68,000. It selectively inhibits chymotrypsin without any effect on trypsin and thrombin. It seems to form a monomolecular compound with chymotrypsin. We will further briefly mention in this group the following proteins:

(*i*) *tryptophan-poor* $\alpha_1$*-glycoprotein:* $s^{1\%} = 3.3$ S; mol. wt., 55,000; 5.5 per cent hexose; 4.5 per cent hexosamine; 3.4 per cent neuraminic acid; 0.3 per cent fucose; 0.39 per cent tryptophan.

(*ii*) *easily precipitable* $\alpha_1$*-glycoprotein:* $s^{1.5\%}$: 3.8 S; it is the fastest postalbumin obtained in soluble starch gel electrophoresis.

(*iii*) *4.6 S postalbumin.* It has electrophoretic and ultracentrifugal properties similar to those of Gc from which it differs by its much higher carbohydrate level (14 per cent hexose; 2.8 per cent hexosamine; 3 per cent neuraminic acid).

(*iv*) *Neuraminic acid lacking* $\beta_1$*-globulin:* $s^{1,5\%} = 2.9$ S; mol. wt., 30,000; 13 per cent hexose; 13 per cent hexosamine; isoelectric point, pH 4.4.

(*v*) $\beta_2$*-glycoprotein I:* $s = 2.9$ S; carbohydrate content = 17 per cent; 4.4 per cent neuraminic acid; mean level ±S.D. = 0.23–0.24 ± 0.04 g per litre.

(*vi*) $\beta_2$*-glycoprotein II:* $s^{1\%} = 3.7$ S; 2.2 per cent hexose; 1.8 per cent hexosamine; 1.5 per cent neuraminic acid; 0.2 per cent fucose; $E_{280\,m\mu}^{1\%,\,1cm} = 11$; it is precipitated by trichloroacetic acid and perchloric acid; serum level, 11 mg per litre.

The neuramino-glycoprotein or 'acid $\alpha_2$-glycoprotein' is of special interest. Some years ago it was isolated by Schultze et al., and more recently Pensky and his co-workers reported upon its C1-esterase inhibitor activity; therefore, it might be postulated that its lack would be responsible for the familial angioneurotic oedema (see above). It has the following properties: 43 per cent carbohydrates with 17 per cent neuraminic acid; $s_{20,\,w}^{0.8\%} = 3.7$ S. As we see, this is the serum protein with the highest neuraminic acid content.

The complexity of the seromucoid family must be clear from what has been said so far; in the following, we will underline their biological importance. Indeed several seromucoids present in the blood serum in very small amounts bind biologically important substances with great affinity and selectivity; one of them is even a hormone.

The thyroxine binding $\alpha$-globulin was first characterized in an indirect way, then obtained in pure form by Gordon et al. [15]. It has the following properties: $s_{c\to 0}^{20,\,w} = 3.9$ S; mol. wt., 58,000; 6.7 per cent hexose; 3.3 per cent glucosamine; 0.7 per cent galactosamine; 2.4 per cent neuraminic acid. Most probably it forms a monomolecular compound with thyroxine and, on this basis, its serum level must be about 11 mg per litre.

As already quoted, albumin and prealbumin also bind thyroxine, but the thyroxine binding $\alpha$-globulin shows by far the greatest affinity. This is well demonstrated by the following data of Woeler and Ingbar:

| | Albumin | Prealbumin | Thyroxine binding $\alpha_1$-globulin |
|---|---|---|---|
| Affinity constant | $6.2\times10^5$ | $2.3\times10^8$ | $1.7\times10^{10}$ |

While tri-iodothyronine, too, is strongly bound by the $\alpha$-globulin, albumin shows only a very weak affinity for this compound and prealbumin is devoid of any binding capacity.

At least two different globulins bind vitamin $B_{12}$ in the human blood serum. Though their existence was indirectly proven already in 1950, they have not yet been obtained from human blood serum in pure form. One is called transcobalamine I and is an $\alpha$-globulin, and the other one is called transcobalamine II and is a $\beta$-globulin. Transcobalamine I has a molecular weight of about 120,000 and transcobalamine II of 36,000. Endogenous vitamin $B_{12}$ is linked to transcobalamine I; the parenterally introduced vitamin appears at first with transcobalamine II, but after 24 h most of it is bound to transcobalamine I. Recently it has been suggested that transcobalamine I, and perhaps also transcobalamine II, are synthesized by polynuclear leukocytes.

We ranged transcobalamines among seromucoids since they have the solubility characters of the latter. Further, a transcobalamine was obtained from hen serum in pure form and was found to be a typical seromucoid with a very low sedimentation coefficient (3.95 S) and very high carbohydrate content (27 per cent). Further, it has $\alpha$-globulin mobility. It must be recalled that hen serum binds about 500 times more vitamin $B_{12}$ than human serum, however, it contains only this $\alpha$-globulin as binding protein.

In 1958 Daughady showed that human blood serum contains an $\alpha$-globulin binding cortisol, corticosterone and progesterone. Slaumwhite and Sternberg (1959) obtained it in pure form and called it transcortin [56]. We report some data concerning rabbit as well as human serum transcortin:

| | Hexose (%) | Hexosamine (%) | Neuraminic acid (%) | Fucose (%) | N (%) | $u \times 10^5$ [cm²/(Volt sec)] | $s^{20,w}_{c\to 0}$ (S) | $D \times 10^{-7}$ (cm²/sec) | $\overline{V}$ | mol.wt. $\times 10^{-4}$ | $E^{1\%1cm}_{274m\mu}$ |
|---|---|---|---|---|---|---|---|---|---|---|---|
| Man | 10.5 | 9 | 4.1 | 1.5 | 12.7 | —4.9 | 3.8 | 6.15 | 0.71 | 5.17 | 6.45 |
| Rabbit | 10.4 | 9.5 | 8.5 | 0.8 | 12.1 | —5.1 | 3.55 | 7.02 | 0.70 | 4.07 | 8.4 |

Its low molecular weight and high carbohydrate content allow us to range it among seromucoids.

The results obtained by Rambert and his co-workers in 1958 concerning a serum protein which would form an unstable chemical bond with sulphate anions entering blood circulation, need confirmation. The same is true for the seromucoid which, according to Bourrillon and his co-workers would bind the gonadotrophic hormone in pregnant mare serum.

The hormone activating erythropoiesis and called therefore erythropoietin was discovered in blood by Carnot and Delfandre in 1906; it was obtained from sheep serum in pure form by White and his co-workers in 1960. It is a typical $\alpha_1$-seromucoid, similar to orosomucoid, however, at least in the case of sheep, it has a higher serin and threonin level and a smaller carbohydrate content. Its chief properties are: isoelectric point, pH 4.5; $u = -5.8 \times 10^{-5}$ cm/(Volt sec); $s = 4.7$ S; mol. wt., 40,000; 8.2 per cent hexose; 6.9 per cent neuraminic acid. But the erythropoietin obtained from rabbit serum in a partially purified state has an even greater neuraminic acid content than orosomucoid (Rambach and his co-workers: 7.7 per cent hexose; 10 per cent hexosamine; 15.6 per cent neuraminic acid).

An inhibitor of hyaluronidase was obtained from human serum by Newman and his co-workers in 1955. It is an $\alpha_1$-globulin with a $s$ of 3.75 S. It would be worth while to check whether the results obtained by these authors concerning its uronic acid content is correct, since uronic acid is absent from all other known serum proteins.

## PROTEINS PRESENT IN BLOOD SERUM IN VERY SMALL AMOUNTS

The inter-$\alpha$-trypsin inhibitor (see section on $\alpha_1$-antitrypsin) was isolated from human serum by Heide and his co-workers and by Steinbuch and his co-workers in 1965. The purified compound is heterodisperse with a 4.4 S, and a 6.4 S component. It may be that the first component originates from the second component by autolysis, since the 6.4 S component turns into the 4.4 S one sponta neously during storage of the serum. At the same time a relatively small peptide fraction appears which alone preserves the trypsin inhibiting capacity. This inhibitory activity is preserved up to 56 °C, a temperature where the other two serum inhibitor components are destroyed. Steinbuch and his co-workers detected $Zn^{++}$ in it; only one ion per molecule is to be found in the native state, but it can bind three zinc ions per molecule during dialysis against a zinc salt.

In 1965 Schoemakers et al. [54] reported to have obtained the Hagemann factor of blood coagulation in a pure state; according to them it is a $\beta_2$-globulin having a rather high carbohydrate content and a molecular weight of 82,000; further it is a protease and there is a relation between the enzyme activity and coagulation. However, a 'purified' Hagemann factor with quite different properties was described somewhat later, in 1969, by Grammens and his co-workers. They spoke about a $\gamma$-globulin, with a mol. wt. of 140,000 and low carbohydrate content, showing no esterase activity. Therefore, the real nature of this highly instable substance remains to be determined.

An $\alpha_2$-globulin was described by MacLarren and his co-workers in 1959; it is invariably present in human blood serum during the last months of pregnancy and after oestrogen administration. It could be detected in the serum of only 18 per cent of young female and male individuals. Its presence in the latter seems to be under the control of an autosomatic dominant gene [29].

Cooperband et al. [9] gave the name of 'immunoregulator $\alpha$-globulin' to a blood serum protein obtained by them. It inhibits the blastogenic effect of phytohaemagglutinin; it is absorbed by lymphocytes and neutralizes the effect of the macrophage migration inhibiting factor.

Purified kallikreins were obtained from human blood serum by Colman et al. [7]. They obtained a mixture of three proteases with different physicochemical characters, but identical immunological ones. Kallikrein I is a slow $\gamma$-globulin (mol. wt., 100,000), kallikrein II a fast $\gamma$-globulin (mol. wt., 163,000) and kallikrein III an $\alpha$-globulin. Kallikreins are zymogens in the native state activated by activated Hagemann factor. Their level in human blood serum is 50–100 mg per litre.

Several proteins present only in trace amounts in blood serum have higher levels in other biological fluids. Their existence was first detected by the study of anti-CSF immune serum. Two of them, the $\beta_{tr}$ and the $\gamma_{tr}$ (tr = trace) were

## *Most important properties of serum proteins*

| | *s* (S) | $\bar{V}$ | *D* (cm²/sec) ($\times 10^7$) | mol.wt. ($\times 10^{-4}$) | Level | |
|---|---|---|---|---|---|---|
| | | | | | Mean value (g/litre) | S. D. |
| *(I) γ-globulins* | | | | | | |
| (1) Kallikrein I | — | — | — | 9.98 | — | — |
| (2) Kallikrein II | — | — | — | 16.3 | — | — |
| (3) C1*q* | 11 | — | — | 39 | 0.1 | — |
| *(II)* $\beta_2$ | | | | | | |
| (4) C6 | 5 | — | — | — | 0.024 | — |
| (5) Properdin | 5–5.3 | — | 2.15 | 22 | — | — |
| (6) Plasminogen | 4.1 | — | — | 8.9 | — | — |
| (7) C-reactive protein | 7.3 | — | — | 12 | — | — |
| (8) $\beta_2$-glycoprotein I | 2.9 | — | — | — | 0.24 | 0.04 |
| (9) $\beta_2$-glycoprotein II | 3.7 | — | — | — | 0.011 | — |
| (10) Hagemann factor | 7.1 | — | — | 8.2 | — | — |
| | 7.7 | 0.724 | 4.45 | 14.2 | — | — |
| *(III)* $\beta_1$ | | | | | | |
| (11) Transferrin | 5.1 | — | 5.5 | 8.5 | 2.8 | 0.24 |
| (12) $\beta_1$C | 9.5 | — | — | — | 1.5 | 0.27 |
| (13) C2 | 5.2 | — | 4 | 11.7 | 0.01 | — |
| (14) C4 | 10 | — | — | — | 0.44 | 0.12 |
| (15) C5 | 8.7 | — | — | — | 0.076 | — |
| (16) Haemopexin | 4.8 | — | — | 8 | 0.75–0.96 | — |
| (17) Transcobalamine II | — | — | — | 3.6 | — | — |
| *(IV)* $\alpha_2$ | | | | | | |
| (18) $\alpha_2$M | 19.6 | 0.73 | 2.4 | 90 | 2–3* | 0.3 |
| (19) Coeruloplasmin | 7.1 | — | — | 14.3 | 0.3 | 0.05 |
| (20) Haptoglobins | — | — | — | 11 | 1.1 | 0.41 |
| (21) Ba-$\alpha_2$, or HS-glycoprotein | 3.6 | — | — | | 0.96 | — |
| (22) Gc | 4.1 | — | — | 5.08 | 0.4–0.7 | — |
| (23) 'Low-molecular-weight' $\alpha_2$ | 2.6 | — | — | — | 0.39 | — |
| (24) 'Tryptophan rich' $\alpha_2$ | 3.4 | 0.71 | — | 4.1 | — | — |
| (25) Neuramino-glycoprotein | 3.7 | — | — | — | — | — |
| (26) Retinol binding protein | 4.6 | — | 6.6 | 6.4 | 0.42–0.48 | 0.02 |
| *(V)* $\alpha_2$-$\alpha_1$ | | | | | | |
| (27) Inter-α-trypsin inhibitor | 6.4 | — | — | — | — | — |
| *(VI)* $\alpha_1$ | | | | | | |
| (28) $\alpha_1$-antitrypsin | 3.5 | — | — | 5.4 | 2.35 | 0.33 |
| (29) Orosomucoid | 2.9–3.5 | 0.67–0.69 | 5.3 | 4–4.5 | 0.9 | 0.15 |
| (30) C1 esterase | — | — | — | 11 | 0.033 | 0.006 |
| (31) $\alpha_1$-X | 3.9 | — | — | 6.8 | — | — |

| | s (S) | $\bar{V}$ | D (cm²/sec) (×10⁷) | mol.wt. (×10⁻⁴) | Level | |
|---|---|---|---|---|---|---|
| | | | | | Mean value (g/litre) | S. D. |
| (32) 'Tryptophan poor $\alpha_1$ | 3.3 | — | — | 5.5 | — | — |
| (33) 'Easly precitable' $\alpha_1$ | 3.9 | — | — | — | — | — |
| (34) 4.6 S post-albumin | 4.6 | — | — | — | — | — |
| (35) Thyroxine binding $\alpha$-globulin | 3.9 | — | — | 5.8 | 0.015 | — |
| (36) Transcobalamine I | — | — | — | 12 | — | — |
| (37) Transcortin | 3.8 | 0.71 | 6.15 | 5.17 | 0.03 | — |
| (38) Hyaluronidase inhibitor | 3.75 | — | — | — | — | — |
| *(VII) Miscellaneous* | | | | | | |
| (39) Albumin | 4.1–5 | 0.73–0.74 | 6.1 | 7.1 | 40.6 | 3.4 |
| (40) LDL + VLDL + chylomicrons | — | — | — | — | male 5.29 | — |
| | | | | | female 4.67 | — |
| (41) HDL | — | — | — | | male 2.84 | — |
| | | | | | female 3.79 | — |
| (42) Prealbumin | 4.2 | — | — | 6.2 | 0.30 | — |

* Strongly depends upon age.
*Symbols:* $s$ = sedimentation coefficient; $D$ = diffusion coefficient expressed in $10^{-7}$ cm²/sec; $\bar{V}$ = partial molecular volume; LDL = low density lipoproteins; VLDL = very low density lipoproteins; HDL = high density lipoproteins.

more thoroughly studied. They are small molecular weight proteins and $\gamma_{tr}$, which is not an immunoglobulin, makes out about 70 per cent of the $\gamma$-band of the CSF electrophoretogram; it is most probably synthesized by brain tissues.

Comparative physiology furnishes even more striking examples of proteins which are only passing through the blood on their way to the excretory organs. Indeed the normal urine of male mice, as well as of male rats contains proteins in great amounts; they are synthesized by the liver and excreted by the kidneys, their blood level remaining always very low.

The same is valid for collagenous substances which can be found in normal human serum in amounts of 30–50 mg per litre. Indeed, their appearance in blood seems to depend upon normal collagen synthesis; a small amount of the newly formed collagen remaining in a soluble state is first absorbed then excreted by the kidneys. It might be supposed that the alkaline polypeptides present in human serum at very low levels originate from nucleoprotein histone metabolism and pass through the blood to be excreted by the kidneys. This is proved by their characteristically alkaline isoelectric point (pH 9–10), their high dibasic amino acid content and by the absence of tryptophan and tyrosine.

Another example from the field of comparative physiology is that of the South Pole fish *Trematomus borchgrevinski*, which lives in waters of —1.9 °C. The blood serum of fish freezes usually at —0.7 °C, whereas that of this fish species freezes at —2 °C. This lowered freezing point mostly depends upon the presence of great amounts of special glycoproteins, a mixture of three isomeric compounds with different molecular weights (10,500; 17,000; 20,500) but of identical composition. This composition corresponds to a simple polymeric form of an oligo-glycopeptide: alanyl-alanyl-threonyl-galactosyl-N-acetyl-glucosamine; threonin is linked to the galactose by a glucoside bond; both terminal amino acids are alanines [10]. The decrease in freezing point is presumably due to a peculiarly strong Donnan effect.

We have not spoken about the unspecific enzymes present in great numbers in blood serum. Probably most of them originate from dissociating tissue cells and only pass through circulation to be excreted by the kidneys or to be caught by the reticuloendothelial system.

## REFERENCES*


1. Alkjaessig, N.: *Biochem. J.* **93,** 171 (1964).
2*a*. Alper, C. A., Popp, R. P., Johnston, R. B. and Rosen, F. S.: *J. Immunol.* **101,** 816 (1968).
2*b*. ibid., **101,** 2182 (1968).
3. Aly, F. W. and Bohner, J.: *Prot. biol. Fluids* **14,** 693 (1966).
4. Barclay, M., Barclay, R. K. and Skipski, V. L.: *Nature* **200,** 362 (1963).
5. Berg, K. and Bearn, A. G.: *J. exp. Med.* **123,** 379 (1966).
6. Bunn, H. F.: *J. Lab. clin. Med.* **70,** 606 (1967).
7. Colman, R. W., Mattler, L. and Sherry, S.: *J. clin. Invest.* **48,** 11 (1969).
8. Connell, G. E., Dixon, G. H. and Smithies, O.: *Nature* **193,** 505 (1962).
9. Cooperband, S. R., Davis, R. C., Schmied, K., and Mannick, J. A.: *J. clin. Invest.* **47,** 22 (1968).
10. De Vries, A. L., Vandenheede, J. and Freeney, R. E.: *J. biol. Chem.* **246,** 305 (1971).
11. Donaldsen, V. H. and Rosen, F. S.: *J. clin. Invest.* **42,** 2204 (1964).
12. Fagerhol, M. K. and Laurell, C. B.: *Clin. chim. Acta* **16,** 199 (1967).
13. Fredrickson, D. S., Levy, R. I. and Lees, R. S.: *New Engl. J. Med.* **276,** 94 (1967).
14. Ganrot, P. O. and Schersten, B.: *Clin. chim. Acta* **15,** 113 (1967).
15. Giorgio, N. A. and Tabachnik, M.: *J. biol. Chem.* **243,** 2247 (1968).
16. Gottschlich, E. C. and Edelman, G. E.: *Proc. nat. Acad. Sci. (Wash.)* **54,** 558 (1965).
17*a*. Gustafson, A., Alaupovic, P. and Furman, R. H.: *Biochemistry* **4,** 596 (1965).
17*b*. ibid., **5,** 632 (1966).
18. Heimburger, N. and Haupt, H.: *Clin. chim. Acta* **12,** 116 (1965).
19. Holtzman, N. A., Naughton, M. A., Iber, F. L. and Gaumnitz, B. M.: *J. clin. Invest.* **46,** 943 (1967).
20. Jamieson, J. A.: *J. biol. Chem.* **240,** 2019 (1965).
21*a*. Jamieson, J. A.: *J. biol. Chem.* **240,** 2914 (1965).
21*b*. id., *Prot. biol. Fluids* **14,** 71 (1966).
22. Jensen, K. B.: *Prot. biol. Fluids* **14,** 677 (1966).
23. Jones, J. W. and Ways, P.: *J. clin. Invest.* **46,** 1151 (1967).
24. Laurell, C. B. and Erickson, S.: *Clin. chim. Acta* **11,** 395 (1965).
25. Lees, R. S. and Hatch, F.: *J. Lab. clin. Med.* **61,** 518 (1963).
26. Levy, R. I. and Fredrickson, D. S.: *Circulation* **34,** Suppl. **111.** 156 (1963).
27. Levy, R. I., Fredrickson, D. S. and Laster, L.: *J. clin. Invest.* **45,** 531 (1966).


* Owing to lack of space only some of the about 1,000 publications consulted for the preparation of the present review could be quoted in the reference list. However, in the text important terms and dates have been included.

28. Levy, R. I., Lees, R. S. and Fredrickson, D. S.: *J. clin. Invest.* **45,** 63 (1966).
29. MacLarren, J. A., Reid, D. E., Kormgres, A. A. and Allen, F. H.: *Vox Sang. (Basel)* **11,** 553 (1966).
30. Mills, G. L. and Wilkinson, P. A.: *Clin. chim. Acta* **8,** 701 (1963).
31. Montgomery, D. A., Weill, D. W. and Dowdle, E. B. D.: *Clin. Sci.* **22,** 141 (1962).
32. Mueller-Eberhard, H. J. and Biro, C.: *J. exp. Med.* **118,** 447 (1963).
33. Mueller-Eberhard, H. J., Calcott, M. A. and Mardiney, M. R.: *Fed. Proc.* **23,** 506 (1964).
34. Nance, W. E. and Smithies, O.: *Nature* **198,** 869 (1963).
35. Nielehn, J. E. and Ganrot, P. O.: *Scand. J. clin. Lab. Invest.* **20,** 113 (1967).
36. Nilsson, U. R. and Mueller-Eberhard, H. J.: *J. exp. Med.* **122,** 277 (1965).
37. Pensky, J., Hinz, C. F., Todd, W. E., Wegwood, R. J., Boyer, J. T. and Lepow, I. H.: *J. Immunol.* **100,** 142 (1968).
38. Peters, T., jr. and Blumenstock, F.: *J. biol. Chem.* **242,** 1574 (1967).
39. Poillon, W. N. and Bearn, A. G.: *Biochim. biophys. Acta (Amst.)* **127,** 407 (1966).
40. Polley, M. J. and Mueller-Eberhard, H. J.: *J. exp. Med.* **128,** 533 (1968).
41. Robbins, J. and Weathers, B.: *Cancer Res.* **26,** 492 (1966).
42*a*. Robbins, K. C. and Summaria, L.: *J. biol. Chem.* **238,** 952 (1963).
42*b*. id., *Immunochemistry* **3,** 29 (1966).
43. Robbins, K. C., Summaria, L., Elwyn, D. and Barlow, G. H.: *J. biol. Chem.* **240,** 541 (1965).
44. Rosen, F. S., Charade, P., Pensky, J. and Donaldsen, V.: *Science* **148,** 957 (1965).
45. Rossing, N. and Andersen, S. B.: *Prot. biol. Fluids* **14,** 319 (1966).
46. Rudman, D., Garcia, L. A., Abell, L. L., Cooke, O. and Akgun, S.: *J. clin. Invest.* **47,** 85 (1968).
47. Rudman, D. and Kelly, T. F.: *Biochemistry* **7,** 3136 (1968).
48*a*. Sándor, G.: *Serum Proteins in Health and Disease.* Chapman, London 1966, p. 178,
48*b*. ibid., p. 233.
48*c*. ibid., p. 240.
49. Sándor, G., Martin, L., Mattern, P., Orley, C., Sureau, B., Berrod, J. and Martin. R.: *Ann. Inst. Pasteur* **113,** 569 (1967).
50. Sándor, G. and Orley, C.: *Ann. Inst. Pasteur* **115,** 803 (1968).
51. Scanu, A.: *J. biol. Chem.* **242,** 711 (1967).
52. Scheinberg, I. H. and Sternlieb, H.: *Lancet* **i,** 1420 (1963).
53. Schmid, K. and Thomson, B. D.: *Endocrinology* **76,** 510 (1967).
54. Schoemakers, J. G. G., Matze, R., Haamers, C. and Zilliken, F.: *Biochim. biophys. Acta (Amst.)* **101,** 166 (1965).
55. Schultze, H. E., Haupt, H., Heide, K. and Heimburger, N.: *Clin. chim. Acta* **8,** 207 (1962).
56. Seal, U. S. and Doe, R. P.: *J. biol. Chem.* **237,** 3136 (1962).
57*a*. Shore, B. and Shore, V.: *Biochemistry* **7,** 2773 (1968).
57*b*. ibid., **7,** 3396 (1968).
58. Slayter, E. M.: *J. molec. Biol.* **14,** 443 (1965).
59. Steinbuch, M., Blatrix, C. and Josso, F.: *Rev. franc. Étud. clin. biol.* **13,** 179 (1968).
60. Vallee, B. L. and Ulmer, D. D.: *Biochemistry* **2,** 1335 (1963).
61. Wermert, H., Masui, H., Radidevich, I. and Werner, S. C.: *J. clin. Invest.* **46,** 1264 (1967).
62. Wolff, O. H.: *Ergebn. inn. Med. Kinderheilk.* **23,** 190 (1965).

CHAPTER 13

# IMMUNOGLOBULINS

by

J. GERGELY



## TERMINOLOGY

The term immunoglobulin designates

1. antibodies
2. proteins without any known antibody activity but structurally and antigenically related to the antibodies.

Immunoglobulins are divided into at least five classes (Table 13-I). These are termed according to the nomenclature recommanded by the WHO as IgG, IgA, IgM, IgD and IgE [5]. Apart from the physiological immunoglobulins there are immunoglobulins produced by certain pathologically proliferated cells (monoclonal gammopathies). These latter are the myeloma proteins, the Waldenström

TABLE 13-I

*Classes of human immunoglobulins*

| | IgG | IgA | IgM | IgD | IgE |
|---|---|---|---|---|---|
| Molecular weight | 150,000 | 180,000<br>500,000 | 950,000 | | 200,000 |
| $s_{20,w}$ (S) | 6.5–7.0 | 7, 10, 13, 15 | 18–20 | 6.2–6.8 | 7.9 |
| Carbohydrate content (%) | 3 | 7.5 | 12 | | 10.7 |
| Heavy chain molecular weight | 53,000 | 64,000 | 70,000 | | 75,000 |
| Light chain molecular weight | | 22,000 | | | |
| Serum concentration in normal adults (mg per 100 ml) | 800–1,600 | 140–420 | 50–190 | 3–40 | 0.01–0.14 |
| Concentration in cord serum (expressed in % of maternal serum level) | 100 | 1 | 10 | | |
| Half-life (days) | 23 | 6 | 5 | 2.8 | |

macroglobulins, the Bence–Jones proteins and the heavy chain disease proteins. Physiological or pathological urinary proteins structurally related to the former are also immunoglobulins. These urinary immunoglobulins have no antibody activity.

## THE STRUCTURE OF IMMUNOGLOBULINS

Studying the structure of immunoglobulins has been made difficult by their heterogeneity which is due to the polyclonal origin of these proteins. Minute amounts of functionally and structurally homogeneous proteins can be isolated from the heterogeneous populations of immunoglobulins only by the use of relatively complicated methods, e.g. immunosorption. The discovery that the structurally homogeneous serum and urinary proteins produced in extreme amounts in monoclonal gammopathies are immunoglobulins led to a favourable turn in the research of immunoglobulin structure. The homogeneity of these latter proteins points to a monoclonal origin. The overwhelming majority of these homogeneous proteins can be regarded as individual members of the physiological population of immunoglobulins. Therefore, the homogeneous proteins produced in monoclonal gammopathies are ideal models for studies on immunoglobulin structure, and an important part of the information available about the structure of immunoglobulins has been derived from the investigation of these proteins.

The studies of Porter [44*a*] and Edelman [10] have been the first steps taken towards the exploration of immunoglobulin structure. Three fragments have been isolated by Porter from rabbit IgG partially hydrolysed by papain. Two of the fragments retained antibody activity. Adopting a different approach, Edelman succeeded in the separation of the polypeptide chains from IgG after cleavage of disulphide bonds, first establishing the involvement of two different polypeptide chains in the IgG molecules. These studies were followed by an intensive research activity resulting in the elucidation of the main structural features of immunoglobulins.

## POLYPEPTIDE CHAINS OF IMMUNOGLOBULINS

Reduction of IgG at neutral pH cleaves the disulphide bridges between the polypeptide chain constituents of the molecule. The chains can be separated by gel filtration in dissociating medium, permitting the isolation of a light (L: mol. wt., 22,000) and a heavy (H: mol. wt., 55,000) component. The IgG molecule is constructed of two heavy and two light chains.

The polypeptide chains are held together by disulphide bridges and by non-covalent binding forces. A pair of a light and a heavy chain is joined by one disulphide bond, and there are disulphide bridges between the two heavy chains, too. The cysteine residue at (or adjacent to) the C-terminal portion of the L chains is involved in the inter-heavy-light-chain bridging. The non-covalent interactions between the polypeptide chains play an important role in stabilizing the conformation of the molecule [8, 12, 16]. The non-covalent bondings are restituted when isolated polypeptide chains are mixed in neutral medium, and a part of the chains are recombined to form four-chain units resembling the native molecule. Recombination may occur between the chains from a single protein (autologous), or between the chains of different immunoglobulins (heterologous); moreover chains from different species can also be recombined. Antibody activity is recovered on recombination [9, 17, 28]. Hence the immunoglobulin polypeptide chains of different origin possess similarly arranged groupings of amino acid residues which are responsible for non-covalent interchain binding forces.

A possible structural relationship between different classes of immunoglobulins was first suggested by Edelman and Benacerraf [11]. Like IgG, IgA and IgM can be cleaved into polypeptide chains by reduction followed by the dissociation of non-covalent binding. Analysis of the isolated polypeptide chains by electrophoresis and immunodiffusion has proved the identity of the L chains and the diversity of the H chains. Likewise proteins of the later discovered IgD and IgE classes have light chains in common with the other classes of immunoglobulins and the structural differences between the classes are carried by the heavy chains. The structural diversity of the heavy chains is reflected by the nomenclature recommanded by the WHO: $\gamma$, $\alpha$, $\mu$, $\delta$ and $\varepsilon$ designate the heavy chains of IgG, IgA, IgM, IgD and IgE, respectively.

## PROTEOLYTIC FRAGMENTATION OF IMMUNOGLOBULINS

As mentioned above, the IgG molecule is split into three fragments by papain and cysteine. The two Fab fragments (mol. wt., 52,000) carry one antigen binding site each. The third fragment (Fc) of human IgG (mol. wt., 49,000) exhibits an electrophoretic mobility greater than that of the Fab. It has no antibody activity, but some of the other biological properties of the IgG molecule such as comple-

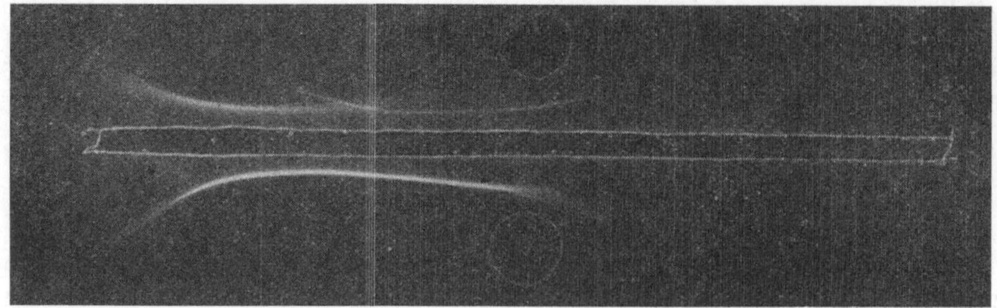

Fig. 13-1. Immunoelectrophoretic patterns of native human IgG (below) and of human IgG digested with papain in the presence of cysteine (above)

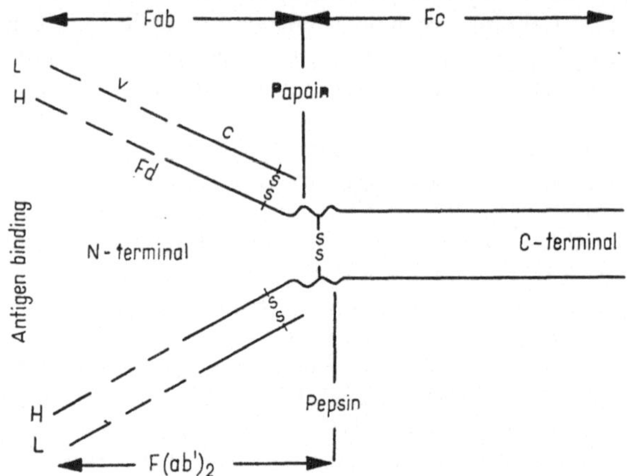


Fig. 13-2. Schematic representation of the human IgG molecule with the sites of papain and pepsin cleavage and the fragments [7]

ment fixation, skin sensitization etc. are associated with this latter fragment (Fig. 13-1) [44*a*].

One part of the IgG molecule is split into smaller peptides on mild peptic proteolysis, while the remaining part which is approximatively of 105,000 molecular weight can act as bivalent antibody like the native protein. This bivalent 5 S fragment $F(ab')_2$ can be cleaved into two 3.5 S fragments (Fab'), which are univalent like the Fab obtained by papain proteolysis. The site of pepsin cleavage is not identical with that of the papain, but they are close by along the heavy chain sequence [52]. Papain acts on some peptide bonds N-terminal while pepsin C-terminal from the inter-heavy-chain disulphide bridges. The heavy chain segment between the sites of cleavage of these two enzymes, called hinge region, is particularly important from both the structural and functional points of view (Fig. 13-2) [26, 36, 40]. Enzymatic splitting of IgM has not provided as useful structural information as that of IgG. An Fab-like fragment (Fab $\mu$) has already been identified. Very little is known about the proteolytic fragmentation of IgA.

Comparison of the isolated polypeptide chains with the fragments obtained by proteolytic cleavage made it possible to outline the structural model of IgG. A structural unit is constituted by four polypeptide chains connected by disulphide bridges and non-covalent bonds. The general structure of immunoglobulins is shown in Fig. 13-3. IgG consists of two heavy and two light chains. The fragment produced by papain cleavage contains the entire light chain and a piece of the heavy chain (Fd), while Fc only contains heavy chain elements. IgM is constructed of five subunits, each consisting of two heavy and two light chains. The subunits are joined by disulphide bridges; as there is only weak non-covalent interaction between the subunits, they can rotate around the disulphide bridges. The molecular weight of the IgM heavy ($\mu$) chains (approx. 70,000) is greater than that of the $\gamma$ chain.

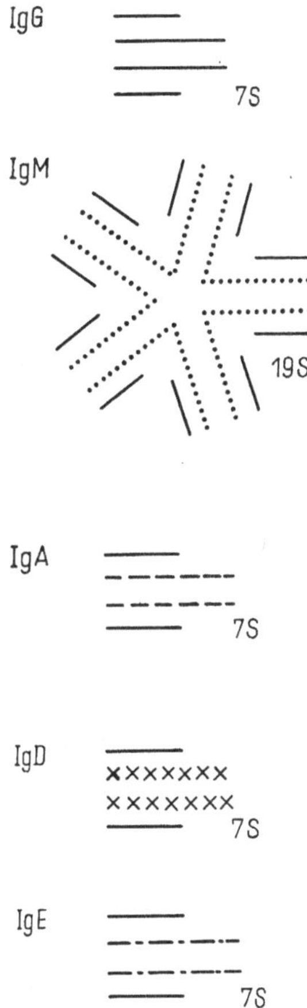


Fig. 13-3. General structure of immunoglobulins

IgA isolated from normal serum is also composed of two heavy and two light chains. Like $\mu$ chains, $\alpha$ chains are somewhat heavier than $\gamma$ chains. The formation of polymers is characteristic for this class of immunoglobulins. IgA is the main immunoglobulin component of exocrine secretions. Secretory IgA is a 11 S protein, thus considerably heavier than the major portion of serum IgA (6.9 S). Secretory IgA is composed of two four-chain IgA molecules linked to a so-called

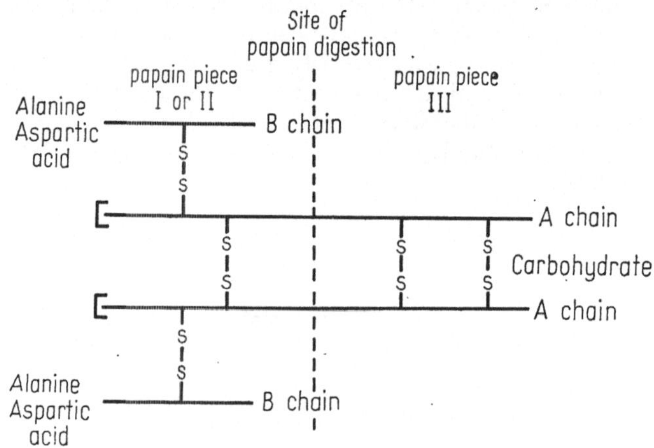


Fig. 13-4. Structural scheme of IgG molecule according to Porter

secretory peptide (S piece) which is produced by epithelial cells [51]. In the polymeric IgA as well in the IgM molecules a new type of polypeptide chains, called J chain has been recently described [29, 37]. The approximate molecular weight of the J chain is 20,000 and it is quite distinct from the S piece as well as from light polypeptide chains of immunoglobulins. Like the other immunoglobulins IgD and IgE are also constructed of two heavy and two light chains. The molecular weight of $\varepsilon$ chains is about 75,000.

Based on the result of reductive and proteolytic cleavage of IgG, Porter constructed the first polypeptide chain model of this protein (Fig. 13-4). A linear model, similar to the original Porter scheme, is shown in Fig. 13-2 with interchain disulphide bridges, presumable sites of papain and peptic cleavage, Fab, Fc and $F(ab')_2$ fragments, as well as intramolecular localization of biological functions. About 93 per cent of the carbohydrate component of IgG is bound to the H chain, two-thirds of this is recovered in the Fc fragment while the remaining third is found in relatively small molecular weight glycopeptides after papain cleavage.

Fab and Fc fragments have a steric structure resembling compact spheric globulae, in contrast to the considerable asymmetry and flexibility of the native IgG. Evidence for this structural correlation was first derived from hydrodynamic investigations of rabbit IgG and fragments. Patterns obtained by electron microscopic studies are consistent with this concept [15]. These investigations gave a figure of 80–120 Å for the long, and a figure of about 34 Å for the short axis. Electron-microscopic observations of ferritin–antiferritin immune complexes have led to the suggestion that when combination with antigens occurs, antibody molecules click open on a hinge point (like the shanks of scissors). This hinge point is located at one end of the molecule and during antigen binding the Y-shaped molecule is extended to twice its original length. Investigations of $F(ab')_2$ fragments permitted the conclusion that the leg of the Y contains the Fc part (Fig. 13-5). The molecular model in Fig. 13-6 has been constructed taking into account these electron-microscopic observations [41, 53].

Electron-microscopic studies of IgM molecules revealed a spider-like structure with five appandages joined together forming a central ring structure. The diameter of the whole molecule is approximately 230–250 Å.

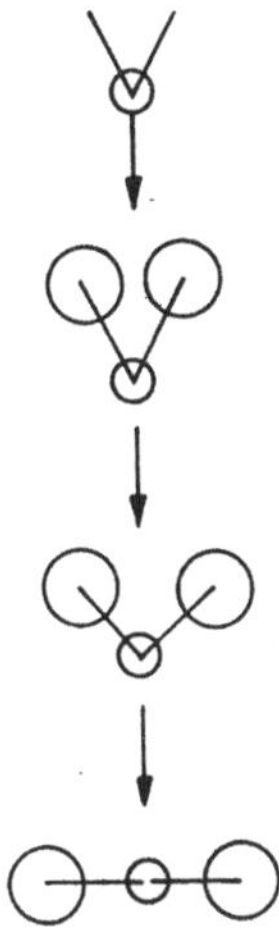

Fig. 13-5. Antigen (o) binding of IgG molecule. Schematic representation based on electron-microscopic patterns (for detailed explanation see text)

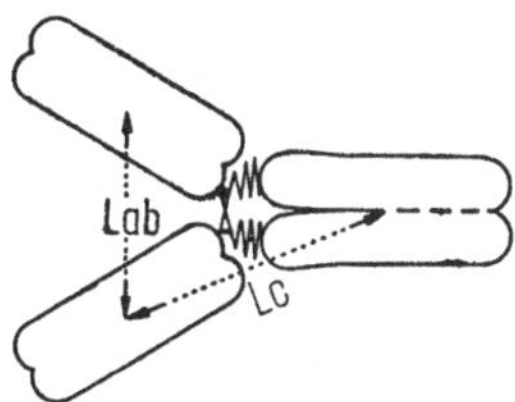


Fig. 13-6. Model of IgG molecule (Charlwood-Utsumi). Distance between the two Fab parts and between the Fab parts and the Fc part is 76 ± 8 Å

## HETEROGENEITY OF IMMUNOGLOBULINS

Study of the biological significance of immunoglobulin heterogeneity is one of the focal problems of immunology. This heterogeneity is the basis of the specificity of the humoral immune response, as only a highly heterogeneous system can correspond adequately to the multitude of antigens. The heterogeneity of immunoglobulins is the consequence of a three-fold variability of their amino acid sequence.

1. Isotypic heterogeneity. All the isotypes are found in each normal individual of a given species.

2. Allotypic heterogeneity, originating from the genetically determined polymorphism of immunoglobulins.

3. Idiotypic heterogeneity or individual antigenic specificity of monoclonal immunoglobulins (antibodies). This level of heterogeneity is related to the variable part of amino acid sequence.

## *Isotipy*

### *Immunoglobulin classes*

Based on differences in the heavy chain structure, immunoglobulins can be divided into at least five classes (IgG, IgA, IgM, IgD and IgE). The class heterogeneity is the most conspicuous expression of the heterogeneity of immunoglobulins. Although the biological significance of the class heterogeneity is not completely understood, there is evidence for the differing functional role of the different immunoglobulin classes in humoral immunity.

### *Immunoglobulin types (sub-classes)*

A further level of isotypic heterogeneity is related to the heterogeneity of antigenic microstructure of the polypeptide chains. Studies of the antigenicity of homogeneous immunoglobulins found in monoclonal gammopathies have led to the discovery of this heterogeneity.

*Light chain types.* Bence–Jones proteins have been grouped into two types according to their antigenic character. The two types are designated as $\varkappa$ (I, K) and $\lambda$ (II, L), respectively. Antigenic determinants, characteristic of the $\varkappa$ and $\lambda$ types are carried by light chains. These are common constituents of all immunoglobulins, accordingly, any type of heavy chain can combine with either $\varkappa$ or $\lambda$ type of light chain. Resulting from the combination of the five types of heavy chains with the two types of light chain ten different types of immunoglobulin can be distinguished:

| Class | Heavy chain type | Light chain type |
|---|---|---|
| IgG | $\gamma_1, \gamma_2, \gamma_3, \gamma_4$ | $\varkappa, \lambda$ |
| IgA | $\alpha_1, \alpha_2$ | $\varkappa, \lambda$ |
| IgM | $\mu_1, \mu_2$ | $\varkappa, \lambda$ |
| IgD | $\delta$ | $\varkappa, \lambda$ |
| IgE | $\varepsilon$ | $\varkappa, \lambda$ |

Two-thirds of the population of IgG molecules belong to the $\varkappa$ type, one-third belongs to the $\lambda$ type under physiological conditions. $\varkappa$ and $\lambda$ determinants do not occur on the same immunoglobulin molecule. The $\varkappa/\lambda$ ratio of the light chains of immunoglobulins A and M is approximately the same as that found in the IgG class. In the IgD class the $\lambda$ type is markedly more frequent than the $\varkappa$ type.

The monoclonally produced immunoglobulins are homogeneous with respect to the light chain type, too; a given myeloma protein, Waldenström macroglobulin or Bence–Jones protein contains only either $\varkappa$ or $\lambda$ type light chains in contrast to the heterogeneous normal immunoglobulins [14, 32*a*, *b*, 35].

A small molecular weight, electrophoretically heterogeneous proteins, antigenically related to the immunoglobulins has been found in the urine of healthy individuals. This protein, called $\gamma_U$ was detected also in the ultrafiltrate of blood serum. The $\varkappa/\lambda$ ratio in these microglobulins, consisting of the light chains of immunoglobulins, is 2 : 1 [2, 50].

The observation that most higher vertebrates possess both $\varkappa$ and $\lambda$ type light chains is significant.

*$\gamma$ chain types.* Evidence have been furnished for minor antigenic differences among heavy chains of IgG. On this basis, four sub-classes of IgG can be distinguished [27]. The heavy chain types are designed as $\gamma_1$, $\gamma_2$, $\gamma_3$, and $\gamma_4$ in the order of their frequency (Table 13-II). All four types are present in the physiological IgG population.

TABLE 13-II

*Sub-classes of IgG*

| Sub-class | $\gamma$ chain type | Relative frequency among myeloma proteins, % |
|---|---|---|
| IgG1 | 1 | 70–80 |
| IgG2 | 2 | 13–18 |
| IgG3 | 3 | 6–8 |
| IgG4 | 4 | 3 |

In normal IgG two populations can be distinguished on the basis of different susceptibility to papain proteolysis. Some 60 per cent of normal IgG are splil by papain into Fab and Fc fragments without adding cysteine or a similar thiot compound to the mixture (papain sensitive population), while the remaining 40 per cent can be split by papain into Fab and Fc fragments only in the presence in an appropriate concentration of a thiol compound (papain resistant population) [25].

IgG 2 and IgG 4 type myeloma proteins are papain resistant, IgG 3 type myeloma proteins are papain sensitive like most of the IgG 1 type myeloma proteins. Testing the papain sensitivity of an IgG myeloma protein may provide therefore some information on the $\gamma$ chain sub-type of the protein.

Sub-class related differences have been found in the susceptibility to tryptic fragmentation of different IgG myeloma proteins too. Immunoelectrophoresis of tryptic digests of IgG results in characteristic patterns corresponding to sub-class specificity so that this procedure can be used for sub-class typing of IgG myeloma proteins [24, 30].

The preparation of sub-class specific antisera is highly complicated; on the other hand, papain- and trypsin-susceptibility can be tested without any special equipment or rare reagent [20, 23, 25].

*α chain types*. By the use of specific antisera the existence of two antigenically distinct types of α chain has been established [18]. An allotypic marker (Am) has been found to be confined on the $\alpha_2$ chains (IgA2 sub-class). IgAs carrying the Am marker have been found to lack the inter-heavy-light-chain disulphide bridge. In such proteins the two light chains are linked by a disulphide bridge, and the light chains are bound to the $\alpha_2$ chains only by non-covalent interaction [34].

*μ chain types*. Two μ chain types could be distinguished by a horse anti-human serum. The serum gives two precipitation lines with a physiological population of IgM, but only one with monoclonal IgMs [1]. Classification of human μ chains into two different sub-classes was also performed by Franklin and Frangione by the use of specifically absorbed rabbit antisera [18].

## *Allotypes*

Human 'gamma-globulin groups', i.e. allotypes were first described by Grubb. The term 'allotype' was constructed by Oudin, who applied it to the polymorphism of rabbit γ-globulins. Allotypes are genetically determined structural variations of proteins. A certain protein can differ in allotypic character in different individuals of the same species. Detection of allotypes in non-human species requires no special technique since immunization of individuals negative for a given allotype with immunoglobulins carrying this allotypic marker results in precipitating antibodies. Human allotypes can be detected by the use of non-precipitating anti-IgG antibodies found in certain human sera. Rh positive erythrocytes sensitized with incomplete anti-Rh antibodies are agglutinated by these human anti-IgG antibodies.

More than twenty allotypes of human immunoglobulins have been discovered (Table 13-III). One group of them, the Gm factors and the ISf factor are localized on the γ chains, these markers are found therefore only in the IgG class. The Inv factors are associated with the ϰ type of light chains, Inv factors are found therefore in all the immunoglobulin classes and Bence–Jones proteins.

The intramolecular localization of some Gm factors have been discovered. Most of them (Gm 1, 2, 5, 14, 22 and 24) are found on the Fc part of the γ chain, Gm 3, 4 and 17 are associated with the Fd part. Gm 3 (and 4) is dependent on the quaternary structure, they are not expressed on isolated γ chain, but only when the γ chain is combined with a light chain. Three of the four γ chain sub-classes are carriers of Gm factors. Gm 1, 2, 3, 4, 17 and 22 are associated with the $\gamma_1$, while Gm 5, 10–16 and 21 with the $\gamma_3$ sub-class. Gm 23 is carried by $\gamma_2$ chains. No allotypic marker has been found on $\gamma_4$ chains. The Gm factors are inherited in definite linkage groups, which have been found characteristically different in different races (Table 13-IV).

Sequence analysis of Bence–Jones proteins has provided evidence for the dependence of the Inv 2 or Inv 3 character on a single amino acid replacement. If the 191st amino acid residue of a ϰ chain is leucine, the chain is Inv 2, if this leucine is replaced by valine, the chain is Inv 3. Likewise a lysine–arginine interchange is determinant for the Oz + or Oz — character of a λ chain [6, 42, 49]. The Oz types are not allotypes; they represent an isotypic heterogeneity of λ chains [13].

TABLE 13-III

*Nomenclature and molecular localization of Gm, ISf and Inv factors*

| WHO nomenclature | Original nomenclature | Molecular localization | | | | |
|---|---|---|---|---|---|---|
| | | H chain | | | | κ chain |
| | | IgG2 | IgG1 | | IgG3 | |
| | | Fc | Fd | Fc | Fc | |
| Gm 1 | Gma | | | x | | |
| Gm 2 | Gm x | | | x | | |
| Gm 3 | Gm $b^w$ or $b^2$ | | x | | | |
| Gm 4 | Gm f | | x | | | |
| Gm 5 | Gm b or Gm $b^1$ | | | | x | |
| Gm 6 | Gm c or like | | | | x | |
| Gm 7 | Gm r | | | | | |
| Gm 8 | Gm 2 | x | | x | | |
| Gm 9 | Gm p | | | x | x | |
| Gm 10 | Gm $b^\alpha$ | | | | x | |
| Gm 11 | Gm $b^\beta$ | | | | x | |
| Gm 12 | Gm $b^\gamma$ | | | | x | |
| Gm 13 | Gm $b^3$ | | | | x | |
| Gm 14 | Gm $b^4$ | | | | x | |
| Gm 15 | Gm s | | | | x | |
| Gm 16 | Gm t | | | | x | |
| Gm 17 | Gm z | | x | | | |
| Gm 18 | Rouen 2 or $R_2$ | x | | x | | |
| Gm 19 | Rouen 3 or $R_3$ | | | | | |
| Gm 20 | Gm z | | | | | |
| Gm 21 | Gm g | | | | x | |
| Gm 22 | Gm y | | | x | | |
| Gm 23 | Gm n | x | | x | | |
| ISf | San Francisco 1 | | | | x | |
| Inv 1 | Inv 1 | | | | | x |
| Inv 2 | Inv a | | | | | x |
| Inv 3 | Inv b | | | | | x |

TABLE 13-IV

*Fixed combinations of Gm factors and their distribution in various races*

| Race | Combination of Gm factors |
|---|---|
| Caucasoid | Gm 1, 2; Gm 3, 5, 13, 14 |
| Negroid | Gm 1, 5, 13, 15; Gm 1, 5, 14; Gm 1, 5, 6 |
| Mongoloid | Gm 1; Gm 1, 2; Gm 1, 13; Gm 1, 3, 5, 13, 14 |

## *Idiotypes*

Homogeneous immunoglobulins possess individual specific antigenic determinants, i.e. antigenic determinants not shared with other homogeneous immunoglobulin populations of the same isotype and allotype. Immunization of rabbits with human myeloma proteins and appropriate absorbtion of the sera can result in antisera not reacting with any protein but the one employed for immunization. The term idiotype was originally proposed by Oudin to designate individual antigenic specificity of rabbit anti-Salmonella antibodies. The idiotypic antigenic determinants are associated with the Fab part of the immunoglobulins [1, 33].

## STRUCTURE OF POLYPEPTIDE CHAINS OF IMMUNOGLOBULINS

### STRUCTURE OF LIGHT CHAINS

Bence–Jones proteins are immunoglobulin light chains in monomeric, dimeric or tetrameric form. Since such proteins can be isolated from urine of myeloma patients in high quantities, Bence–Jones proteins are indispensable model substances for the structural study of light chains. Sequence studies of Bence–Jones proteins have been in progress since 1960 and the entire sequence of a number of them has been published. Light chains of mouse myeloma proteins have also been studied for amino acid sequence. The results show the heterogeneity of the primary structure of immunoglobulins thus providing starting points for various concepts on the evolution of immunoglobulins.

Human and murine immunoglobulin light chains are composed of an approximately identical number (213–218) of amino acids. Comparison of different light chain sequences has led to the conclusion that the N-terminal half of the light chain sequence is variable, i.e. each chain possesses a particular amino acid sequence, while the C-terminal half of the sequence is identical within a given isotype. (In the constant sequence of human $\varkappa$ chains the only variation is a valine–leucine replacement associated with the Inv allotypes.) Not every amino acid residue is variable in the N-terminal half, there are regions with constant amino acid sequence.

The complete amino acid sequence of a $\varkappa$ type Bence–Jones protein (Ag) is shown in Fig. 13-7. This protein was studied by Putnam et al. [48]. As indicated on the figure there are only 48 variable positions. Intrachain disulphide bonds form two loops within the light chains, each loop contains about sixty amino acid residues. One of the two loops is found within the constant half, the other within the variable half of the polypeptide chain. The $\varkappa$ and $\lambda$ chains contain cysteine residues in homologous position. Four cysteine residues form the two intrachain disulphide bonds, and a further cystein residue is involved in the disulphide bond joning the light chain to the heavy chain. This latter cysteine is the C-terminal amino acid in $\varkappa$ chains, while in $\lambda$ chains it is situated adjacent to the C-terminal amino acid. In certain Bence–Jones proteins two light chains are joined by a disulphide bridge formed by cysteine residues at, or next to, the C-terminal position (Fig. 13-8). Light chains are remarkably symmetrical; splitting at the point between the constant and variable portions would result in two halves of approximately identical size.

Comparison of constant and variable sequences of human and mouse $\varkappa$ and $\lambda$ chains revealed considerable homologies, e.g. in the constant region of mouse and human K chains 58 per cent of the amino acid residues are identical, 29 per cent

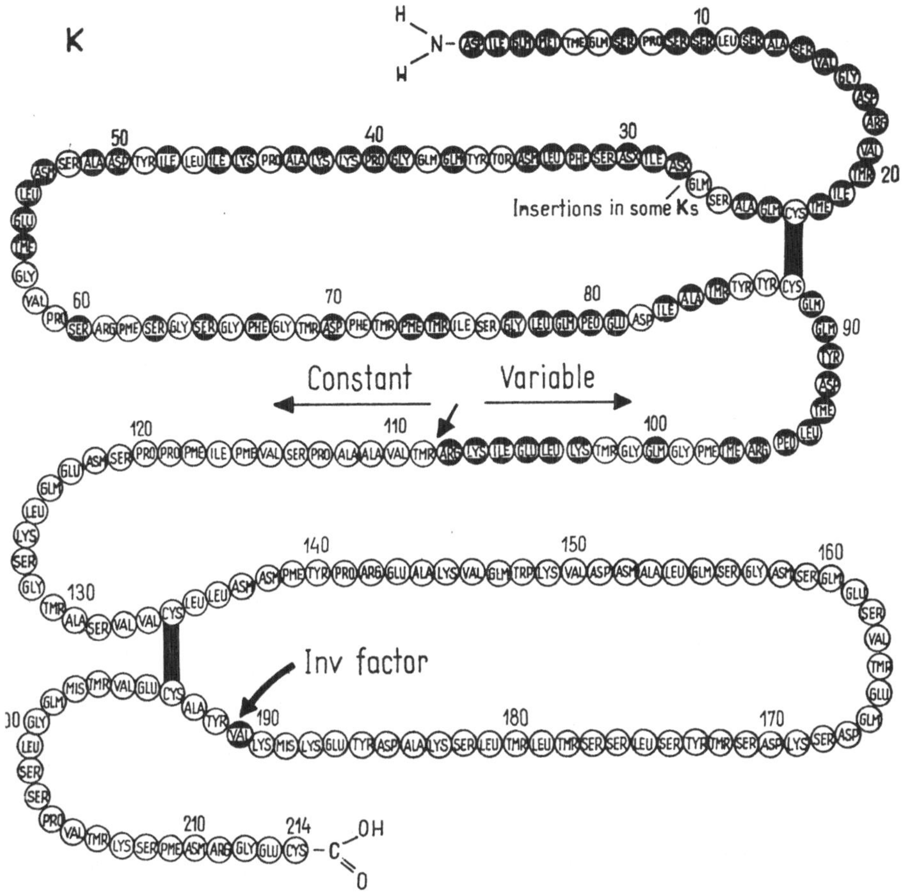

Fig. 13-7. Primary structure of ϰ chain according to Putnam. Variable positions are indicated by dark, constant positions by white circles

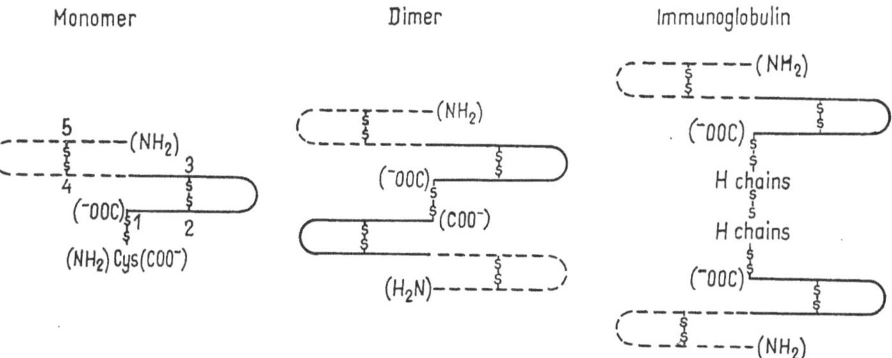


Fig. 13-8. Monomeric and dimeric forms of light chains (Bence-Jones proteins) and binding of light chains to heavy chains (according to Milstein)

can be converted to the other by a single nucleotide base change, and 13 per cent can be converted by two base changes. Similar base change frequencies have been found by comparison of proteins known to be related by evolution (haemoglobins, cytochrome Cs, insulins etc.). The degree of homology between human $\varkappa$ and human $\lambda$ chains is similar to that found between mouse $\varkappa$ and human $\varkappa$ chains. There is a region where the number of identical residues is higher than 70 per cent for mouse and human or for human $\varkappa$ and human $\lambda$ chains [47, 48].

Comparison of the variable regions of various Bence–Jones proteins permitted the subdivision of light chains into sub-groups. The degree of homology between light chains of the same sub-group is markedly higher than between light chains of different sub-groups. Three such sub-groups can be distinguished in the $\varkappa$ chains and four in the $\lambda$ chains. (There are $\varkappa$ or $\lambda$ type-specific stretches of amino acid sequence within the variable half of the light chains, too.)

## STRUCTURE OF HEAVY CHAINS

Investigation of the primary structure of heavy chains is more difficult than that of light chains. Heavy chains are roughly twice as long as light chains. There are several classes and sub-classes of heavy chains while only two types of light chains. Complete amino acid sequence of myeloma protein $\gamma$ chains has already been published. Like light chains, heavy chains are composed of an N-terminal variable region and a C-terminal constant region. The relative homogeneity of the C-terminal portion has been suggested by the early investigations of Porter. This was confirmed by peptide analyses of the Fc-fragment and partial sequence studies.

Studies of the N-terminal half of heavy chains have yielded evidence for a variable region within this part of the chain. Among the first 100 amino acid residues (starting with the N-terminal residue) 20 were found variable by comparison of heavy chain fragments obtained by BrCN cleavage [45]. Like $\varkappa$ and $\lambda$ chains, heavy chains could be divided into sub-groups on the basis of the degree of homology within the variable region. These variable sequence sub-groups are not related to classes or sub-classes of heavy chains. A striking similarity between light and heavy chains is the existence of loops formed by intrachain disulphide bonds. Each loop contains about 60 amino acids. Two loops are on the Fc and two on the Fd piece of the $\gamma$ chains, and two loops on the variable region of the Fd piece [38, 44*b*, 45].

## STRUCTURAL HOMOLOGIES BETWEEN HEAVY AND LIGHT CHAINS

A surprisingly high degree of homology has been found by amino acid sequence analysis between heavy and light chains.

Cysteine residues are situated in homologous positions and the sequences around cysteine residues show very high degrees of homology, not only when different polypeptide chains are compared, but also when comparing different regions of the same polypeptide chain. Thus four homology regions are defined in $\gamma$ chains and two in $\varkappa$ or $\lambda$ chains. Three of the homology regions of $\gamma$ chains belong to the constant sequence while the fourth to the variable sequence. These observations based on sequence comparison of immunoglobulin polypeptide chains provide the basis for theories on the molecular evolution of immunoglobulins. A primordial gene, equivalent to a peptide of mol. wt. 12,000 is supposed to be the common ancestor of immunoglobulin genes. Resulting from an unequal crossing over, a new fused gene emerged, the ancestral light chain gene. This precursor gene underwent another fused duplication to give the heavy chain gene. The more ancient heavy chain is the $\mu$ chain (Fig. 13-9).

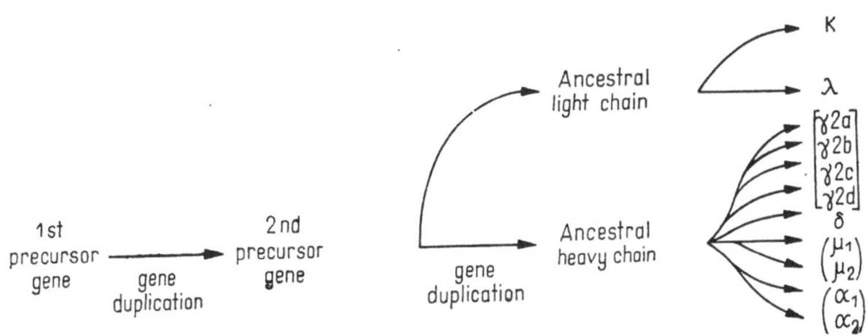


Fig. 13-9. Presumed scheme of molecular evolution of immunoglobulin polypeptide chains

## CONNECTIONS BETWEEN STRUCTURE AND FUNCTION OF IMMUNOGLOBULINS

The structural bases of immunoglobulin function have been investigated following the accumulation of knowledge on immunoglobulin structure. Most of the data have been derived from studies on IgG.

### THE ANTIGEN BINDING SITE

The part of immunoglobulin surface which specifically binds the corresponding antigenic determinant is called antigen binding site or active site. Studies on fragments produced by limited proteolytic cleavage made it evident that the antigen binding site of IgG is localized on the Fab part of the protein. As the Fab fragment contains the entire light chain and a piece of the heavy chain the participation of both chains in the antigen binding seems probable.

Sequence data indicating the existence of constant and variable regions within the light and heavy polypeptide chains are highly significant for the active site problem. The variable region is located on the N-terminal stretch of both polypeptide chains; thus presuming the localization of the active site on the variable region seems reasonable. Experimental data finding slight but significant differences in the amino acid composition of antibodies of different specificities are coherent with this concept. Three regions of the light chains, classed as 'hypervariable', extensively vary in sequence. Although the available sequence data on heavy chains are still insufficient for this sort of comparison one can suggest the existence of regions also in the variable part of heavy chains which are more heterogeneous than the rest of the chains. Several investigations proved that the hypervariable regions are the major constituents of the antigen combining site. Many other amino acid residues throughout the variable region are probably also involved in the determination of antibody specificity, although perhaps indirectly by affecting the overall tertiary structure of the Fab fragment. The question whether the light or the heavy chain is more important in the antigen binding cannot be answered directly: some experiments point to the decisive role of the light chain, others demonstrate the importance of the heavy chain and there are also data suggesting the participation of both polypeptide chains. The observation that the presence of a hapten promotes the recombination of the heavy and light chains of the corresponding antibody is highly interesting [46].

Antibodies of the IgG class are bivalent. Four polypeptide chain units of antibodies of other immunoglobulin classes also seem bivalent, only the IgM antibodies exhibit a different reactivity. IgM antibodies have been found pentavalent, hence the four-chain IgM subunits seem to be univalent. This fact does not necessarily mean that IgM subunits have only one antigen binding site. It is possible that only one of the active sites can bind the antigen due to steric hindrance. IgG antibodies may also be virtually univalent, e.g. the so-called incomplete haemagglutinins. Experimental evidence indicates that these IgG antibodies have, in fact, two antigen binding sites, but only one of them can bind the corresponding antigenic determinant on the erythrocyte surface.

## STRUCTURAL ASPECTS OF FUNCTIONAL PROPERTIES OTHER THAN ANTIBODY SPECIFICITY

The antibody function of immunoglobulins is—strictly speaking—the specific binding of antigens. Besides immunoglobulins are carriers of further biological functions such as tissue binding, complement fixation, reaction with rheumatoid factor and placental passage. These functional properties show no direct antigen specificity and are thus called non-specific functions.

### *Tissue binding*

Studying the skin sensitizing property of Fab and Fc fragments from IgG antibodies it has been found that only the Fc fragment can sensitize the guinea pig skin, while the Fab fragment (the fragment carrying antibody specificity) is inactive in this respect. The antibody specificity and the skin sensitizing capacity is associated with different parts of the antibody molecule. This explains the early observation that treatment of antibodies with pepsin destroys their skin sensitizing capacity [43].

There are antibodies possessing specific binding property for certain cells. These cytophilic antibodies are attached to the receptors of the corresponding cells by their Fc piece. Thus the cytophilic antibody fixed to the cell surface is still able to react with the corresponding antigen.

Under physiological conditions a great number of protein molecules are adsorbed to erythrocyte surface. IgG is the most firmly bound of all the plasma proteins. About 10,000–30,000 incomplete anti-D antibodies can be attached by specific antigen–antibody interaction to the surface of an Rh (D) positive erythrocyte, while the number of IgG molecules adsorbed by non-antibody type binding is about 200,000. IgG fixed by this type of binding is not detectable by antiglobulin reaction, in contrast to specifically bound antibodies. The reason for this difference may be sought for in the fixed steric orientation of specifically bound incomplete antibodies attached to the erythrocyte surface by their combining site (on the Fab part) thus rendering the Fc part accessible for the antiglobulin reagent. (Antiglobulin sera have mostly anti-Fc activity.) IgG adsorbed by non-antibody type binding is presumably attached by its Fc part or without any fixed steric orientation [22].

IgG molecules easily undergo aggregation. Isolation procedures, storage or mild heating may cause aggregation resulting in the formation first of 9–10 S dimers and then of larger aggregates. This process is accompanied by changes in conformation exposing new antigenic determinants (being in hidden position in the native protein). Aggregation thus may also affect the functional properties of IgG (see complement fixation and rheumatoid factor binding). Structural differences in the Fc part and in the so-called hinge region of IgG are important with respect to some non-antibody type functions, e.g. the papain resistant portion of IgG is preferentially adsorbed on the erythrocyte surface (non-antibody type binding) [19, 21].

### *Reaction with the complement system*

Antibodies of the IgG and IgM classes have been found to react with complement.

The complement fixing capacity of IgG is associated with the Fc part of the protein. Aggregated Fc fragment has been found anti-complementary in contrast to the Fab fragment. Antibodies react with complement when they are combined with antigen. At least two molecules of IgG antibodies must be situated in close proximity for complement fixation, as revealed by electron-microscopic studies of the haemolysis following the reaction of erythrocytes with IgG haemolysins and complement. One single IgM molecule, bound to antigen is sufficient for complement fixation. Combination with antigen presumably induces a change in steric conformation of the IgM molecule bringing the complement fixing sites of the subunits in a position suitable for the reaction with the first component of the complement system. The site of IgG combining with the first component of the complement system seems to be located on the CHII homology region, i.e. on the N-terminal half of the Fc part of the molecule, as suggested by the experiments of Kehoe and Fougereau [31]. These authors succeeded in isolating an H chain fragment from a mouse IgG2, a myeloma protein, by BrCN-cleavage which represented the aforementioned region of the H chain and retained some complement fixing capacity.

Not all IgGs react equally with complement. Guinea pig IgG can be electrophoretically separated into two fractions. The $\gamma_1$ fractions having a higher anodic mobility does not fix complement, while the slower $\gamma_2$ does. Human IgG sub-classes differ in complement fixing capacity too. Proteins of the IgG1 and IgG3 sub-classes react strongly with complement, proteins of the IgG2 sub-class react weakly, while those of the IgG4 sub-class do not bind complement [39].

### *Placental passage of immunoglobulins*

Placenta serves as a selective filter for plasma proteins. The only class of immunoglobulins which can pass from maternal to fetal circulation is IgG. A convincing evidence for this fact is the almost complete absence of IgG from the blood of newborns of agammaglobulinaemic mothers. IgG production is first detectable 3 to 5 weeks after birth. IgG of the newborn is always identical with the maternal IgG in its Gm properties. The infant's own Gm phenotype can be determined only after the elimination of the maternal IgG. Concerning the structural basis of placental passage, it has been found that isolated Fc fragments can pass into rabbit foetuses from mothers like native IgG, while Fab fragments can pass to a far lesser extent. In conclusion, transplacental passage of IgG is thought to depend upon some structural properties of the Fc part [3, 4].

### *Other functional properties depending on the Fc part of IgG*

Rheumatoid factor is an anti-IgG antibody reacting with certain antigenic determinants of IgG. These determinants are hidden in the native protein and are only exposed by certain changes in conformation. Such conformational alteration can be induced by heat aggregation. Antigenic determinants reacting with the rheumatoid factor are located on the Fc part of IgG. The Fc part of IgG also plays a decisive role in the regulation of the catabolism of the protein. An isolated Fc fragment is eliminated markedly more slowly than the Fab or $F(ab')_2$ fragments and only slightly more fastly than native IgG. Injection of homologous IgG or its Fc fragment significantly increase the turnover of endogenous IgG, while no such effect has been observed after administration of the Fab fragment.

## PARAPROTEINS

The term paraprotein designates relatively homogeneous protein found in blood and urine (sometimes in extreme quantities) of patients suffering from plasmocytome, Waldenström macroglobulinaemia or related diseases. According to the original definition of Apitz, proteins differing from their normal counterparts by structure, and not found in normal individuals are paraproteins. Another definition taking the immunoglobulin concept into account states that paraproteins are pathologic immunoglobulins with structural abnormalities, defective with respect to functional properties. The main difference between paraproteins and immunoglobulins produced under physiological conditions are (*i*) the antigenic deficiency of paraprotein in comparison with the corresponding class of normal immunoglobulins; (*ii*) the existence of individual antigenic determinants of paraproteins.

Paraproteins can display both antigenic deficiency and antigenic excess when compared with their normal counterparts. Antisera produced against normal immunoglobulins are more likely to reveal antigenic deficiency of paraproteins while individual specificity of paraproteins can be detected by the use of antisera produced against isolated paraproteins.

Structural abnormality is considered to be the most important characteristic of paraproteins by both of the aforementioned concepts. However, it is extremely difficult to answer the question whether paraproteins are in fact structurally abnormal proteins.

TABLE 13-V

*Characteristics of physiological IgG and IgG myeloma proteins*

| | Physiological IgG | IgG myeloma proteins |
|---|---|---|
| Electrophoresis | Broad, diffuse zone | Narrow, discrete zone |
| Antibody activity | Directed against various antigens | Monospecific, or unknown |
| Light chain type | $\varkappa : \lambda$ ratio $= 2 : 1$ | Either $\varkappa$ or $\lambda$ |
| Heavy chain type | $\gamma_1$, $\gamma_2$, $\gamma_3$, $\gamma_4$ all present | One of the four types |
| Origin | Multiclonal | Monoclonal |

Characteristics of physiological IgG and IgG myeloma proteins are summarized in Table 13-V showing the structural and functional heterogeneity of normal IgG in contrast to the homogeneity of myeloma proteins. Each myeloma protein is produced by a malignantly proliferated clone of immunoglobulin forming cells (monoclonal protein), and thus myeloma proteins can be regarded as single members of the heterogeneous population of normal immunoglobulins. This concept has been supported by the discovery of antibody activity of numerous monoclonal immunoglobulins in recent years. In conclusion, paraproteins are more likely structurally normal products of malignant cell populations than proteins with structural abnormalities. However, the possibility that the structural genes responsible for immunoglobulin synthesis in some of the malignant immunocytes are altered cannot be completely excluded either.

## REFERENCES


1. Backhausz, R.: *Ann. immunol. hung.* **11,** 123 (1969).
2. Berggard, I. and Edelmann, G. M.: *Proc. nat. Acad. Sci. (Wash.)* **49,** 33 (1963).
3. Brambell, F. W. E.: *Lancet* **ii,** 1087 (1966).
4. Brambell, F. W. R., Hemmings, W. A., Oakley, F. R. S. and Porter, R. R.: *Proc. roy. Soc. (Edinb.)* **151**B, 160 (1963).
5. *Bull. Wld Hlth Org.* **30,** 447 (1964).
6. *Bull. Wld Hlth Org.* **33,** 721 (1965).
7. Cohen S. and Milstein, C.: *Advanc. Immunol.* **7,** 1 (1967).
8. Cohen, S. and Porter, R. R.: *Advanc. Immunol.* **4,** 287 (1964).
9. Dorrington, K. J., Zarlengo, M. H. and Tanford, C.: *Proc. nat. Acad. Sci. (Wash.)* **58,** 996 (1967).
10. Edelman, G. M.: *J. Amer. chem. Soc.* **81,** 3155 (1959).
11. Edelman, G. M. and Benacerraf, B.: *Proc. nat. Acad. Sci. (Wash.)* **48,** 1035 (1962).
12. Edelman, G. M. and Gall, W. E.: *Ann. Rev. Biochem.* **38,** 415 (1969).

13. Ein, D.: *Proc. nat. Acad. Sci. (Wash.)* **60,** 982 (1968).
14. Fahey, J. L.: *J. Immunol.* **91,** 448 (1963).
15. Feinstein, A. and Rowe, A. J.: *Nature* **205,** 147 (1965).
16. Fleishman, J. B.: *Ann. Rev. Biochem.* **35,** 836 (1966).
17. Franek, F. and Nezlin, R. S.: *Biokhimiya (Moscow)* **28,** 193 (1963).
18. Franklin, E. C. and Frangione, B.: *J. Immunol.* **99,** 810 (1967).
19. Gergely, J., Árky, I. and Medgyesi, G. A.: *Vox Sang. (Basel)* **12,** 252 (1967).
20. Gergely, J., Fudenberg, H. H. and Erna van Loghem: *Immunochemistry* **7,** 1 (1970).
21. Gergely, J., Horváth, E., Medgyesi, G. A. and Puskás, É.: *Vox Sang. (Basel)* **14,** 161 (1968).
22. Gergely, J., Medgyesi, G. A. and Horváth, E.: *Vox Sang. (Basel)* **11,** 724 (1966).
23. Gergely, J., Medgyesi, G. A. and Stanworth, D. R.: *Immunochemistry* **4,** 369 (1967).
24. Gergely, J., Medgyesi, G. A., Wang, A. C. and Fudenberg, H. H.: *Immunochemistry* **9,** 589 (1972).
25. Gergely, J., Stanworth, D. R., Jefferis, R., Normansell, D. E., Henney, C. S. and Pardoe, G. I.: *Immunochemistry* **4,** 101 (1967).
26. Givol, D. and DeLorenzo, F.: *J. biol. Chem.* **243,** 1886 (1968).
27. Grey, H. M. and Kunkel, H. G.: *J. exp. Med.* **120,** 253 (1964).
28. Grey, H. M. and Mannik, M.: *J. exp. Med.* **122,** 619 (1965).
29. Halpern, M. S. and Koshland, M. E.: *Nature* **228,** 1276 (1970).
30. Jerry, L. M., Kunkel, H. G. and Grey, H. M.: *Proc. nat. Acad. Sci. (Wash.)* **65,** 557 (1970).
31. Kehoe, J. M. and Fougereau, M.: *Nature* **224,** 1212 (1969).
32*a*. Korngold, L. and Lipari, R.: *Cancer* **9,** 183 (1956).
32*b*. ibid., **9,** 262 (1956).
33. Kunkel, H. G., Killander, J. and Mannik, M.: *Acta med. scand.* **179,** Suppl. 445, 63 (1966).
34. Kunkel, H. G. and Prendergast, R. A.: *Proc. Soc. exp. Biol. (N. Y.)* **112,** 190 (1966).
35. Mannik, M. and Kunkel, H. G.: *J. exp. Med.* **117,** 213 (1963).
36. Medgyesi, G. A. and Gergely, J.: *Immunochemistry* **6,** 768 (1969).
37. Mestecky, J., Zikan, J. and Butler, W. T.: *Science* **171,** 1163 (1971).
38. Milstein, C.: *FEBS Symposium* **15,** 43 (1969).
39. Müller-Eberhard, H. J.: *Ann. Rev. Biochem.* **38,** 389 (1969).
40. Nisonoff, A., Wissler, F. C., Lipman, L. N. and Woernley, D. L.: *Arch. Biochem. Biophys.* **89,** 230 (1960).
41. Noelken, M. E., Nelson, C. A., Buckley, E. C. and Tanford, C.: *J. biol. Chem.* **240,** 218 (1965).
42. Oudin, J.: *Proc. roy. Soc. Ser. B.* **166,** 207 (1966).
43. Óváry, Z. and Karush, F.: *J. Immunol.* **86,** 146 (1961).
44*a*. Porter, R. R.: *Biochem. J.* **73,** 119 (1959).
44*b*. id., *FEBS Symposium* **15,** 13 (1969).
45. Press, E. M. and Piggot, P. J.: *Cold Spr. Harb. Symp. quant. Biol.* **32,** 45 (1967).
46. Pressman, D. and Grossberg, A. L.: *The Structural Basis of Antibody Specificity.* Benjamin Inc., New York 1968.
47. Putnam, F. W.: *FEBS Symposium* **15,** 21 (1969).
48. Putnam, F. W., Titani, K., Wikler, M. and Shinoda, T.: *Cold Spr. Harb. Symp. quant. Biol.* **32,** 9 (1967).
49. Steinberg, A. G.: *Prog. med. Genetics* **2,** 1 (1962).
50. Takatsuki, K. and Osserman, E. F.: *J. Immunol.* **92,** 100 (1964).
51. Tomasi, T. B., Tan, E. M., Solomon, A. and Prendergast, R. A.: *J. exp. Med.* **121,** 101 (1962).
52. Utsumi, S. and Karush, F.: *Biochemistry* **4,** 1766 (1965).
53. Valentine, R. C. and Greene, N. M.: *J. molec. Biol.* **27,** 615 (1967).

CHAPTER 14

# SKIN SENSITIZING ANTIBODY, REAGINIC ANTIBODY. BLOCKING ANTIBODY. HOMOCYTOTROPIC ANTIBODY

by

E. RAJKA

Completed by

L. KESZTYŰS



## SKIN SENSITIZING ANTIBODY, REAGINIC ANTIBODY

After the discovery of the Ig classes, several experiments were performed to identify the skin sensitizing antibody (reagin), i.e. the antibody which fixes to tissue cells of the same species so that, on subsequent combination with antigen, an immediate hypersensitivity reaction (type I reaction) occurs. Initially it was believed that reagin belonged to the IgA class, but skin hypersensitivity, weal and flare reactivity could be demonstrated with the Prausnitz–Küstner (P–K) test also in connection with other Ig classes, even with IgG regarded as immunochemically pure [52].

Ishizaka et al. [28*c*] were the first to isolate by various purification and fractionation procedures a new class of Ig, whose properties corresponded in every respect to those of reagin [28*c*]. They demonstrated that the reaginic antibody is contained by a single Ig fraction which differs in its antigenicity from IgG, IgA, IgM and IgD and is sedimented in the ultracentrifuge between the mono- and polymeric forms of IgA, at a 8.2 S coefficient. 0.001–0.002 $\mu$g (1–2 ng) N of this protein, in given cases even $10^{-5}$–$10^{-6}$ $\mu$g N, was sufficient to sensitize passively human skin analogously to the P–K reaction. The new Ig is probably present in IgA as an impurity [27*a*]. The reaginic antibody, which was chiefly found in the sera of patients with ragweed pollenosis, was named IgE. It possesses light (L) and heavy (H) chains like all other Ig classes [28*a*]. Apart from serum, the IgE occurs in sputum (respiratory fluid) and nasal secretion as well. Against the earlier view [26*a*], IgE has been detected in colostrum and urine from both healthy and allergic subjects. Colostral and serum IgEs are of an equal molecular size [31*b*].

Precipitation of IgE (with rabbit antiserum) depresses the skin sensitizing activity of allergic patients' sera; this is an additional proof of the association of the reaginic antibody with IgE [27*b*]. The *in vivo* reaginic activity of IgE can be demonstrated by provoking passive cutaneous anaphylaxis (PCA) in monkeys, or by the Schultz–Dale reaction on monkey ileum or lung specimen; anti-IgE serum eliminates the activity of IgE under such conditions, too [65]. Soluble antigen (ragweed allergen) + IgE conjugate can elicit a weal and flare reaction on human skin [27*b*]. Anti-IgE is itself urticariogenic, serving as a direct proof of the presence of IgE on target cells of normal subjects [28*d*].

A research team in Uppsala demonstrated in the serum of a patient with paraproteinaemic myeloma a monoclonal paraprotein antibody [32], which behaved in every respect like a reagin. They originally named the protein IgND, using the initials of the patient for designation. The substance had only a $\lambda$-type light chain. As it was found in comparative studies that neither IgE, nor IgND corresponded to any of the known Ig classes, the two kinds of antibody have been regarded as identical and have uniformly been termed as IgE at the WHO immunological conference held in Lausanne in February 1968. In the meantime a second myeloma patient with IgE in serum has been described [46] whose serum responded to monkey IgE antiserum in the same manner as Johansson's myeloma IgND and the IgE of atopic allergic patients [28*a*, 30*a*].

The main properties of IgE can be characterized as follows [7]: mol. wt. 190,000–200,000 as calculated from the sedimentation constant. This high value can be attributed to the heavy $\varepsilon$ chain which has the mol. wt. of 72,500. The formula of IgE is $\varepsilon_2\varkappa_2$, or $\varepsilon_2\lambda_2$. Its carbohydrate content being relatively high, 11.5 per cent, it is a $\gamma_1$-glycoprotein. It is thermolabile and on digestion with papaine, several intermediate fragments can be separated, some of which resemble the Fc fragment. Digestion with pepsin yields a more homogeneous $F(ab')_2$ fragment, comprising the antigenic determinants of the IgE class. Studies of the skin sensitizing capacity of the different fragments have shown that only the heavy $\varepsilon$ chain and the Fc fragments are active [31*b*]. The latter, moreover, can passively sensitize human leukocytes and monkey lung tissue in a reversed-type reaction, indicating that IgE combines with the target cell through the Fc portion of the molecule [26*b*].

Immunochemically, IgE agglutinates red blood cells coated with the homologous allergen, indicating that the antibodies are bivalent. They do not, however, possess a complement fixing capacity. The reaction of allergen + IgE (direct) or IgE + anti-IgE (reversed) on target cells releases histamine from human leukocytes and both histamine and SRS-A from monkey lung, probably by a mechanism based on changes in enzymatic sequence [27*c*]. Contact with the homologous antigen of lung specimens gained by pneumectomy and sensitized passively with the serum of a donor with ragweed allergy caused the release of a third factor (ECF-A), which exerted a selective chemotactic action on human eosinophilic cells. The immunoglobulin mediator of ECF-A release also proved to be an IgE [35].

IgE is also present in normal serum. Swedish investigators give its geometric mean level as 160 ng per ml in children and 330 ng per ml in normal adult population [8*d*]. High IgE levels (2,500–3,000 ng per ml) weigh in favour of the diagnosis of allergy—chiefly in asthma and other atopic diseases—, but specific desensitization, e.g. in pollenosis, causes reduction of the concentration by one half or more [26*a*]. Individuals with concentrations less than 15 ng per ml are considered to be IgE deficient.*

* According to recent findings, human serum Ig levels should not be measured in mg per ml or ng per ml, because the results obtained in the different laboratories

Distinction should nevertheless be made between prolonged and rapid (rush) desensitization. A marked fall of the IgE level occurs in the former case; in rush desensitization, rise of the IgE was observed 2–4 weeks after the beginning of the procedure and it was attributed to a booster effect. The rise in serum reagin in the case of rapid desensitization may be associated with increased clinical tolerance to the allergen, i.e. with a rapid decrease of skin sensitivity to the latter [8*b*].

At our present state of knowledge, it can be generally accepted that at high concentrations of serum IgE, the skin test is usually positive, although it may be negative in certain cases, and further that in immediate hypersensitivity, the antigen binding capacity of IgE is related with the passive skin sensitizing capacity of the IgE containing serum and that this P–K reaction can be blocked by the non-antibody myeloma-protein of Johansson and Bennich [28*c*, 56]. Simple correlations do not, however, exist, as e.g. the serum of children with birch allergy usually contains 15 times more circulating IgE than the serum of children with dandelion allergy [8*c*]. Using a new *in vitro* model consisting of human skin slices passively sensitized by antigen-specific IgE raises the possibility that adenyl cyclase-cyclic AMP system exerts an inhibitory (a regulatory) effect on IgE-mediated hypersensitivity in human skin [70].

Interestingly, newborn and even premature infants respond to passively transferred adult reagins in the P–K reaction, but do not show a positive cutaneous response to anti-IgE. Accordingly, the immediate hypersensitivity mechanism of newborn infants can be regarded as competent, while the skin-fixed IgE is insufficient for a reaction with anti-IgE. Against earlier findings [8*d*], the average IgE level of cord serum from newborns is only 2.1 I.U. per ml, whereas maternal post-partum levels are as high as 205 I.U. per ml. Apparently, newborn infants only possess 1 per cent of the adult IgE level. This correlates well with the fact that no allergic disease occurs in newborn babies. Infants older than 6 weeks may nevertheless occasionally show characteristic allergic signs indicating a corresponding rise in their serum IgE level to 5.5 I.U. per ml on the average. Six months old babies already possess an average serum IgE level of 57.6 I.U. per ml. The extraordinary variation of serum IgE known in adults can already be observed at this age: the post-partum IgE level of 35 mothers varied between 19 and 810 I.U. per ml, that of seventeen 6-month-old babies between 4.1 and 458 I.U. per ml. Standard deviations of the IgE levels are thus much greater than with other classes of Ig. In adults, this may naturally be due to allergic sensitization, but a separate genetic control of the basal IgE level cannot be excluded either. As yet there is no evidence of the transplacental passage of IgE [4, 39].

IgE is synthesized by plasma cells, above all in lymph nodes, at a turnover rate of 2–3 days. IgE producing plasma cells chiefly occur in the respiratory and

by various techniques are not comparable in this manner. It has been recommended to use instead the International Reference Preparation for each class of Ig, and express the results in International Units (I.U.) per ml relative to the reference standard. It is hoped that this proposal will be generally accepted from the beginning of 1972, ensuring the uniformity of measurements. The appropriate standards available for IgE is the Standard Reference Serum (code No. 68/341) of the World Health Organization, 1.0 ml of which contains 9,346 I.U. IgE. Instructions for obtaining the reference preparation are outlined in papers of reference Nos 18, 25 and 63.

gastrointestinal tracts. No IgE containing cells have been found in bone marrow, oesophagus, pulmonary parenchyma, liver, thyroid gland, kidney and parotis of humans and monkeys [64]. The distribution of the IgE producing plasma cells can account for the finding that nasal polyp fluids from positive skin test reactors occasionally contain more reagin than the patient's serum, indicating a primary local nasal allergy [17]. IgE is fixed to basophilic leukocytes; neither other granulocytes, nor small lymphocytes carry IgE [27c].

Extraction of pure monoclonal IgE has made the preparation of a specific antiserum possible which can be used for the detection of IgE antibody with the *in vitro* radioisotope or radioallergosorbent techniques [66] if the appropriate allergen is combined with insoluble Sephadex or cellulose particles, or co-polymerized with ethylchloroformate during incubation with the test serum [33, 59]. Radioisotope-labelled IgE antiserum added to the suspension will be bound by the particles if the IgE and the allergen are corresponding. It could thus be demonstrated that although the IgE level increases 6-fold in allergic asthma [31*a*], it does not rise as long as the intradermal and provocative tests are negative. The same applies to pollenosis in which the IgE level is as a rule high if the skin test is positive [8*a*]. The known marked rise of the IgE level in certain parasitic infections is probably not permanent, declining with the elimination of the infestation, because apart from cases with a personal and/or family history of allergy, increased production of IgE is a temporary phenomenon [34, 53]. Not only the rise, but also the fall of the IgE level can signify disease. Deficiency of IgE can be observed in family members of patients suffering from ataxia-teleangiectasia (65 per cent), suggesting a genetic control of the disease [9]. In sera from asthmatic patients sensitive to ricinus seeds, IgE antibodies could be demonstrated with Coombs' red-cell-linked antigen + anti-globulin reaction, using specific anti-IgE serum as anti-globulin serum [16]. Human IgE is demonstrable in monkey skin by the immunofluorescent technique if the skin specimens are incubated with reagin containing (ragweed) serum and treated afterwards with dye-labelled anti-IgE globulin. Reaginic antibodies become fixed to mast cells in the monkey skin [24]. The relatively simple immunofluorescence test can also be carried out *in vitro* for routine clinical examination [12]. An additional method of human IgE demonstration is based on the phenomenon that rat peritoneal mast cells incubated in serum from patients with pollen allergy undergo a characteristic cytopathic change if the corresponding antigen, or anti-human IgE, or anti-$\varkappa$ serum is added to the system. No cytopathic effect occurs if normal serum is used instead of the allergic patients' serum. The physical properties of the cytopathic factor of allergic patients' sera are identical with those of the IgE-type reagins: the sedimentation rate is 7.8–8.7 and exposure at 56 °C for 60 min inactivates both the reaginic and cytopathic effects. Chromatography of sera from pollenosis patients on DEAE-Sephadex column reveals a similar distribution. The method can detect IgE concentrations lower than 10 ng per ml [49].

It is difficult to compare the values obtained by the different methods. If the radioallergosorbent test is used, deviations may arise from the heterogeneity of the commercial allergen preparations, because even 100 to 1,000-fold concentration differences may occur in allergen extracts produced by the same firm [31*a*]. It has also been postulated that a fraction of the reaction between anti-IgE and myeloma protein IgE is idiotypic, and other cross-reacting antigens may also be present in the test serum, because Ig molecules from different classes may possess similar variable regions [29]. The *in vitro* quantitation of IgE against specific antigens has been difficult because of the small amount of such antibody in serum. Only part of the total IgE would be antibody against a particular antigen. To overcome this difficulty, Zeiss et al. [68] employed a solid phase radioimmunoassay for the quantitation of human IgE against ragweed antigen E.

The majority of reagin containing sera can be stored at low temperature for several months without loss of activity, some sera, however, rapidly loose strength. According to Augustin [3], apart from the valency committed to bind antigen, IgE contains an additional valency to a common cellular constituent, which accounts for its adhesive tendency; reagin becomes fixed to tissues also in the P–K reaction, whereas the group specific for the allergen remains unbound. Thus reagins do not act toward the release of the mediators unless they are bound to cells or shock tissue at the time of encounter with the antigen. Since, however, circulating reagins are also present in the blood, they can be demonstrated by passive transfer. The fixing of reagins to cells accounts for their persistence at the site of the P–K transfer for several days or weeks, during which time the allergic reaction can be repeatedly elicited.

Reagins from patients suffering from a spontaneous atopic disease are generally not demonstrable by precipitation or agar gel diffusion, while precipitins do occur in induced sensitization, e.g. in rabbits injected with pollen. Reagins giving a positive P–K reaction with a pollen fraction differing from the reagin forming component of hay fever pollen allergy can also be induced in normal subjects by injection of e.g. ambrosia pollen. Antigens other than pollen (serum, ascaris extract, certain drugs) are more efficient inducers of reagin formation.

The blood reagin level is not conclusive of allergic reactivity in immediate hypersensitivity, although a parallelism undoubtedly exists between skin reactivity and circulating antibody level. Both the circulating and cell-fixed reagins encounter the allergen, but in the tissues a smaller amount of reagin is usually available for the reaction; cell-fixed reagin amounts only to about 25–50 per cent of humoral reagin. If, however, sera from allergic patients are transfused into normal subjects, the reagins disappear from the circulation within a few hours, becoming fixed to cells of the skin, conjunctiva and mucous membranes.

## BLOCKING ANTIBODY*

A parallelism may or may not exist between the serum IgE level and the intensity of the immediate-type allergic process. For instance, in rush desensitization, the serum IgE level rises, while the intensity of the skin tests tends to diminish owing to the improvement of tolerance of the organism towards the allergen. The fact that after specific pollen treatment, provocation of a reaction on skin and conjunctiva requires 5–10 and 100 times as much allergen, respectively, as before treatment, also suggests the role of an inhibitory antibody [42*a*].

The term 'blocking antibody' proposed by Cooke [14*b*], has been used to desig-

* Blocking antibodies [58] playing a role in the immunological enhancement of cell-mediated transplantation and tumour immunity are not discussed under this heading.

nate those inhibitory antibodies which occur in skin reactions related with allergic processes or diseases, whence their role should clearly be differentiated from the serological concept of inhibition [67]. In neutralization tests, the sera of specifically treated patients require more pollen allergen for the reaction than the sera of untreated patients; at a stable reagin level this means the increase of tolerance to the allergen in the treated subjects [55*a*]. Maunsell [44] proposed a more simple procedure for the demonstration of the blocking antibody: sera from specifically treated pollenosis patients incubated with the pollen antigen for 1 h at 37 °C will elicit a weaker reaction than reagin containing sera from untreated patients plus the allergen; both sera are applied to the skin of hay fever patients or to normal skin passively sensitized with reaginic serum. The minimal concentration (threshold) required to elicit a positive reaction can be established by the appropriate variation of the mixture. Since unlike reagin, blocking antibodies have no affinity to cells and disappear from the passively sensitized site relatively soon, application of pollen extract 48 h after passive sensitization may already elicit a positive reaction [38].

The inhibitory factor is a true antibody which can be separated from reagin. Electrophoretically, reagin is the more mobile of the two; the blocking antibody migrates with IgG. The sera of allergic patients contain both reagin and blocking antibody, whereas sera of pollen-treated non-allergic subjects contain as a rule exclusively blocking antibodies; the latter also occur in cows with pollen allergy [15]. Blocking antibodies inhibiting the histamine releasing effect of IgE on human leukocytes have been found in nasal secretions not only of individuals sensitive to, or immunized against, inhalatory allergens, but also in those of normal subjects; it follows that all persons exposed to environmental inhalatory (pollen) allergens can produce nasal blocking antibodies [60].

Blocking antibodies are highly specific; separate kinds of blocking antibodies are formed to each pollen fraction; cross-reactions with various pollen extracts are nevertheless frequent. Blocking antibodies are relatively thermostable [42*a*] and, unlike reagins, they pass the placental barrier, to judge from their presence in cord blood and infant blood [55]. The initial observations of Cooke were later confirmed by Harley, who called the inhibitory factor 'reaction inhibitory substance' [21]. Blocking antibodies are demonstrable by complement fixation reaction or, if the allergic condition is atopic, by haemagglutination test. The haemagglutinin demonstrated in pollinosis has been regarded as the blocking antibody [54]. The serum level of blocking antibodies is usually low, about 0.1–1 $\mu$g per ml, as assessed by the haemagglutination technique.

Initially it was supposed that the blocking antibodies formed during treatment with pollen are related with clinical immunity [42*b*] and treatment was accordingly conducted in conformity with the decrease in skin reactivity [1*a*, *b*]; attempts were even made to treat hay-fever patients with serum of normal patients which contained blocking antibody due to treatment with pollen [13]. It was, however, soon found that blocking antibodies can scarcely be regarded as the carriers of immunity and their titer is no indicator of a successful therapy [14*a*], in brief, desensitization is unrelated to blocking antibody. The appearance of the latter is probably only an accompanying phenomenon of repeated antigenic stimuli. Thus clinical improvement is clearly unrelated to the rise of the haemagglutinin titre [2].

The precise role of blocking antibodies is still a matter of dispute [41], because there is a relatively weak correlation between their serum levels and the clinical results of desensitization. It seems, nevertheless, certain that specific desensitization stimulates not only the synthesis of IgE antibodies, but also of antibodies belonging to other Ig classes. Certain authors have postulated that one important function of blocking antibodies is to interfere with reagin synthesis [57]. This could in fact account for the phenomenon that in prolonged desensitization, the initial increase of IgE production is followed by the fall of the serum IgE level [43]. The immediate favourable results of rush desensitization are, however, not explicable by this mechanism. According to contemporary knowledge, reagin and blocking (*in vivo* neutralizing) antibodies are coexistent, but nothing more can be said about their relationship until investigations into the fundamental regulation of the immune response yield more information in this respect, too [51].

## HOMOCYTOTROPIC ANTIBODY

Atopic allergic conditions occur not only in humans but also in animals (cows, dogs, etc.). Atopic allergy (seasonal pollen dermatitis) was first observed in dogs [47, 48]. Apart from the human skin sensitizing antibody, i.e. from reagin (IgE), which cannot be passively transferred to the skin of species other than man and monkey, the anaphylactic antibodies [10] or, according to the recent terminology, homocytotropic antibodies (HCA) [6] of animals (dogs, rabbits, etc.) also possess skin sensitizing properties. Human reagin (IgE) and HCA are not identical [37], although in addition to skin sensitization, they have several other properties in common: both are thermolabile [69] and passively transferable with serum, chiefly by passive cutaneous anaphylaxis (requiring higher concentrations of animal than of human serum, though) and neither can pass across the placenta, to judge from mouse experiments [50]. Experimental observations suggest that the functional and structural type of HCA varies with the species. Rhesus monkeys injected i. v. with 2,4,6-trinitrophenyl-haemocyanin produced HCA separable into two components, a thermolabile and a thermostable immunoglobulin [1*c*]. Rats synthesize two kinds of HCA, one of which possesses a molecular structural portion identical with, or at least similar to, human IgE [40]. Rats infected with the nematode *Nippostrongylus brasiliensis* have particularly high serum HCA levels [10*a*, 36, 55*a*].

The results in an experimental situation in the rat, a species in which it has been shown that reaginic antibodies belong to an antigenically distinct Ig class 'rat IgE' whose biological function is comparable to the human IgE, show that there is no direct quantitative relationship between the size of skin reactions and the level of specific circulating reaginic antibody [30*a*].

Like human IgE, HCA persists at the passively sensitized site for a relatively long time, 48 h at the least [23]. The HCAs of rabbit and rat resemble one another in respect of electrophoretic mobility, molecular size and chemical (2-mercaptoethanol) sensitivity [45]. Guinea pig and mouse HCAs differ from the homologous antibody responsible for passive cutaneous anaphylaxis. HCA is regularly encountered in dogs (canine IgE) [47]; under appropriate experimental conditions, the canine IgE induces in dogs a bronchial secretion without eosinophilia [11]. The distribution of IgE in canine skin was studied by immunofluorescence. The antibody was found to be associated exclusively with mast cells and to be largely cytoplasmically located. It is the only canine antibody with a homocytotropic affinity for mast cells [20*a*].

HCA formed to various proteins (ovalbumin) chiefly in alum-precipitated form as well as in atopic-type sensitization with ascaris antigens or other enteral parasitic infections of sheep [23] and rat [20] constitutes an independent Ig (antibody) category and can be differentiated from IgA and IgG by adsorption [19]; it is demonstrable in homologous hosts by passive cutaneous anaphylaxis, using the dye Evans blue and by isotope ($^{131}$I) technique as well [23]. The thermostable HCA synthesized by guinea pigs in response to purified dextran becomes fixed to the skin through the Fc fragment. Differences in fixing have been attributed to certain delicate, probably allotypic structural variations of the Fc portion, because the structure of the Fc is complementary to the loci which the antibody (the Fc) becomes fixed to in the skin [5]. Antibodies of this kind temporarily appear in the blood of rabbits after foot-pad immunization (e.g. with dinitrophenyl-bovine $\gamma$-globulin), disappearing after a few days or weeks [69]. The administration of bovine serum albumin (in complete Freund's adjuvant) is, however, followed by the formation of a persistent skin sensitizing antibody, which is thermostable, fixes C and migrates like a slow $\gamma$-globulin [22]. Administration of a low dose (0.1 $\mu$g) of ovalbumin (in Al/OH/$_3$ gel) to mice induces a persistent high-level synthesis of homocytotropic and IgGI antibodies, but when high doses (100 $\mu$g) are given, only the IgG1 production increases and reagin synthesis is low and temporary. It has been supposed that reagins have a higher avidity to antigen than other Ig classes. Thus the originally reagin forming cell population also responds to low doses of antigen, while high antigen doses stimulate the synthesis of additional classes of Ig (e.g. IgM) as well, which then probably suppress the formation of reagins [61]. The recent experimental results are consistent with the view that macrophages may feedback control an early event which determines reagin response [62*c*]. Bovine HCA can be separated into a thermostable and a thermolabile component [62*a*, *b*].

The severity of passive cutaneous anaphylaxis due to HCA containing rabbit serum (rabbit IgE-globulin) can be reduced by 50 per cent by adsorption to anti-FcND antiserum, which is specific for human IgE (IgND monoclonal antibody). Accordingly, the rabbit HCA is an Ig class of the rabbit analogous with human IgE [69]. Hyperimmune 7 S-type rabbit sera completely inhibit HCA [26*b*].

An inhibitory antibody, reminiscent of human blocking antibodies which suppresses passive cutaneous anaphylaxis and intravenously induced systemic anaphylaxis, has also been demonstrated in animals (dogs) [47].

## REFERENCES

1*a*. Albus, G.: *Z. ges. exp. Med.* **95**, 703 (1935).
1*b*. ibid., **95**, 710 (1935).
1*c*. Amkraut, A. A., Malley, A. and Begley, D.: *Int. Arch. Allergy* **44**, 369 (1973).
2. Arbesman, C. E., Kantor, S. Z., Rapp, D. and Rose, N. R.: *J. Allergy* **31**, 342 (1960).
3. Augustin, R., O'Sullivan, S. A. and Conolly, R. C.: *Acta allergol. (Kbh.)* **21**, 430 (1966).

4. Basaral, M., Orgel, H. A. and Hamburger, R. N.: *J. Immunol.* **107,** 794 (1971).
5. Battisto, R. J., Budman, D. and Freedman, R.: *J. exp. Med.* **134,** 381 (1971).
6. Becker, E. L. and Austen, K. F.: *J. exp. Med.* **124,** 379 (1966).
7. Bennich, H. H., Ishizaka, K., Johansson, S. G. O., Rowe, D. S., Stanworth, D. R. and Terry W. P.: *Immunology* **15,** 323 (1968).
8*a*. Berg, T. and Johansson, S. G. O.: *Int. Arch. Allergy* **36,** 219 (1969).
8*b*. ibid., **41,** 434 (1971).
8*c*. ibid., **41,** 452 (1971).
8*d*. id., *Acta paediat. scand.* **58,** 513 (1969).
9. Biggar, D., Lapointe, N., Ishizaka, K., Meuwissen, H., Good, R. A. and Frommel, D.: *Lancet* **ii,** 1089 (1970).
10. Bloch, K. J.: *Prog. Allergy* **10,** 84 (1967).
10*a*. Block, K. J., Ohman, J. L., Waltin, J. and Cygan, R. W.: *J. Immunol.* **110,** 197 (1973).
11. Booth, B. H., Talbot, C. H. and Patterson, R.: *Int. Arch. Allergy* **40,** 639 (1971).
12. Centifanto, Y. M. and Kaufman, H. E.: *J. Immunol.* **107,** 608 (1971).
13. Cohen, M. B. and Friedman, J.: *J. Allergy* **16,** 121 (1945).
14*a*. Cooke, R. A.: *J. Allergy* **15,** 212 (1944).
14*b*. id., In *Allergy in Theory and Practice.* Saunders, Philadelphia 1947.
15. Cooke, R. A., Menze, A. E. O., Kessler, W. R. and Myers, P. A.: *J. exp. Med.* **101,** 177 (1955).
16. Coombs, R. R. A., Hunter, A., Jonas, W. E., Bennich, H., H., Johansson, S. G. O. and Panzani, R.: *Lancet* **i,** 1115 (1968).
17. Donovan, R., Johansson, S. G. O., Bennich, H. H. and Soothill, J. F.: *Int. Arch. Allergy* **37,** 154 (1970).
18. *Eur. J. Immunol.* Editorial, **1,** 224 (1971).
19. Freeman, M. J., Braley, H. C., Kaplan, A. M. and McArthur, W. P.: *Int. Arch. Allergy,* **36,** 530 (1969).
20. Goose, J. and Blair, A. M. J. N.: *Immunology* **16,** 749 (1969).
20*a*. Halliwell, R. E. W.: *J. Immunol.* **110,** 422 (1973).
21. Harley, D.: *Fortschr. Allergielehre* **1,** 185 (1939).
22. Henson, P. M. and Cochrane, C. G.: *J. exp. Med.* **129,** 153 (1969).
23. Hogarth-Scott, R. S.: *Immunology* **16,** 543 (1969).
24. Hubscher, T., Watson, J. I. and Goodfriend, L.: *J. Allergy* **43,** 186 (1969).
25. *Immunochemistry.* Editorial, **8,** 991 (1971).
26*a*. Ishizaka, K.: *J. Amer. med. Ass.* **211,** 2090 (1970).
26*b*. id., *Folia allergol.* **17,** 384 (1970).
27*a*. Ishizaka, K. and Ishizaka, T.: *J. Allergy* **37,** 169 (1966).
27*b*. id., *J. Immunol.* **101,** 68 (1968).
27*c*. id., *Ann. Allergy* **28,** 189 (1970).
28*a*. Ishizaka, K., Ishizaka, T. and Hornbrock, M. M.: *J. Immunol.* **97,** 75 (1966).
28*b*. ibid., **98,** 490 (1967).
28*c*. id., *J. Allergy* **37,** 121 (1966).
28*d*. ibid., **42,** 320 (1968).
29. Ishizaka, K., Tomioka, H. and Ishizaka, T.: *J. Immunol.* **105,** 1459 (1970).
30. Ito, K., Wicher, K. and Arbesman, C. E.: *Int. Arch. Allergy* **39,** 178 (1970).
30*a*. Jarrett, E. E. E. and Stewart, D. C.: *Immunology* **24,** 37 (1973).
31*a*. Johansson, S. G. O.: *Lancet* **ii,** 951 (1967).
31*b*. id., In *VII. Internat. Congr. Allerg. Firenze, 1970.* Excerpta Medica Internat. Congr. Series No. 211, 17.
32. Johansson, S. G. O. and Bennich, H. H.: *Immunology* **13,** 381 (1967).
33. Johansson, S. G. O., Bennich, H. H. and Berg, T.: *Int. Arch. Allergy* **41,** 443 (1971).
34. Johansson, S. G. O., Melbin, T. and Vaniquist, B.: *Lancet* **i,** 1118 (1968).
35. Kay, A. B. and Austen, K. F.: *J. Immunol.* **107,** 899 (1971).
36. Keller, R.: *Int. Arch. Allergy* **37,** 197 (1970).
37. Kindt, T. J. and Todd, C. W.: *J. exp. Med.* **130,** 859 (1969).
38. Langner, R. H. and Kern, R. A.: *J. Allergy* **10,** 1 (1938).
39. Levine, B. B.: Sheldon Memorial Lecture. Amer. Acad. Allergy. Chicago, Febr. 1971.
40. Liakopoulous, A. and Perelmutter, L.: *J. Immunol.* **107,** 131 (1971).

41. Lichtenstein, L. M., Norman, P. S. and Winkenwerder, W. L.: *Amer. J. Med.* **44,** 514 (1968).
42a. Loveless, M. H.: *J. Immunol.* **38,** 25 (1940).
42b. ibid., **47,** 165 (1943).
42c. id., *J. Allergy* **15,** 311 (1944).
43. Malley, A. and Perlman, F.: *J. Allergy* **43,** 59 (1969).
44. Maunsell, K.: *Lancet* **ii,** 199 (1946).
45. McAninch, J. R. and Patterson, R.: *Immunology* **18,** 91 (1970).
46. Ogawa, M., Kochwa, S., Smith, Ch., Ishizaka, K. and McIntyre, O. R.: *New Engl. J. Med.* **281,** 1217 (1970).
47. Patterson, R.: *Progr. Allergy* **13,** 332 (1969).
48. Patterson, R., Roberts, M. and Pruzansky, J. J.: *J. Immunol.* **102,** 455 (1969).
49. Perelmutter, L. and Liakopoulou, A.: *Int. Arch. Allergy* **40,** 481 (1971).
50. Prouvost-Dannon, A. and Bianghi, R.: *Int. Arch. Allergy* **38,** 648 (1970).
51. Ptak, W. and Pryjma, J.: *Eur. J. Immunol.* **1,** 408 (1971).
52. Radermecker, M.: *Acta allergol. (Kbh.)* **24,** 1 (1969).
53. Rosenberg, E. B., Whalen, G. E., Bennich, H. H. and Johansson, S. G. O.: *New Engl. J. Med.* **283,** 1148 (1970).
54. Sherman, W. B. and Portnoy, J.: In *Mechanism of Hypersensitivity.* Ed. by Shaffer, J. H., LoGrippo, G. A. and Chase M. W. Churchill, London 1959, p. 89.
55. Sherman, W. B., Stulla, A. and Cooke, R. A.: *J. Allergy* **11,** 225 (1940).
55a. Smith, S. R., Hwang, A., Eichelberger, J. and Randell, P.: *Int. Arch. Allergy* 382 **44,** (1973).
56. Stanworth, D. R., Humphrey, J. H., Bennich, H. H. and Johansson, S. G. O.: *Lancet* **ii,** 330 (1967).
57. Stannegård, Ö. and Bellin, L.: *Immunology* **18,** 775 (1970).
58. Takasugi, M. and Klein, E.: *Immunology* **21,** 675 (1971).
59. Tannenbaum, M. and Goodfriend, L.: *Int. Arch. Allergy* **41,** 778 (1971).
60. Turk, A., Lichtenstein, L. M. and Norman, P. S.: *Immunology* **19,** 85 (1970).
61. Vaz, E. M., Vaz, N. M. and Levine, B. B.: *Immunology* **21,** 11 (1971).
62a. Wells, P. W. and Eyre, P.: *Vet. Rec.* **87,** 173 (1970).
62b. id., *Immunochemistry* **9,** 88 (1972).
62c. White, G. J. and Hölm, U. S.: *J. Immunol.* **110,** 327 (1973).
63. WHO Expert Committee on Biological Standardization. *Wld Hlth Org. techn. Rep. Ser.* No. 463. 1971.
64. Wicher, K., Ishizaka, T. and Arbesman, C. E.: *In VII. Internat. Congr. Allergol. Firenze, 1970.* Excerpta Medica Internat. Congr. Series No. 211, 17.
65. Wicher, K., Kobamashi, S., Arbesman, C. E. and Ishizaka, K.: *J. Allergy* **41,** 74 (1968).
66. Wide, L., Bennich, H. H. and Johansson, S. G. O.: *Lancet* **ii,** 1105 (1967).
67. Wiener, A. S.: *Ann. Allergy* **10,** 535 (1952).
68. Zeiss, C. R., Pruzansky, J. J., Patterson, R. and Roberts, U.: *J. Immunol.* **110,** 414 (1973).
69. Zwaifler, N. J. and Robinson, J. O.: *J. exp. Med.* **130,** 907 (1969).
70. Yamamoto, S., Greaves, U. W. and Fairley, U. W.: *Immunology* **24,** 77 (1973).

CHAPTER 15

# COMPLEMENT

by

Z. CSIZÉR



## INTRODUCTION

It was already shown by Bordet in 1898 that haemolytic sera, like the bactericidal sera studied by Buchner, are inactivated by heating for 30 min at 56 °C. He proved that heat did not affect the haemolytic antibody itself but a non-specific thermolabile factor which caused the lysis of red cells having been sensitized by the specific haemolysin [11]. This non-specific, thermolabile factor, which is present in all normal, unheated sera, was termed alexine by Buchner and complement by Ehrlich. Now the latter name is generally accepted.

The term 'complement' (C) is applied to a complex system present in normal serum and tissue fluids. The complement system, activated characteristically by antigen–antibody interaction within the body, mediates a number of biologically significant events. It consists of 11 blood serum proteins which altogether represent about 10 per cent of the human serum globulin fraction. In the presence of antigen–antibody complexes the complement proteins have membrane damaging or cytolytic activity. In addition to cytolysis, complement may cause release of histamine (H) from mast cells, contraction of smooth muscles, capillary permeability changes, chemotactic attraction of polymorphonuclear leukocytes, retention of leukocytes by immune adherence, mobilization of leukocytes from bone marrow, effects of a kinin-like substance, enhancement of phagocytosis and intracellular digestion, and promotion of blood coagulation. Because of these various activities, the biological role and significance of complement may vary iron protection against microbial infection to mediation of immunological injury. Activation of C by the antigen–antibody complex cannot be considered the only possibility. An alternate pathway that may lead to the activation of the complement system has been presented [8].

## NOMENCLATURE [48, 65]

The components of complement (C) are designated numerically and in the order of their reaction they are as follows [8]: C1, C4, C2, C3, C5, C6, C7, C8 and C9. C1 consists of three sub-components, called C1q, C1r, C1s. E is used for erythrocyte, S for a single site of initiation of C fixation, and A for antibody to cell surface antigens. The components enumerated after EAC denote a state of reactivity. For instance, EAC1423 or EAC1–3 represent the complex produced by the reaction of the first 4 complement components. E* is used for damaged cell, and the cell membrane lesion at a site of complement fixation is denoted S*. Complement components that have acquired enzymatic activity are indicated by placing a bar above the numerals which refer to the components in which the activity resides, e.g. $C\overline{42}$ denotes the activity described as C3 convertase. Fragments of components produced during complement fixation reaction by peptide-bond cleavage are denoted by small letters. For example, the two fragments of C3 are called C3a and C3b. Complement component that has lost a defined activity is designated with the letter 'i'.

## PROPERTIES OF HUMAN COMPLEMENT COMPONENTS

During the past two decades C research has experienced an explosive development. The isolation of the complement components, some in a high state of purity, the partial elucidation of the reaction mechanism, the development of quantitative analytical methods and the recognition of the sequential fragmentation of the complement components have been the most important achievements. For the purification of complement components different combinations of CM-, DEAE- and TEAE-cellulose chromatography, gel filtration (Sephadex G-100 and G-200), chromatography on hydroxyapatite, and preparative block electrophoresis have been generally used. As a result of these extensive investigations some of the properties of the individual complement components are known at present and these are listed in Table 15-I.

Due to difficulties in identifying and measuring complement components, it is so far uncertain which cells or tissues synthesize them. To the study of the synthesis of complement components by individual cells, a modified haemolytic plaque assay technique was developed. Columnar epithelial cells of the small intestine were found to be the only cells of guinea pig capable of producing haemolytic plaques [19]. Isolated segments of human colon, and to a lesser extent ileum, were capable of synthesizing haemolytically active C1 [18]. C3 and C4 have been shown to be formed in macrophages [56], but human C3 has been shown to be produced by the parenchymatous cells of the liver [1*a*]. C2 is thought

TABLE 15-I

*Properties of human complement components*

| | C1 complex | C1q | C1r | C1s | C4 | C2 |
|---|---|---|---|---|---|---|
| Serum concentration ($\mu$g per ml) | | 190 | | 22 | 430 | 25–30 |
| Sedimentation coefficient (S) | 18 | 11.1 | 7.0 | 4.0 | 10.0 | 5.5 |
| Approximate mol. wt. | | 388,000 | 168,000 | 79,000 | 240,000 | 117,000 |
| Electrophoretic mobility | | $\gamma_2$ | $\beta$ | $\alpha_2$ | $\beta_1$ | $\beta_2$ |
| Carbohydrate (%) | | 15 | | | 14 | |
| Reactive SH | | | | | | 1–2 |
| Isoelectric focusing (pI) | 4.99 | | | | 6.40 | 5.52 |
| Thermolability (56 °C, 30 min) | + | + | + | + | — | + |

| | C3 | C5 | C6 | C7 | C8 | C9 |
|---|---|---|---|---|---|---|
| Serum concentration ($\mu$g per ml) | 1,200 | 75 | 55–65 | | $<10$ | $<10$ |
| Sedimentation coefficient (S) | 9.5 | 8.7 | 5.7 | 5–6 | 8.0 | 4.5 |
| Approximate mol. wt. | 185,000 | 206,000 | 125,000 | 100,000 | 150,000 | 79,000 |
| Electrophoretic mobility | $\beta_1$ | $\beta_1$ | $\beta_2$ | $\beta_2$ | $\gamma_1$ | $\alpha$ |
| Carbohydrate (%) | 2.7 | 19 | | | | |
| Reactive SH | 1–2 | | | | | |
| Isoelectric focusing (pI) | 5.75 | 4.10 | 6.00 | 5.59 | 5.60<br>6.50 | 4.72 |
| Thermolability (56 °C, 30 min) | — | + | — | — | + | + |

to be produced by macrophages, but perhaps by other cells, too. C3 exists in different allotypic forms, distinguishable by their net surface charge at pH 8.6. Up to now eight C3 phenotypes have been observed of the 15 predicted ones [2, 6].

## REACTION SEQUENCE OF COMPLEMENT COMPONENTS

### INTERACTION OF NATIVE COMPLEMENT COMPONENTS

In their native form complement proteins are inactive, though, some of them exhibit affinity for each other, and the consequent reversible interactions are functionally significant. The three sub-components of C1 occur in serum as a $Ca^{++}$ dependent complex. The complex dissociates into the sub-components C1q, C1r, C1s, in the absence of $Ca^{++}$ and re-forms when the three proteins are mixed in the presence of $Ca^{++}$. Having been activated, the complex of C1 triggers the complement chain reaction. Native C4 and C2 enter into reversible interaction and these two proteins constitute the precursors of an enzyme having an essential function in the complement reaction. Similarly, C5, C6, and C7 can enter into reversible association, this interaction is not yet fully understood. Recent experiments have shown that under physiological conditions C5, C6, and C7 react independently and consecutively in immune haemolysis [9]. It is not possible to choose between the hypotheses of sequential action and functional unit of C5, C6, and C7 since experimental data in support of each have been obtained. Recently it has been shown that C5 may act through both alternative pathways. Furthermore, native C5 may adsorb non-specifically to cell-surface receptors of unsensitized erythrocytes [21*b*].

## INTERACTION OF C1q WITH IMMUNOGLOBULINS

The classical mechanism of complement activation begins with the interaction of C1 with antigen–antibody complexes or immunoglobulin aggregates. C1 recognizes IgG1, IgG2, IgG3, and IgM through its sub-component C1q. The C1 binding site is located in the Fc portion of the heavy chain of these immunoglobulins. IgG4, IgA, IgD, and probably IgE do not bind complement. IgG4 does not bind complement, but it may be cytophilic antibody. According to recent findings the properties of complement fixation and cytophilic binding can reside in the same antibody molecule, but there seems to be no functional relationship between them [60]. It is assumed that the C1 fixation site is revealed only upon distortion of the antibody molecule by combination with the antigen. A single IgM antibody molecule attached to the surface of a red cell can activate complement and lyse the cell, i.e. one molecule suffices to establish a complement fixing site. The IgM molecules are probably distorted by the combination with the antigen and therefore one molecule of IgM can be sufficient to initiate complement activation [13]. In contrast to IgM antibodies, about 4,000 IgG molecules are required to cause cell lysis with complement. In that case the IgG molecules get crowded on the cell surface, two antibody molecules become attached side by side on the same surface, activating the complement system. Two adjacent molecules of IgG antibody are needed to establish a complement fixing site and initiate the effects of complement, probably because of the distortion of their Fc portions [33]. The affinity of C1q for the Fc portion of IgG sub-groups varies according to IgG3 $>$ IgG1 $>$ IgG2. The binding sites of non-aggregated, monomeric IgG and 7S sub-unit of IgM have similar affinity for C1. The higher polymers of IgM are more efficient in C1 fixation [4]. Conformational changes accompanying the aggregation of immunoglobulins may permit firmer binding of C1q.

## ACTIVATION AND BINDING OF COMPLEMENT COMPONENTS [8, 44*a*, *b*]

Interactions of native complement components cause biochemical or biological activities not yet known. The sites which are responsible for the various activities of complement require activation. At least two functional sites may be distinguished: (*i*) a combining region which is reactive with immunoglobulins, complement proteins or biological membranes, and (*ii*) a region through which the various complement proteins manifest their specific roles in the complement chain

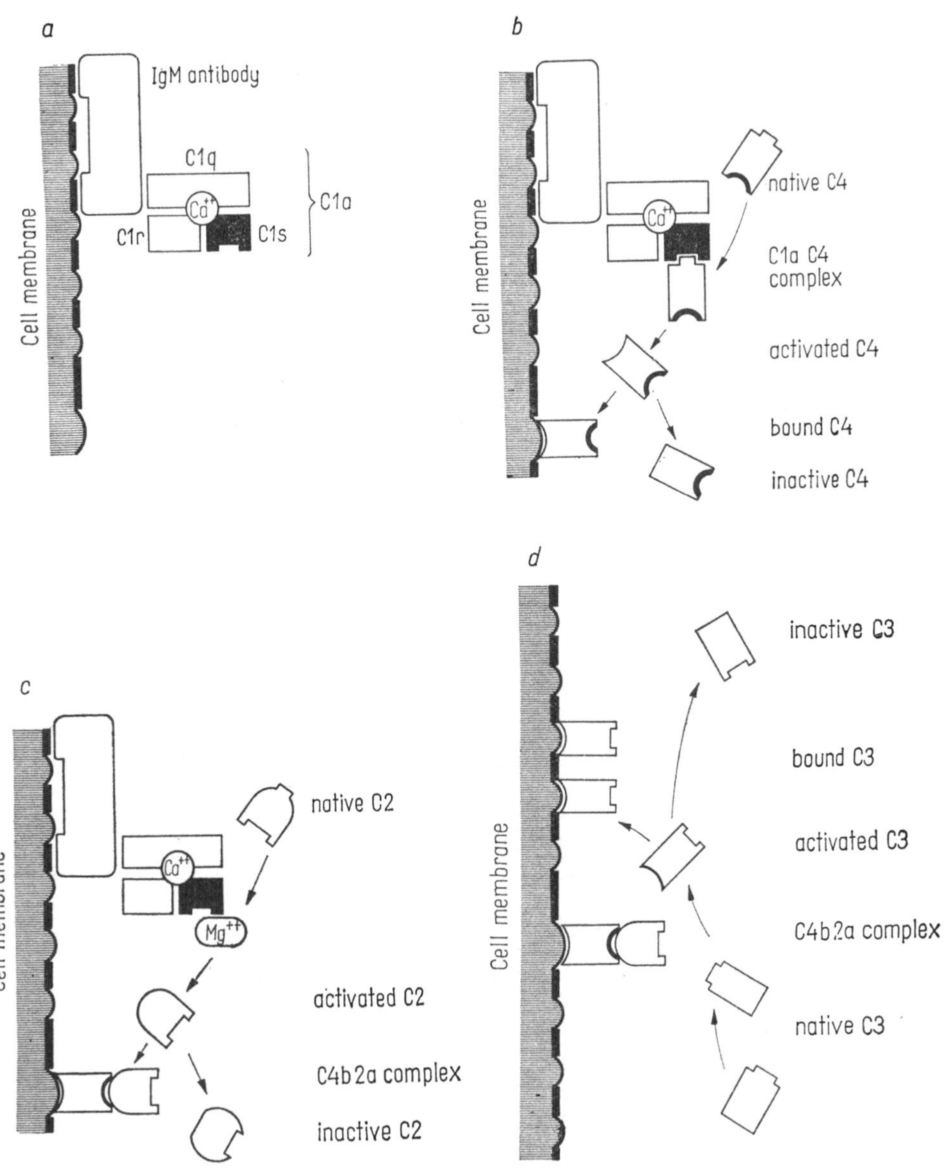


Fig. 15-1*a-d*. Schematic representation of activation and binding of complement components from C1 to C3

reaction. We can generally say that during the activation of a complement component fragmentation occurs. The low molecular weight fragment possesses the biological activity and a small proportion of the high molecular weight fragment binds to the receptors of cells, while a larger proportion of it becomes inactivated in the fluid phase.

In the C1 complex, the C1q sub-component recognizes and reacts with antigen–antibody complex directly without any activation. This combination activates C1r, and this sub-component activates the C1s proesterase to an active esterase. Activated C1 then catalyses binding of C4 to the cell surface or to an antigen–antibody complex. The activating enzyme of C2 that enables the molecule to become bound to its cell surface acceptor is C1 esterase. C1 esterase activates C4 and C2 by their cleavage into two fragments, and this activation requires $Mg^{++}$. The enzymatically active complex, C4b2a, which is capable of initiating C3–C9 consumption, is called C3 convertase. C3 is converted by the active, cell-fixed C42 complex to an active form which attaches to the adjacent cell membrane. C3 convertase acts on C3, cleaving it into two fragments, C3a and C3b. Subsequently, the C3b fragment becomes bound to the cells (Fig. 15-1). The fragmentation of C3 may proceed further, possibly by action of adventitious proteolytic enzymes [55]. Little is known so far about the activation and binding of the next three components. C5 is cleaved upon activation by C4b2a3b (C3 depend-

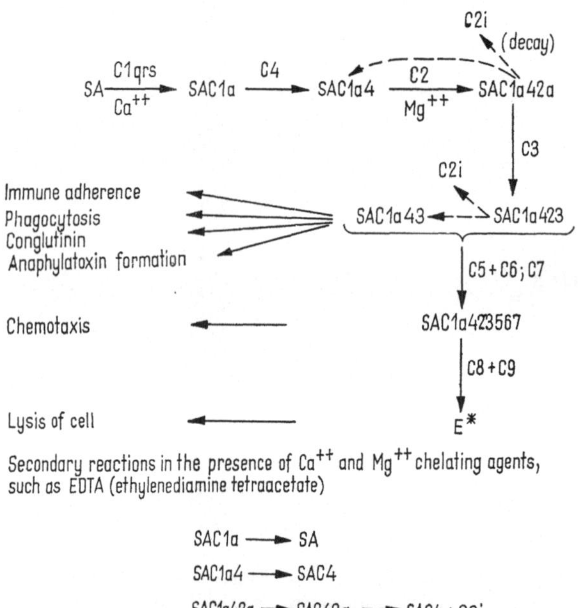


Fig. 15-2. The reaction sequence of complement activation and binding (from Humphrey and White) [31]. S, single site of initiation of complement fixation; A, antibody; C2i, haemolytically inactive C2a; E, erythrocyte; E*, damaged erythrocyte

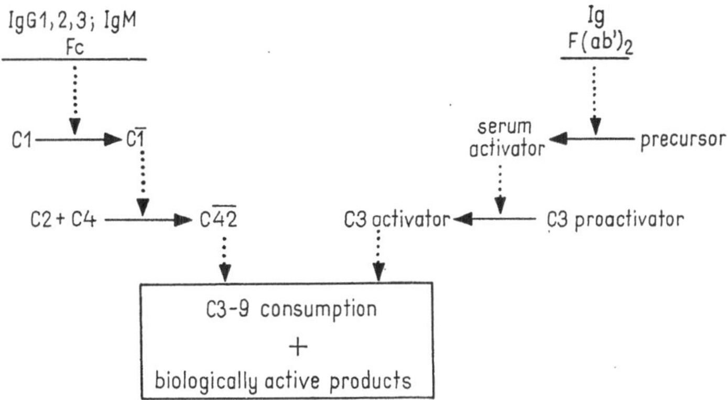


Fig. 15-3. Diagram of two distinct mechanisms of complement activation (from Götze and Müller-Eberhard) [23]

ent peptidase) sites into C5a and C5b. A small portion of C5b fragments becomes firmly bound directly to the cell membrane. The half-life of the EAC1–5 intermediate complex is very short. Then, C6 and C7 interact with fixed C5 in an unknown manner. C5, C6, and C7 components appear to act together, but recently there is some evidence to show that the transformation of EAC1–3 to EAC1–7 consists of three independent and consecutive reaction steps. The cell membrane is still intact at this stage. In the next reaction step, C8 is taken up by the cell surface. Cell-fixed C5, modified by C6 and C7, may activate C8, which produces a low-grade lysis in absence of C9, i.e. actually causes membrane damage. C9 becomes specifically attached to the target cells and aggravates this lesion, possibly through interaction with the cell-fixed C8 [26] (Fig. 15-2).

Recently, data for an alternative mechanism of complement activation have accumulated omitting C1, C2, and C4 and postulating activation of a so far unidentified serum enzyme, C3 proactivator convertase (C3PA convertase), which transforms the C3 proactivator (C3PA), a protein of human serum, to its enzymatically active form [23]. The antibody independent activation of the complement system starting with C3 can be attained by means of naturally occurring plant or bacterial polysaccharides (zymosan, agar, inulin, and various lipopolysaccharides of Gram-negative bacteria) or aggregates of certain immunoglobulins (aggregated IgA and IgG proteins) which interact with C3PA. The polysaccharides and immunoglobulin aggregates may play some role as activating substances of C3PA convertase, which cleaves C3PA into fragments a and b. This reaction is $Mg^{++}$ dependent. The C3 activator, fragment a of C3PA, can cleave C3 into C3a and C3b, i.e. this pathway further on leads to consumption of C3–C9. The C3 activator system has several features in common with the properdin system (Fig. 15-3). It has not been known up to now whether bypass- and properdin systems use the same serum factors. C3PA is regarded to be identical with factor B of the properdin system and with the glycine-rich $\beta$-glucoprotein. Factor A of the properdin system and the purified properdin factor seem to be necessary for the mediation of bypass-reaction [1, 35*b*].

In animals with hereditary defects of the C system, a circumscribed gap in the classical reaction chain can be compensated by the bypass mechanism of C3 activation [8]. This means that C does not only play a role in the classical immune reactions but also in various fields of general defense.

## INHIBITORS OF COMPLEMENT

Complement activation and binding can be inhibited *in vitro* by chelating agents, such as, citrate or EDTA, with complex $Ca^{++}$ and $Mg^{++}$; by heat inactivation of the heat-labile components (C1, C2, C5, C8, and C9); C4 and C3 are demolished by ammonia or hydrazine; the esterase enzymes of complement proteins are destroyed by alkyl phosphonates, which combine with the active sites and block them; the aromatic amino acid derivatives restrain the formation of the heat-stable intermediate from EAC1a42a. Effect of trypsin, streptokinase and other enzymes on complement components in normal human serum has been widely examined [40*a*, *b*].

Serum inhibitor of C1 esterase, a protein normally found in the serum of several species including man, is the best-characterized naturally occurring inhibitor. It inactivates C1, either fixed or in free solution. It is a heat-labile $\alpha_2$-neuraminoglycoprotein which blocks the C1 esterase activity on the complex EAC14, preventing formation of the complex EAC142 [41]. However, physiologically it may be more significant as an inhibitor of plasma kallikrein and PF/Dil [43]. Incubation of C1s with plasmin, trypsin, or lysosomal enzymes of human polymorphs diminish the esterase activity by proteolytic cleavage. At injured tissue sites a control mechanism is thought to prevent the continuation of complement chain reaction [58]. C2a may be released into the fluid phase during the decay of EAC1a42a. The free C2a becomes haemolytically inactive (C2i). This process may play an important role by inhibiting the spontaneous intravascular activation of complement sequence. C3 inactivator (KAF) is a heat-stable $\beta_1$-globulin of serum which does not affect native C3 but diminishes the haemolytic and immune adherence activity of fixed C3 [39]. The alternate pathway is essentially a C3b-feedback pathway which is normally controlled by the activity of KAF [47*a*]. The heat-labile C6 inactivator ($\beta_2$-globulin) inactivates fixed C6 enzymatically. Its biological role is not known [57]. Human serum contains a heat-labile 11 S $\alpha_2$-globulin, an inactivator of the anaphylatoxins C3a and C5a.

## BIOLOGICAL ACTIVITIES OF COMPLEMENT

### LESIONS OF BIOLOGICAL MEMBRANES DUE TO COMPLEMENT

When cells are lysed by antibody and complement, characteristic and uniform bubbles, pits or holes are disclosed by electron microscopy, using the negative staining technique. The diameter of the lesions in the membrane is about 103 Å with human complement [31]. The pattern of holes is usually circular but sometimes it is asymmetric and surrounded by a clear ring. Similar holes are seen in red cells, tumour cells or Gram-negative bacteria affected by complement (Fig.

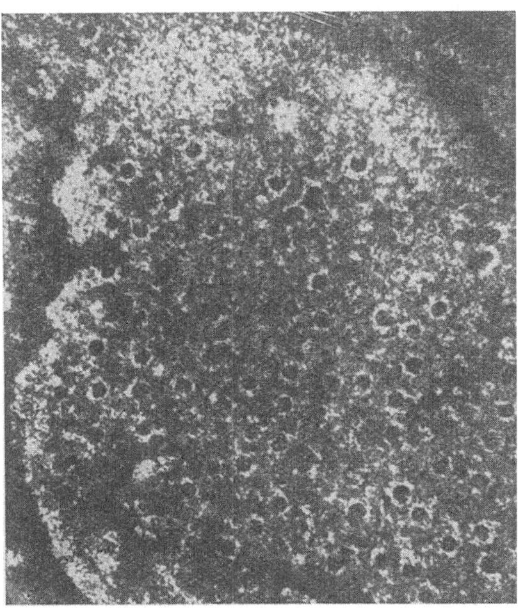

Fig. 15-4. Effect of antibody and human complement on *Shigella shigae*. ×250,000 (from Humphrey and White) [31]

15-4). These lesions are probably due to micelle formation in the surface lipid layers of different biological membranes and visualized as holes within them [30*b*]. Complement system activated by antibody in the absence of C9 has been shown to damage lipid membranes, but not to make holes in them [35]. Probably, C9 aggravates these lesions by impairing the osmotic regulation of the membrane, i.e. after the complement sequence from C1 to C8, only C9 makes electron-microscopically visible holes [26]. In the case of red cells this leads to uptake of water due to the Donnan effect and the resulting swelling causes more serious membrane damage [24]. In nucleated cells disorganization of the internal environment leads to rupture of lysosomes and death (lysis) without swelling. According to the several examinations on Gram-negative bacteria the target of the bactericidal antibody–complement system is the cell wall lipopolysaccharide. The killed bacteria are rendered susceptible to the lytic effect of lysozyme. According to recent findings, typical holes are formed when liposomes (aqueous dispersions of vesicles with walls of one or more stable bimolecular lipid layers containing Forssman antigen) are damaged by complement activated by the antigen-antibody complex or in the reactive lysis systems (involving attachment to erythrocyte membranes or other hydrophobic surfaces of a C567 complex which interacts with C8 and C9) [59]. No lesions were seen before the addition of C8 and C9 in the reactive lysis system or when C6-deficient serum was used in the conventional antibody mediated system. Since liposomes are composed only of lipids, the substrate of the terminal components of complement seems to be of lipid nature [28]. Experiments with pure lecithin liposomes suggests that the substrate is presumably phospholipid [38]. These findings indicate that C8 and C9 act on a lipid substrate of the biological membranes to form characteristic micellar structures, and this is responsible for the irreversible cell damage [36*c*]. The extent of any chemical changes should be very small, for such changes have not yet been detected [32]. According to recent data, C5b, C6 and C7 form a triangular complex, and the central area of this complex represents the binding site of C8. Six molecules of C9 associate to this formation composing a decamolecular complex which may be responsible for the membrane damage [35*a*]. On the other hand, it was shown that during the complement reaction sequence, the lesions first became visible in the non-lytic intermediate complex EAC14235 and their number was unaffected when lysis was induced by C6–9 [50]. These studies of complement action on biological membranes may be useful for the investigation of the biological membrane structure [42*c*].

It was found that alternate complement pathway mediated cell damage and lysis inefficiently or not at all. On the other hand, bypass mechanism can mediate bactericidal and phlogistic reactions even in the unimmunized animal with generation of biological products of inflammatory activity, i.e. this mechanism appears to play a major role in inflammatory reactions and protection against bacterial invasion. These data indicate that the classical and alternate complement pathways have different immunopathological potential [41*a*, 50*a*].

## *One-hit theory of immune haemolysis*

The isolation of purified complement components enables us to study the reaction mechanisms between the complement components. The earliest successful work was the quantitative measurement of C2 with the intermediate EAC14 complex [14]. It was found that titration curves showing the percentage of cells in the state EAC142a as a function of C2 concentration were concave to the abscissa. This shape is characteristic of the titration curve of a one-hit (single-hit), non-cumulative (successive hits constitute independent events) process. According to the one-hit theory, the production of one S* is necessary and sufficient for lysis of a red cell [42*a*, *b*]. Applying the Poisson distribution for the quantitative treatment of dose-response data of individual complement components, the results were expressed in terms of number of effective molecules or as site forming units. For instance, it was found that 400 molecules of C4 represented one effective molecule. Using radioactive labelling, it was shown that only about 20 of the 400 C4 molecules became fixed to the cells, the others remained unbound and underwent inactivation [21*a*]. According to further findings a single cell-fixed molecule of C1 and C5 may correspond to an effective molecule [17]. In contrast, of C2 and C3 more than 1,000 molecules are needed for the production of one effective molecule [20, 49]. Direct observation of electron micrographs and counting of the holes associated with complement dependent lysis of red cells yielded values close to those predicted (a predicted number of active site of EAC142 per cell were treated with an excess of later complement components). Therefore, there is little doubt that the holes represent the sites of lesion in the erythrocyte membrane produced by complement, and that the one-hit theory has been proved by direct observation [12, 30*a*].

## CONGLUTININ (K) AND IMMUNOCONGLUTININ (iK) [36*b*, 37]

Conglutinin is a unique and natural constituent of the serum of many (but not all) Bovidae. The characteristic activity of conglutinin is to combine firmly, but reversibly, in the presence of $Ca^{++}$ with conglutinogen, a polysaccharide determinant, or more properly reactant, occurring, for example, in yeast cells. It also combines, in the presence of $Ca^{++}$, with the carbohydrate moiety of fixed C3 from several species, but this reaction requires an additional serum factor, the conglutinogen activating factor (KAF) distinct from the components of haemolytic C. Conglutination, i.e. agglutination of complement-coated particles by conglutinin, is based on this reaction. The active reactant of zymosan was identified as a mannan–peptide conjugate. It has been reported that N-acetyl-D-glucosamine specifically inhibits the conglutination of alexinated particles. It is possible to perform specific mixed conglutination reactions between complement-coated particles and zymosan in the presence of conglutinin. For these reasons, it is probable that similar carbohydrate groups are responsible for the conglutinogen character of fixed C3 and yeast cells. KAF reacts with fixed C3 in the conglutination reaction making this reactive with conglutinin and reducing its haemolytic and immune adherence activities (C3 inactivator) [39]. The analogy of conglutinin with C-reactive protein and properdin is obvious on the basis of their non-immunoglobulin nature, requirement for $Ca^{++}$ or $Mg^{++}$ ions, and reactivity with specific polysaccharides. They belong to the same type of the immunological phenomenon. The phenomenon of conglutination provides a useful serological tool for demonstrating fixation of C. (The term conglutination is used for the reactions of both conglutinin and immunoconglutinins.)

Immunoconglutinins (iKs), antibodies against C are directed toward antigenic determinants which are hidden in the native complement components and become accessible upon their fixation to antigen–antibody complexes. Unlike conglutinin, their reactions are not dependent on $Ca^{++}$, nor do they react with yeast. None of the iKs studied so far show the specificity to be expected of antibody to conglutinogen, so it seems that conglutinogen and immunoconglutinogens have separate determinants. Two classes of immunoconglutinins are to be distinguished. Whereas iso- and heterostimulated immunoconglutinins are first of IgM and then of IgG antibody type, autostimulated immunoconglutinins (formed in response to antigenic stimulation by the animal's own complement) are invariably of the IgM type and remains so even after repeated stimulation. They appear to be directed against fixed C3 and C4 and possibly other components [36*a*]. The biological significance of immunoconglutinins is not clear. Immunoconglutinins appear to belong to the same class of immunological substances as the rheumatoid factor. Both are groups of predominantly IgM antibodies, and appear to be directed against the products of an immunological reaction. There is some evidence that they play a role in enhancing the opsonization of virulent bacteria by clumping the antibody-coated and complement-fixed organisms. On the other hand, the involvement of these factors in the complement dependent allergic reactions (allergic cytotoxicity and Arthus reaction) may be disadvantageous to the host.

## IMMUNE ADHERENCE AND PHAGOCYTOSIS

Immune adherence (the attachment of antigen–antibody–complement complexes to the surface of platelets and erythrocytes of many species but not to platelets of Primates) is an extremely sensitive *in vitro* reaction for measuring antigen, antibody and complement activity. As little amounts as 0.005 $\mu g$ of ovalbumin [61], 0.001 $\mu g$ of human serum albumin [45*a*] or, in general, 0.0005 to 0.005 $\mu g$ antibody nitrogen are clearly detectable by this reaction. The reaction can be detected by direct microscopic observation, haemagglutination, platelet agglutination, clearance techniques, or by the use of labelled reagents. Immune adherence does not occur in the absence of C and depends upon the attachment of C3 to the complexes. It was shown that at least 60 to 100 fixed C3 molecules per cell are needed for the reaction [22]. Immune adherence is a temperature dependent process, which does not require divalent cations and seems to be an active process, perhaps enzymatic in nature. Erythrocytes from most human donors are reactive, but some persons have been found to have non-reactive erythrocytes. It has been suggested that a specific receptor is present on the surface of the red cells of most humans and other Primates. (It is possible that non-Primate platelets have the same surface receptors.) Human red cells are rendered non-reactive by the action of proteolytic enzymes. On the other hand, mucopeptides split from human, but not from non-Primate, erythrocytes by proteolytic enzymes inhibit the immune adherence reaction, i.e. appear to contain the specific receptor [45*b*].

Apart from the usefulness of the phenomenon as a very sensitive indicator of the presence of antibody, it was shown that *in vitro* phagocytosis of complexes by human polymorphs was enhanced when they were attached to human erythrocytes. The finding that immune adherence to monkey red cells occurred *in vivo* suggests that this reaction may play a role in aiding phagocytosis [46]. It was found that antigen–antibody complexes treated with C would attach to lymphocytes (but only a small portion of them), plasma cells as well as to macrophages and confer on them the ability to take up intact antigen after washing [62]. It is possible that in this case attachment occurred to a receptor similar to or identical with the immune adherence receptor. The same complement components as those required for the immune adherence were sufficient to promote phagocytosis (C1, C4, C2 and C3). The detailed mechanism of phagocytosis is not known [45*c*]. In the absence of serum the engulfment of inert particles by phagocytes takes place vigorously. On the other hand, phagocytosis of particles, such as bacteria, is undoubtedly promoted by specific antibodies (opsonins) or by other serum factors that appeared to be distinct from conventional antibody [29]. Nevertheless, the opsonizing effect of antibodies seems to be potentiated by complement (probably up to C3). IgM antibodies are much more effective than IgG antibodies in promoting phagocytosis, similarly to the relative effectiveness of IgM and IgG antibodies in sensitizing red cells for lysis by complement [51].

The receptors on neutrophils (and also those on monocytes and macrophages) which allow adherence to C3 are different from those which permit adherence to antibodies. Recently it has been shown that C3 has the greatest importance in immune adherence, phagocytosis, and release of constituents form neutrophils

$\beta$-glucuronidase from the primary and alkaline phosphatase from the secondary, granules) [27].

## CHEMOTAXIS OF NEUTROPHIL POLYMORPHONUCLEAR LEUKOCYTES [63*b*]

The interaction of antigen with antibody and complement *in vivo* (in the Arthus-type reactions) or in a special chamber for measuring the migration of polymorphs through a Millipore filter showed that a powerful chemotactic substance was released. By using serum from C6 deficient rabbits as a source of complement, and supplementing this with purified later C components it was found that activation as far as C7 is required for the formation of leukocyte chemotactic factor. This is a macromolecular product and is denoted C567 [64]. The chemotactic factor activates a proesterase in the cell membrane of polymorphonuclear leukocytes. Recently, materials of low molecular weight with chemotactic activity have been shown to be formed *in vitro* when activation occurs as far as C3 and at the stage of C5. The fragments of C3 and C5, C3a and C5a, have chemotactic and anaphylatoxin activities [10, 53, 63*a*]. These two activities reside in different regions of C3a and C5a [10]. It is still an open question whether complement activation represents the normal physiologically important mechanism of chemotaxis [45*c*].

## ANAPHYLATOXIN

Anaphylatoxin is a substance which is able to release histamine from mast cells and which thereby causes smooth muscle contraction and changes in capillary permeability. Both manifestations of anaphylatoxin activity are inhibited by anti-histamines. Systemically, it may cause anaphylactic shock. C3a, a fragment of C3 is one of the two known anaphylatoxins and in addition it has chemotactic activity [15, 22]. Anaphylatoxin and chemotactic activities reside in different regions of C3a [10]. In addition to C3 convertase (C42), also trypsin, plasmin ($\beta_1$-globulin, which can also activate C1s to C1 esterase), thrombin, and the C3 inactivator are capable of cleaving C3. The other known anaphylatoxin is C5a, a sub-component of C5 [15, 53]. The two anaphylatoxins were found to differ in their biological specificities; a segment of guinea pig ileum (anaphylatoxin is usually assayed by measuring the extent of contraction of a segment of guinea pig ileum) which has been rendered unresponsive to C3a by repeated application of this material retains full responsiveness to C5a and *vice versa*. Perhaps, C3a and C5a react with different receptors of smooth muscles. They may be chemically distinct but have some common structures, since both are inactivated by the same inhibitor of human serum. The physiological role of anaphylatoxins is not clear, and the involvement of complement in the anaphylaxis mediated by homocytotropic antibodies remains an open question.

## PROMOTION OF BLOOD COAGULATION AND OTHER BIOLOGICAL ACTIVITIES

Immune complexes, aggregated $\gamma$-globulin and cell wall products of Gram-negative bacteria can initiate and accelerate normal blood coagulation. Blood taken from C6 deficient rabbits shows defective clotting without lacking in any of the classical factors of coagulation. Addition of physiological amounts of isolated human or rabbit C6 normalizes the coagulation. The consumption of 10 to 15 per cent of C6 has been shown during coagulation, therefore, C6 seems to play some role in the normal coagulation mechanism of human blood. It cannot be exluded that intravascular coagulation, often accompanying immune diseases in man, is mediated by complement [3].

Besides participation in normal blood coagulation, C6 seems to be required for the detoxification of endotoxic lipopolysaccharides of Gram-negative bacteria by serum. The detoxifying capacity of C6 deficient rabbit serum is markedly reduced but can be normalized by addition of isolated human C6 [34].

Immunological tolerance develops when an immune response is regulated by the presence of antigen–antibody complexes in a relative antigen excess. Induction of immunological tolerance requires the presence of a functioning C system, indicating the presence of complement fixing antigen–antibody complexes. It was reported that administration of an inhibitor of complement, e.g. vitamin A, together with a tolerance inducing dose of antigen, which normally results in tolerance induction, resulted in immunity rather than tolerance [7, 54]. The tolerance induction in C4 deficient guinea pig showed that intact classical complement pathway is not necessary for tolerance induction [16*a*].

Mobilization of leukocytes from the bone marrow was observed when guinea pig femur was perfused with supernatants of the reactions of antigen–antibody complexes. Leukocyte-mobilizing factor (LMF) was found only in the presence of C1, C4, C2 and C3. The administration of LMF was followed by a peripheral leukocytosis [23].

After the depletion of plasma complement *in vivo* by a protein of cobra venom, hypersensitivity reactions depending upon neutrophil participation, for example in acute nephrotoxic nephritis, were markedly inhibited [16]. The antibody mediated C activation is known to initiate tissue damage in other immune lesions, e.g. in the Arthus reaction [5]. On the other hand, it seems clear that the acute inflammatory response is related to the non-immunological generation of a C3 cleavage product in the model of experimental myocardial infarcts, and of a C5 derived inflammatory mediator in the tick-bite lesion [7*a*].

The connection of biologically active fragments split off from early C factors during activation with kinin-like substances has not been exactly defined. The split off fragments release kinins or have such activity themselves. Effects of kinin-like substance was observed in the reaction mixture of C1, C4 and C2 [44*b*].

## COMPLEMENT IN HUMAN DISEASE [25, 52]

The complement fixation technique as a classical indicator of antigen–antibody reaction *in vitro* has been used since the beginning of this century. (For detailed information see Chapter 22.)

The rapid development witnessed in the understanding of the structure, function and biological significance of complement and the improvement of diagnostic possibilities by the new methods employed in the clinical laboratories allow now a better insight into the pathology of disorders of the complement system. It has become possible to measure the total amount of the haemolytic complement by haemolytic assay or the amounts of the individual complement components by radial immunodiffusion (Mancini) technique or by the technique of reaction intermediates. Only a short list of human diseases caused or accompanied by some disorders of the C system will be given below.

*Congenital complement deficiencies:* C1q deficiency in thymic alymphoplasia or agammaglobulinaemia, C2 deficiency, functional C3 deficiency, C5 deficiency, lack of $\alpha_2$-globulin inhibitor of C1 esterase in hereditary angioneuritic oedema.

*Elevated complement level:* acute rheumatic fever, rheumatoid arthritis, acute polyarthritis, degenerative joint disease, systemic lupus erythematosus without active renal disease, polyarteritis nodosa, dermatomyositis, acute gouty arthritis, Reiter's syndrome, active phases of obstructive jaundice, acute myocardial infarction, sarcoidosis, thyroiditis, ulcerative colitis, typhoid fever, diabetes, some cases of renal allograft rejection.

*Depression of complement level:* acute post-streptococcal glomerulonephritis, chronic membranoproliferative glomerulonephritis, Goodpasture's syndrome, systemic lupus erythematosus with renal involvement, some cases of renal allograft rejection, rheumatoid synovial fluid, hepatitis, haemolytic anaemia, cryoglobulinaemia, paroxysmal nocturnal haemoglobinuria, subacute bacterial endocarditis, myasthenia gravis.

## REFERENCES


1. Alper, C. A., Goodkofsky, I. and Lepow, I. H.: *J. exp. Med.* **137,** 424 (1973).
1a. Alper, C. A., Johnson, A. M., Birtch, A. G. and Moore, F. D.: *Science* **163,** 287 (1969).
2. Alper, C. A. and Propp, R. P.: *J. clin. Invest.* **47,** 2181 (1968).
3. Arroyave, C. M. and Müller-Eberhard, H. J.: *Immunochemistry* **8,** 995 (1971).
4. Augener, W., Grey, H. M., Cooper, N. R. and Müller-Eberhard, H. J.: *Immunochemistry* **8,** 1011 (1971).
5. Austen, K. F.: *Johns Hopk. Med. J.* **128,** 57 (1971).
6. Azen, E. A. and Smithies, O.: *Science* **162,** 905 (1968).
7. Azar, M. M. and Good, R. A.: *J. Immunol.* **106,** 241 (1971).
7a. Berenberg, J. L., Ward, P. A. and Sonenshine, D. E.: *J. Immunol.* **109,** 451 (1972).
8. Bitter-Suermann, D.: *Klin. Wschr.* **50,** 277 (1972).
9. Bitter-Suermann, D., Hadding, U., Melchert, F. and Wellensiek, H. J.: *Immunochemistry* **7,** 955 (1970).
10. Bokisch, V. A., Müller-Eberhard, H. J. and Cochrane, C. G.: *J. exp. Med.* **129,** 1109 (1969).
11. Bordet, J.: *Ann. Inst. Pasteur* **12,** 688 (1898).
12. Borsos, T., Dourmashkin, R. R. and Humphrey, J. H.: *Nature (Lond.)* **202,** 251 (1964).
13. Borsos, T. and Rapp, H. J.: *Science* **150,** 505 (1965).
14. Borsos, T., Rapp, H. J. and Cook, C. T.: *J. Immunol.* **87,** 330 (1961).
15. Cochrane, C. G. and Müller-Eberhard, H. J.: *J. exp. Med.* **127,** 371 (1968).
16. Cochrane, C. G., Müller-Eberhard, H. J. and Aikin, B. J.: *J. Immunol.* **105,** 55 (1970).
16a. Cohen, B. E., Green, I. and Davie, J. M.: *J. Immunol.* **110,** 608 (1973).
17. Colten, H. R., Borsos, T. and Rapp, H. J.: *Science* **158,** 1590 (1967).

18. Colten, H. R., Gordon, J. M., Borsos, T. and Rapp, H. J.: *J. exp. Med.* **128,** 595 (1968).
19. Colten, H. R., Gordon, J. M., Rapp, H. J. and Borsos, T.: *J. Immunol.* **100,** 788 (1968).
20. Cooper, N. R.: *Fed. Proc.* **27,** 314 (1968).
21*a*. Cooper, N. R. and Müller-Eberhard, H. J.: *Immunochemistry* **5,** 155 (1968).
21*b*. id., *J. exp. Med.* **132,** 775 (1970).
22. Dias da Silva, W., Eisele, J. W. and Lepow, I. H.: *J. exp. Med.* **126,** 1027 (1967).
23. Götze, O. and Müller-Eberhard, H. J.: *J. exp. Med.* **134,** 90s (1971).
24. Green, H., Barrow, P. and Goldberg, B.: *J. exp Med.* **110,** 699 (1959).
25. Hadding, U.: *Hautarzt* **23,** 1 (1972).
26. Hadding, U. and Müller-Eberhard, H. J.: *Immunology* **16,** 719 (1969).
27. Henson, P. M.: *J. exp. Med.* **134,** 114s (1971).
28. Hesketh, T. R., Dourmashkin, R. R., Payne, S. N., Humphrey, J. H. and Lachmann, P. J.: *Nature (Lond.)* **233,** 620 (1971).
29. Hirsch, J. G. and Strauss, B.: *J. Immunol.* **92,** 145 (1964).
30*a*. Humphrey, J. H. and Dourmashkin, R. R.: *Ciba Found. Symp. Complement.* Ciba AG., Basel 1965, p. 175.
30*b*. id., *Adv. Immunol.* **11,** 75 (1969).
31. Humphrey, J. H. and White, R. G.: *Immunology for Students of Medicine.* 3rd ed. Blackwell, Oxford, 1970, p. 195.
32. Inoue, K. and Kinsky, S. C.: *Biochemistry* **9,** 4767 (1970).
33. Ishizaka, T., Ishizaka, K., Borsos, T. and Rapp, H. J.: *J. Immunol.* **97,** 716 (1966).
34. Johnson, K. J. and Ward, P. A.: *Fed. Proc.* **30,** 356 (1971).
35. Knudson, K. C., Bing, D. H. and Kater, L.: *J. Immunol.* **106,** 258 (1971).
35*a*. Kolb, W. P., Haxby, J. A., Arroyave, C. M. and Müller-Eberhard, H. J.: *J. exp. Med.* **135,** 549 (1972).
35*b*. König, W., Bitter-Suermann, D., Dierich, M. and Hadding, U.: *Immunochemistry* **10,** 431 (1973).
36*a*. Lachmann, P. J.: *Immunology* **11,** 263 (1966).
36*b*. id., *Adv. Immunol.* **6,** 479 (1967).
36*c*. Lachmann, P. J., Bowyer, D. E., Nicol, P., Dawson, R. M. C. and Münn, E. A. *Immunology* **24,** 37 (1973).
37. Lachmann, P J. and Coombs, R. R. A.: *Ciba Found. Symp. Complement.* Ciba AG., Basel 1965, p. 242.
38. Lachmann, P. J., Munn, E. A. and Weissmann, G.: *Immunology* **19,** 983 (1970).
39. Lachmann, P. J. and Müller-Eberhard, H. J.: *J. Immunol.* **100,** 691 (1968).
40*a*. Laurell, A.-B.: *Acta path. microbiol. scand.* **72,** 139 (1968).
40*b*. ibid., **77,** 291 (1969).
41. Lepow, I. H., Naff, G. B. and Pensky, J.: *Ciba Found. Symp. Complement.* Ciba AG., Basel 1965, p. 74.
41*a*. May, E. J., Green, I. and Frank, M. M.: *J. Immunol.* **109,** 595 (1972).
42*a*. Mayer, M. M.: *Immunochemical Approaches to Problems in Microbiology.* Rutgers University Press, New Brunswick 1961, p. 268.
42*b*. id., *Ciba Found. Symp. Complement.* Ciba AG., Basel 1965, p. 4.
42*c*. id., *Immunochemistry* **7,** 485 (1970).
43. Miles, A. A. and Wilhelm, D. L.: *Brit. J. exp. Path.* **36,** 71 (1965).
44*a*. Müller-Eberhard, H. J.: *Adv. Immunol.* **8,** 1 (1968).
44*b*. id., *Ann. Rev. Biochem.* **38,** 389 (1969).
45*a*. Nelson, D. S.: *Adv. Immunol.* **3,** 131 (1963).
45*b*. id., *Ciba Found. Symp. Complement.* Ciba AG., Basel 1965, p. 222.
45*c*. id., *Macrophages and Immunity.* North-Holland, Amsterdam 1969, p. 99.
46. Nelson, R. A.: *Proc. roy. Soc. Med.* **49,** 55 (1956).
47. Nelson, R. A., Jensen, J., Gigli, I. and Tamura, N.: *Immunochemistry* **3,** 111 (1966).
47*a*. Nicol, P. A. E. and Lachmann, P. J.: *Immunology* **24,** 259 (1973).
48. Nomenclature of Complement. *Immunochemistry* **7,** 137 (1970).
49. Polley, M. J. and Müller-Eberhard, H. J.: *J. exp. Med.* **128,** 533 (1968).
50. Polley, M. J., Müller-Eberhard, H. J. and Feldman, J. D.: *J. exp. Med.* **133,** 53 (1971).

50a. Root, R. K., Ellman, L. and Frank, M. M.: *J. Immunol.* **109,** 477 (1972).
51. Rowley, D. and Turner, J. J.: *Nature (Lond.)* **210,** 496 (1966).
52. Schur, P. H. and Austen, K. F.: *Ann. Rev. Med.* **19,** 1 (1968).
53. Shin, H. S., Snyderman, R., Friedman, E., Mellors, A. and Mayer, M. M.: *Science* **162,** 361 (1968).
54. Sinclair, N. R. and Chain, P. L.: *Nature (Lond.)* **234,** 104 (1971).
55. Spitzer, R. E., Stitzel, A. E., Pauling, V. L., Davis, N. C. and West, C. D.: *J. exp. Med.* **134,** 656 (1971).
56. Stecher, V. J., Morse, J. H. and Thorbecke, G. J.: *Proc. Soc. exp. Biol. (N.Y.)* **124,** 433 (1967).
57. Tamura, N. and Nelson, R. A., jr.: *J. Immunol.* **99,** 582 (1967).
58. Taubman, S. B. and Lepow, I. H.: *Immunochemistry* **8,** 951 (1971).
59. Thompson, R. A. and Lachmann, P. J.: *J. exp. Med.* **131,** 629 (1970).
60. Thrasher, S. G. and Cohen, S.: *J. Immunol.* **107,** 672 (1971).
61. Turk, J. L.: *Immunology* **1,** 305 (1958).
62. Uhr, J. W.: *Proc. nat. Acad. Sci. (Wash.)* **54,** 1599 (1965).
63a. Ward, P. A.: *J. Immunol.* **101,** 818 (1968).
63b. id., *J. exp. Med.* **134,** 109s (1971).
64. Ward, P. A. and Becker, E. L.: *J. exp. Med.* **125,** 1001 (1967).
65. WHO: *Bull. Wld Hlth Org.* **39,** 935 (1968).

CHAPTER 16

# DEVELOPMENT OF HUMAN IMMUNOLOGICAL FUNCTIONS: IMMUNOLOGICAL MATURATION

by

M. KOLTAY

Completed by

P. OSVÁTH



## INTRODUCTION

The development of adaptive immunity coincides with the appearance of organized lymphatic structures during both phylogenesis and ontogenesis [52, 53, 88, 89]. In the course of human embryogenesis the lymphoid organs appear in the following sequence: thymus, spleen, lymph nodes and the lymphoid tissue of the intestine. After the 3rd–6th months of pregnancy the foetus is capable of independent adaptive immunological processes (Fig. 16-1) [6, 77, 88].

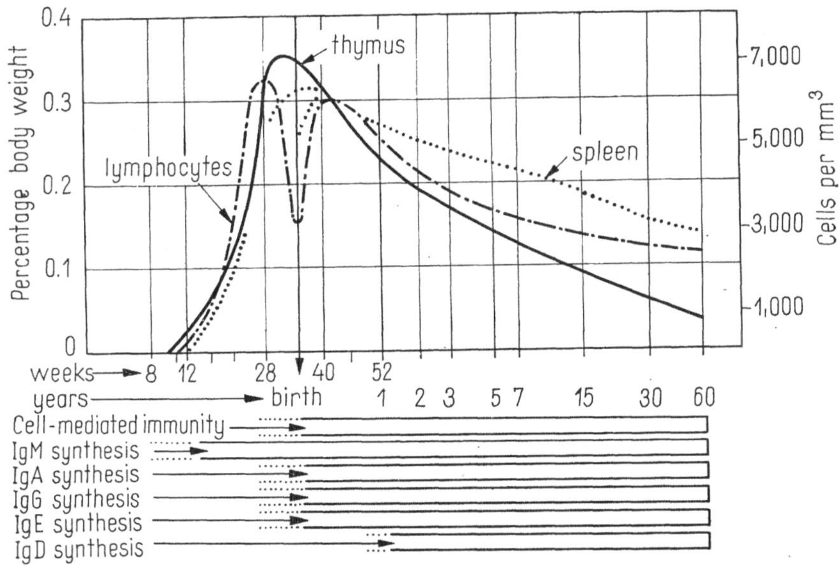


Fig. 16-1. Development of cell-mediated and humoral immunity in the foetus and newborn

## DEVELOPMENT OF CELL-MEDIATED IMMUNITY

The ability for cell-mediated immune responses appears already during intrauterine life in man [6, 88]. Thus tuberculosis immunization with BCG vaccination can be performed in newborns, just like at later ages, not only in mature but also in premature newborns [45]. Delayed-type skin sensitization with natural substances [124] or with chemicals such as dinitrofluorobenzone is possible in most newborns [132]. Although the intensity of delayed skin reactions in young babies is often lower than at later ages [6], this may be due to local factors rendering the infant's skin less suitable for the development of such reactions [120]. In fact, the passive transfer of the ability to give a delayed hypersensitivity reaction from the mother to the foetus should be possible not only by means of the 'transfer factor', but also because leukocytes are able to pass through the human placenta during intrauterine life [32, 137].

It has been possible to demonstrate 'chimaerism' of cells of maternal karyotype in consequence of transplacentally transmitted cells in two cases. This caused a graft versus host reaction resulting in premature delivery. Such cases are considered to be exceptional [42]. However, it is well known that foetal erythrocytes can pass the placental barrier especially in cases of complicated delivery [91] and artificial abortion [21]. The antibodies directed against these erythrocytes may cause a haemolytic disease of the newborn in the following pregnancy [33]. There is ample evidence that foetal leukocytes can also pass the placenta and so there are antibodies reacting with tissue (HL-A) antigens of the foetus in the maternal sera of mice [67] and humans [66]. According to our present knowledge, it is not yet clear whether these cytotoxic antibodies may damage the foetus or may even cause its rejection. In most cases the foetus is protected by the reduction of cell-mediated immune response during pregnancy [103].

*Transplantation immunity*, in which cell-mediated immune processes play likewise a decisive role, probably also develops during intrauterine life in mammals [88]. According to experiments carried out on sheep, the foetus is completely tolerant to skin homografts during the first half of pregnancy, but during the second half rejection ensues similarly as in adult animals [117]. The period of the development of the human transplantation immunity is not known. In any case, the newborn is able to recognize the histoincompatibility of skin homografts [40, 100].

Investigations of the immunological responsiveness of the cellular type revealed that foetal lymphocytes are able to react to PHA with blast transformation from the 14th–16th week of intrauterine life [68, 82, 98]. The lymphocytes of newborns and premature infants display a transformation ability similar to that observed in adults [78, 94*a*, 96, 99]; actually they even show an increased tendency to spontaneous transformation as compared with later ages [78, 94*a*, *b*, 102]. Thus the overall results of lymphocyte studies indicate that newborns, infants and children should be regarded as competent from the point of view of cell-mediated immunity.

*Immunological tolerance* is an immunological response consisting of the development of specific non-reactivity of the lymphoid tissues to a given antigen capable in other circumstances of inducing cell-mediated or humoral immunity. The tolerance to foreign antigens is well established in foetal life. Nevertheless, even in newborn animals, only thymectomy can contribute to a higher than adult degree of immunological tolerance [37]. In humans early feeding with cow's milk does not prevent, but rather enhances the development of allergic symptoms in atopic children [65]. In animal experiments the tissue antigens are well tolerated until delivery in mother–child relation and the other way round [9]. There is not sufficient evidence supporting the hypothesis that human newborns tolerate foreign antigenic configurations without reaction. However, the syndrome of neonatal rubella gives an example of the complexity of this question: there are high levels of IgM-type antibodies and, in spite of this, the virus can persist in the cells for several months [25, 112], i.e. a cellular immunological tolerance coexists with high humoral immunological reactivity.

There is another example of the possible role of neonatal immunological tolerance in illnesses at a later age: human milk often contains cytomegalovirus (17 per cent) [56], which may cause not only the typical illness during infancy, but also haemolytic anaemia with positive Coombs' reaction in the case of immunological tolerance in older children. This possibility has also been shown in newborn mice infected with CCM virus [41]. The DNS of the cytomegalovirus may be incorporated into the nucleus and repressed there; in the case of derepression it can cause cancer of the breast in the adult [56].

## DEVELOPMENT OF HUMORAL IMMUNITY

Independent immunological responsiveness of the humoral type is evidenced by plasmocytosis and by the appearance of specific humoral antibodies in human foetuses suffering from congenital syphilis and toxoplasmosis [34, 115, 116]. The active immunoglobulin synthesizing ability of foetal immunologically competent cells has been proved by means of immunofluorescent and immunochemical techniques [23, 50, 87, 133]. The humoral antibodies produced during intrauterine life are mostly of IgM type, although low concentrations of antibodies of IgA and IgG types may also be found [83, 92, 133].

Nevertheless, under normal conditions the healthy foetus produces antibodies only in slight amounts, since the antigen stimulus necessary to this is absent [57]. Namely, the intact placenta protects the foetus against the majority of antigens during intrauterine life creating a situation similar to that of the germ-free animals. At the same time the foetus and the newborn display considerable passive humoral immunity of maternal origin.

*Passive humoral immunity* is present in all mammalian animals of newborn age, however, the way of the transportation of the maternal antibodies differs with the animal species and is in close connection with the structure of the placenta (Fig. 16-2). Where the foetal and maternal blood circulations are separated by several layers, passive immunity is acquired from the colostrum in which antibodies are present in high concentrations; these antibodies are then absorbed from the intestinal tract without decomposition. Thus immunity only develops immediately after birth. If, however, the barrier is thinner between the two circulations, antibodies can pass directly through the placenta into the circulation of the foetus or are excreted into the amniotic fluid wherefrom they enter

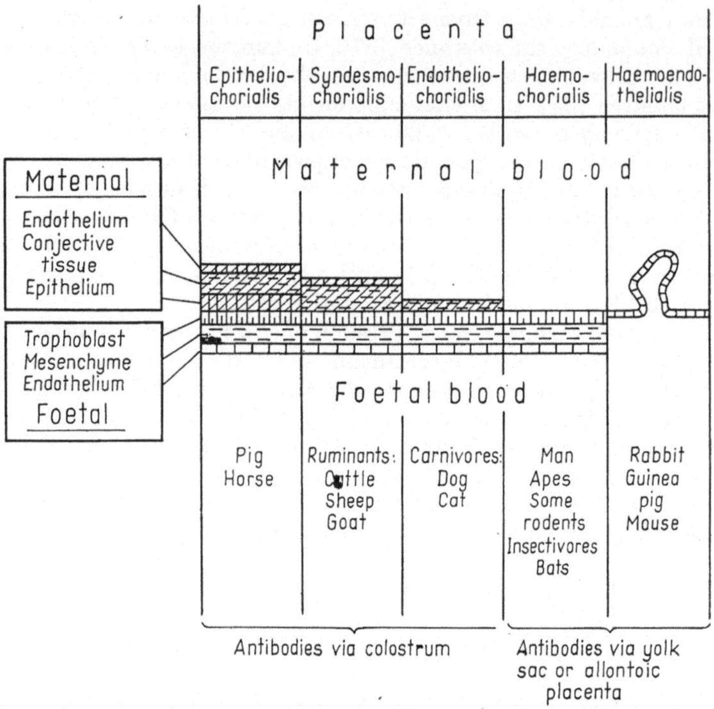


Fig. 16-2. Transfer of maternal antibodies to the foetus in different animal species

the foetal intestinal tract and are absorbed. The different ways of passive immunization can exist side by side [13, 92, 96].

In man systemic passive immunity of newborn children is exclusively diaplacentar. Transfer of maternal antibodies into the foetus starts relatively early during the 3rd month of pregnancy. However, transport of immunoglobulins is most active during the last weeks owing to an increased permeability of the placenta in this phase [49*b*]. As the placenta is permeable only to IgG-type immunoglobulins, the foetus is supplied only with these antibodies [51, 92, 135]. Thus transfer is both selective and active. Namely, permeability does not depend on the size of the molecule; for instance, IgA molecules which are of similar size or the much smaller albumin, glycoprotein and transferrin molecules do not or hardly ever pass the placenta [51]. Selective transfer depends on a structure linked to the Fc fragment of the IgG molecule called the 'placental transfer site' [6, 49*a*, *b*, 51]. The actual IgG concentration of the serum of the foetus and of the newborn is determined first of all by the length of the gestation period [60, 140]. Since this connection is of a logarithmic character, lower values should be expected in premature infants [59, 60, 125, 140]. The human placenta itself does not produce immunoglobulins [30].

According to comparative investigations of maternal and cord blood samples, the IgG level of the mature newborn is identical with that of the mother or may occasionally be somewhat higher [28, 49b, 59, 92]. The IgG of maternal origin, the half-life of which is about 33 days longer than in later ages of life [14], is gradually metabolized in the first postnatal months. At the same time, independent IgG production starts only slowly during the first quarter of infancy. Owing to this fact and to the expansion of plasma volume taking place during this time [27, 131], the actual IgG level of the sucklings decreases at the age of 3–5 months; this is usually described as *physiological hypogammaglobulinaemia*. The decrease is generally mild and mostly unnoticed clinically [72, 74]. However, in about 10 per cent of the cases, it facilitates the development of infections. Physiological hypogammaglobulinaemia can be more severe in premature newborns [60]. The IgG production and level gradually increase during the second half of infancy, but reach the average adult values only at the age of 3–4 years [5, 18, 24, 43, 59, 64, 106, 123, 138].

Other immunoglobulins do not pass the intact placenta. In spite of this, IgM is present in nearly all newborn infants. However, its concentration only amounts to 5–10 per cent of the average adult level [18, 28, 29, 73, 120, 122, 127, 139]. A higher IgM level found in newborn infants indicates a probable intrauterine infection. Such a connection can also be demonstrated, apart from congenital syphilis, in the congenital rubella syndrome and in cytomegalia [3, 4, 84, 108, 114, 121]. The IgM level quickly increases already during early infancy under the effect of antigenic stimuli coming from the environment. The average adult value is reached by the end of infancy or somewhat later [18, 28, 106, 122, 123, 139].

Humoral immune response is thus possible even in the newborn; nevertheless there are certain characteristics distinguishing them from the reactions of later infancy, childhood and adult age. The primary humoral immune response induced by a single large dose of antigen is biphasic in adults but also in children. In the beginning IgM-type antibodies are only formed, but this is followed by the apperance of IgG within a few days; only the latter type is produced later on. The sequence of events is the same in newborns and in young infants; however, the period of IgM production is 4–5 times longer [6, 88, 119]. The importance of the ability of newborn infants to produce IgM can be evaluated in different ways. It gives some protection against the endotoxins of Gram-negative bacteria [6, 86], pneumocystis Carinii [75] and, in contrast to IgG, it enhances the secondary response to repeated antigenic stimuli [85].

IgA occurs in newborn infants less frequently than IgM and its concentration is also lower, amounting only a hundredth of the adult level [127]. IgA can regularly be detected first in the secretions at the age of two weeks and in the blood somewhat later. Its concentration reaches the average adult level only by the age of 14 years [5, 29, 64, 73, 106, 122, 123, 139].

The lowest normal values of IgA are under 15 mg per cent until the age of three years, and this may contribute to the frequency of respiratory infections, for this immunoglobulin, attached to a 'T' piece, is secreted to the mucosal surfaces and plays a role in protection against viral infections [95]. However, only half of the patients suffering from frequent respiratory infections had defective IgA levels in the serum [97]. Higher protection against viral infections (influenza, Sabin live poliomyelitis virus) can be achieved with vaccines given through the mucosa, because of the local protection afforded by the secretory IgA. The lack

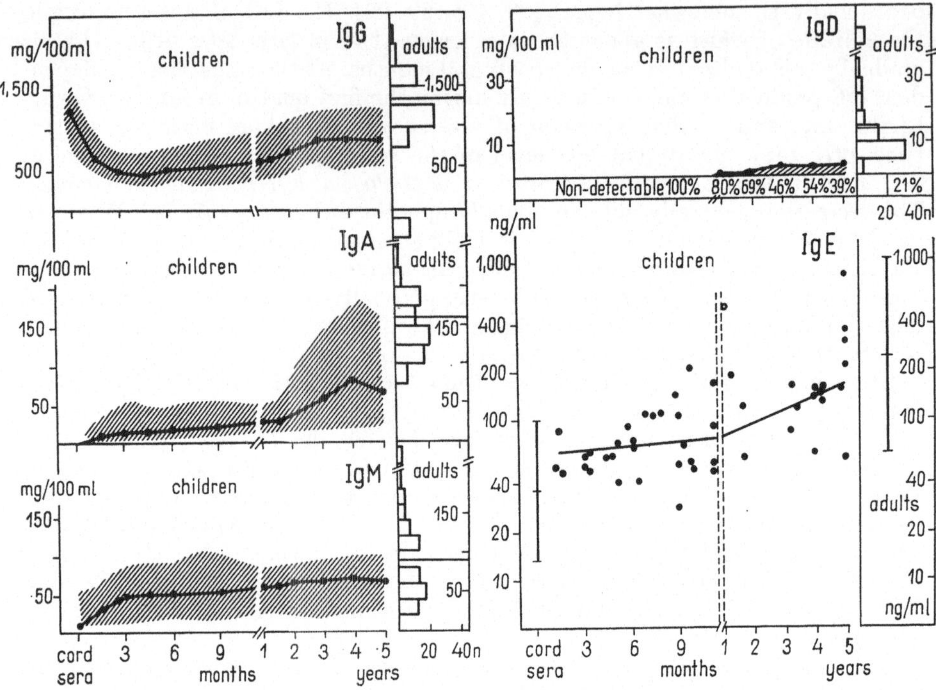


Fig. 16-3. Comparison of the quantitative relations of the different immunoglobulin classes in children and adults

of IgA coincides with the presence of precipitating antibodies against bovine proteins and with milk allergy in consequence of the enhanced absorption of undegraded protein molecules [22, 129]. Thus, the association of frequent respiratory infections and milk allergy can equally be explained by the lack of secretory immunoglobulin in these cases.

It is well known that certain serotypes of *E. coli* cause 'dyspepsia' only during infancy. This might be explained by the lack of capacity to form antibodies directed against the B antigen of bacteria, as revealed by passive haemagglutination studies [93, 105]. However, it is not clear whether these antibodies rendering protection against diarrhoea at an older age are of IgA type or not.

IgD cannot be detected in newborns [64, 127], as it first appears at about the age of seven months [64, 111]. Serum IgD is lacking ($< 1$ mg per cent) in 20 per cent of healthy children as it is absent in a similar ratio among adults. Average IgD concentration is only 20 per cent of the adult level at the age of 5 years [107].

On the other hand, about 15 per cent of the adult IgE concentration can regularly be found at newborn age. IgE concentration gradually increases during infancy and at the age of 3 years it is about half of the adult level [63*a*, *b*].

Serum IgE levels display a very high variability: according to the data of Kumar et al. [76] the normal level in children may be 20–475 ng per ml, the mean value being 143 ng per ml. Only 25 per cent of asthmatic children have an IgE level above S. D. 2, i.e. 700 ng per ml. This might be explained by the high affinity and quick adsorption of IgE molecules to the surface of mast cells [81]. In 'intrinsic asthmatics' having normal IgE values Assem et al. [12] could achieve histamine release from basophil leukocytes by means of adding anti-IgE globulin. Most pollen-allergic asthmatic children have an elevated IgE level only during the season [19]. High IgE levels are almost always found in atopic dermatitis and ascaridiasis patients [17]. However, studies in twins have shown that also hereditary factors determine the IgE levels besides the environment [54].

The quantitative relations of the different immunoglobulins are demonstrated in Fig. 16-3.

## IMMUNOLOGICAL CONSTELLATION OF NEWBORNS AND INFANTS

Although the function of thymus dependent (T) lymphocytes representing the bulk of circulating immunologically competent cells is complete in the newborn, the role of the thymus changes during postnatal life.

The antigen of thymus cells can first be identified in the structures of the third and fourth branchial clefts in the second month of foetal life. It is the central organ of immune system during intrauterine life and initiates the production of immunologically competent cells, which get into the circulation and become deposited in different organs [61].

Lymphocytes contained by the bursa of Fabricius in fowls (in man intestinal Peyer's patches) (B cells) change their antigenicity and biological properties: they become antibody secreting cells (ASC) and function independently of the thymus during extrauterine life. However, even the production of thymus dependent (T) cells is gradually transferred to the bone marrow in postnatal life [1, 136]. The bone marrow produces the precursors of the antigen reactive cells (ARC) which will be 'educated' in the thymus to become immunologically competent. Defective cellular immunity can, therefore, be reconstituted by transplantation of bone marrow [7, 46]. Such a restricted function of thymus can also be produced with the filtrate of the organ containing 'ICIF' (immunocompetence inducing factor): this can transform the cells originating from the bone marrow.

The two systems are linked through the ability of T cells (helper cells) to co-operate with B cells in the production of some antibodies. The ability of T cells to give cell-mediated hypersensitivity reactions and to co-operate in antibody production accounts for the association often seen between the two phenomena.

One of the peculiarities of the humoral immune response of young infants is that not all antigens are uniformly immunogenic at all ages [6, 77, 88, 118, 119, 120]. The active immune response of newborn and young infants also depends on the passive immunity of maternal origin [120]. Immunity can hardly or not at all be induced to antigens which against antibodies of maternal origin are present in high titres in newborn infants [6, 38, 49*b*, 79, 120].

In contrast with previous views, it has no direct influence on the immune state whether the infant receives natural or artificial nutrition. Mother's milk and mainly the colostrum are undoubtedly very rich in antibodies and immunoglobulins [10], mostly in IgA; the amount of IgM is also significant, whereas only minimal concentrations of IgG can be found [15, 80]. Most IgA molecules in milk are present in polymerized form and contain the 'secretory (transport) piece', i.e. are of exocrine or secretory type [16, 130]. The level of polymerized (secretory) IgA increases in the last trimester of pregnancy, the highest levels being reached at the time of delivery (12.8–70 $\mu$g per ml, normal: 5 $\mu$g per ml) [126]. Most of the IgA is probably not actively transported from the blood to the milk, but is locally produced in the mucosa of the mammary gland [10, 130]. The concentration of humoral antibodies in the colostrum is the highest on the first day of lactation decreasing rapidly thereafter, and from the fourth day it is stabilized at a rather low level [15, 80]. The mode of action of the immunoglobulins in the human milk is not clear. Although the immunoglobulins of the milk are highly resistant to decomposing processes in the intestinal tract probably owing to their polymerized state [70*a*], antibodies are not absorbed in human newborn infants, in contrast to certain animal species, but are passing through the intestinal canal and excreted with the faeces [10, 16, 26, 58, 69, 128]. In agreement with this, there is no considerable difference between the immunoglobulin levels of the sera of breast-fed and artificially nourished infants [8, 92], whereas the faeces of the former contains antibacterial and antiviral antibodies in considerable concentrations [70*a*, *b*]. Accordingly, the humoral antibodies of the colostrum and mother's milk only exert a passive protecting effect against enteral bacteria and viruses in the gastrointestinal tract [10, 48]. This mechanism may also be involved in warding off the potential danger of a physiological bacterial invasion of the intestinal tract and in the scanty settlement of the physiological flora of the bowels.

The actual immunoglobulin antibody level of the individual strongly depends on environmental factors especially during newborn and infant life, but also later. Under normal circumstances bacterial invasion from the environment already starts on the first day of life: the bacterial floras of the intestinal and upper respiratory tracts gradually develop constituting the first intensive antigenic stimulus. The effect of the environment is shown by the observation that in newborns kept under semisterile conditions where the development of the physiological bacterial flora is slower, the increase of the serum IgM level is also considerably slower [113]. On the other hand, there is no difference between the responses of mature and premature newborns kept in the same environment [31, 55, 110, 119]. Thus antibody concentration is proportional to that of extrauterine life [110], and independent of the length of gestation.

## THE ROLE AND DEVELOPMENT OF NON-SPECIFIC IMMUNE PROCESSES

The specific immune response of the organism offering an effective protection against different infections depends on the protective and functional immunity, but in vertebrates it is, in addition, closely linked with a number of heterogeneous mechanisms summarized under the term 'non-specific immunity' [36, 49*b*, 62]. Such mechanisms include the action of lysozyme or interferon, phagocytosis as well as chemical and physical barriers to infection.

*The phagocytic activity* of leukocytes can be observed in man already in the first half of intrauterine life; however, this activity seems to be lower during infancy than at later ages. This temporary insufficiency of phagocytosis [11] which may be caused by the low level of the opsonins [90], shows a gradual increase after the end of infancy. The phagocytic activity is found to be lower in premature than in mature newborns in proportion to the difference in gestation [36, 90]. On the other hand, the bactericidic activities of leukocytes are similar in the newborn and at later ages [104].

The C3 component of the *complement system* can be found in man already at the end of the first trimester of foetal life owing to an active synthesis in the liver [44]. It is not sure whether or not C3 passes through the placenta [2, 20, 101]. The C activity also shows a connection with the length of gestation [39, 109]; this activity of mature newborn infants amounts to about half of that in adult age [20, 35]. However, already in the first weeks of life a C activity near that of adults can be present [36, 47, 87]. The C3 level of 3–6 months old infants is the same as in adults [39]. The age-related changes of different C factors are not necessarily parallel with one another [71]. *Properdin* is a globulin, present in normal serum, which plays a part in the lysis of Gram-negative bacteria in the presence of complement and $Mg^{++}$ ions. It is probably not produced during intrauterine life, nor does it pass through the placenta. Thus it is either absent in newborns or is present in a very low concentration and the adult level is reached at about the age of 2 years [71, 134].

Of the other non-specific immune mechanisms, *interferon* seems to be decreased in newborn age, whereas *lysozyme* activity is either normal or increased [36].

## REFERENCES


1. Abdou, N. I. and Richter, M.: *Advanc. Immunol.* **12,** 202 (1970).
2. Adinolfi, M. and Gardner, B.: *Acta paediat. scand.* **56,** 450 (1967).
3. Aiuti, F., Umgari, S., Turbessi, G. and Serra, G. B.: *Helv. paediat. Acta* **21,** 66 (1966).
4. Alford, C. A., Schaefer, J., Blankenship, W. J., Straumfjord, J. V. and Cassady, G.: *New Engl. J. Med.* **277,** 437 (1967).
5. Allansmith, M., McClellan, B. H., Butterworth, M. and Maloney, J. R.: *J. Pediat.* **72,** 276 (1968).
6. Altemeier, W. A. and Smith, R. T.: *Pediat. Clin. N. Amer.* **12,** 663 (1965).
7. Amman, A. J., Meuwissen, H. J., Good, R. A. and Hong, R.: *Clin. exp. Immunol.* **7,** 343 (1970).
8. Amman, A. J. and Stiehm, E. R.: *Proc. Soc. exp. Biol. (N.Y.)* **122,** 1098 (1966).
9. Anderson, J. M.: *Nature* **206,** 786 (1965).
10. Ansaldi, N.: *Minerva pediat.* **20,** 1906 (1968).
11. Argyris, B. F.: *J. exp. Med.* **128,** 459 (1968).
12. Assem, E. S. K., Turner-Warwick, M., Cole, P. and Shaw, K. M.: *Clin. Allergy* **1,** 353 (1971).
13. Atkins, H. J. B.: *Brit. med. J.* **1,** 187 (1958).
14. Barandum, S., Stampfli, K., Spengler, G. H. and Riva, G.: *Helv. med. Acta* **26,** 111 (1959).
15. Bardare, M. and Cislaghi, G. V.: *Minerva pediat.* **20,** 1519 (1968).
16. Bellanti, J. A.: *Amer. J. Dis. Child.* **115,** 239 (1968).
17. Bennich, H. and Johansson, S. G. O.: *Advanc. Immunol.* **13,** 1 (1971).
18. Berg, T.: *Acta paediat. scand.* **58,** 229 (1969).
19. Berg, T. and Johansson, S. G. O.: *Int. Arch. Allergy* **41,** 434 (1971).

20. Bläker, F., Fischer, K. and Witte, P.: *Dtsch. med. Wschr.* **94,** 1978 (1969).
21. Boda, D., Osváth, P., Godó, B., Gellén, J. and Szontágh, F.: *Orv. Hetil.* **109,** 1631 (1968).
22. Buckley, R. H. and Dees, S. C.: *New Engl. J. Med.* **281,** 465 (1969).
23. Buffe, D. and Burtin, P.: *Ann. Inst. Pasteur* **112,** 468 (1967).
24. Collins-Williams, C., Toft, B., Generoso, L. and Moscarello, M.: *Canad. med. Ass. J.* **96,** 1510 (1967).
25. Cooper, L. Z., Green, R. H., Krugman, S., Giles, J. O. and Mirick, G. S.: *Amer. J. Dis. Child.* **110,** 408 (1966).
26. Crabbé, P. A., Bazin, H., Eyssen, H. and Heremans, J. F.: *Int. Arch. Allergy* **34,** 362 (1968).
27. Csorba, S.: *Z. Kinderheilk.* **99,** 263 (1967).
28. Csorba, S., Kávai, M. and Jezerniczky, J.: *Acta paediat. Acad. Sci. hung.* **10,** 53 (1969).
29. Csorba, S., Kávai, M. and Karmazsin, L.: *Acta paediat. Acad. Sci. hung.* **8,** 405 (1967).
30. Dancis, J., Braverman, N. and Lind, J.: *J. clin. Invest.* **36,** 398 (1957).
31. Dancis, J., Osborn, J. J. and Kunz, H. W.: *Pediatrics* **12,** 151 (1953).
32. Desai, R. G. and Creger, W. P.: *Blood* **21,** 665 (1963).
33. Editorial: *Lancet* **ii,** 958 (1972).
34. Eichenwald, H. F. and Schinefield, H. R.: *J. Pediat.* **63,** 870 (1963).
35. Ewald, R. A., Williams, J. H. and Bowden, D. H.: *Vox Sang. (Basel)* **6,** 312 (1961).
36. Fiandino, G.: *Minerva pediat.* **20,** 1891 (1968).
37. Filipp, G. and Boross, B. von: *J. Allergy* **39,** 167 (1967).
38. Fink, C. W. and LoSpalluto, J.: *J. Pediat.* **65,** 1083 (1964).
39. Fireman, P., Zuchowski, D. A. and Taylor, P. M.: *J. Immunol.* **103,** 25 (1969).
40. Fowler, R., jr. Schubert, W. K. and West, C. D.: *Ann. N. Y. Acad. Sci.* **87,** 403 (1960).
41. Fudenberg, H. H.: In *Immunobiology.* Ed. by Good, R. A. and Fischer, D. W. Sinauer, Stamford 1971.
42. Fudenberg, H. H., Good, R. A., Goodman, H. C., Hitzig, W., Kunkel, H. G., Roitt, I. M., Rosen, F. S., Rowe, D. S., Seligmann, M. and Soothill, J. R.: *Pediatrics* **47,** 927 (1971).
43. Fulginiti, W. A., Sieber, O. F. jr., Claman, H. N. and Merrill, D.: *J. Pediat.* **68,** 723 (1966).
44. Furuyama, M., Yoshioka, H. and Oguni, Ch.: *Helv. paediat. Acta* **26,** 220 (1971).
45. Gaisford, W.: *Brit. med. J.* **2,** 1164 (1955).
46. Gatti, R. A., Allan, H. D., Meuwissen, H. J., Hong, R., and Good, R. A.: *Lancet* **ii,** 1366 (1968).
47. Gewurz, H., Pickering, R. J., Clark, D. S., Page, A. R., Finstad, J. and Godd, R. A.: In *Immunologic Deficiency Diseases in Man.* Ed. by Bergsma, D. and Good, R. A. The National Foundation, New York 1968, p. 396.
48. Gindra, J. J., Gothefors, L., Hanson, L. A. and Winberg, J.: *Acta paediat. scand.* **61,** 587 (1972).
49*a*. Gitlin, D.: *Pediatrics* **34,** 198 (1964).
49*b*. id., *Acta paediat. scand.* **172,** Suppl. 60 (1967).
50. Gitlin, D. and Biasucci, A.: *J. clin. Invest.* **48,** 1433 (1969).
51. Gitlin, D., Kumate, J., Urrusti, J. and Morales, O.: *J. clin. Invest.* **43,** 1938 (1964).
52. Good, R. A., Finstad, J., Gewurz, H., Cooper, M. D. and Pollara, B.: *Amer. J. Dis. Child.* **116,** 477 (1967).
53. Good, R. A. and Papermaster, W. W.: *Advanc. Immunol.* **4,** 1 (1964).
54. Hamburger, R. N. and Barezel, N.: *J. Allergy Clin. Immunol.* **49,** 91 (1972).
55. Haworth, J. C., Norris, M. and Dilling, L.: *Arch. Dis. Childh.* **40,** 243 (1965).
56. Hayes, K., Danks, D. M., Gibas, H. and Jack, I.: *New Engl. J. Med.* **287,** 172 (1972).
57. Heremans, J. F.: *Curr. Top. Microbiol. Immunol.* **45,** 131 (1968).
58. Heremans, J. F., Crabbé, P. A. and Masson, P. L.: *Acta med. scand.* **179,** Suppl. 445; 84 (1966).

59. Hitzig, W. H.: *Die Plasmaproteine in der klinischen Medizin.* Springer, Berlin 1963.
60. Hobbs, J. R. and Davis, J. A.: *Lancet* **i,** 757 (1967).
61. Irvine, W. J.: *Modern Trends in Immunology.* Vol. II. Ed. by Cruickshank, R. and Weir, D. M. Butterworth, London 1967, p. 250.
62. Janeway, C. A.: *Arch. Dis. Childh.* **41,** 358 (1966).
63*a*. Johansson, S. G. O.: *Int. Arch. Allergy* **34,** 1 (1968).
63*b*. id., *Proc. roy. Soc. Med.* **62,** 971 (1969).
64. Johansson, S. G. O. and Berg, T.: *Acta paediat. scand.* **56,** 572 (1967).
65. Johnstone, D. E. and Dutton, A. M.: *New Engl. J. Med.* **274,** 735 (1966).
66. Kaiser, G., Keserű, T., Piukovich, I. and Hetyey, P.: *Orv. Hetil.* **113,** 17 (1972).
67. Kaliss, N.: *Proc. Soc. exp. Biol. (N.Y.)* **129,** 83 (1968).
68. Kay, H. E. M., Wolfendale, M. M. and Playfair, J. H. L.: *Lancet* **ii,** 804 (1966).
69. Keller, R., Dwyer, J. E. and D'Amodio, M.: *Pediatrics* **43,** 330 (1969).
70*a*. Kenny, J. F., Boesman, M. J. and Michaels, R. H.: *Pediatrics* **39,** 202 (1963).
70*b*. id., *J. Pediat.* **67,** 943 (1965).
71. Koch, Fr., Schultze, H. E. and Schwick, G.: *Klin. Wschr.* **36,** 17 (1958).
72. Koltay, M.: Clinical, immunological and experimental studies of antibody deficient states. Thesis. Szeged 1964.
73. Koltay, M., Backhausz, R., Bátory, G. und Virág, I.: *Z. Immun.-Forsch.* **130,** 368 (1966).
74. Koltay, M. and Ébrey, P.: *Ann. paediat. (Basel)* **201,** 296 (1963).
75. Koltay, M. and Ilyés M.: *Acta paediat. scand.* **55,** 489 (1966).
76. Kumar, L., Newcomb, R. W., Ishizaka, K., Middleton, E. and Hornbrook, M. M., jr.: *Pediatrics* **47,** 848 (1971).
77. Lamy, M., Seligman, M., Nézelof, C. and Griscelli, C.: *Minerva pediat.* **18,** 799 (1966).
78. Leikin, S., Mochir-Fatemi, F. and Park, K.: *J. Pediat.* **72,** 510 (1968).
79. Levi, J. M., Krautzov, F. E., Levova, T. M. and Fomenko, G. A.: *Immunology* **16,** 145 (1969).
80. Liberatori, J., La Vecchia, L., Papa, G., Ambrosino C. and Ansaldi, N.: *Minerva pediat.* **20,** 1959 (1968).
81. Lichtenstein, L. M. and de Bernardo, R.: *Int. Arch. Allergy* **41,** 56 (1971).
82. Matsaniotis, N., Economou-Mavrou, C. and Tsenghi, O.: *Arch. Dis. Childh.* **42,** 549 (1967).
83. Matsen, J. M., Heimlich, E. M. and Busser, R. J.: *Ann. Allergy* **25,** 607 (1967).
84. McCracken, G. H. and Schienefeld, H. R.: *Pediatrics* **36,** 933 (1965).
85. Metzger, H.: *Advanc. Immunol.* **12,** 57 (1970).
86. Michael, J. G. and Rosen, F. S.: *J. exp. Med.* **118,** 619 (1963).
87. Mikhailova, Z. M. and Mikheeva, G. A.: *Pediatriia (Moscow)* **46/1,** 47 (1967).
88. Miller, J. F. A. P.: *Brit. med. Bull.* **22,** 21 (1966).
89. Miller, J. F. A. P. and Davies, A. J. S.: *Ann. Rev. Med.* **15,** 23 (1964).
90. Miller, M. E.: *J. Pediat.* **74,** 255 (1969).
91. Mollison, P. L. and Walker, W.: *Lancet* **i,** 429 (1952).
92. Muralt, G.: *Helv. med. Acta* **29,** Suppl. 42 (1962).
93. Neter, E., Westphal, O., Lüderitz, R. M., Gino, E. and Gorzinsky, E. A.: *Pediatrics* **16,** 801 (1955).
94*a*. Nicola, P.: *Minerva pediat.* **20,** 668 (1968).
94*b*. ibid., **20,** 1807 (1968).
95. Ogra, P. L. and Karzon, D. T.: *Pediat. Clin. N. Amer.* **17,** 385 (1970).
96. Oppenheim, J. J.: *Fed. Proc.* **27,** 21 (1968).
97. Osváth, P., Ilyés, M., Koltay, M. and Bernátsky, M.: *Gyermekgyógy. (Budapest)* **22,** 500 (1971).
98. Papiernik, M.: *Path. europ.* **4,** 75 (1969).
99. Pentycross, C. R.: *Clin. exp. Immunol.* **5,** 213 (1969).
100. Ponzone, A., Zanetti, D., Fabris, C., De Sanctis, C. and Malandra, C.: *Minerva pediat.* **20,** 2005 (1968).
101. Propp, R. P. and Alper, C. A.: *Science* **162,** 672 (1968).
102. Pulvertaft, R. J. V. and Pulvertaft, I.: *Lancet* **ii,** 892 (1966).
103. Purtilo, D. T., Hallgren, H. and Yunis, E. J.: *Lancet* **i,** 769 (1972).

104. Quie, P. G.: *J. Pediat.* **75,** 533 (1969).
105. Ralovich, B., Hajdi, Gy. and Bognár, Sz.: *Gyermekgyógy. (Budapest)* **22,** 506 (1971).
106. Rauer, U. and Freund, R.: *Mschr. Kinderheilk.* **117,** 559 (1969).
107. Relyveld, E. H.: *Rev. franç. Allerg.* **9,** 219 (1969).
108. Remington, J. S., Miller, M. J. and Brownlee, I.: *Pediatrics* **41,** 1082 (1968).
109. Ritchie, J. H., Aronson, S., Milkovich, L. and Yerushalmi, J.: *Israel. J. med. Sci.* **5,** 439 (1969).
110. Rothberg, R. M.: *J. Pediat.* **75,** 391 (1969).
111. Rowe, D. S., Crabbé, P. A. and Turner, M. W.: *Clin. exp. Immunol.* **3,** 477 (1968).
112. Schimke, R. N., Bolano, C. and Kirkpatrick, C. H.: *Amer. J. Dis. Child.* **118,** 626 (1969).
113. Schneegans, E., Heumann, G., Muralt, G., Butler, E. and Geisert, J.: *Sem. Hop. Paris* **44,** 2410 (1968).
114. Scotti, A. T. and Logan, L.: *J. Pediat.* **73,** 242 (1968).
115. Silverstein, A. M.: *Nature (Lond.)* **194,** 196 (1962).
116. Silverstein, A. M. and Lukes, R. J.: *J. lab. Invest.* **11,** 918 (1962).
117. Silverstein, A. M., Prendergast, R. A. and Kramer, K. L.: *J. exp. Med.* **119,** 2 (1964).
118. Silverstein, A. M., Uhr, J. W. and Kramer, K. L.: *J. exp. Med.* **117,** 799 (1963).
119. Smith, R. T., Eitzman, D. V., Catlin, M. E., Wirtz, E. O. and Miller, B. E.: *Pediatrics* **33,** 163 (1964).
120. Sterzl, J. and Silverstein, A. M.: *Advanc. Immunol.* **5,** 337 (1967).
121. Stiehm, R. E., Amman, A. J. and Cherry, J. D.: *New Engl. J. Med.* **275,** 971 (1966).
122. Stiehm, R. E. and Fudenberg, H. H.: *Pediatrics* **37,** 715 (1966).
123. Stoop, J. W., Zegers, B. J. M., Sander, P. C. and Ballieux, R. E.: *Clin. exp. Immunol.* **4,** 101 (1969).
124. Straus, H. W.: *J. Allergy* **2,** 137 (1931).
125. Thom, H., McKay, E. and Gray, D. W.: *Clin. Sci.* **33,** 433 (1967).
126. Thompson, R. A. and Asquist, P.: *Clin. exp. Immunol.* **7,** 491 (1970).
127. Toivanen, P., Rossi, T. and Hirvonen, T.: *Experientia (Basel)* **25,** 527 (1969)
128. Tomasi, T. B., jr. and Czerwincki, D. S.: In *Immunologic Deficiency Diseases in Man.* Ed. by Bergsma, D. and Good, R. A. The National Foundation, New York 1968, p. 270.
129. Tomasi, T. B., jr. and Katz, L.: *Clin. exp. Immunol.* **9,** 3 (1971).
130. Tomasi, T. B., jr., Solomon, E. M. and Prendergast, R. A.: *J. exp. Med.* **121,** 101 (1965).
131. Trevorrow, V. E.: *Pediatrics* **24,** 764 (1959).
132. Uhr, J. W., Dancis, J. and Neuman, C. G.: *Nature* **187,** 1130 (1960).
133. Van Furth, R., Schnit, H. R. E. and Hijmans, W.: *J. exp. Med.* **122,** 1173 (1965).
134. Vendramini, R., Calapas, G. G., Callegaro, A. and Gallo, E.: *Boll. Ist. sieroter. milan.* **39,** 14 (1960).
135. Wahlquist, B.: *Advanc. Pediat.* **10,** 305 (1958).
136. Waksman, B. H.: In *Immunobiology.* Ed. by Good, R. A. and Fischer, D. W Sinauer, Stamford 1971.
137. Walknowska, J., Conte, F. A. and Grumbach, M. M.: *Lancet* **i,** 1119 (1969).
138. Washburn, C. T.: *Bull. Johns Hopk. Hosp.* **118,** 40 (1966).
139. West, C. D., Hong, R. and Holland, N. H. *J. clin. Invest.* **41,** 2054 (1962).
140. Yeung, C. Y. and Hobbs, J. R.: *Lancet* **i,** 1167 (1968).

CHAPTER 17

# CHEMICAL MEDIATORS OF IMMEDIATE HYPERSENSITIVITY. THE ROLE OF MAST CELLS IN THE ANTIGEN-ANTIBODY REACTION

by

B. CSABA and Å. NILZÉN



The symptoms of anaphylactic and allergic reactions are due to chemical factors, the so-called biological mediators or shock substances, which are released when an antigen combines with its specific antibody. Histamine and 5-hydroxytryptamine (5-HT) are the two most important substances of this kind. The fact that also slow reacting substances of anaphylaxis (SRSA), acetylcholine, choline, heparin, hyaluronic acid, bradykinin, kallidine, leukotaxin, the permeability factors, the substance P, etc. may appear in variable concentration in the anaphylactic shock of the different species, explains the great variety of symptoms observable in the anaphylaxis and allergy of the different species.

Certain biological mediators have also been demonstrated in mast cells. These cells undergo marked morphological damage in anaphylactic shock. Convincing quantitative relationships between the mast cell population and the tissue concentration of certain mediator substances (histamine, 5-HT, hyaluronic acid, SRS-A, etc.) have been established. These findings directed attention to the role of the mast cells.

Essentially, research work on mediators dates back to the beginning of the century when investigators dealt almost exclusively with the role of histamine. As from the 'thirties and 'forties, a steadily increasing number of communications were published to show that also other mediators were involved in anaphylactic and allergic processes. Several pharmacologically active substances were described as being released or synthesized in anaphylactic shock; histamine in 1932, acetylcholine in 1935, SRS in 1940, plasma kinin in 1950 and serotonin in 1955. In the chapter which follows these biologically active compounds and the role of mast cells will be discussed.

## HISTAMINE

by Å. NILZÉN

### INTRODUCTION

The role of histamine both in physiological and in pathological processes has been the subject of intensive research for decades. Histamine was synthesized by Windaus and Vogt in 1907 [100] and some of its pharmacological characteristics were described by Dale and Laidlaw in 1910 [20]. Since then attempts have been made to elucidate the pharmacological effects of histamine. The effect of histamine on the cardiovascular system, the bronchi, the sensory nerves and the exocrine glands has been investigated. A good survey of previous literature concerning these subjects is given in the *Handbook of Experimental Pharmacology* [79*d*].

The biological role of histamine has, however, not yet been clarified. The measuring of the amount of histamine in different tissues has not significantly increased our understanding of the importance of histamine. An indication of its role has been gained through the determination of the amount of histamine in an organ before and after a reactive process in a tissue, but this does not tell us much about the metabolism of histamine as a whole.

### THE STORING AND SYNTHESIZING OF HISTAMINE IN TISSUES

The histamine content in a tissue is dependent on the capability of the tissue to form and store histamine and possibly also on the ability of the cells to take up exogenously added histamine. In most tissues histamine is stored in special cells, the mast cells [79*a*, *c*] and in the blood it is stored in the basophilic leukocytes [31]. There is, however, histamine both in the epidermis and in the cells of the gastrointestinal tract, where there are no mast cells. The presence of histamine has also been demonstrated in brain tissue in spite of the absence of mast cells. The way in which histamine is stored in these tissues is unknown. The high metabolism of histamine in the intestine seems, however, to indicate that a special storing mechanism is not necessary. On the other hand, experiments have established that the bound histamine under different conditions is found in highly constant quantities in tissues [43], which indicates a special mechanism of storing in most tissues.

It seems very likely that mast cells and basophilic leukocytes store and synthesize histamine with the help of the enzyme histidine decarboxylase. This enzyme has been found in the peritoneal mast cells of rats [8, 85*a*] as well as in the mastocytoma of dogs [57*a*]. *In vitro* experiments have shown the presence of histidine decarboxylase in man in the gastric mucosa [8, 45], in the blood [57*b*] and in the lungs [56]. These findings seem to suggest that the essential requirement for the synthesizing of histamine in man has been found [84].

By means of radioactive technique it has been demonstrated in man that exogenous histamine is not taken up, at least not for any considerable length of time, since all radioactivity is found in the urine after 24–28 h [68, 86].

There are, however, some investigations which show that normal mast cells of rat passively take up and bind histamine to their granules [15, 33]. Of special interest to the discussion concerning the taking up and the storing of histamine is the fact that the taking up of radioactive histamine by the peritoneal mast cells of rats is proportional to the incubation period and to the extracellular histamine concentration and that the release both of exogenous and endogenous histamine through the use of compound 48/80 occurs in equal proportions [15, 72]. In view of these results it is not unreasonable to suggest that exogenous histamine could be taken up and stored by mast cells.

In two cases of urticaria pigmentosa, the mast cells were shown to form radioactive histamine from added $^{14}$C-L-histidine. This indicates also that mast cells in man not only store but also form histamine [57*c*].

For the understanding of the mechanism of histamine formation the study of the histamine synthesizing capacity of rats during anaphylactic shock elicited by egg white is of considerable importance. The results are expressed in terms of $^{14}$C-histamine formed *in vitro* from $^{14}$C-histidine by a given amount of tissues. The conclusion is that there is no correlation between elevation of histamine forming capacity in anaphylactic shock and the number of mast cells in the investigated tissue [46*a*].

The physiological role of histamine has been much debated during the last few years and the literature makes it evident that stored histamine is believed to play a significant role in anabolic events, such as the growth of capillaries and also in reparable tissue reactions in certain neoplastic diseases [44, 78]. It is also apparent that induced histamine, allegedly synthesized in the cells of the vascular system, is considered to be part of the control of microcirculation in order to ensure a sufficient blood flow through the tissues [85*b*].

## THE RELEASE OF HISTAMINE

This discovery that histamine releasing substances cause degranulation of mast cells [79*a*] has led to the assumption that degranulation is necessary to the release of histamine [78].

A number of data from experiments concerning the release of histamine through the influence of liberators have been presented in recent years [6, 8, 9, 17*a*, 22, 26, 34*b*, 42, 51, 79*b*, 93].

## HISTAMINE IN ALLERGIC REACTIONS

The symptoms which appear in a sensitized person after the addition of allergen, in so-called immediate hypersensitivity, are most probably caused by pharmacologically active substances, released in antigen–antibody reactions. These substances seem to be released from various cells. Histamine is one of the main mediators, and this survey will only deal with the role of histamine in immediate hypersensitivity and in a number of reactions of similar nature. Only in passing will certain experimental investigations be mentioned which are of importance in the understanding of the activity of histamine. References to the relevant literature will be given.

## ANAPHYLAXIS AND HISTAMINE

The part played by histamine in anaphylactic reactions in different animal species is very well documented in the literature. The guinea pig is the animal which has perhaps been most studied as to anaphylaxis, and the investigations seem to prove that histamine plays a decisive role in mediating the symptoms in the antigen–antibody reaction [1]. Histamine has been detected *in vivo* in blood in anaphylactic reactions [18*a*]. Isolated sensitized organs and systems of organs have frequently been used to demonstrate the release of histamine in anaphylactic reactions, e.g. lungs [2, 4, 11, 14, 17*b*, 29, 34*a*, 35, 36, 102] and skin [11, 25, 66*a*, 99, 101*b*].

In recent years we have learnt much about the mechanism of anaphylactic histamine release from mast cells in experiments using mast cell systems of guinea pig, rat and mouse [11, 65, 66*b*, 75, 96]. That also basophils from sensitized guinea pigs are capable of releasing histamine has been suspected ever since it was demonstrated that the number of basophil leukocytes increases during sensitization and that the number of circulating basophils decreases when shock is elicited [80*b*].

Recently, elegant experiments have demonstrated that basophils from the bone marrow in sensitized guinea pigs release up to 90 per cent of their histamine after challenge with antigen [32].

It has been established that degranulation of mast cells in the lung occurs when histamine is released [21, 67]. The release of histamine in the different organs of the guinea pig shows one peculiarity. Anaphylactic reactions cause a relatively small release in the intestine. The mast cells of the intestine suffer very little or no damage at all from the anaphylactic shock. In the uterus, however, which, like the intestine, contains a large number of mast cells, a considerable release of histamine occurs and degranulation of mast cells takes place [10, 87*a*].

The release of histamine begins early in the course of anaphylactic shock, during which an increased amount of histamine in the blood can be noticed. This increase is, however, of very short duration [59, 97]. The amount of histamine in the plasma of guinea pigs is very high during shock [28, 59, 89].

The levels of histamine and histaminase released into the blood of guinea pigs during anaphylactic shock increase rapidly within the first minute after the antigen injection. Then there is little increase for the next 5–6 min. It has been pointed out that the concentration of histamine during anaphylactic shock is greater in plasma than in whole blood.

The discovery that histamine is not only released in anaphylaxis, but is also formed [46*b*] seems to be of importance in understanding some of the reactions in anaphylaxis in humans, among others the delayed and prolonged symptoms sometimes occurring in drug allergy.

The role of histamine in anaphylactic reaction in species other than the guinea pig must be considered very important. Many investigations have been carried out. References of the literature, both previous and recent, are given in *Pathogenese und Therapie allergischer Reaktionen* (Ferdinand Enke Verlag, Stuttgart 1966, pp. 445–456).

No investigations of the part played by histamine in anaphylactic shock in man have for natural reasons been made. However, anaphylactic reactions in man cause symptoms like urticaria, angioneurotic oedema and bronchospasm, on account of which investigations of the role of histamine in these diseases could also be of relevance to anaphylaxis.

## HISTAMINE IN CERTAIN ALLERGIC AND RELATED REACTIONS

Histamine has long been considered to play a decisive role in the development of symptoms of immediate allergic reactions. This view is based on investigations showing increased histamine excretion in the urine, changes in the amount of histamine in blood plasma, histamine release from sensitized tissues incubated or perfused with specific antigen. The already classical experiment of Katz (1942) [49*a*, *c*] is one of the best examples which shows that sensitized tissues in contact with actual allergen release histamine. Since then a large number of experiments have been conducted in order to demonstrate that histamine is the main mediator in immediate allergic reactions. In this connection it has also been shown that, by using relatively specific antihistamine substances, the blocking of the histamine receptors also considerably prevents the development of certain symptoms.

Interesting research concerning the role of histamine in allergic reactions in man has been carried out in recent years. Even though it was possible relatively early to show, through direct or indirect evidence, that histamine is released from a sensitized tissue [69*a*], it was only at the beginning of the 'fifties that more convincing *in vitro* experiments were carried out [58].

A sensitized tissue releases histamine after the administration of specific allergen. An example of this is that sensitized bronchial tissue releases histamine if actual allergen is added [88].

There is reason to believe that a large portion of the histamine in blood is contained in the leukocytes [18*b*]. The basophil leukocytes seem to be an important storage place for histamine [31]. The basophil leukocytes in man are evidently capable of synthesizing histamine just as the tissue mast cells [57*b*].

Plasma contains under normal conditions insignificant amounts of histamine or no histamine at all [58].

Histamine release from the leukocytes takes place when specific antigen is incubated with the blood from allergic persons [50]. That histamine release occurs from blood cells has been established by many investigators [49*b*, 54*a*]. The histamine release from blood cells in atopic persons after the administration of specific allergen has been studied for several years. In this connection both whole blood and suspensions of leukocytes have been used [3, 7*a*, 55, 63, 64, 70, 71, 76*a*].

It is of interest to note that inhalants release more histamine than do foodstuffs. This corresponds to the fact that extracts of inhalants produce larger weals at skin tests than do extracts of foodstuffs [70]. The author of this survey has made such observations, too, and has also noted, which is perhaps still more surprising, that benzylpenicillin and benzylpenicilloyl polylysine (PPL), when added to whole blood, do not to any great extent release histamine to plasma, not even in patients who give a very strong skin test.

If fragments of monkey lungs passively sensitized with human allergic sera are challenged with specific antigen, histamine release follows. This method seems to be very sensitive and may permit the detection of reagin in the sera of allergic patients not detectable in the Prausnitz–Küstner test [30, 61].

It has been shown that rabbit and guinea pig antibodies (anti-IgE globulin) specific for IgE produce weals in normal humans and monkeys, whereas antibodies specific for other immunoglobulins fail to give such reactions [40]. The pathomechanism is considered to be a reversed allergic reaction against cell-fixed normal IgE [39]. Rabbit antibodies specific for human IgE release histamine from leukocytes in atopic subjects, but antibodies for other immunoglobulin classes do not. The sensitivity of leukocytes to anti-IgE is increased by passive sensitization with reaginic serum containing high concentration of IgE. Anti-IgE releases histamine from human lung tissue [73]. The results of these experiments show that the interaction between tissue or cell-fixed IgE and anti-IgE results in histamine release.

Histamine release before and after specific antiallergic treatment has also been studied [90*a*]. During specific treatment a progressive increase was found in the concentration of allergen required to release a significant part of the total amount of histamine [76*b*].

It has been stated that serum from allergic subjects inhibits the antigen induced release of histamine from sensitive human leukocytes. Such an effect of normal serum has not been observed [54*b*]. It has also been demonstrated that serum from patients who have undergone specific treatment shows a higher antigen neutralizing activity, as measured by the amount of histamine released, than does serum from untreated individuals [54*b*].

The histamine release from whole blood also seems to decrease after hyposensitization [7*b*].

The amount of allergen that has to be added to induce the histamine release from leukocyte suspensions from allergic donors is very small. A quantitative study has been made [53] and judging from the allergen dose-response curve as small an amount as $2.6 \times 10^{-6}$ $\mu$g per ml is sufficient to release 50 per cent of the histamine amount in a leukocyte suspension.

The finding that leukocyte histamine is released *in vitro* by crude staphylococcal antigen supernatants containing protein antigen A or by electrophoretically separated protein antigen A is of interest from the point of view of bacteriological allergy. Pre-incubation of antigens with antigen A precipitin containing sera blocked the release [60].

The mechanism of the release in allergic reactions may be the same as in anaphylaxis [38, 87*b*].

It is likely that the released histamine comes from the basophils and tissue mast cells. Indirect proofs of this have been presented in many studies [80*a*, 81, 91].

It has been suggested that histamine release in man may be followed by an increased formation of histamine [58].

It may be of interest to refer to some works concerning histamine research in connection with some special diseases.

So-called physical allergy, i.e. skin reactions mainly of urticarial type, has a complex aetiology [77]. As early as 1924 Lewis and Grant [52] suggested that histamine mediates these symptoms. (For literature up to 1959 see [24, 69*a*, 77].)

In cold urticaria increased amount of histamine in plasma has been observed during exposure to cold [37, 82]. However, increase of the histamine level in whole blood seems to occur in both healthy and in cold hypersensitive persons after cold exposure [24]. During cold exposure a degranulation of the basophil leukocytes takes place in the blood [41]. An increased amount of excreted histamine and 1-methylimidazol-4-acetic acid has been found [94].

An interesting observation is that if a bulla is produced by means of carbon dioxide in the skin of normal persons and in persons with cold urticaria [27], the histamine amount is considerably increased in the cold sensitive patients [47]. It can be postulated that more histamine is released in persons with cold urticaria than in healthy persons during cold exposure—especially in the tissue exposed to cold.

In urticaria factitia, and dermographism, it has been demonstrated that the histamine amount decreases markedly in the weals [69*a*, 74, 101*a*]. This seems to prove that histamine has been released and eliminated from the affected skin.

During muscular work there is a significant increase in the histamine content of blood and plasma and the number of leukocytes also increases [23].

In urticaria provoked by physical exercise the blood histamine increases considerably [90*b*].

It has been shown that during muscular work the plasma histamine level fluctuates during the first few minutes in both healthy persons and in patients with chronic urticaria as well as in persons with urticaria provoked by exercise. A marked increase in the histamine content was noted in both urticaria provoked by exercise and in chronic urticaria.

As demonstrated by Fig. 17-1, the histamine content is normalized after a few minutes following the end of work. However, after about one hour an increase in the plasma level can be observed. This phenomenon is so characteristic that it can be regarded as a sign of normal histamine metabolism. In this respect there is a marked difference between healthy persons and those with urticaria [69*b*].

### *Urticaria*

It has already been mentioned that histamine plays a decisive role in the pathogenesis of urticaria. Here we only mention that urticaria can be elicited by injection of histamine liberators.

It is of interest in this connection that some workers have reported good therapeutical effect after injection of histamine liberators [94, 95, 96, 97]. In chronic urticaria patients the systemic effect of polymyxin B, a histamine liberator, was more pronounced than in patients suffering from varicose ulcers, psoriasis, etc. [101*a*].

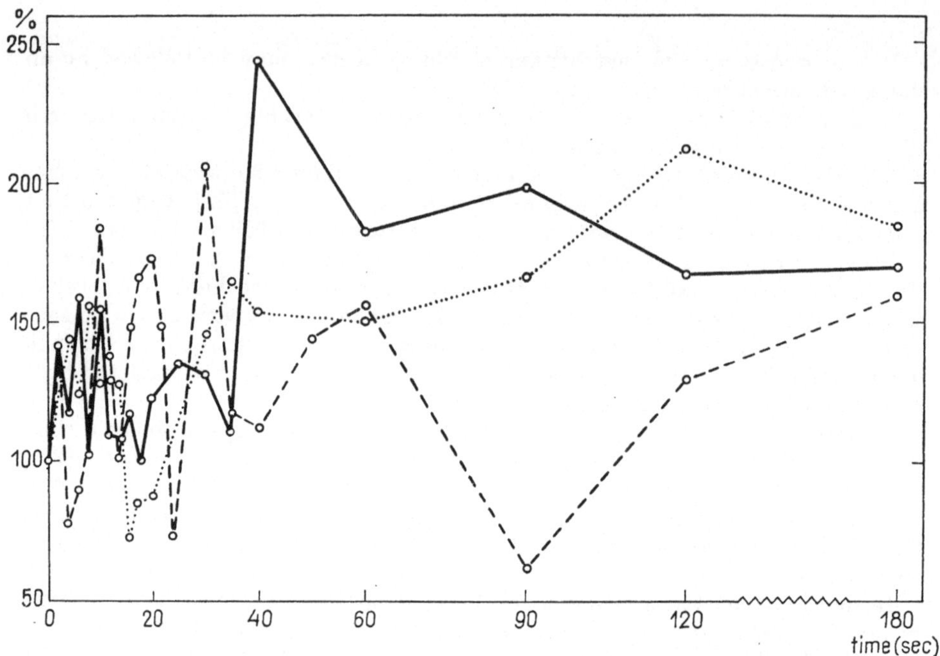


Fig. 17-1. The histamine level in serum during and after muscular exercise. During the first 24 min the patients and controls are cycling on a test-cycle. Every 6th minute the load is increased: 300 kpm,* 600 kpm, 900 kpm and 1200 kpm. The histamine amount before the beginning of the experiments is called 100 per cent
Broken line, healthy persons; solid line, patients with chronic urticaria; dotted line, patients sensitive to heat and/or muscular work

## *Asthma*

Experimental asthma is relatively easy to produce in guinea pigs. The symptoms can be elicited with inhalation of homologous antigen. In sensitized guinea pigs these symptoms resemble human bronchial asthma [48]. It is of special interest to note that corticosteroids inhibit experimental asthma in guinea pigs passively sensitized with ovalbumin [27]. Bronchoconstriction after application of histamine aerosol could, however, not be demonstrated [62]. Similar observations have been made by a number of research workers [36, 62]. Antihistamine protects guinea pigs against bronchoconstriction, resulting from inhalation of histamine aerosol [34*a*].

The role of histamine in spontaneous asthma in man seems to be of hardly any importance. Some research workers have noted increased histamine in plasma [16, 50, 88, 92]. There are, however, investigations demonstrating no increase of histamine in plasma [5, 83]. On the other hand, it has long been known that asthma patients are more sensitive than healthy persons to inhaled histamine [19, 35, 98].

* kilopondmeter

Histamine aerosol has been used to study pulmonary ventilation in healthy and asthmatic subjects. As an example of this the research concerning $N_2$ clearance can be mentioned. It has been able to prove objectively that asthmatic persons are more sensitive to inhaled histamine than are healthy subjects. The reason for this increased sensitivity is discussed with reference to experiments with different drugs. Hexamethonium, a ganglion blocking preparation, reduces the sensitivity. This suggests that a nervous mechanism is responsible for the increased reactivity [13].

In this connection it is of interest to note that patients suffering from byssinosis do not show hypersensitivity to inhaled histamine. The fact that byssinotic textile workers are not hypersensitive to histamine suggests that repeated bronchoconstriction in itself does not lead to histamine sensitization of bronchial smooth muscle [12].

## REFERENCES


1. Albanus, L. and Winqvist, G.: *Acta haemat. (Basel)* **26,** 365 (1961).
2. Alberty, J. and Huurrekorpi, L.: *Acta allerg. (Kbh.)* **14,** 386 (1959).
3. Arsdel, P. P. van, Middleton. E., Sherman, W. B. and Buchwald, H.: *J. Allergy* **29,** 429 (1958).
4. Bartosch, R., Feldberg, W. and Nagel, E.: *Pflügers Arch. ges. Physiol.* **231,** 616 (1933).
5. Beall, G. N. and Ohanian, S. H.: *J. Allergy* **34,** 8 (1963).
6. Benditt, E. P. and Lagunoff, D.: *Progr. Allergy* **8,** 195 (1964).

7*a*. Bergquist, G. and Nilzén, A.: *Acta allerg. (Kbh.)* **23,** 363 (1968).

7*b*. ibid., **24,** 261 (1969).

8. Bloom, G. D., Fredholm, B. and Haegermark, Ö.: *Acta physiol. scand.* **71,** 270 (1967).
9. Bloom, G. D. and Haegermark, Ö.: *Exp. Cell. Res.* **40,** 637 (1965).
10. Boréus, L. O.: *Acta physiol. scand.* **52,** 320 (1961).
11. Boréus, L. O. and Chakravarty, N.: *Acta physiol. scand.* **48,** 315 (1960).
12. Bouhuys, J. B.: *Amer. Rev. Dis.* **95,** 89 (1967).
13. Bouhuys, A., Jönsson, S., Lindell, S. E., Lundgren, C., Lundin, G. and Ringquist, T. R.: *Clin. Sci.* **19,** 79 (1960).
14. Brocklehurst, W. E.: *J. Physiol.* **151,** 416, (1960).
15. Cabut, M. and Haegermark, Ö.: *Acta physiol. scand.* **68,** 206, (1966).
16. Cerqua, S.: *Minerva med.* **27,** 542 (1936).

17*a*. Chakravarty, N.: *Acta physiol. scand.* **48,** 133 (1960).

17*b*. ibid., **48,** 146 (1960).

18*a*. Code, C. F.: *Amer. J. Physiol.* **127,** 78 (1939).

18*b*. id. *Physiol. Rev.* **32,** 47 (1952).

19. Curry, J. J.: *J. clin. Invest.* **25,** 785 (1946).
20. Dale, H. H. and Laidlaw, P. P.: *J. Physiol.* **41,** 318 (1910).
21. Diamant, B.: *Acta physiol. scand.* **55,** 11 (1962).
22. Diamant, B. and Uvnäs, B.: *Acta physiol. scand.* **53,** 315 (1961).
23. Dunér, H. and Pernow, B.: *Scand. J. clin. Lab. Invest.* **10,** 394 (1958).
24. Dunér, H., Pernow, B. and Sterky, G.: *Acta allerg. (Kbh.)* **15,** 417 (1960).
25. Emmelin, N., Kahlson, G. S. and Lindström, K.: *Acta physiol. scand.* **2,** 78 (1941).
26. Fawsett, D. W.: *J. exp. Med.* **100,** 217 (1954).
27. Feinberg, S. M. and McIntire: *J. Allergy* **24,** 302 (1953).
28. Giertz, J., Hahn, F., Hahn, H. and Schmutzler, W.: *Klin. Wschr.* **40,** 598 (1962).
29. Giertz, H., Hahn, F., Opferkerch, N. and Schmutzler, W.: *Arch. exp. Path. Pharmakol.* **242,** 42 (1961).
30. Goodfriend, L., Kovacs, B. A. and Rose, B.: *Int. Arch. Allergy* **30,** 511 (1966).

31. Graham, H. T., Lowry, O. H., Wheelwright, F., Lenz, M. A. and Parish, H. H.: *Blood* **10,** 467 (1955).
32. Greaves, M. W. and Burdis, B. D.: *Int. Arch. Allergy* **34,** 313 (1968).
33. Green, J. P.: *Fed. Proc.* **26,** 211 (1967).
34*a*. Halpern, B. N.: *Arch. int. Pharmacodyn.* **68,** 339 (1942).
34*b*. id., *Proc. 3rd. Int. Congr. Allerg.* Ed. by Halpern, B. N. and Holtzer, A. Flammarion, Paris 1958, p. 351.
35. Herxheimer, H.: *Int. Arch. Allergy* **2,** 27 (1951).
36. Herxheimer, H. and Rosa, L.: *J. Physiol. (Lond.)* **118,** 7 (1952).
37. Hidelmann, G., Preuss, E. G. and Kaiser, W.: *Dtsch. med. Wschr.* **82,** 284 (1957).
38. Högberg, B. and Uvnäs, B.: *Acta physiol. scand.* **48,** 133 (1960).
39. Ishizaka, K. and Ishizaka, T.: *J. Immunol.* **100,** 554 (1968).
40. Ishizaka, T., Ishizaka, K., Johansson, G. O. and Bennich, H.: *J. Immunol.* **102,** 884 (1969).
41. Juhlin, A. and Shelly, G.: *J. Amer. med. Ass.* **177,** 371 (1961).
42. Juhlin, L.: *Arch. Derm. (Chicago)* **88,** 771 (1963).
43. Kahlson, G.: *Lancet* **i,** 67 (1960).
44. Kahlson, G. and Rosengren, E.: *Physiol. Rev.* **48,** 155 (1968).
45. Kahlson, G., Rosengren, E., Svahn, D. and Thunberg, R.: *J. Physiol. (Lond.)* **167,** 45 (1963).
46*a*. Kahlson, G., Rosengren, E. and Thunberg, R.: *J. Physiol. (Lond.)* **172,** 188 (1964).
46*b*. id., *Lancet* **i,** 782 (1966).
47. Kaiser, W. and Preuss, E. G.: *Allergie u. Asthma* **14,** 18 (1968).
48. Kallos, P. and Pagel, W.: *Acta med. scand.* **91,** 2192 (1937).
49*a*. Katz, G.: *Science* **91,** 221 (1940).
49*b*. id., *J. Pharm. exp. Ther.* **72,** 22 (1941).
49*c*. id., *Proc. Soc. exp. Biol. (N.Y.)* **49,** 272 (1942).
50. Katz, G. and Cohen, S.: *J. Amer. med. Ass.* **117,** 1782 (1941).
51. Lagunoff, O. and Benditt, E.: *J. exp. Med.* **112,** 571 (1960).
52. Lewis, T. and Grant, R. T.: *Heart* **11,** 209 (1924).
53. Lichtenstein, L. M.: *Mechanism of Allergic Histamine Release from Human Leukocytes. Biochemistry of the Acute Allergic Reactions.* Blackwell Scientific Publications, Oxford and Edinburgh 1966.
54*a*. Lichtenstein, L. M. and Osler, A. G.: *J. exp. Med.* **120,** 507 (1964).
54*b*. id., *J. Immunol.* **96,** 169 (1966).
55. Lichtenstein, L. M., Piao King, T. and Osler, A. G.: *J. Allergy* **38,** 174 (1966).
56. Lilja, B., Lindell, S. E. and Saldeen, T.: *J. Allergy* **31,** 492 (1960).
57*a*. Lindell, S. E., Rorsman, H. and Westling, H.: *Experientia (Basel)* **15,** 31 (1959).
57*b*. id., *Acta allerg. (Kbh.)* **16,** 216 (1961).
57*c*. id., *Acta derm.-venereol. (Stockh.)* **40,** 277 (1961).
58. Lindell, S. E. and Westling, H.: *Histamine Metabolism in Man. Handbook of Experimental Pharmacology.* Springer, Berlin–Heidelberg–New York 1966, p. 734.
59. Logan, G. B.: *J. Allergy* **40,** 207 (1967).
60. Martin, R. R. and White, A.: *J. Immunol.* **102,** 437 (1969).
61. Mc Gerity, J. L., Arbesman, C. E. and Wicher, K.: *J. Allergy* **43,** 200 (1969).
62. Mendes, E.: *Acta allerg. (Kbh.)* **11,** 181 (1957).
63. Middleton, E. and Sherman, W. B.: *J. Allergy* **31,** 441 (1960).
64. Middleton, E., Sherman, W. B., Fleming, W. and Arsdel, P. P. van: *J. Allergy* **31,** 448 (1960).
65. Mongar, J. L.: *J. Physiol. (Lond.)* **135,** 320 (1957).
66*a*. Mongar, J. L. and Schild, H. O.: *J. Physiol. (Lond.)* **118,** 461 (1952).
66*b*. ibid., **135,** 301 (1957).
67. Mota, I. and Vugman, I.: *Nature* **177,** 427 (1956).
68. Nilsson, K., Lindell, S. E., Schayer, R. W. and Westling, H.: *Clin. Sci.* **18,** 313 (1959).
69*a*. Nilzén, Å.: *Acta derm.-venereol. (Stockh.)* **27,** Suppl. 17. (1947).
69*b*. To be published.
70. Noak, J. W.: *J. Allergy* **26,** 385 (1955).

71. Noak, J. W. and Brand, A.: *J. Allergy* **25,** 210 (1954).
72. Nordlander, N. B.: *Acta med. scand.* **157,** 235 (1957).
73. Paul, W. and Weir, D. M.: *Clin. exp. Immunol.* **5,** 311 (1969).
74. Pellerat, M. and Murat, M.: *Ann. Derm. Syph. (Paris)* **6,** 76 (1946).
75. Provost–Danon, A., Silva Lima, M. and Queiroz, Javierre, M.: *Life Sci.* **5,** 289 (1966).
76*a*. Pruzansky, J. J. and Patterson, R.: *J. Allergy* **38,** 315 (1966).
76*b*. ibid., **39,** 44 (1967).
77. Rajka, E.: In *Allergie und allergische Erkrankungen.* Vol. II. Ed. by Rajka, E. Akadémiai Kiadó, Budapest 1959, p. 602.
78. Riley, J. F.: *Ann. N. Y. Acad. Sci.* **103,** 164 (1963).
79*a*. Riley, J. F. and West, G. B.: *J. Physiol. (Lond.)* **120,** 528 (1953).
79*b*. id., *J. Path. Bact.* **69,** 269 (1955).
79*c*. id., *Arch. Derm. (Chicago)* **74,** 471 (1956).
79*d*. id., The Occurrence of Histamine in Mast Cells. In *Handbook of Experimental Pharmacology.* Springer, Berlin, 1966, Vol. 18/1. p. 116.
80*a*. Rorsman, H.: *Acta derm.-venereol. (Stockh.)* **37,** 121 (1957).
80*b*. id., *Acta Allergy* **17,** 36 (1962).
81. Rorsman, H. and Rosengren, E.: *Acta derm.-venereol. (Stockh.)* **38,** 377 (1958).
82. Rose, B.: *Histamine, Hormones and Hypersensitivity.* Recent Progr. Hormone Res. Vol. VII. Academic Press, New York 1952, p. 384.
83. Rose, B., Rusted, I. and Fownes, J. A.: *J. clin. Invest.* **29,** 113 (1950).
84. Rotschild, Z. and Schayer, R. W.: *Biochem. biophys. Acta (Amst.)* **30,** 23 (1958).
85*a*. Schayer, R. W.: *Amer. J. Physiol.* **186,** 199 (1956).
85*b*. ibid., **202,** 66 (1962).
86. Schayer, R. W. and Cooper, J. A.: *J. appl. Physiol.* **9,** 481 (1956).
87*a*. Schild, H. O.: *J. Physiol.* **95,** 393 (1939).
87*b*. id., *Mechanism of Anaphylaxis. III. Congr. Int. Allerg. Paris* (1958).
88. Schild, H. O., Hawkins, D. F., Mongar, J. and Herxheimer, H.: *Lancet* **ii,** 376 (1951).
89. Schmutzler, W., Giertz, H. and Hahn, F.: *Int. Arch. Allergy* **22,** 69 (1963).
90*a*. Serafini, U.: *J. Allergy* **19,** 256 (1948).
90*b*. id., *Gazz. int. Med. Chir.* **55,** 341 (1951).
91. Shelley, W. B. and Juhlin, L.: *Blood* **19,** 208 (1962).
92. Sicuteri, F., Michelacci, S. and Franchi, G.: *Int. Arch. Allergy* **22,** 408 (1913).
93. Singleton, E. M. and Clark, S. L.: *Scand. J. clin. Lab. Invest.* **14,** 1744 (1965).
94. Tham, R.: *Scand. J. clin. Lab. Invest.* **18,** 603 (1966).
95. Ungar, G. and Damgaard, E.: *J. exp. Med.* **101,** 1 (1955).
96. Uvnäs, N. and Thon, I. L.: *Exp. Cell Res.* **23,** 45 (1961).
97. Waalkes, T. P., Weissback, H., Bozicevich, J. and Udenfriend, S.: *J. clin. Invest.* **36,** 1115 (1957).
98. Weiss, S., Robb, G. P. and Blumgart, H. L.: *Amer. Heart J.* **4,** 664 (1929).
99. Westerholm, B.: *Acta physiol. scand.* **61,** 195 (1964).
100. Windaus, A. and Vogt, W.: *Ber. dtsch. chem. Ges.* **40,** 3691 (1907).
101*a*. Zachariae, H.: *Acta derm.-venereol. (Stockh.)* **43,** 214 (1963).
101*b*. id., *Skin Histamine.* Munksgaard, Copenhagen 1965.
102. Ängård, E., Bergqvist, U., Högberg, B., Johansson, K., Thon, I. L. and Uvnäs, B.: *Acta physiol. scand.* **59,** 97 (1963).

## OTHER MEDIATORS. MAST CELLS

by B. CSABA

### 5-HYDROXYTRYPTAMINE

Although this vasoconstrictor, contained in the blood and involved in coagulation, was described at the end of the last and at the outset of the present century already [18, 163], it was not identified until its synthesis at the beginning of the 'fifties [77]. 5-HT was found to be identical with enteramine and serotonin [51, 137, 139, 140]. It was demonstrated by *in vitro* tests in 1955 that, as a result of an antigen–antibody reaction not only histamine but also 5-HT was released from rabbit platelets [84*b*]. This phenomenon was shortly thereafter demonstrated *in vivo*, too [173]. Since then, numerous experiments have been carried out in order to elucidate the pathogenic role played by 5-HT in anaphylactic shock.

Most species store the largest amount of 5-HT in the mucosal enterochromaffin cells of the gastrointestinal tract [52, 53], while considerable quantities have been observed in the platelets [84*a*], in different parts of the brain and of the spleen. Smaller amounts of the substance have been described in the liver, kidney and lung. The rat skin abounds in 5-HT [133*a*]: more than 50 per cent of the total amount is to be found there. It has further been proved that in the majority of species (guinea pig, dog, man, cattle, horse, rabbit, pig, hamster, cat), 5-HT is not concentrated in the tissue mast cells. There is hardly any 5-HT in the lung of rats, mice and rabbits [168]. Concentration of the 5-HT in the gastrointestinal tract of humans has been found to be proportional to the distribution of argyrophil cells [141].

5-HT is a product of tryptophan metabolism. It is enzymatically decarboxylized and, after undergoing desamination, excreted in the form of 5-hydroxyindole acetic acid (5-HIAA) [167]. There are detailed publications and monographs on the biological function of 5-HT in the various species, its pharmacological and pathophysiological actions, its antagonists and release [51*b*, 51*c*, 63, 78, 131*a*, 131*b*, 158, 165]. Their detailed discussion would go beyond the scope of this chapter.

Considering that the results of *in vivo* and *in vitro* experiments with 5-HT are not analogous, the mediator role and the significance of this substance have still not been completely elucidated. The ability of 5-HT to contract smooth muscles varies from species to species. The isolated colon of the rat and its uterus in oestrus are particularly sensitive to serotonin. So are the bronchiolar muscles of the cat and the rat, less so those of the guinea pig and the dog, whereas human and rabbit bronchioles are highly resistant [15*c*, 131*a*, 168].

Certain authors do not regard 5-HT as a mediator in the anaphylactic shock of dogs [3, 28, 152] and attribute this function only to histamine because they have failed to observe either a release of 5-HT or the elevation of its blood level. On the other hand, Japanese authors registered the presence of increased amounts of the substance in the portal vein of dogs in anaphylaxis [157*a*]. The anaphylactic reactions of the dog are only very slightly mitigated by lysergic acid diethylamide-25 (LSD-25) [157*b*]. 5-HT induces bronchiospasm [19, 42, 113] and pulmonary hypertension [148] in the dog, a phenomenon worthy of note because these symptoms are present in anaphylaxis, too [23].

Release of 5-HT has further been observed in the anaphylactic shock of cats [48, 157*b*], which presumably intensifies the liberation of histamine. The lung and blood platelets of the cat and dog contain comparatively large amounts of 5-HT.

Herxheimer [81] provoked a shock similar to anaphylaxis in guinea pigs by making them inhale 5-HT aerosol, and failed to prevent it by LSD. Other authors [132] succeeded in preventing the classical anaphylactic shock of guinea pigs by the intravenous administration of LSD. Release of 5-HT from the intestine and spleen of anaphylactic guinea pigs has also been described [47]. It is now currently agreed upon that, in addition to histamine, 5-HT too may be involved in the anaphylaxis of guinea pigs [152]; its role is, however, secondary [29, 174]. The amount of 5-HT in the lung of guinea pigs is very small [174]. Some authors found it to be increased in this organ during anaphylactic shock [93], while others made no such observation [49, 147]. It is a significant fact that anaphylactic shock does not change the concentration of 5-HT in the blood [86]. The various Schultz–Dale test findings are likewise contradictory. Some authors [57] think it improbable that 5-HT would be released during this reaction of the ileum [57] because it also occurs in the presence of LSD and 2-bromolysergic acid ethylamide (BOL); others found [65] that anaphylactic contraction of the ileum could not be inhibited unless the Tyrode solution contained not only antihistamine but also atropine and LSD. Accordingly, they postulate the participation of three mediators in the Schultz–Dale reaction of the guinea pig ileum, namely histamine, 5-HT and acetylcholine.

In the anaphylactic shock of rabbits both histamine and 5-HT are released from the platelets in the presence of $Ca^{++}$ ions *in vivo* as well as *in vitro*. The platelets of rabbits contain great amounts of 5-HT (7.5 $\mu$g per $10^9$ platelets) [173]. While the plasma concentration of amines becomes higher, the amount of histamine and 5-HT decrease in the whole blood along with the decreasing platelet count. The amount of amines in the lung exhibits a simultaneous temporary increase, a phenomenon due to the antigen–antibody reaction giving rise to the formation of leukocytic thrombi in the platelets, which become arrested in the pulmonary vessels [171*a*]. All these changes can be produced also by the intravenous administration of glycogen [172] but not in rabbits pretreated with heparin [87, 183]. The latter inhibits the absorption of 5-HT added to the platelets *in vitro* and prevents at the same time the clotting of intravascular blood and the formation of thrombi. Nevertheless, certain authors do not ascribe much significance to 5-HT in the pathogenesis of anaphylactic reactions of rabbits and in the production of allergic vascular lesions [26, 104, 105*a*, *b*] because pretreatment with reserpine, which depletes the tissues of 5-HT, fails to prevent the lethal shock and allergic vascular lesions following administration of egg-white. The antagonists of 5-HT such as LSD, dihydroergotamine and chlorpromazine are likewise ineffective. Intestinal hyperperistalsis in rabbit anaphylaxis may nevertheless be caused by the release of 5-HT [111].

Opinions are divided also concerning the role of 5-HT in the anaphylactic shock of rats. It is difficult to assess the experimental data available and to draw conclusions since rats and mice are fairly resistant to the effects of anaphylaxis, histamine and 5-HT. Investigators have long tried to reduce the resistance of these animals e.g. by adding vaccine (BPV) to the animals' diet [154], adrenalectomy [38, 58, 182], hypophysectomy [116], employment of Freund's adjuvant [108], application of cold stress [183], and treatment with thyroxine [133*b*, 160]. BPV is now usually administered by the intraperitoneal route. It is the cell wall of the microorganism which contains the sensitizing agent [125, 128]. Other bacterial preparations have no effect.

According to Sanyal and West [152] neither histamine nor 5-HT should be regarded as mediator substances in the anaphylactic shock of rats because shock can be induced also in animals whose skin and intestines have been depleted of histamine and 5-HT by pretreatment with reserpine and 48/80. Rat uterus responds only to comparatively large doses of histamine but contracts intensively in anaphylaxis [96]. Although the uterus of rats in oestrus is highly sensitive to 5-HT, this substance does not seem to contribute to the anaphylactic contraction since it takes place in the presence of LSD as well and also because no 5-HT is demonstrable in the blood plasma of shocked rats, while antihistamines markedly inhibit the development of shock [118]. Also, rats pretreated with reserpine and injected with specific 5-HT antagonists develop passive cutaneous anaphylaxis (PCA) [16].

In contrast, there are also data available indicating that 5-HT is a mediator in the anaphylactic shock of rats. It has been found [64*a*] that on addition of antigen, the suspension of cells taken from the peritoneum of sensitized rats releases histamine and 5-HT. Considerable amounts of 5-HT are released by the small intestine after perfusion with antigen, and also by minced pieces of sensitized uterine tissue. Experimenting with the isolated skin and the perfused hind leg of rats, Halpern et al. [75] found that the kinetics of histamine and 5-HT release were more or less the same no matter whether it was caused by anaphylactic shock or dextran. The optimum concentration of the antigen is highly important for the release of 5-HT from the isolated peritoneal cell suspension of rats [64*b*]. An anaphylactic response of isolated cells will only occur, i.e. mediators will only be released, at a certain antigen–antibody ratio. If this is so, experiments investigating the mediator function of 5-HT in rat anaphylaxis should be devised accordingly. The theory is gaining ground that kinins [36] are the principal mediators in the anaphylactic shock of rats, while also histamine and 5-HT contribute to the development of the shock syndrome [33]. In rat anaphylaxis the additive role of histamine and 5-hydroxytryptamine is also of importance since after the administration of *Bordetella pertussis* vaccine the resistance of rats to the toxic effect of histamine and 5-HT decreases [32*a*].

Changes in 5-HT metabolism during anaphylactic shock in rats have proved that 5-HT is probably one of the active mediators of rat anaphylaxis besides the kinins [32*b*].

The anaphylactic mediators of mice require likewise further elucidation. That 5-HT is involved in the pathogenesis of the mouse anaphylactic shock syndrome has been observed in some, and disproved by other, experiments. Isolated mouse uterus is undoubtedly extremely sensitive to 5-HT: even doses less than 5 ng per ml induce contraction. Besides, BPV considerably increases the sensitivity of mice to active and passive anaphylactic shock as also to 5-HT [100]. The Schultz–Dale reaction is inhibited in these animals by 5-HT antagonists, e.g. by LSD and reserpine [56]. Pretreatment with 5-HT antagonists like BOL, LSD or chlorpromazine and with reserpine, which accelerates the excretion of 5-HT, affords protection against anaphylactic shock even *in vivo* [67, 166]. Lethal doses of 5-HT provoke symptoms similar to those of anaphylactic shock [124]. Capillaries of the mouse are 100 to 150 times more sensitive to 5-HT than to histamine; it has been demonstrated [76] that passive cutaneous anaphylaxis is caused by the simultaneous release of histamine and 5-HT and by their interaction. The combined administration of antihistamine and LSD prevents anaphylactic shock in the mouse. On the other hand, previous removal of histamine and 5-HT from the tissues by reserpine and 48/80 [171*b*] or treatment with BOL and mepyramine (i.e. the antagonists of the two amines) will not prevent lethal anaphylactic shock.

Accordingly, neither of these amines seems to play a decisive role in mouse anaphylaxis. The blood and tissue 5-HT levels of mice died in anaphylactic shock are not markedly changed [171*b*]. While a simultaneous release of histamine, bradykinin and SRS has been observed during the first minutes of acute anaphylactic shock [107], no increase in the concentration of 5-HT was found in the blood of mice that had died of the shock. Mastocytomatous mice, which excrete much 5-HIAA, do not become more sensitive to systemic anaphylaxis [110], and the mastocytoma has no effect on the course of anaphylaxis [41].

5-HT is not regarded as a pathogenic factor in human allergy [79] and bronchiolar myospasm [15*c*]. Japanese authors [157*a*] found increased 5-HT levels in the blood and increased amounts of 5-HIAA in the urine of patients suffering from penicillin allergy. Urinary output of 5-HIAA remains unchanged in cases of hay fever [22]. UML (1-methyl lisergic acid), a specific 5-HT antagonist, has yielded satisfactory results in the treatment of asthmatic and allergic patients [8, 69, 74]. Serotonin concentration was measured in nasal allergy and was found significantly higher than in the controls [73].

Local injections of 5-HT were given to 12 subjects using the skin-window technique. Eosinophilia was found in the cellular exudate during the first hours. The cells probably contain substances which neutralize serotonin [181].

From the conflicting evidence the conclusion may be drawn that 5-HT acts undoubtedly as a mediator substance in certain species or certain tissues, and, together with other mediators, contributes to the development of symptoms following the combination of antibody with antigen. Further information regarding its function and significance is expected to be gained from future studies.

## ACETYLCHOLINE (CHOLINE)

Went and Lissák [109, 176*a*, *b*, *c*] were the first to report the involvement of acetylcholine and choline in anaphylactic shock. After perfusing the isolated heart of sensitized guinea pigs with homologous antigen, they found choline in the perfusate. They further demonstrated that, in shock, the amount of choline decreased in the heart, while the concentration of histamine remained unchanged. Reaction to allergen perfusion was completely inhibited by atropine. The pharmacological effects of acetylcholine: vasodilation, decrease in blood pressure, intensified lacrimation, salivation and secretion of gastric and pancreatic juice, enhanced oesophageal, gastric, intestinal, vesical and cholecystic mobility, uterine contraction, bronchiospasm, etc. closely resemble certain symptoms of anaphylaxis and allergy. Thus the theory has been advanced that increased release of acetylcholine following strong nervous stimuli plays a decisive role in allergic phenomena [35*a*, *b*]. The sites of all urticarial (and so also allergic urticarial) inflammations are surrounded by a zone of reflex hyperaemia presumably induced by acetylcholine.

Some investigators went as far as to conclude that acetylcholine is the only shock substance of all allergic phenomena [175]. Anaphylactic shock developed and caused a decrease in the activity of liver cholinesterase in white mice, indicating the pathogenetic role of this substance [37]. Although acetylcholine has been propounded as mediator in the Schultz–Dale reaction of guinea pigs [65] beside histamine and 5-HT, we hesitate to accept it as an important mediator substance because it is not released in amounts that would be sufficient for the production of anaphylactic and allergic reactions; nevertheless, it has a modifying effect on other mediator substances.

## HEPARIN AND HYALURONIC ACID

Heparin was prepared from dog liver in 1916: hence its name [112]. To be found in the metachromatic granules of mast cells, heparin is contained also in the lung and in various other tissues. That histamine and heparin form a complex in mast cells was described already in 1948 [66]. Heparin presumably binds histamine and 5-HT in the mast cells only at pH less than 7.0 [98*b*]. No bond is formed if pH is changed towards the neutral zone or if a higher salt concentration is present. There is a parallelism between mast cell count and the amount of hyaluronic acid in several normal and pathological tissues [6*a*]; under the influence of hormones, the mast cells secrete hyaluronic acid, the precursor of heparin [6*b*].

Heparin has an anticoagulant effect: it inactivates thrombin, inhibits the conversion of prothrombin into thrombin and prevents the agglutination of thrombocytes. In dogs in anaphylaxis and peptone shock, histamine and heparin are simultaneously released by the liver and, as a result, the clotting time is considerably prolonged [145, 147]. It has been repeatedly confirmed that the number of mast cells diminishes in the liver of dogs in cases of anaphylactic or peptone shock and that heparin and histamine are released at the same time [120, 121].

Heparin does not aggravate the shock symptoms, moreover it mitigates the damage of the capillary endothelial cells by inhibiting thrombocyte agglutination. Besides, it prevents the extravascular coagulation of plasma proteins exudated from the capillaries. Following pretreatment with heparin no thrombocytic-leukocytic thrombi will be formed in the pulmonary vessels of rabbits in anaphylactic shock [171]. The Arthus phenomenon is also mitigated by heparin [106]. Heparin pretreatment prevents the liberation of 5-HT from the platelets of anaphylactic rabbits; the platelet count and the serum 5-HT level are not reduced, neither are the urinary 5-HIAA and plasma 5-HT levels increased [88]. The liver of anaphylactic guinea pigs releases heparin which gets into the plasma and—according to recent observations—releases histaminase. Heparin is, thus, the mediator of histaminase and moderates anaphylactic manifestations not only by its anticoagulant effect but also by the liberation of enzymes which cause the decomposition of histamine [68]. Release of heparin presumably gives rise to similar phenomena in other species as well, although its effects may be less pronounced [98*c*].

## SLOW REACTING SUBSTANCE A (SRSA)

By perfusing guinea pig lungs and incubating egg yolks with cobra venom. Feldberg and Kellaway [54] prepared a substance which caused the slow contraction of smooth muscles. It has been termed slow reacting substance to distinguish it from histamine and acetylcholine giving rise to rapid contraction. According to a subsequent statement of these authors, a substance similar to SRS, appeared *in vitro* in the perfusate of the anaphylactic guinea pig lung [97]. It was then Brocklehurst [15*a*, *d*] who provided direct and definitive evidence to show that in anaphylactic shock there appears in the lung of guinea pigs—apart from histamine—a mediator substance which is pharmacologically different from all substances known so far and elicits a slow reaction of ileum. Brocklehurst called it SRSA (slow reacting substance of anaphylaxis), indicating by this term that the substance is released as a result of the antigen–antibody reaction and that it is different from other compounds of the SRS group.

The chemical properties of SRS, which is formed under the effect of cobra venom lecithinase A correspond to those of unsaturated fatty acids [170]. Although attempts at a chemical identification of the SRS released in anaphylaxis have been unsuccessful so far, experiments with partially purified SRSA show that the compound is lipid [15*e*], acidic and contains sialic acid both in free state and bound by glycosides. SRSA would, thus, represent a mixture of neuraminic acid and glycoside [24]. It has been suggested furthermore that SRSA may be a permeability factor [130*b*] because only combined diethylcarbamazine (Hetrazan), mepyramine maleate and methysergid are able to inhibit the PCA reaction, whereas the antigen induced release of SRSA is considerably diminished by Hetrazan alone.

SRSA is obtained by perfusion of isolated rabbit, monkey and human lungs in anaphylactic shock [15*d*], but is released in goats even *in vivo* [138]. In sheep, the specific antagonist to histamine and 5-HT did not influence the anaphylactic response to egg albumen. Sodium meclofenamate, an antagonist of bradykinin and SRSA, had a marked inhibitory effect on egg albumen anaphylaxis [4]. Some authors suggested that SRS is stored in mast cells [169] and that the concentration of histamine and SRSA is closely correlated with the mast cell count [14*a*], but these statements have not been confirmed [15*b*, 138]. According to a recent theory, not mast cells but polymorphonuclear leukocytes ensure the optimum release of SRSA. An eosinophil leukocyte chemotactic factor of anaphylaxis (ECFA) was demonstrated in actively or passively sensitized guinea pig lung, which was also accompanied by the release of both histamine and SRSA. SRSA and ECFA could also be separated by gel filtration [95, 130*a*]. However, the release of histamine and SRSA mediated by rat IgE is dependent on the participation of the mast cell but does not require the presence of circulating polymorphonuclear leukocyte (PMN) or an intact complement system, thus differing from the PMN and complement-dependent pathway of SRSA release mediated by the IgGa antibodies of hyperimmune serum [129]. Release of these substances has been demonstrated in the anaphylactic shock of mice, too [107]. The antigen-induced release of SRSA in anaphylaxis of rats pretreated with IgE is markedly influenced by agents which act to increase or decrease the levels of cellular cyclic-AMP. For example, depletion of cellular cyclic-AMP through direct $\alpha$-adrenergic stimulation with norepinephrine enhances IgE-mediated SRSA release. The $\alpha$-adrenergic blocking agent phenoxybenzamine prevents the enhancement of SRSA release activated with norepinephrine and enhances the inhibition produced with epinephrine [101]. The prostaglandins, $PGE_1$ and $PGE_2$, effectively inhibit the IgE and IgGa mediated release of SRSA in the rat in a dose-response fashion. Indirect evidence did not establish that an increase in tissue cyclic-AMP levels and no synergism between $PGE_1$ and dietyhlcarbamasine or disodium chromoglycate was demonstrable [101].

On being reinjected with the antigen, slices of guinea pig lung release SRSA and histamine only if the animal has been sensitized with 7S IgG1 antibody. None of the amines is released after sensitization with 7S IgG2 antibody, whereas IgG antibodies of the rabbit or rat antiserum or their sub-classes are responsible for the release of anaphylactic SRSA [162] in the rat.

The largest amounts of SRSA are released in the lung, followed by the aorta and the great veins [15*d*]. It has no effect on the bronchial muscles of the guinea pig, dog, rabbit, and cat, but contracts the ileum of guinea pigs, the jejunum of rabbits, the colon of rats and the rectal caecum of fowls. Since human bronchioles are particularly sensitive to SRSA, it may play a significant role in bronchial asthma [15*e*]. Its effect is prolonged, and it does not cause tachyphylaxis. Recent investigations have shown [117] that, in the rat, antibodies of the class IgG1 are responsible for the release of SRSA.

No specific antagonist of SRSA has been found so far and, therefore, it is rather difficult to evaluate the significance of this substance as a pathogenic factor in allergic and anaphylactic conditions.

## ACTIVE POLYPEPTIDES AND OTHER MEDIATORS

Essentially, two large groups of polypeptides belong under this heading; one of them, the group of kinins, comprises peptides of the bradykinin-kallidin type. They stimulate the smooth muscles, produce vasodilatation, increase capillary permeability, induce the accumulation and migration of leukocytes and cause strong pain by stimulating the corresponding nerve fibres [46]. The other group comprises vasoactive polypeptides which have no such strictly circumscribed pharmacological mediator effect in inflammatory processes. Substances belonging to this group are oxytocin, vasopressin, substance P, angiotensin, further polypeptides which do not occur in mammals but are frequently used in experiments and clinical practice, such as eledoisin, phylokinin, physalaemine. It should be noted that this grouping is quite arbitrary.

So far, Rocha E Silva [144] has been the only author who tried to establish a consistent nomenclature for the biologically active polypeptides. He recommended 'kinin hormones' as a collective term including (*i*) angiotensin, bradykinin and kallidin which originate from the plasma; (*ii*) substance P which originates from the intestinal wall and the central nervous system; (*iii*) urokinin, colostrokinin, vespakinin, scorpiokinin and other related compounds derived from diverse sources. This grouping serves the purpose to distinguish kinins from neural hormones, i.e. from oxytocin and vasopressin.

A hypotensive substance was found in human urine already in 1909 [2], and later another in the pancreatic juice [134]. Also Frey and his associates [59, 60, 61] prepared similar substances from urine, blood plasma and other tissues. Since the greatest amounts were found in the pancreas, these vasoactive agents —supposed to be identical irrespective of origin—were termed kallikrein (kallikreas = pancreas). But a few years later Werle et al. [177] discovered that kallikrein is an enzyme releasing a smooth muscle stimulating substance from plasma proteins. It was first called DK *(darmkontrahierende Substanz)* and is now known as kallidin. Rocha E Silva et al. [146] demonstrated a hypotensive polypeptide with smooth muscle stimulating action in the blood of dogs treated with trypsin or snake venom. This was called bradykinin.

The amino acid structure of kinins is schematically illustrated below (synonyms are given in brackets):

*Bradykinin*

(kallidin I, kallidin-9, kinin-9, nonapeptide)

N-terminal Arg$^1$-Pro$^2$-Pro$^3$-Gly$^4$-Phe$^5$-Ser$^6$-Pro$^7$-Phe$^8$-Arg$^9$ C-terminal

*Kallidin*

(kallidin II, lysil-bradykinin, kinin-10, decapeptide)

Lys$^1$-Arg$^2$-Pro$^3$-Pro$^4$-Gly$^5$-Phe$^6$-Ser$^7$-Pro$^8$-Phe$^9$-Arg$^{10}$

*Methionyl-lysil-bradykinin*

(methionylkallidin, kinin-11, undecapeptide, hendecapeptide)

Met$^1$-Lys$^2$-Arg$^3$-Pro$^4$-Pro$^5$-Gly$^6$-Phe$^7$-Ser$^8$-Pro$^9$-Phe$^{10}$-Arg$^{11}$

*Phylokinin** (Erspamer and Anastasi) [52]

Arg$^1$-Pro$^2$-Pro$^3$-Gly$^4$-Phe$^5$-Ser$^6$-Pro$^7$-Phe$^8$-Arg$^9$-Ileu$^{10}$-Tyr$^{11}$ $HSO_3$

*Eledoisin*** (Erspamer) [51*c*]

Met$^1$-Leu$^2$-Gly$^3$-Ileu$^4$-Phe$^5$-Ala$^6$-Asp$^7$-Lys$^8$-Ser$^9$-Pro$^{10}$-Pyr$^{11}$

*Physalaemin** (Erspamer and Anastasi) [52]

Met$^1$-Leu$^2$-Gly$^3$-Tyr$^4$-Phe$^5$-Lys$^6$-Asp$^7$-($NH_2$)-Pro$^8$-Asp$^9$-Ala$^{10}$-Pyr$^{11}$

Kinins derive from $\alpha_2$-globulin of the mammalian plasma. This precursor substance is termed kininogen, kallidinogen or prokinin. Kininogen is a glycoprotein that has been prepared from human plasma in three structural varieties. Several proteolytic enzymes are known (kallikrein, trypsin, plasmin) which can split kinins from kininogens. Kallikreins, the most important kininogenases, have been isolated from urine, pancreas and plasma. From heat-acid-denatured horse plasma, plasmin released mainly methionyl-lysilbradykinin and small amounts of bradykinin and kallidin. Plasma kallikrein released only bradykinin from this substrate. Trypsin released mainly bradykinin and kallidin [62]. Angiotensin and eledoisin have independent receptor sites in the wall of the aorta and pulmonary artery of the rabbit. The contracting effect of tested kinins has another mechanism than the contractions produced by noradrenalin [135].

* Phylokinin and physalaemin were prepared from the skin of a South American frog species.

** Eledoisin was prepared from the salivary gland of molluscs.

There are several excellent monographs dealing with kinins [50, 99*a*, 164] a detailed discussion of which would exceed the scope of this chapter.

The function of kinins is still inadequately known but there are observations to show that polypeptides of the bradykinin type may be involved in various pathological processes such as pancreatitis, toxaemia caused by burns, asthma, pulmonary oedema, gout, rheumatoid arthritis, osteo-arthritis, foreign body granuloma, hereditary angioneurotic oedema, carcinoid syndrome, certain transfusion reactions, pain caused by wasp bite, etc. [40, 99*b*].

Bradykinin-like activity in systemic anaphylaxis and in the peptone shock of dogs was first observed by Beraldo [12]. The plasma kinins appear to qualify from a pharmacodynamic point of view for perpetuating the hypotension during the later phase in canine anaphylaxis, when blood histamine levels have returned to near normal [180]. The presence of considerable amounts of plasma kinin during anaphylactic shock was subsequently found in the blood of sensitized guinea pigs, rats and rabbits [17]. The concentration of bradykininogen is markedly reduced in the plasma of rabbits during anaphylactic shock [39, 104] but not in the plasma of anaphylactic dogs and guinea pigs [25]. Perfusion of sensitized guinea pig lung with antigen is immediately followed by the appearance of kallikrein in the perfusate [89]. ε-aminocaproic acid, an inhibitor of trypsin-like enzymes which participate in the production of plasma kinin, notably counteracts the development of anaphylaxis in mice [184]. The effect of body temperature and some mediator antagonists on anaphylactic shock in mice showed that kinins play a significant role in anaphylaxis in mice, and that 5-HT also participates in the development of the shock syndrome [31]. Cellulose sulphate, while diminishing the plasma level of bradykininogen by some 80 per cent, inhibits also PCA. It reduces moreover the rate at which bradykinin is released by the plasma *in vitro* under the effect of the antigen–antibody complex [149]. Cellulose sulphate influences the level of bradykininogen without activating the anaphylatoxin system. Not only histamine and SRSA, but also bradykinin has been observed to be released in the anaphylactic shock of mice, while the level of bradykinogen became 30 per cent lower in the plasma during the first minutes following the reinjection of antigen [107]. Bradykinin is the principal mediator in the anaphylactic shock of rats, too [36]. It is interesting to note that the sensitivity of rats to exogenous proteases (trypsin, pronase) was not influenced by BPV treatment. Acid protease activity of serum was increased during active and heterologous passive anaphylactic shock. The neutral protease levels were markedly elevated only in BPV pretreated rats undergoing severe, active anaphylactic shock. The elevated serum levels of these enzymes indicate lysosomal damage during anaphylaxis [30].

Kinins are presumably involved also in the pathogenesis of bronchial asthma. If intravenously administered to non-sensitized guinea pigs, bradykinin gives rise to marked bronchoconstriction [27], which could be prevented by acetylsalicylic acid and epinephrine. Administered to asthmatic patients in the form of aerosol, bradykinin has been found to reduce vital capacity, to produce bronchiospasm and dyspnoea, while similar doses had no effect on non-asthmatic individuals [80]. The presence of kinins has been demonstrated in skin perfusates after provocation with the sensitizing allergen [115]. The concentration of kinins rose tenfold in the blood of patients during acute asthmatic attack [1].

The foregoing data justified the conclusion that kinins are among the pathogenic factors of allergic and anaphylactic reactions. The human skin and lung contain much protease; since the capillaries are damaged by allergic reactions and thus plasma proteins (including $\alpha_2$-globulins) may gain access to the cells thus furnishing the substrate for bradykinin formation which is also facilitated by the proteolytic activity increased by antigen–antibody reaction. Of course, this theory has still to be verified by further experiments.

Antigen–antibody reaction inducing intensified proteolysis, leads to the formation of secondary endogenous stimulants, the so-called permeability factors (PF). There are two kinds of PF in the human plasma [92]: one of them, moving with the $\gamma$-globulins, resembles kallikrein, the other resembles $\beta$-globulin. Human serum kallikrein and PF are, however, clearly distinguishable on the basis of their electrophoretic motility, chromatographic features, ultracentrifugal sedimentation and kinin liberation [91]. Menkin [114] described a number of substances and termed them in accordance with their most characteristic properties as leukotaxin, necrosin, pyrexin, etc. (leukotaxin increases capillary permeability like $\alpha$- and $\beta$-globulin of plasma). Although attempts to demonstrate any function of these endogenous substances in antigen–antibody reaction have been unsuccessful, it is nevertheless probable that they affect the clinical manifestation of allergic reactions.

## THE ROLE OF MAST CELLS IN ANTIGEN-ANTIBODY REACTION

It was Ehrlich [44*a*, *b*] who first described the morphological features and staining properties of mast cells about a hundred years ago. He affirmed that these cells were found in the connective tissues and contained metachromatic granules. The nature of these granules and the function of mast cells remained long obscure until Jorpes et al. [90] demonstrated that mast cells contain heparin. This discovery was believed to explain the function of mast cells. Since they abound around the vessels, their function seemed to be the synthesis of heparin for the prevention of intravascular blood clotting. Accordingly, they were also called heparinocytes. Riley and West [143*a*, *b*] stated that mast cells contained not only heparin but histamine as well and the tissues containing many mast cells abounded also in histamine. Graham et al. [71, 72] demonstrated the presence of histamine in the basophils of the blood. It was then proved by Ehrich [43] that the basophils of the blood and the mast cells of the tissues have the same function. His experiments revealed a strict parallelism between the number of basophils circulating in the blood of man, cat, guinea pig and rabbit on the one hand, and the histamine concentration in the blood on the other. Basophil leukocytes from the bone marrow of sensitized guinea pigs liberated their histamine on incubation *in vitro* with the specific antigen at 37 °C, pH 7.8 and in the presence of $Ca^{++}$ ions [161]. No such correlation seems to exist in respect of eosinophils and neutrophils.

Also other substances than heparin and histamine have been described as the normal constituents of mast cells. There are reports [6*a*] to show that a striking parallelism exists in various healthy and morbid tissues between the mast cell count and the amount of hyaluronic acid. Mast cells secrete hyaluronic acid, a precursor of heparin under hormonal control. The mast cells of the rat were found to contain moreover 5-HT [11], further histidine decarboxylase [153], a chymotrypsin-like enzyme [9] and 5-HTP decarboxylase [103]. A chymotrypsin-like protease has been found in rat mast cells which resembles pancreatic chymotrypsin bound to heparin [94]. Recently unsaturated fatty acids, phosphatide cholines, SRS and also enzymes resembling phosphatidase A and chymotrypsin have been described in the mast cells of cats, guinea pigs and rats [5].

The binding of metals has also been described among the functions of mast cells. They are, according to this concept, involved in calciphylaxis, calcergy and the local fixation of haematogenic particles (iron, lead, carbon) including also microbes, toxins, pigments and malignant cells [155].

There are several excellent monographs available on the morphology, physiology and pathology, constituents, etc. of the mast cells [10, 34, 98*d*, 142, 150, 155, 178*a*].

Large numbers of mast cells are present in the subcutaneous connective tissue, the pleura, mesentery, scrotum and uterus of mammals. Besides, they are found in the loose connective tissues around the minor vessels of homoiotherms while being practically absent from the central nervous system. Parenchymatous organs contain, as a rule, few mast cells (except for the liver of dogs and the lung of cats and bovines), whereas the capsule of such organs abounds in mast cells. There are few mast cells in the tissues of rabbits but many basophils in their blood. Certain tissues (e.g. those of the gastrointestinal tract, the gastric mucosa, the epidermis) contain much histamine but comparatively few mast cells. Mobilizable histamine is stored in the mast cells. It is supposed that intracellular histamine is not chemically bound but is contained in a diffusible form in the mitochondrial fraction, wherefrom it is released due to some lytic effect connected with the damage of the membranes of granules, or to the disintegration of intracellular granules. While histamine releasing organic compounds act both on the intracellular particles and on intact mast cells, antigen releases the histamine of intracellular granules only in sensitized tissues with unimpaired cellular structure.

Fragmentation of mast cells, caused by peptone, and the resulting release of heparin have been proposed to explain the alteration of these cells in the anaphylactic shock of humans and several animal species as well as the prolongation of clotting time in peptone shock [82, 179].

Heparin is released together with histamine in the liver of dogs during anaphylactic and peptone shock and both substances are supposed to originate from the same cell [121, 147]. The liver mast cell count is decreased simultaneously. Injection of antigen into sensitized animals after the administration of chemical histamine liberators (48/80; D-tubocurarine) does not elicit anaphylactic shock. If, on the other hand, antigen is reinjected some 15 to 17 days after the administration of 48/80, anaphylactic shock will result and there will be intensive histamine release. It follows that the regeneration of degranulated mast cells takes 2 to 3 weeks. This permits the assumption that mast cells store not only histamine, but also antibodies (on their surface).

Although the symptoms of anaphylactic shock vary in the different species, it is common that the mast cells release pharmacologically active substances which produce the shock syndrome. The alterations of mast cells in anaphylaxis has been studied most frequently in the guinea pig and the rat.

The guinea pig lung contains numerous mast cells in the walls of alveoli, around the bronchioles and in the pleura [122]. In anaphylactic shock, they become disintegrated, lose their metachromatic granules and are reduced in number. The amount of histamine in the lung decreases at the same time. Antihistamines are unable to prevent the damage of mast cells. The bulk of histamine released in anaphylaxis in the guinea pig originates from mast cells which, in addition to storing histamine, also fix antibodies on their surface [118*c*]. If the nasal mucosa of sensitized guinea pigs is treated with increasing doses of antigen, discharge of mast cells and the increase in the intensity of shock symptoms proceed at the same rate [13].

Each mast cell of the various guinea pig tissues (aorta, trachea, uterus, jejunum) contains 21–34 picogram (pg $= 10^{-12}$ g) histamine [14*b*], of which 12 to 16 picogram is liberated at the 'disappearance' of the cell. The quantity of histamine contained in the mast cell is approximately the same irrespective of species and tissue [142]. Only mast cell tumours are exceptions in this respect: their mastocytes contain 1,290 picograms of histamine [20].

Notwithstanding the above data, anaphylactic shock is more than the damage of mast cells. Forssman's antibody produces lethal anaphylaxis in guinea pigs without damaging the mast cells or liberating histamine. Mast cells are impaired only if it is on their surface that the antigen reacts with the reversibly adsorbed antibody [85]. Lethal doses of the antigen–antibody complex produce in the guinea pig neither mast cell damage nor histamine release [118*b*].

In rats both mast cell damage and histamine release have been observed in anaphylactic shock [98*a*]. *In vitro* reaction of the peritoneal mast cells of sensitized rats with homologous antigen damages these cells in a characteristic way. 48/80 and antigen–antibody reaction have the same effect on the mesenteric mast cells of the rat, namely swelling, disintegration and disruption [83]. The release of histamine, heparin and granule protein from rat mast cells treated with compound 48/80 *in vitro* showed that the ratio of heparin to granule protein was similar in discharged granules and granules remaining in the cell after compound 48/80 treatment. The principal mechanism of histamine release induced by 48/80 involves an initial discharge of histamine containing granules, followed by an exchange of histamine in the granules for cations in the extracellular medium [55]. Beside histamine presumably also 5-HT is released due to the antigen–antibody reaction, irrespective of the role played by the two amines in rat anaphylaxis [159]. Isolated peritoneal mast cells of rats sensitized with horse serum and BPV retain their reactivity with the specific antigen even after repeated washings. This is possible only if antibodies are absorbed onto the mast cells and if the antigen–antibody reaction takes place on the cell surface [119]. Employing ferritin antigen it was possible to demonstrate by electron micrographs that in PCA, elicited 24 to 72 h after sensitization, the ferritin accumulated exclusively on the surface of mast cells [123]. Certain investigators suggested that antibodies were formed within the mast cells [70] because reinjection of the antigen still produced mild anaphylactic shock after depleting the sensitized mast cells with 48/80 or polymyxin. However, based on a critical review of the literature dealing with mast cells, Keller [98*c*] reached the conclusion that mast cells are damaged in anaphylaxis because antigen–antibody reaction occurs on their surface. The reaction depends on temperature, pH, ionic strength and requires the presence of complement.

Rat mast cells undergo ultrastructural change in the course of anaphylactic histamine release; the centrally placed granules become swollen, while the peripheral granules become smaller and their electron density increases [21]. Detection of human IgE antibody as an agent of producing rat mast cell degranulation was possible if rat mast cells were passively sensitized with the rye grass pollen sensitive subject's serum and challenged with a monospecific rabbit antimyeloma IgE antiserum [102]. IgGa antibodies, in contrast to IgE antibodies, mediated the antigen induced release of histamine from rat peritoneal mast cells without a latent period and without binding firmly to target cells, while in IgE-mediated reactions two steps could be distinguished: preparation of target cells with antibody and challenge with antigen [7*a*, *b*].

The mast cells of mice also contain histamine, heparin and 5-HT [143*c*]. However, only by prolonged treatment (31 days) with 48/80 is it possible to drain the histamine content of the tissues, and even then to 50 per cent only, whereas in the rat a treatment of short duration suffices to reduce the amount of histamine considerably. The number of mast cells, their production and morphological alterations, have nothing to do with anaphylactic phenomena [45, 166]. It is more or less generally agreed upon that in mouse anaphylaxis 5-HT and histamine are not released by the mast cells but emerge from other sources, nor does it seem probable that only these two amines function as mediator substances. Anyway, mast cells are not important factors in the allergic reactions in the mouse. In immediate hypersensitivity electron-microscopic alterations (swelling without vacuolation; rupture of the perigranular membrane; loss of electron density; aggregation of individual granules) have nevertheless been observed in the mast cells of mice, which are different from those induced by 48/80 [127]. Histamine is thought to be released from the mast cells of mice only when there are reagin-type antibodies present [136*a*]. *In vitro* immune damage of mouse peritoneal mast cells and release of histamine were produced by the addition of antimouse serum or antimouse rabbit $\gamma$-globulin at 37 °C which does not depend upon complement action [136*b*]. The antigen–antibody ratio is regarded to be important in passive sensitization of the mast cells as well as for histamine release. The antibodies are not adsorbed to mast cells until after the antigen–antibody reaction has run its course [126].

No decay of the mast cells in the skin of cats has been observed during anaphylactic shock [178*b*].

As regards humans, the bronchial connective tissue of patients suffering from bronchial asthma contains less mast cells and they are more degranulated than those in healthy individuals [151*a*, *b*]. The degree of mast cell impairment shows a direct relation with the severity of asthma. It is probable that in cases of bronchial asthma histamine is released by the mast cells of the bronchial connective tissue. Antihistamines have no effect on degranulation ensuing upon 48/80 treatment, on the decrease in mast cell count or on the process of histamine release, but neutralize the effect of already released and circulating histamine in the tissue receptors [151*c*].

Basophilic leukocytes undergo degranulation in patients suffering from penicillin and drug allergy as also in rabbits sensitized with various antigens if allergen finds repeated access to, or antigen is reinjected into, the organism. Shelley [156] coined the term 'indirect basophil degranulation test' for this phenomenon which is suitable for the detection of circulating antibodies in any kind of allergic disease.

Although the function of mast cells has not been clarified so far, they undoubtedly contribute to anaphylactic manifestations. Mast cells, similarly to other kinds of cells, undergo damage due to the antigen–antibody reaction because they fix antibodies, and this leads to the release of various intracellular mediator substances and enzymes.

## REFERENCES


1. Abe, K., Wattanabe, N., Kumagai, N., Mouri, T., Seki, T. and Josinaga, K.: *Experientia (Basel)* **23,** 626 (1967).
2. Abeolus, J. E. and Bardier, E.: *C. R. Soc. Biol. (Paris)* **66,** 511 (1909).
3. Akcasu, A. and West, G. B.: *Int. Arch. Allergy* **16,** 326 (1960).
4. Alexander, F., Eyre, P., Head, K. W. and Sanford, J.: *J. comp. Path.* **80,** 19 (1970).
5. Anggard, E., Berquist, U., Högberg, B., Johansson, R., Thon, I. L. and Uvnäs, B.: *Acta physiol. scand.* **59,** 97 (1963).

6*a*. Asboe-Hansen, G.: *Int. Rev. Cytol.* **33,** 399 (1954).

6*b*. id., *Amer. J. Med.* **26,** 470 (1959).

7*a*. Bach, M. K., Bloch, K. J. and Austen, K. F.: *J. exp. Med.* **133,** 752 (1971).

7*b*. ibid., **133,** 772 (1971).

8. Ballestero, L. H. and Zmud, B. S.: *Prensa méd. arg.* **48,** 89 (1961).
9. Benditt, E. P.: *Fed. Proc.* **15,** 507 (1956).
10. Benditt, E. P. and Lagunoff, D.: *Progr. Allergy* **8,** 195 (1964).
11. Benditt, E. P., Wong, R. L., Arose, M. and Roeper, E.: *Proc. Soc. exp. Biol. (N.Y.)* **90,** 303 (1955).
12. Beraldo, W. T.: *Amer. J. Physiol.* **163,** 283 (1950).
13. Boreus, L. O.: *Acta physiol. scand.* **48,** 431 (1960).

14*a*. Boreus, L. O. and Chakravarty, N.: *Acta physiol. scand.* **48,** 315 (1960).

14*b*. id., In *Experientia (Basel)* **16,** 192 (1960).

15*a*. Brocklehurst, W. E.: *J. Physiol. (Lond.)* **120,** 16 (1953).

15*b*. id., *Proc. III. Internat. Congr. Allerg.* Paris-Flammarion, 1958, p. 361.

15*c*. id., In *5-Hydroxytryptamine.* Ed. by Lewis, G. P. Pergamon Press, New York 1958, p. 172.

15*d*. id., *J. Physiol. (Lond.)* **151,** 416 (1960).

15*e*. id., *Progr. Allergy* **6,** 539 (1962).

16. Brocklehurst, W. E., Humphrey, J. H. and Perry, W. L. M.: *J. Physiol. (Lond).* **150,** 485 (1960).
17. Brocklehurst, W. E. and Lahiri, S. C.: *J. Physiol. (Lond.)* **160,** 15 (1962).
18. Brodie, T. G.: *J. Physiol. (Lond.)* **26,** 48 (1900).
19. Bulle, P. H.: *Fed. Proc.* **18,** 1472 (1958).
20. Cass, R., Riley, J. F., West, G. B., Head, K. W. and Stroul, W. W.: *Nature* **174,** 318 (1954).
21. Chakravarty, N., Gusefson, G. T. and Pihl, E.: *Acta path. microbiol. scand.* **71,** 233 (1967).
22. Christensson, B. and Ekwall, B.: *Acta allerg. (Kbh.)* **15,** 425 (1960).
23. Cirstea, M.: *J. Physiol. (Paris)* **52,** 847 (1960).
24. Cirstea, M., Niculescu, V., Rusovici, L. and Suhaciu, G.: *Int. Arch. Allergy* **32,** 105 (1967).
25. Cirstea, M., Suhaciu, G. and Butulescu, J.: *Arch. Int. Physiol.* **73,** 231 (1965).
26. Cohen, S. G. and Sapp, T. M.: *J. Allergy* **31,** 248 (1960).
27. Collier, H. O. J.: In *International Symposium on Hypotensive Peptides, Florence, 1965.* Ed. by Erdős, E. G., Back, N., Sicuteri, F. and Wilde, A. F. Springer, New York 1966, p. 305.
28. Csaba, B.: The role of histamine and 5-hydroxytryptamine in experimental anaphylaxis. Thesis. Debrecen 1965.

29. Csaba, B., Kassay, L. and Gomba, Sz.: *Kísérl. Orvostud.* **18,** 35 (1966).
30. Csaba, B. and Muszbek, L.: *Acta allerg. (Kbh.)* **27,** 55 (1972).
31. Csaba, B. and Tóth, S.: *Int. Arch. Allergy* **40,** 316 (1971).
32*a*. Csaba, B. and Went, M.: *Acta physiol. Acad. Sci. hung.* **39,** 369 (1971).
32*b*. id., *Int. Arch. Allergy* **43,** 25 (1972).
33. Csaba, B. and West, G. B.: *Int. Arch. Allergy* **33,** 99 (1968).
34. Csaba, G.: Data to the regulation of mast cell formation. Thesis. Budapest 1968.
35*a*. Danielopolu, D.: *Rev. Immunol.* **11,** 382 (1947).
35*b*. id., *Schweiz. med. Wschr.* **78,** 567 (1948).
36. Dawson, W., Starr, M. S. and West, G. B.: *Brit. J. Pharmacol.* **27,** 249 (1966).
37. Derkakh, V. V.: *Sborn. Nauk Rab. Khar'kov Med. Inst.* **79,** 130 (1969).
38. Dews, P. B. and Code, C. F.: *J. Immunol.* **70,** 199 (1953).
39. Diniz, C. R. and Carvalho, I. F.: *Ann. N. Y. Acad. Sci.* **104,** 77 (1963).
40. Dolovich, J., Back, N. and Arbesman, C. E. *J. Allergy* **41,** 103 (1968).
41. Donaldson, R. M., jr., Malkiel, S. and Gray, S. J.: *Proc. Soc. Exp. Biol. (N.Y.)* **103,** 261 (1960).
42. Douglas, W. W. and Toh, C. C.: *J. Physiol.* (*Lond.*) **120,** 311 (1953).
43. Ehrich, W. E.: *Science* **118,** 603 (1953).
44*a*. Ehrlich, P.: *Arch. mikr. Anat.* **13,** 263 (1877).
44*b*. id., *Arch. Anat. Physiol. (Lpz.)* **3,** 166 (1879).
45. Einbinder, J. M., Walzer, R. A. and Nelson, C. T.: *J. Immunol.* **93,** 165 (1964).
46. Elliot, D. F., Horton, E. W. and Lewis, G. P.: *J. Physiol. (Lond.)* **153,** 473 (1960).
47. Engelhardt, G.: *Naunyn-Schmiedberg's Arch. exp. Path. Pharmak.* **238,** 99 (1960).
48. Engelhardt, G. and Roser, F.: *Naunyn-Schmiedberg's Arch. exp. Path. Pharmak.* **230,** 90 (1957).
49. Engelhardt, G. and Schwabe, U.: *Naunyn-Schmiedeberg's Arch. exp. Path. Pharmak.* **239,** 170 (1960).
50. Erdős, E. G.: *Advanc. Pharmacol.* **4,** 1 (1966).
51*a*. Erspamer, V.: *Arzneimittel-Forsch.* **2,** 253 (1952).
51*b*. id., *Pharmacol. Rev.* **6,** 425 (1954).
51*c*. id., *Arzneimittel-Forsch.* **3,** 151 (1961).
52. Erspamer, V. and Anastasi, A.: In *International Symposium on Hypotensive Peptides. Florence, 1965.* Ed. by Erdős, E. G., Back, N., Sicuteri, F. and Wilde, A. F. Springer, New York 1966.
53. Erspamer, V. and Asero, B.: *Nature* **169,** 800 (1952).
54. Feldberg, W. and Kellaway, C. H.: *J. Physiol. (Lond.)* **94,** 187 (1938).
55. Fillion, G. M. B., Slorach, S. A. and Üvnas, B.: *Acta physiol. scand.* **78,** 547 (1970).
56. Fink, M. A.: *Proc. Soc. exp. Biol. (N.Y.)* **92,** 673 (1956).
57. Fink, M. A. and Gardner, C. E.: *Proc. Soc. exp. Biol. (N.Y.)* **97,** 554 (1958).
58. Flaschman, D. H.: *J. infect. Dis.* **38,** 461 (1926).
59. Frey, E. K.: *Arch. klin. Chir.* **142,** 663 (1926).
60. Frey, E. K., Kraut, H. and Schultz, F.: *Naunyn-Schmiedeberg's Arch. exp. Path. Pharmak.* **158,** 334 (1930).
61. Frey, E. K. and Werle, E.: *Klin. Wschr.* **12,** 600 (1933).
62. Gapantuk, E. and Henriques, O. B.: *Biochem. Pharmacol.* **19,** 2091 (1970).
63. Garattini, S. and Valzelli, L.: *Serotonin.* Elsevier Publishing Co., Amsterdam, London, New York 1965.
64*a*. Garcia-Arocha, H.: *Canad. J. Biochem. Physiol.* **39,** 403 (1961).
64*b*. id., *Proc. int. Union. Physiol. Sci.* **2,** Abstr. 596 (1962).
65. Geiger, W. B. and Alpers, H. S.: *J. Allergy* **30,** 316 (1959).
66. Gerendás, M., Csefkó, J. and Udvardy, M. D. F.: *Nature* **162,** 257 (1948).
67. Gershon, M. D. and Ross, L. L.: *J. exp. Med.* **15,** 367 (1962).
68. Giertz, H., Hahn, F., Krull, P. and Albert, U.: *Int. Arch. Allergy* **33,** 306 (1968).
69. Girard, J. P.: *Helv. med. Acta.* **28,** 476 (1961).
70. Gözsy, B. and Kátó, L.: *Int. Arch. Allergy* **21,** 138 (1962).
71. Graham, H. T., Lowry, O. H., Wahl, N. and Priebet, M. K.: *J. exp. Med.* **102,** 307 (1955).
72. Graham, H. T., Wheelwright, F., Parish, H. H., Marks, A. R. and Lowry, O. H.: *Fed. Proc.* **11,** 350 (1952).

73. Habib, J. A., Belal, A., El Garem, A., El Lozy, M., Hafisa, M., El Banna and Toporsada, H.: *Acta allerg. (Kbh.)* **26,** 39 (1971).
74. Hajós, M. K.: *Acta allerg. (Kbh.)* **17,** 358 (1962).
75. Halpern, B.-N., Liacopoulos-Briot, M., Spicak, V., Nevau, T., Perramant, M. F. and Branellec, A.: *Arch. int. Pharmacodyn.* **147,** 431 (1964).
76. Halpern, B. N., Neveu, T. and Spector, S.: *Brit. J. Pharmacol.* **20,** 389 (1963).
77. Hamlin, K. E. and Fischer, F. E.: *J. Amer. chem. Soc.* **73,** 5007 (1951).
78. *Handbook of Experimental Pharmacology*. Ed. by Erspamer, V. Vol. 19. Springer, Berlin–Heidelberg–New York 1966.
79. Herxheimer, A. and Schachter, M.: *J. Physiol. (Lond.)* **145,** 34 (1959).
80. Herxheimer, A. and Stresemann, E.: *J. Physiol. (Lond.)* **158,** 38 (1961).
81. Herxheimer, A.: *J. Physiol. (Lond.)* **128,** 435 (1955).
82. Holmgren, H. and Wilander, O.: *Z. mikr-anat. Forsch.* **42,** 242 (1937).
83. Högberg, B. and Uvnäs, B.: *Acta physiol. scand.* **48,** 133 (1960).
84*a*. Humphrey, J. H. and Jaques, R.: *J. Physiol. (Lond.)* **124,** 305 (1954).
84*b*. ibid., **128,** 9 (1955).
85. Humphrey, J. H. and Mota, I.: *Immunology* **2,** 31 (1959).
86. Inoue, T. and Kuriaki, K.: *C. R. Soc. Biol. (Paris)* **151,** 1470 (1957).
87. Johansson, S. A.: *Acta physiol. scand.* **50,** 95 (1960).
88. Johansson, S. A.: *Opuscula med.* **5,** 112 (1960).
89. Jonasson, O. and Becker, E. L.: *J. exp. Med.* **123,** 509 (1966).
90. Jorpes, J. E., Holmgren, H. and Wilander, O.: *Z. mikr.-anat. Forsch.* **42,** 279 (1937).
91. Kagen, L. J.: *Brit. J. exp. Path.* **45,** 604 (1964).
92. Kagen, L. J., Leddy, J. P. and Becker, E. L.: *J. clin. Invest.* **42,** 1353 (1963).
93. Kato, R., Mariani, L. and Valzelli, L.: *Atti Soc. lombarda. Sci. med.-biol.* **13,** 297 (1958).
94. Kawiak, J., Vensel, W. H., Komender, J., and Barnard, E. A.: *Biochim. biophys. Acta (Amst.)* **235,** 172 (1971).
95. Kay, A. B., Stechschulte, D. J. and Austen, F.: *J. exp. Med.* **133,** 602 (1971).
96. Kellaway, C. H.: *Brit. J. exp. Path.* **11,** 72 (1930).
97. Kellaway, C. H. and Trethewie, E. R.: *Quart. J. exp. Physiol.* **30,** 121 (1940).
98*a*. Keller, R.: *Int. Arch. Allergy* **11,** 328 (1957).
98*b*. id., *Arzneimittel-Forsch.* **8,** 390 (1958).
98*c*. id., *Experientia (Basel)* **18,** 286 (1962).
98*d*. id., *Tissue Mast Cells in Immune Reactions*. Karger, Basel 1966.
99*a*. Kellermeyer, R. W. and Richard, C. G.: *New Engl. J. Med.* **279,** 802 (1968).
99*b*. ibid., **754,** 859 (1968).
100. Kind, L. S.: *Bact. Rev.* **22,** 173 (1958).
101. Koopman, W. J., Orange, R. P. and Austen, K. F.: *Proc. Soc. exp. Biol. (N.Y.)* **137,** 64 (1971).
102. Korotzer, J. L., Haddad, Z. H. and Lopada, A. F.: *Immunology* **20,** 545 (1971).
103. Lagunoff, D., Lam, K. B., Roeper, E. and Benditt, E. P.: *Fed. Proc.* **16,** 363 (1957).
104. Lecomte, J.: *C. R. Soc. Biol. (Paris)* **155,** 1411 (1961).
105*a*. Lecomte, J. and Fischer, P.: *C. R. Soc. Biol. (Paris)* **151,** 1279 (1957).
105*b*. id., *Arch. int. Physiol. Biochem.* **66,** 50 (1958).
106. Lecomte, J. and Hughes, J.: *Arch. Allergy* **5,** 367 (1954).
107. Lima, A. O.: *Int. Arch. Allergy* **32,** 46 (1967).
108. Lipton, M. M., Stone, S. H. and Freund, J.: *J. Immunol.* **77,** 453 (1956).
109. Lissák, K. and Went, S.: *Naunyn-Schmiedeberg's Arch. exp. Path. Pharmak.* **180,** 466 (1936).
110. Malkiel, S. and Hargis, B. J.: *J. Allergy* **31,** 513 (1960).
111. Marcelle, R. and Lecomte, J.: *C. R. Soc. Biol. (Paris)* **153,** 1889 (1959).
112. McLean, J.: *Amer. J. Physiol.* **41,** 250 (1916).
113. Medakovic, M.: *Acta med. iugoslav.* **12,** 293 (1958).
114. Menkin, V.: *Science* **123,** 527 (1956).
115. Michel, B., Russel, T., Winkelmann, R. K. and Gleich, G. J.: *J. clin. Invest.* **47,** 68 (1968).
116. Molomut, N.: *J. Immunol.* **37,** 113 (1939).

117. Morse, H. C., Block, K. J. and Austen, K. F.: *J. Immunol.* **101,** 658 (1968).
118*a*. Mota, I.: *Brit. J. Pharmacol.* **12,** 453 (1957).
118*b*. id., *Nature* **191,** 572 (1961).
118*c*. id., *Int. Rev. Cytol.* **15,** 363 (1963).
119. Mota, I. and Dias da Silva, W.: *Nature (Lond.)* **186,** 245 (1960).
120. Mota, I., Ferri, A. G. and Junqueira, L. C. U.: *Acta halmat. (Lpz.)* **15,** 409 (1956).
121. Mota, I., Junqueira, L. C. W., Beraldo, W. T. and Ferri, A. G.: *Nature (Lond.)* **173,** 547 (1954).
122. Mota, I. and Vugman, I.: *Nature (Lond.)* **177,** 427 (1956).
123. Movat, H. Z., Lovett, C. A. and Taichman, N. S.: *Nature (Lond.)* **212,** 851 (1966).
124. Munoz, J.: *Proc. Soc. exp. Biol. (N.Y.)* **95,** 328 (1957).
125. Munoz, J., Rib. E. and Larson, C. L.: *J. Immunol.* **83,** 496 (1959).
126. Nelson, M., Vaz, N. M. and Ovary, Z.: *J. Immunol.* **100,** 1014 (1968).
127. Nelson, R. L., Katz, H. I. and Zelickson, A. S.: *Ann. Allergy* **26,** 281 (1968).
128. Niwa, M.: *J. Biochem. (Tokyo)* **51,** 222 (1962).
129. Orange, R. P., Stechschulte, D. J. and Austin, K. F.: *J. Immunol.* **105,** 1087 (1970).
130*a*. Orange, R. P., Valentine, M. D. and Austin, K. F.: *Science* **157,** 318 (1967).
130*b*. id., *Proc. Soc. exp. Biol. (N.Y.)* **127,** 127 (1968).
131*a*. Page, J. H.: *Physiol. Rev.* **34,** 563 (1954).
131*b*. ibid., **38,** 277 (1958).
132. Pallotta, A. J. and Ward, J. W.: *J. Pharmacol. exp. Ther.* **119,** 174 (1957).
133*a*. Parratt, J. R. and West, G. B.: *J. Physiol. (Lond.)* **137,** 169 (1957).
133*b*. id., *Int. Arch. Allergy* **16,** 288 (1960).
134. Petroff, J. R.: *Z. ges. exp. Med.* **44,** 641 (1925).
135. Popovic, J., Kovalak, V., Smyk, L. and Blaskova, I.: *Folia Fac. Med. Univ. Comenianae Bratislav* **6,** 205 (1968) (read 1970).
136*a*. Prouvost-Danon, A., Peixoto, J. M. and Javierre, M. Q.: *Immunology* **15,** 271 (1968).
136*b*. ibid., **18,** 749 (1970).
137. Rand, M. and Reid, G.: *Nature (Lond.)* **169,** 801 (1952).
138. Rapp, H. J.: *J. Physiol. (Lond.)* **158,** 35 (1961).
139. Rapport, M. M., Green, A. A. and Page, I. H.: *J. biol. Chem.* **176,** 1243 (1948).
140. Reid, G. and Rand, M.: *Aust. J. exp. Biol. med. Sci.* **29,** 401 (1951).
141. Resnick, E. H. and Gray, S. J.: *Gastroenterology* **41,** 119 (1961).
142. Riley, J. F.: *The Mast Cells.* Livingstone, Edinburgh, 1959.
143*a*. Riley, J. F. and West, G. B.: *J. Physiol. (Lond.)* **119,** 44 (1953).
143*b*. ibid., **120,** 528 (1953).
143*c*. id., *Arch. int. Pharmacodyn.* **102,** 304 (1955).
144. Rocha E Silva, M.: *Ann. N. Y. Acad. Sci.* **104,** 190 (1963).
145. Rocha E Silva, M. and Aronson, M.: *Brit. J. exp. Pathol.* **33,** 577 (1952).
146. Rocha E Silva, M., Beraldo, W. T. and Rosenfeld, G.: *Amer. J. Physiol.* **156,** 261 (1949).
147. Rocha E Silva, M., Scroogieg, A. E., Fidlar, E. and Jacques, L. B.: *Proc. Soc. exp. Biol. (N.Y.)* **64,** 141 (1947).
148. Rose, J. C.: *J. clin. Invest.* **36,** 924 (1957).
149. Rotschild, A. M.: In *Proceedings of the 3rd International Pharmacological Meeting.* Vol. 7. Ed. by Ariens, E. J. Pergamon Press, New York 1968.
150. Sagher, F. and Even-Paz, Z.: *Mastocytosis and the Mast Cell.* Karger, Basel–New York 1967.
151*a*. Salvato, G.: *Allergie u. Asthma* **6,** 23 (1960).
151*b*. id., *Int. Arch. Allergy* **18,** 348 (1961).
151*c*. id., *Acta allerg. (Kbh.)* **18,** 529 (1963).
152. Sanyal, R. K. and West, G. B.: *J. Physiol. (Lond.)* **144,** 525 (1958).
153. Schayer, R. W.: *Amer. J. Physiol.* **186,** 199 (1956).
154. Seegal, B. C. and Khorazo, D.: *Arch. Path.* **7,** 827 (1929).
155. Selye, H.: *The Mast Cells.* Butterworth, London 1965.
156. Shelley, W. B.: *J. Amer. med. Ass.* **184,** 171 (1963).
157*a*. Shibusawa, K., Tokuzawa, K., Kishi, S., Kajiya, Y., Kasuga, H. and Fujiwara, S.: *Gunma J. med. Sci. (Japan)* **7,** 91 (1958).

157*b*. ibid., **7**, 101 (1958).
158. Shore, P. A.: *Pharmacol. Rev.* **14,** 531 (1962).
159. Sjoerdsma, A., Waalkes, T. P. and Weissbach, H.: *Science* **125,** 1202 (1957).
160. Spencer, P. S. J. and West, G. B.: *Brit. J. Pharmacol.* **17,** 137 (1961).
161. Starr, M. S.: *Int. Arch. Allergy* **37,** 376 (1970).
162. Stechschulte, D. J., Austin, F. K. and Bloch, K. J.: *J. exp. Med.* **125,** 127 (1967).
163. Stevens, L. T. and Lee, F. S.: *Johns Hopk. Biol. Studies* **3,** 99 (1884).
164. *Structure and Function of Biologically Active Peptides: Bradykinin, Kallidin and Congeners.* Ed. by Erdős, E. G., Whipple, H. E. and Silverzweig, S. *Ann. N. Y. Acad. Sci.* **104,** 1–464 (1963).
165. Telford, J. M. and West, G. B.: *Int. Arch. Allergy* **23,** 29 (1963).
166. Tokuda, S. and Weiser, R. S.: *J. Immunol.* **86,** 292 (1961).
167. Udenfriend, S., Titus, E., Weissbach, H. and Peterson, R. E.: *J. biol. Chem.* **219,** 335 (1956).
168. Udenfriend, S. and Waalkes, T. P.: In *Mechanism of Hypersensitivity. Intern. Symposium.* Ed. by Safter, J. H., LoGrippo, G. A. and Chase, M. W. Little Brown, Boston, Massachussets 1959, pp. 219–226.
169. Uvnäs, B. and Thon, I. L.: *Exp. Cell Res.* **18,** 512 (1959).
170. Vogt, W.: *J. Physiol. (Lond.)* **136,** 131 (1956).
171*a*. Waalkes, T. P. and Coburn, H.: *J. Allergy* **30,** 394 (1959).
171*b*. ibid., **31,** 151 (1960).
172. Waalkes, T. P., Coburn, H. and Bethesda, A. B.: *J. Allergy* **31,** 395 (1960).
173. Waalkes, T. P., Weissbach, H., Bozicevich, J. and Udenfriend, S.: *J. clin. Invest.* **36,** 1115 (1957).
174. Weissbach, H., Waalkes, T. P. and Udenfriend, S.: *Science* **125,** 235 (1957).
175. Wenner, W. F. and Buhrmester, C. C.: *J. Allergy* **9,** 85 (1937).
176*a*. Went, S. and Lissák, K.: *Naunyn-Schmiedeberg's Arch. exp. Path. Pharmak.* **179,** 609 (1935).
176*b*. ibid., **179,** 616 (1935).
176*c*. ibid., **182,** 509 (1936).
177. Werle, E., Götze, W. and Keppler, A.: *Biochem. Z.* **289,** 217 (1937).
178*a*. West, G. B.: *J. Pharm. Pharmacol.* **11,** 513 (1959).
178*b*. id., *Lancet* **i,** 1332 (1964).
179. Wilander, O.: *Skand. Arch. Physiol.* **81,** Suppl. 15 (1938).
180. Wilkens, H. J. and Back, N.: *Arch. int. Pharmacodyn. Ther.* **190,** 14 (1971).
181. Wolf-Jurgensen, P. and Henningsen, S. T.: *Acta allerg. (Kbh.)* **25,** 48 (1970).
182. Wyman, L. C.: *Amer. J. Physiol.* **89,** 356 (1929).
183. Zilberstein, R. M.: *Nature* **185,** 249 (1960).
184. Zweifach, B. W., Nagler, A. L. and Troll, W.: *J. exp. Med.* **113,** 437 (1961).

CHAPTER 18

# SUPPRESSION OF IMMUNOPATHOLOGICAL EFFECTS

by

G. GY. PETRÁNYI



## POSSIBLE MODES OF SUPPRESSION OF IMMUNOPATHOLOGICAL EFFECTS

Therapeutic inhibition of the natural or pathological immune response is called immunosuppression. Before discussing the immunosuppressive interventions, it seems to be necessary to review the immunological processes which can be interfered with most efficiently.

1. Recognition of antigen and uptake of information with the participation of macrophages as well as T and B lymphocytes (see Chapter 8). The encounter and contact of lymphocyte receptors with antigen are the most important events of this stage. These may be influenced at the following points:

(*a*) Antigen-specific treatment [110]. (*i*) Antigen avoidance. This measure, when possible, is highly effective in reaginic allergy, contact sensitivity, and drug reactions. It requires precise identification of the antigen. (*ii*) Antigen administration. Desensitization is sometimes effective in atopic disease and in some forms of contact dermatitis. In view of the complexities of interactions between the different systems, the administration of antigen alone or combined with short courses of immunosuppressive treatment, is likely to be valuable. The dangers of exacerbation of symptoms must be considered. (*iii*) Antibody administration. The suppression of antibody response to foetal cells by antibody administered to mothers with rhesus-incompatible babies has been very effective. This approach is likely to be applied more widely and preliminary attempts have been made in certain transplant situations.

(*b*) Inhibition of the access of the antigen to immunological centres by surgical intervention, e.g. by transection of lymph vessels, removal of regional lymph nodes, etc.

(*c*) Inhibition of the antigen-seizing capacity of macrophages and of their participation in the processing of antigen (by RES blockade, anti-macrophage serum treatment, and selective destruction of macrophages by isotope-labelled antigen or silicon powder).

(*d*) At the level of antigen reactive cells and their receptors, immunosuppressive effects can be achieved in two ways: (*i*) general destruction (by cytotoxic drugs, irradiation or thymectomy) of all clones capable of giving immune response or selective elimination of the clone reacting with the antigen in question (induction of tolerance by repeated administration of small amounts of the antigen or by combination of this therapy with drug treatment); (*ii*) prevention of the contact of the receptors with the antigen by blocking the receptors. In this way, the cells become unsuitable for activation. Such a blockade can be achieved by treatment with anti-lymphocyte serum or with a specific activator, e.g. phytohaemagglutinin.

2. The immune response can be most efficiently inhibited at the stage when antigen-specific immune clones are developing, i.e. in the phase of proliferation. There are many agents inhibiting mitotic activity and DNA synthesis, e.g. X-ray irradiation, alkylating agents, antimetabolites and antimitotic cytostatic drugs.

3. Efferent branch of the immune reaction.

(*a*) Both the humoral and the cell-mediated immune responses can be inhibited by reducing the number and the activity (protein synthesis including immunoglobulin synthesis, metabolic activity) of the immunocytes participating in the reaction. Most of the lymphotoxic agents (X-ray, cytotoxic drugs, hormones) as well as some surgical interventions (splenectomy, drainage of the thoracic duct) act in this way.

(*b*) The cell-mediated immune response can be inhibited by attacking the effector cells in two ways, viz., by coating the antigen receptors (with anti-lymphocyte serum) or by blocking the foreign tissue antigens, which is one of the most promising immunosuppressive interventions and may be brought about by treatment with the 'protective' or 'enhancing' factor (antigen–antibody complex).

(*c*) Various other factors necessary in immune phenomena can also be eliminated, e.g. the C3 complement component, histamine or inflammatory agents can be blocked.

The great variety of processes which might be inhibited call for different surgical, chemotherapeutic, radiological and immunological methods of intervention.

The numerous attempts with combined drug treatment are difficult to survey and evaluate. In this chapter, therefore, the methods and drugs appearing to be of little importance are not mentioned. The great variety of possible immunosuppressive methods also indicate that none of the methods is perfect. In addition, each of the interventions has a number of side-effects in addition to its interference with the immune response.

## IMMUNOSUPPRESSIVE INTERVENTIONS

Of the methods of immunosuppression used with success under experimental conditions, only few can be applied in human therapy. As all of them have anti-inflammatory effects, any detectable therapeutic benefit is not necessarily achieved by immunosuppression [110]. The immunosuppressive action of such agents differs from species to species.

The efficiency of immunosuppressive interventions may be estimated on the basis of animal experiments and/or clinical testing. The experimental response to be suppressed is usually induced with bacterial antigens (e.g., *S. typhi*, other salmonellae, *E. coli*) serum albumin (human or bovine), haemocyanin, heterologous (human, sheep, duck) erythrocytes, peptides of low molecular weight or hapten–protein conjugates. The immune response induced by antigens can be followed by titrating the serum antibody or estimating the number of antibody forming cells in the spleen. The effects on the cell-mediated immune response can be estimated by following the delayed hypersensitivity reaction, by the skin grafting, by the graft-versus-host reaction and by transplanting various organs and tumours [44, 57, 80, 88]. Any drug needs to be tested in monkey and, as far as possible, in man. *In vitro* tests that correlate with the prevention of skin graft rejection include the rosette test, opsonization, mixed lymphocyte culture and lymphocytotoxic activity [110, 122*a*].

According to Makinodan et al. [57], none of the numerous tests may serve as a reliable yardstick for measuring the effect of an immunosuppressive intervention. This is because the manifestation of immunosuppressive effects is influenced by other factors, such as (*i*) species, age, sex, immunological status, possible disease of the experimental subject (animal or man); (*ii*) characteristics of specific immune processes that have occurred prior to the test (immunological history, primary or secondary immune response, etc.); (*iii*) mode of administration of the antigen and of its metabolization; (*iv*) qualitative and quantitative properties of the test antigen; (*v*) peculiarities and sensitivity of the test method.

## IMMUNOSUPPRESSION WITH DRUGS

In this chapter only unequivocally immunosuppressive drugs will be dealt with. The general properties (dose dependence, toxicity, specific and selective therapeutic effects, possibility of induction of tolerance, etc.) of the groups of drugs are discussed in a separate subchapter. The clinical application and the schemes of administration will be only briefly mentioned and the reader is referred to the second, clinical, volume of the present work.

### *Alkylating agents*

Alkylating agents, i.e. drugs showing a very strong affinity to nucleophilic groups of negative charge (phosphate, amino, SH amidazol, carboxyl, etc. groups) exert an injuring effect on DNA, and conglomerate proteins and amino acids [88*c*]. They injure all kinds of cells, to the greatest extent those with high DNA-synthesis and cell-division rates. Alkylating agents are most active in the premitotic phase G-2 [88*c*]. The most important representative of this group of agents is cyclophosphamide.

Cyclophosphamide (Endoxan), a mustard-derivative of relatively low toxicity, is capable of suppressing antibody production induced by either bacterial antigens or by sheep erythrocytes [81, 86, 94, 106]. It is almost equally effective if administered before or after immunization, yet, has the strongest effect if administered on the first or second day following the antigenic stimulus [85].

In mice, rats and rabbits, survival of allogenic grafts is substantially prolonged by Endoxan [8*d*, 97], but the drug has no effect on the cell-mediated immune response of guinea pigs [8*c*]. In graft-versus-host models, Endoxan prevents the secondary disease [8*f*, 54]. In skin grafting experiments carried out in the H-3 system, Nouza [72] found cyclophosphamide to be the most effective immunosuppressive drug, as effective as irradiation. The immunosuppressive effect of Endoxan is very specific: this drug has the highest therapeutic index and, if appropriately administered, it is even able to induce tolerance [85]. Recent studies indicated that the effect of cyclophosphamide on the B lymphocytes was more severe and long lasting than the effect on the T cell compartment [96*a*].

Numerous other alkylating agents (Melphalan, Myleran, chlorambucil, Leukeran, dimesyl-erythrite—R-74—and TEM) have been found immunosuppressive, but the effect of these drugs is less general: they affect only certain immune responses [8*d*, 48, 72, 76]. Some of these drugs have been applied with success in treating certain clinical syndromes, e.g. R-74 in myositis of autoimmune origin [79]. Side-effects of cyclophosphamide include dizziness, nausea, vomiting, alopecia. mucosal ulceration, hepatotoxicity, and skin pigmentation.

### *Antimetabolites*

Of the immunosuppressive agents, antimetabolites have received the greatest attention in recent years. There is a group of antimetabolites which, by inactivating or substituting enzymes responsible for different steps of purine and pyrimidine synthesis, inhibit DNA and RNA synthesis [8*d*, 44*b*, 88*c*].

6-mercaptopurine (purinethol, Leopurine) inhibits the synthesis of adenine and guanine from inosinic acid [8*d*, 88*c*]. The drug has been found immunosuppressive in many systems, but contradictory data have also been published. Post-immunization administration of 6-mercaptopurine in a single dose or in several doses substantially inhibits antibody response [85, 90, 106]. IgG production is inhibited most significantly [11]. On the other hand, pre-immunization administration of the same drug strongly stimulates antibody production [15, 106].

The effect of 6-mercaptopurine on cell-mediated immunity also seems to be variable. In some experiments [8*d*], the drug inhibited the skin-grafting reaction, whereas other experiments have led to negative results [8*d*, 54], or resulted in stimulation [72, 88*b*]. In spite of the inconsistent experimental results, 6-mercaptopurine has been reported to have an excellent effect in the treatment of diseases of allergic or autoimmune origin. Schwartz and Dameshek [89*b*] and Gyula Petrányi [78] were the first to introduce the drug with success in the therapy of autoimmune diseases of the haemopoietic system and in lupus nephritis respectively.

Nowadays, azathioprine (Imuran), the imidazol derivative of 6-mercaptopurine, is the best-known immunosuppressive drug. Its immunological effect is equal to that of 6-mercaptopurine, and its therapeutic index is even higher [30]. Due to its suppressive effect on cell-mediated immunity, Imuran is mainly used in organ transplantation, since it seems to have a selective action on T lymphocytes. Murray et al. [70], who carried out renal transplantation in a thousand dogs found Imuran preferable to 22 other drugs. Imuran is administered as a basal treatment in the clinical practice to prevent rejection crisis after renal and other organ transplantations as well as in the therapy of some autoimmune diseases [64, 69].

There are numerous further antimetabolites whose immunosuppressive effect is due to their inhibiting purine and pyrimidine synthesis. However, none of these exceed 6-mercaptopurine in effectivity. 5-fluorouracil, 5-bromouracil, 6-azauridine, 5-thioguanine as well as cytosine arabinoside, are the most important representatives of this group [8*d*, 38, 39, 41, 88*c*, 93]. The major side-effects of 6-mercaptopurine and azathiopurine include alopecia, anaemia, leukopenia, hepatic toxicity, pancreatitis, oesophagitis and stomatitis.

Amethopterin (Methotrexate) is an antimetabolite with a different mechanism of action. Being an inhibitor of the enzyme dehydrofolic acid reductase, it is an antagonist of folic acid, and thus interferes with thymidine synthesis [111]. Methotrexate inhibits antibody production, especially if administered on the second day following the antigenic stimulus [8*a*]. Also the tuberculin sensitivity of the mouse and the reaction of the guinea pig skin grafts were inhibited [8*b*, 82, 105]. Berenbaum [8*b*] has pointed out as an advantage of the drug that its toxic effects can be abolished by an immediate administration of folic acid without flaring up the transplantation reaction. The use of Methotrexate in renal transplantation experiments on dogs led to inconsistent results [42]. In the clinical practice, the drug is used in the prevention of the secondary disease following bone-marrow transplatation and in the therapy of some autoimmune diseases [44*a*, 60].

### *Antibiotics*

Among antibiotic drugs, actinomycin C and D, azaserine and mitomycin possess an immunosuppressive activity. These drugs, like alkylating agents and ionizing radiation, seem to injure the end-product of DNA synthesis [8*d*, 72, 97].

It is still unclear how actinomycin acts in animal experiments on antibody production (is it a selective inhibitor of DNA-dependent messenger-RNA synthesis?) [24]. There is no doubt that it inhibits the transplantation immune reaction [54, 72]. The teams led by Calne and co-workers [17] and Murray et al. [70] applied actinomycin C with success in controlling the rejection crisis after experimental renal transplantation and in preventing rejection. The major side-effects of this agent are bone marrow depression, nausea, vomiting, and stomatitis. Based on animal experiments, subtoxic doses of actinomycin D are administered, in combination with prednisolone, also to man in connection with renal transplantation [70, 92]. Azaserine (an inhibitor of nucleutide synthesis?) can also be administered mainly as the drug of basal treatment in the course of renal transplantations both for experimental animals and man [67]. The major side-effects of azaserine include delirium, coma, stomatitis and jaundice.

### *Alkaloids*

In this group of drugs, Vinblastine, Vincristine and the podophyllotoxin derivative Proresid (podophyllinic acid ethylhydrazide) deserve mention. All these drugs act by stopping mitosis in the metaphase. Vinblastine's inhibit effect on antibody production is mainly utilized in after-treatment [106]. Cell-mediated immune response can be inhibited only moderately [76]. Proresid has been proved to possess favourable immunosuppressive activity both in animal experiments and in the clinical practice [6, 99].

### *Hormones*

Corticosteroid derivatives are known to be anti-inflammatory and to induce a lympholytic effect, but their mode of action in prolonging allograft survival is very complex. High local concentration of cortisone may produce stabilization of cell and lysosomal membranes, and this inhibits target cell damage by attacking lymphocytes. It is interesting that in the thymus a corticosteroid sensitive peripheral lymphocyte population and a resistant one exist. Their use in allergic and autoimmune diseases as well as in connection with organ transplantations is dealt with in detail in another chapter of this book (Chapter 43 in Volume 2). The side-effects of prolonged corticosteroid therapy include severe pancreatitis, peptic ulceration, aseptic bone necrosis, hyperglycaemia, withdrawal arthritis, Cushingoid features, cataract formation, hypertension, acne, and demineralization of bone.

### *Biologically active substances*

There are numerous biologically active substances under study for immunosuppressive effect. The properties, effects and points of attack of these substances are variable, in some cases not quite clear. Concanavaline A is a pure protein prepared from *Canavalia ensiformis*. The drug which is known to agglutinate red cells and stimulate mitotic activity, substantially inhibits the development of delayed hypersensitivity. Its use has proved to be favourable in the course of skin transplantation tests [55, 59].

Of the tumoricidal substances described recently, L-asparaginase has been found to be immunosuppressive [18, 45, 88*d*]. The enzyme, the function of which is depletion of asparaginase and which was discovered in the serum of the guinea pig, inhibits lymphoma. In connection with their inhibitory effect on cell-mediated immunity, the antiserotonin drug cinaserine [2'(3-dimethylamino propylthiol)cinnemanilide] and the neuraminidase prepared from *Vibrio comma* deserve attention [2, 51].

The purified cobra venom contains a factor which inhibits the C3 and C9 components of the complement and thus affects the antigen–antibody reaction. It is able, to some extent, to prevent the Arthus reaction and the rejection of enxografts [91].

The Mowbray factor, an immunosuppressive ribonuclease enzyme in the $\alpha_2$ fraction of the serum [68], may be classified in this group of drugs.

## POSSIBILITIES OF THE USE OF IONIZING RADIATION

Benjamin and Sluka [7] were the first to recognize the effect on the immune apparatus of ionizing radiation. The effect of this kind of radiation is due to its injuring and destroying DNA. The immunological effects of radiation have been excellently reviewed by several authors [20, 58, 100, 101]. We only wish to point out the following characteristics in this chapter:

1. The humoral immune response is definitely blocked by radiation administered before the antigenic stimulus. Immunocytes which are in the proliferative stage are already resistant to radiation. Consequently, the secondary immune response can hardly be influenced by irradiation. The different radiosensitivity of different immune phenomena and of the cells taking part in them is best shown by the fact that lymphocytes stimulated *in vitro* resist even 2,400 R, whereas non-stimulated lymphocytes are killed by 180 R [87].
2. Several steps of the immune reaction may be blocked by ionizing radiation. Fatal doses inhibit the antigen uptake, the phagocytosis and the production of lymph-node opsonins. Immunosuppression is, however, mostly due to the antimitotic effect of radiation. As the lymphoid system is made of tissues which show a very high cell division rate, numbers of the cells taking part in the immune response may be radically reduced by radiation.
3. If lethal irradiation is administered in divided doses, the cellular immune reaction will not be blocked. Appropriately administered irradiation substantially prolonged the survival of skin grafts in mice and rabbits. Animals surviving due to the effect of bone marrow treatment even became incapable of specific response (see below). For this reason, irradiation is often utilized in bringing about immunologically indifferent or non-reactive test animals, which having been reconstituted by bone marrow treatment, are mainly used in transfer experiments [8*d*, 21].

The following methods are available for the practical use of ionizing radiation [46, 47]:

1. *Whole body irradiation.* To achieve an immunosuppressive effect, a single lethal dose (600–1,200 R) must be administered. Such large doses give rise to fatal injuries in the bone marrow and in the mucous membranes even if attempts are made to prevent the damage of the haemopoietic organs by bone marrow treatment. Whole body irradation was the only measure used in the early attempts at organ transplantation, but it is no longer applied today [16, 46].

2. *Local irradiation.* Irradiation of the graft may be performed following organ transplantation. According to some authors, this may be favourable for the survival of the graft [20, 47, 73], while others [61] failed to confirm the immunosuppressive significance of this intervention.

Extracorporeal irradiation of blood and of thoracic duct lymph appears to be a very successful method, due to a decrease in circulating lymphocytes on the one hand, and to a reduction in the number of perifollicular lymphocytes in the lymph nodes and in the spleen, on the other. Extracorporeal irradiation of the blood, a procedure free of side-effects, has been introduced into clinical practice in connection with organ transplantation [19].

3. *Selective irradiation of the lymphatic system with radioisotopes.* Attempts have been made to irradiate the lymphoid system by using isotopes ($^{198}$Au, $^{206}$Bi, $^{90}$Ittrium chelate) accumulating in lymphoid organs. Some results have undoubtedly been achieved (e.g. an increase in the survival time of skin grafts), but a general toxic effect is unavoidable. The method has not been introduced into clinical practice [47].

4. The use of *isotope-labelled antigen* is an interesting new attempt. Ada and Byrt [1], using a mixed lymphocyte population and an antigen labelled with a strongly radioactive isotope preparation, succeeded in selectively killing the cells taking part in the corresponding immune response, i.e. mainly those that had reacted with the radioactive antigen.

## SURGICAL INTERVENTIONS

Surgical ablation of immunologically component tissue (e.g. thymectomy, splenectomy, or thoracic duct drainage) is effective in certain experimental diseases, and has also been tried in human beings [110].

The survival of skin grafts can be prolonged by removal of the regional lymph node or intersection of the lymph vessels connecting the graft with the lymph node. However, the result of such interventions is only transient because recanalization soon allows the information to be taken up and thus the immune reaction to ensue [53].

In case of weak H incompatibility, McGregor and Gowans [62] succeeded in achieving, in contrast to the 16-day survival of the control grafts, a 300-day survival of skin grafts in rats by chronic drainage of the thoracic duct, i.e. continuous removal of lymphocytes. The method proved to be effective also in the case of strong H incompatibilities. Drainage of the thoracic duct for immunosuppressive purposes has been attempted in man, too. Four- or five-day drainage substantially reduced the delayed hypersensitivity reaction and increased the survival time of allogenic grafts two- to three-fold. The circulating small lymphocytes substantially decreased in number [103]. However, the results were not so outstanding when this method was applied to supplement medicinal immunosuppression in renal transplantation [28].

Experimental splenectomy, applied in the therapy of autoimmune diseases, inhibits antibody production, and if it is combined with thymectomy and drug therapy, a moderate inhibition of the cellular response can also be achieved [56,

108]. The beneficial effect of splenectomy in haemolytic anaemia may well not be immunosuppressive [110].

Thymectomy failed to reduce the immune reaction in adults, except in combination with other treatments. It should be noted that, in adult age, the regeneration of the injured lymphoid system, similarly to the processes taking place during intrauterine life, becomes thymus dependent again [52, 108].

## IMMUNOLOGICAL METHODS

The object of immunosuppression is to achieve a specific, long-lasting unresponsiveness to a well-defined antigen. The procedures referred to above give rise to unresponsiveness for short periods of time and, besides their specific action, often reduce the general immunoreactivity of the organism. Induction of specific unresponsiveness needs immunological interventions. Although this question is dealt with elsewhere (Chapter 5), it seems to be necessary to outline some methods here, in order to render the understanding of the methods of induction of immunotolerance easier.

1. *The functional blockade of the RES* (reticuloendothelial system) is a method which has been used with success for a long time. Antibody production can be most effectively reduced with carbon, colloidal iron, or oil emulsion. The effect is based on the inhibition of the afferent branch of the immune reaction, i.e. of the uptake of information. The time and sequence of administration of the active substance and of the antigen is of great importance. In some cases, the former must be administered 24–48 h before the antigen.

In other cases, e.g. with PVP (polyvinylpyrrolidone), thorotrast, Chinese ink, an opposite effect, i.e. stimulation of the immune response, can be observed. Inhibition of the cellular response has been successful also by silica powder, which kills macrophages selectively [84].

2. Specific immunological unresponsiveness may be induced, first of all, by *small or large doses of the antigen* itself (see Chapter 5). More recently, attempts have been made to induce tolerance to H antigens by the administration of chemical preparations obtained from tissues and transplantation antigens, or whole blood 'microtransfusions', especially in connection with organ transplantation. Combination of antigen treatment with the administration of immunosuppressive drugs provides more favourable conditions for inducing tolerance [22, 71, 88c].

3. It has been well known for a long time that immune response can be inhibited with doses of *homologous antibody* given simultaneously with the antigen. The characteristics of the blocking of the humoral immune response to various antigens (sheep erythrocytes, bacterial antigens, serum albumin, etc.) by passively administered antibodies are summarized in the following.

The specific effect of antibody treatment is bound to the Fab fragment of the antibody molecule. To achieve a suppressive effect, the antibody must be administered simultaneously with the antigen or within 24 h. The production of early antibodies is easier to suppress than that of late antibodies. The inhibition is due to a decrease in the number of antibody forming cells, while the antibody yield per cell remains unchanged. Immunological memory cannot be influenced by antibody treatment. 'Late antibodies' of high affinity are more effective than 'early antibodies' of low affinity. It is highly probable that the passive antibodies act by binding the antigen [111]. The mechanism of this process is described in detail in Chapter 11.

There is experimental evidence suggesting that, besides antibody production, the cell-mediated immune response can also be suppressed by antibody treatment. Such an effect was demonstrated in connection with delayed hypersensitivity as well as in the course of renal transplantation in rats [83].

Treatment with protective antibodies (enhancing factor; antibody–antigen complex) deriving from allogeneic donors also seems to be promising. In some cases of renal transplantation in rats, the method yielded excellent results [35].

4. The therapy with *heterologous anti-lymphocyte serum* (ALS) also belongs to the immunological methods. In view of its importance and clinical use, a separate chapter has been devoted to this method (see Chapter 19).

5. The *specific anti-allotype serum* exerts its immunosuppressive effect by its binding to the receptor of the lymphocyte. Like ALS treatment this intervention is non-specific [111].

6. The procedures aimed at the *inhibition of the graft-versus-host reaction* are used with success in clinical practice in connection with bone marrow transplantation. The immunologically competent cells, i.e. those capable of developing a graft-versus-host reaction, are removed by sucrose-gradient centrifugation or by filtration on a glass-bead column covered by the specific antigen [23, 107, 111]. *In vitro* pre-incubation of bone marrow cells with antigens (e.g. erythrocytes) from the recipient seems to be an interesting idea. The pretreated bone marrow will then show a reduced immune reactivity (induction of tolerance *in vitro*) if exposed to antigen. The mechanism of the phenomenon is unknown [13, 104*b*].

## CHARACTERISTICS OF IMMUNOSUPPRESSION

### GENERAL TOXIC EFFECTS

The dose-response curve of most cytostatic drugs and irradiation techniques used for immunosuppressive purposes is extraordinarily steep. According to experimental evidence, in mammals there is little difference between the tumoricidal and immunological doses of the drugs. Clinical observations have suggested that this rule is valid also for man.

As regards the acute symptoms of toxicity, the impairment of the bone marrow and of the mucous membranes is prominent. Besides bone marrow depression, which is reflected by all the laboratory tests, ulcers in the oral mucosa, gastrointestinal ulcers, jaundice, alopecia and subjective symptoms, such as nausea, diarrhoea, emesis, paresthesia, weakness, delirium and coma may occur [34, 64]. Besides acute toxicity, late symptoms may also occur due to cumulative effects. Among these, late bone marrow lesions are the most important which may lead to conditions favouring malignancy. The function of the liver, kidneys, lungs, central nervous system and of the gonads may be disturbed. Foetal injuries may also occur as a consequence of intensive treatment during the first trimenon of pregnancy [50].

To avoid toxic symptoms and to increase the difference between the immunological and toxic doses, combined therapy has been initiated. Combined administration of ALS and Imuran and/or prednisolone is the most favourable combination. Applying this combination, the dose of both drugs can be reduced below the toxic threshold without reducing the immunosuppressive effect. In some cases even a stimulation of the latter has been observed [32, 33, 65, 93, 96]. In order to prevent a rejection crisis, combined administration of prednisolone and actinomycin C has appeared to be favourable. This therapy, if added to a basal therapy with Imuran or Azaserine, is thought to be the most effective drug combination [64].

Under experimental conditions, e.g. in the treatment of experimental allergic encephalomyelitis, combinations in which one of the components is not immunosuppressive in itself (duazomycin, epinephrine and propiomazine) may also be favourable [43, 109].

## EFFECTS DEPENDING ON TIMING AND ON THE DOSE OF THE IMMUNOSUPPRESSIVE AGENT

Immunosuppressive interventions exert their optimum effect only if administered at the most favourable time relative to the introduction of the antigen [85, 95*a*]. According to Berenbaum [8*e*], single large doses of ionizing radiation and Busulphan are most effective if given immediately before the introduction of the antigen; antimetabolites, nitrogen mustard, TEM, cyclophosphamide and actinomycin, on the other hand, are most effective if administered on the day before, or 4–5 days after, giving the antigen. A drug given at any time except the optimum is in general ineffective.

Dose dependence is another characteristic of the immunosuppressive effect. For instance, Endoxan, R-74 and Myelobromol (dibromomannite) have the same effect if given in single doses amounting to 5, 10 and 20 per cent of the $LD_{50}$, respectively [77].

Immunosuppressive agents may stimulate antibody production (augmentation) depending on the dose and the time of administration. This has been demonstrated in connection with the administration of most of the drugs (Endoxan, 6-mercaptopurine, uracyl mustard, 5-fluoro-2-deoxyuridine, cytosine arabinoside, dibromodulcitol, actinomycin D, hydrocortisone) and irradiation [5, 15, 25, 40, 85]. Augmentation of cell-mediated immune response has also been claimed. In these cases the survival of skin grafts was reduced [72, 88*c*]. Augmentation of the immune response is probably based on release of nucleic acids from the cells killed by the cytostatic drugs. Uptake of the nucleic acids may raise the number of antigen reactive cells and enhance their proliferation [88*c*].

However, the phenomenon of augmentation of antibody production must be judged carefully. For instance, immunosuppressive treatment may postpone the start of the proliferative phase of the immune response. In such cases, the whole antibody response may be shifted in time and even the decline will be delayed. It may occur that the serum antibody titre is measured only once, at a time when the immune response of control animals is already declining while the treated animals have just reached the peak of the titre curve. In such a case, augmentation is only apparent. In other cases, the reason of the augmentation of the serum titre (19 S antibodies) is unknown; hydrocortisone treatment may, e.g. augment the antibody response without any excess increase in the antibody forming cells [5].

## CIRCUMSTANCES OF THE SPECIFIC IMMUNOSUPPRESSIVE EFFECTS

In spite of their non-specific toxic effect on general reactivity, immunosuppressive drugs can be applied for specific inhibition of well-defined immune responses [89*a*]. This specific effect can be understood taking into consideration that among the different antigens affecting the organism there is probably only one or very few which are active at the time when the drug's activity is at its highest level. Borel used pikryl chloride to sensitize guinea pigs which had already been sensitized by o-chlorobenzyl chloride. 6-mercaptopurine administered simultaneously with pikryl chloride prevented delayed hypersensitivity to this substance, but failed to alter the reactivity to o-chlorobenzyl chloride [10]. Hersch et al. [43] examined the immune response of leukaemic patients to different antigens administered during a five-day period of amethopterin treatment. The suppression of the antigen given 24 h after the start of the treatment was complete. To the antigens given one and two days after the end of the treatment, the immune response was partially suppressed or unaltered, respectively [43]. These two examples are sufficient to throw light on the possibility of a specific effect and on the importance of the time factor in this respect.

## SELECTIVE EFFECTS

Three types are known:

1. The immune responses to various antigens given simultaneously are influenced differently by the same treatment. According to both experimental and clinical experience, the immune response directed to the stronger, more foreign, i.e. more immunogenic, antigen is less effectively inhibited than that directed to a weaker antigen [29, 43]. This is valid not only for drugs, but also for X-ray irradiation and other kinds of immunological treatment (e.g. ALS treatment) [58, 66].
2. There are drugs which interfere more strongly with the cell-mediated immune response than with the humoral response and the other way round. For instance, the cell-mediated response can be selectively blocked by 6-mercaptopurine or a combination of dibromodulcitol and dibromomannitol without impairing the humoral response [12, 76].
3. A further possibility of selective action is selectivity in respect of immunoglobulin classes. It has been demonstrated both experimentally and clinically that amethopterin, 6-mercaptopurine, Imuran, Endoxan, and cortisone inhibit, first of all, the production of IgG antibodies. IgM production may, at the same time, remain unaltered. Moreover, in such cases the production of IgM antibodies may persist for unusually long periods of time [5, 9, 11, 31, 88*c*]. These phenomena have called attention to the regulatory role of the IgG antibodies, i.e. to their negative feed-back effect (see Chapter 11).

The selective effect of immunosuppressive interventions suggests that the different cell populations taking part in the immune response have different drug sensitivities. According to Schwartz [88*c*], this also indicates that the cell-mediated response and the production of IgM and IgG antibodies are bound to different cell populations.

## POSSIBILITY OF INDUCTION OF IMMUNOLOGICAL TOLERANCE

Attempts to induce specific immunological tolerance by the combination of antigen and drug treatment as well as X-ray irradiation were started in the late nineteen fifties. Schwartz and Dameshek [89*a*] induced specific tolerance to human serum albumin (HSA) by simultaneous administration of HSA and 6-mercaptopurine. The specific tolerance persisted for several months. At the same time, the animals gave the usual response to other antigens (e.g. to bovine serum albumin). Tolerance even to particulate antigens, such as sheep erythrocytes, tumour cells, skin and renal grafts, which lasted for longer or shorter periods was brought about by combined treatment. In these experiments, the following drugs were used: cyclophosphamide, amethopterine, 6-mercaptopurine and cytosine arabinoside [27, 36, 37, 63, 95*b*, 104*a*, 105, 112]. Attempts were also made with X-ray irradiation. The following characteristics of the chemotherapeutic induction of immunological tolerance were established from these experiments [88*c*]:

1. Immunological tolerance can be brought about in adult animals and humans by combined administration of cytotoxic drugs and antigen.
2. The tolerance is very specific, affecting only the antigen which was administered simultaneously with the drug(s). A normal response can be induced by any other antigen. The drug-induced tolerance is biologically indistinguishable from the tolerance inducible in the neonatal age.
3. The strength and duration of the tolerance depends on the dose of the drug and on the quantity of the antigen administered during the period of drug treatment.
4. In transplanting allografts the degree of H incompatibility is an important factor. The weaker the H conditions, the greater the probability of a successful tolerance.

The induction of tolerance is still in an experimental phase. The initial successes in connection with organ transplantation are especially promising [74].

## EVALUATION OF TESTS SERVING FOR MEASURING IMMUNOSUPPRESSIVE EFFECTS

The success of immunosuppressive interventions depends on several factors, primarily on the course of the immune reaction to be influenced and on the goal to be achieved [98]. In the case of organ transplantation this is e.g. prevention of rejection symptoms, whereas in that of an autoimmune disease, clinical remission. However, other, non-immunological processes may also influence the clinical picture of autoimmune diseases which may be responsible for incomplete clinical remission (except in cases when the patient is not treated with the drug of choice indicated in that specific form of autoimmune disease). In conditions of uncleared aetiology treatment may fail due to the lack of participating immune processes in the pathomechanism of the disease. In such cases, the outcome of the immunosuppressive treatment may elucidate the aetiology [75]. In view of these, attempts have been made to measure the immunosuppressive effect by various tests.

Among others, the following tests have been applied: measuring of the natural serum antibody titre, e.g. to isohaemagglutinogen, *E. coli*, streptolysin; delayed hypersensitivity reaction (to BCG, PPD, monilia, etc.); primary immune response (to haemocyanin, heterologous erythrocytes, etc.). However, the results of none of the applied tests have shown any correlation with the immunosuppressive effect manifesting itself in clinical remission [261].

Recently the changes in spontaneous blast transformation of lymphocytes or in that induced by PHA, specific antigen, or allogeneic lymphocytes as well as changes in the uptake of thymidine by lymphocytes in cultures have been measured *in vitro* during immunosuppressive therapy [14, 49, 79, 102, 110]. Measuring the inhibition with sheep erythrocytes of spontaneous rosette formation by lymphocytes also appears to be a useful method [3, 4], along with the leukocyte migration test and the cytotoxic effects of lymphocytes [110]. However, as mentioned above, there is little hope to find a test which would yield an appropriate indicator of the impacts affecting the actual immune response to the specific antigen. *In vitro* or *in vivo* tests for the observation of the specific antigen and of the reacting cells seem to be the best approximation.

## SUPPRESSION OF THE EFFECTS OF THE ANTIGEN–ANTIBODY REACTION

Antihistamines, corticosteroids, and disodium cromoglycate are of value for the symptomatic treatment of reaginic disease and some other forms of immunopathological disease. The use of other agents is less clearly established, but has given promising results. Such drugs may produce only transient suppression of symptoms while they are given; lasting improvement—as sometimes happens with corticosteroids or cyclophosphamide in the steroid-sensitive nephrotic syndrome—may result from breaking a vicious circle of disease [110].

## REFERENCES


1. Ada, G. L. and Byrt, P.: *Nature (London)* **222,** 1291 (1969).
2. Ambinder, E. P., Schwartz, G. H., Rubin, A. L. and Stenzel, K. H.: *Transplantation* **7,** 147 (1969).
3. Bach, J. F., Dardenne, M. and Fornier, C.: *Nature (London)* **222,** 998 (1969).
4. Bach, J. F., Dormont, J., Dardenne, M. and Belner, H.: *Transplantation* **8,** 265 (1969).
5. Benczur, M., Petrányi, G. Gy. and Alföldy, P.: *Orv. Hetil.* **112,** 183 (1971).
6. Benczur, M. and Szántó, L.: *Orv. Hetil.* **110,** 595 (1969).

7. Benjamin, E. and Sluka, E.: *Wien. klin. Wschr.* **21,** 311 (1908).
8a. Berenbaum, M. C.: *Lancet* **ii,** 1363 (1964).
8b. id., *Biochem. Pharmacol.* **2,** 29 (1962).
8c. id., *Transplantation* **3,** 671 (1965).
8d. id., *Brit. med. Bull.* **21,** 140 (1965).
8e. id., In *Immunity, Cancer and Chemotherapy. Basic Relationship on the Cellular Level.* Ed. by Mihich, E. Academic Press, New York 1967, p. 217.
8f. id., In *Symp. Tissue and Organ Transplantation.* Ed. by Mihich, E. *J. Clin. Path.* **20,** Suppl. 471 (1967).
9. Blinkoff, R. C.: *Fed. Proc.* **23,** 190 (1964).
9a. Blomgren, H. and Andersson, B.: *Cell. Immunol.* **1,** 545 (1971).
10. Borel, Y.: cited by 88c.
11. Borel, Y., Fanconnet, M. and Mischer, P. A.: *J. exp. Med.* **122,** 263 (1965).
12. Borel, Y. and Schwartz, R. S.: *J. Immunol.* **92,** 754 (1964).
13. Bortin, M. M. and Rimm, A. A.: *J. Immunol.* **102,** 1042 (1969).
14. Bozsóky, S.: In *Transplantatiós Immunológia (Immunology of Transplantation).* Ed. by Petrányi, Gy. Petrányi, G. Gy., Benczúr, M. and Jánossy, Gy. Akadémiai Kiadó, Budapest 1971, p. 295.
15. Börzsönyi, M. and Connors, T. A.: *Neoplasma* **16,** 393 (1969).
16. Calne, R. Y.: *Brit. J. Surg.* **48,** 384 (1961).
17. Calne, R. Y., Wheeler, J. H., Horn, B. A. and Path, M. S.: *Brit. med. J.* **1,** 154 (1965).
18. Chakravarty, A. K. and Friedman, H.: *Science* **167,** 869 (1970).
19. Chanana, A. D., Brecher, G., Croncite, E. P., Joel, D. and Schnappauf, H.: *Radiat. Res.* **27,** 330 (1966).
20. Cronkite, E. P. and Chanana, A. D.: In *Human Transplantation.* Ed. by Rapaport, J. I. and Dausset, J. Grune and Stratton, New York 1968, p. 423.
21. Davie, W. E. and Cole, J. L.: *Science* **140,** 483 (1963).
22. De Weck, D. L. and Frey, J. R.: In *The Immune Response and its Suppression.* Ed. by Sorkin, E. Antibiotica et Chemotherapia, Vol. 15. Karger, Basel 1969, p. 110.
23. Dicke, K. A., Tridente, G. and van Bekkum, P. W.: *Transplantation* **8,** 422 (1969).
24. Dietrich, F. M.: *Int. Arch. Allergy* **29,** 313 (1966).
25. Dobbs, J., Rivero, J., Sabb, F. and Lee, S. L.: *Immunology* **14,** 213 (1968).
26. Dóbiás, Gy., Perényi, É. and Nábrádi, J.: In *Transplantatiós Immunológia (Immunology of Transplantation).* Ed. by Petrányi, Gy., Petrányi, G. Gy., Benczúr, M. and Jánossy, Gy. Akadémiai Kiadó, Budapest 1971, p. 335.
27. Dukor, P. and Dietrich, F. M.: In *Organtransplantation.* Ed. by Heymer, A. und Ricken, D. Schattauer, Stuttgart 1969.
28. Dumont, A. E.: In *Human Transplantation.* Ed. by Rapaport, F. I. and Dausset J. Grune and Stratton, New York 1968, p. 482.
29. Elek, G., Földes, I., Tóth, F. and Vandra, E.: In *Transplantatiós Immunológia (Immunology of Transplantation).* Ed. by Petrányi, Gy., Petrányi, G. Gy., Benczúr, M. and Jánossy, Gy.: Akadémiai Kiadó, Budapest 1971, p. 149.
30. Elion, G. B. and Hitchings, G. H.: *Fed. Proc.* **18,** 221 (1959).
31. Eliott, E. V. and Sinclair, N. R.: *Immunology* **15,** 643 (1968).
32. Feldman, J. D.: *Arch. intern. Med.* **123,** 713 (1969).
33. Floerscheim, G. L.: *Transplantation* **8,** 392 (1969).
33a. Fournier, C., Bach, M. A., Dardenne, M. and Bach, J. F.: *Transpl. Proc.* **5,** 523 (1973).
34. Frei, E.: *Fed. Proc.* **26,** 918 (1967).
35. French, M. E. and Batchelor, J. R.: *Lancet* **ii,** 1103 (1969).
36. Frisch, A. W. and Davies, G. H.: *J. Lab. clin. Med.* **68,** 103 (1966).
37. Gordon, R. O., Wade, M. E. and Mitchell, M. S.: *J. Immunol.* **103,** 233 (1969).
38. Gray, G. D., Mickelson, M. M. and Crim, J. A.: *Transplantation* **6,** 805 (1968).
39. Gray, G. D. and Perper, R. J.: *Transplantation* **7,** 183 (1969).
40. Haines, F. R., Johnson, A. G. and Petering, H. G.: *Fed. Proc.* **26,** 934 (1967).
41. Harris, J. E. and Hersh, E. M.: *Cancer Res.* **28,** 2432 (1968).
42. Hechtman, H. B., Blumenstock, A. D., Thomas, E. and Ferrebee, J. W.: *Ann. Surg.* **159,** 119 (1964).

43. Hersch, E. M., Carbone, P. P., Wong, V. and Freirich, E. J.: *Cancer Res.* **25,** 1177 (1965).
44*a*. Hitchings, G. H. and Elion, G. B.: *Pharmacol. Rev.* **15,** 365 (1963).
44*b*. id., *Ann. N. Y. Acad. Sci.* **129,** 799 (1966).
45. Hobik, H. P.: *Naturwissenschaften* **56,** 217 (1969).
46. Hume, D. M., Magee, J. H. and Kaufman, H. M. jr., Rittenburg, M. S. and Prout, G. R., jr.: *Ann. Surg.* **158,** 608 (1963).
47. Hume, D. M. and Wolf, J. S.: *Transplantation* **5,** 1174 (1967).
48. Humphreys, R. S., Glynn, J. P. and Goldin, A.: *Transplantation* **1,** 65 (1963).
49. Jánossy, Gy. and Ónody, K.: In *Transplantatiós Immunológia (Immunology of Transplantation).* Ed. by Petrányi, Gy., Petrányi, G. Gy., Benczúr, M. and Jánossy, Gy. Akadémiai Kiadó, Budapest 1971, p. 103.
50. Karnofsky, D. A.: *Fed. Proc.* **26,** 925 (1967).
51. Kirchner, H.: *Lancet* **ii,** 747 (1964).
52. Kisken, W. A.: *Arch. Surg.* **92,** 386 (1966).
53. Lambert, B. P., Frank, H. A., Bellman, S. and Farnsworth, D.: *Transplantation* **3,** 62 (1965).
54. Lemmel, E. M. and Nouza, K.: *Folia Biol. (Prague)* **12,** 253 (1966).
55. Leon, M. A. and Schwartz, H. J.: *Proc. Soc. exp. Biol. (N.Y.)* **131,** 735 (1969).
56. Leonard, L. and McHutchinson, G.: *Transplantation* **3,** 343 (1965).
57. Makinodan, I., Albright, J. F., Perkinson, E. H. and Nettesheim, R.: *Med. Clin. N. Amer.* **49,** 1596 (1965).
58. Makinodan, T. and Genzogian, N.: In *Radiation, Protection and Recovery.* Ed. by Hollaender, A. Pergamon Press, Oxford 1960.
59. Markowitz, H., Person, D. A., Gitnick, D. L. and Ritts, R. E., jr.: *Science* **163,** 476 (1969).
60. Mathe, G., Amiel, J. L. and Niemetz, J. L.: *Blood* **20,** 119 (1962).
61. McCornick, J. R. and Egdhal, R. A.: *Transplantation* **4,** 100 (1966).
62. McGregor, D. D. and Gowans, J. L.: *Lancet* **i,** 629 (1964).
63. McLaren, A.: *Transplant. Bull.* **28,** 479 (1961).
64. Merrill, J. P.: In *Human Transplantation.* Ed. by Rapaport, F. T. and Dausset, J. Grune and Stratton, New York 1968, p. 61.
65. Mitchell, R. M., Sheil, A. C., Stafsky, A. C. and Murray, J. E.: *Transplantation* **4,** 323 (1966).
66. Monaco, A., Wood, M. L. and Russel, P. S.: *Ann. N. Y. Acad. Sci.* **129,** 190 (1966).
67. Mosely, V. R., Scheil, A. G., Mitchell, R. M. and Murray, J. E.: *Transplantation* **4,** 678 (1966).
68. Mowbray, J. F., Boylston, A. W., Milton, J. D. and Weksler, M.: In *The Immune Response and its Suppression.* Ed. by Sorkin, E. Antibiotica et Chemotherapia, Vol. 15, Karger, Basel 1969, p. 384.
69. Murray, J. E.: *Transplantation* **2,** 147 (1966).
70. Murray, J. E., Sheil, A. G., Moseley, R., Knight, P., McGaric, J. and Dammin, G. J.: *Ann. Surg.* **160,** 449 (1964).
71. Nossal, G. J. V.: *Circulation* **39,** 5 (1969).
72. Nouza, K.: *Folia biol. (Prague)* **12,** 266 (1966).
73. Ono, K., Lindsey, E. S. and Creeck, O., jr.: *Transplantation* **7,** 176 (1969).
74. Owens, E. R.: *Nature (London)* **219,** 970 (1968).
75. Patakfalvi, A., Horváth, T. and Jávor, T.: In *Transplantatiós Immunológia (Immunology of Transplantation).* Ed. by Petrányi, Gy., Petrányi, G. Gy., Benczúr, M. and Jánossy, Gy. Akadémiai Kiadó, Budapest, 1971, p. 331.
76. Petrányi, G. Gy.: Comparative study of the immunosuppressive effect of cyto-static drugs in immunological models. Thesis. Budapest 1968.
77. Petrányi, G. Gy.: In *Transplantatiós Immunológia (Immunology of Transplantation).* Ed. by Petrányi, Gy., Petrányi, G. Gy., Benczúr, M. and Jánossy, Gy. Akadémiai Kiadó, Budapest 1971, p. 119.
78. Petrányi, Gy.: *Acta med. Acad. Sci. hung.* **20,** 387 (1964).
79. Petrányi, Gy., Szegedi, Gy. and Kakuk, Gy.: In *Transplantatiós Immunológia (Immunology of Transplantation).* Ed. by Petrányi, Gy., Petrányi, G. Gy., Benczúr, M. and Jánossy, Gy. Akadémiai Kiadó. Budapest 1971, p. 359.

80. Potel, J.: *Arzneimittel-Forsch.* **15,** 527 (1965).
81. Potel, J. and Broch, N.: *Arzneimittel-Forsch.* **15,** 659 (1965).
82. Prichard, R. W. and Hayer, D. M.: *Amer. J. Pathol.* **38,** 325 (1961).
83. Rowley, D. A., Fitch, F. W., Axelrod, M. A. and Pierce, C. W.: *Immunology* **16,** 549 (1969).
84. Sabet, I., Newlin, C. and Friedman, H.: *Immunology* **16,** 433 (1969).
85. Santos, C. W.: *Fed. Proc.* **26,** 907, (1967).
86. Santos, C. W. and Owens, A. W.: *Blood* **20,** 11 (1962).
87. Schrek, R. and Stefani, S.: *J. Nat. Cancer Inst.* **32,** 507 (1964).
88*a*. Schwartz, R. S.: *Progr. Allergy* **9,** 246 (1965).
88*b*. id., *Fed. Proc.* **26,** 914 (1967).
88*c*. id., In *Human Transplantation*. Ed. by Rapaport, F. T. and Dausset, J. Grune and Stratton, New York 1968, p. 440.
88*d*. id., *Nature (London)* **224,** 275 (1969).
89*a*. Schwartz, R. and Dameshek, W.: *Nature (London)* **183,** 1682 (1959).
89*b*. id., *Blood,* **19,** 483 (1962).
90. Schwartz, R., Stock, J. and Dameshek, W.: *Proc. Soc. exp. Biol. (N.Y.)* **99,** 164 (1958).
91. Shin, H. S., Gewuzz, H. and Snydermann, R.: *Proc. Soc. exp. Biol. (N.Y.)* **131,** 203 (1969).
92. Starzl, Th. E., Marchioro, T. L., Faris, T. D., Hutt., M. P., Carey, T. A. and Ogden, D. A.: *Ann. N. Y. Acad. Aci.* **129,** 598 (1966).
93. Starzl, Th. E. and Porter, K. A.: In *Human Transplantation*. Ed. by Rapaport, F. T. and Dausset, J. Grune and Stratton, New York 1968, p. 489.
94. Stender, H. S., Stranch, B. and Winter, H.: *Strahlentherapie* **115,** 175 (1961).
95*a*. Sterzl, J.: In *Immunity, Cancer and Chemotherapy. Basic Relationship on the Cellular Level.* Ed. by Mihich, E. Academic Press, New York 1967, p. 71.
95*b*. id., In *The Immune Response and its Suppression*. Ed. by Sorkin, E. Antibiotica et Chemotherapia. Vol. 15, Karger, Basel 1969, p. 135.
96. Stewart, P. B. and Cohen, V.: *Science* **164,** 1082 (1969).
96*a*. Stockman, D. G., Heim, R. L., South, M. A. and Trentin, J. J.: *J. Immunol.* **110,** 277 (1973).
97. Sutton, W. R., Hagen, F. W., Griffith, B. W. and Preston, S. W.: *Arch. Surg.* **87,** 840 (1963).
98. Swanson, M. A. and Schwartz, R. S.: *New Engl. J. med.* **277,** 163 (1967).
99. Szántó, L., Görgényi, F., Benczur, M., Ligetiné, Reviczky, A., Bányai, B., Lőrincz, G. and Gömöri, B.: *Orv. Hetil.* **110,** 182 (1969).
100. Taliafferro, W. H. and Taliafferro, L. G.: *J. Immunol.* **66,** 181 (1951).
101. Taliafferro, W. H., Taliafferro, L. G. and Jaroslav, B. N.: *Radiation and Immune Mechanism*. Academic Press, New York 1964.
102. Tennenbaum, J. I., Pierre, St. and Cerilli, G. J.: *Transplantation* **6,** 986 (1968).
103. Tunner, W. S., Carbone, P. P., Blaylock, W. K. and Irvin, G. L.: *Surg. Gynecol. Obstet.* **121,** 334 (1965).
104*a*. Uphoff, D. E.: *Transplant. Bull.* **28,** 116 (1961).
104*b*. id., *Nature (London)* **222,** 1089 (1969).
105. Uphoff, D. E. and Pitkins, L.: *Blood* **20,** 113 (1962).
106. Uyeki, E. M.: *Exp. Haematol.* **12,** 17 (1967).
107. Van Bekkum, D. W.: In *Bone-Marrow Conservation, Culture and Transplantation*. Int. Atomic Energy Agency, Vienna, 1969.
108. Veith, F. J., Luch, R. J. and Murray, J. E.: *Surg. Gynecol. Obstet.* **121,** 299 (1965).
109. Vogel, C. L. and Calabresi, P.: *Proc. Soc. exp. Biol. (N.Y.)* **131,** 251 (1969).
110. WHO Scientific Group: *Clinical Immunology*. WHO, Geneva 1972, p. 42.
111. Wigzell, H.: In *The Immune Response and its Suppression*. Ed. by Sorkin, E. Antibiotica et Chemotherapia. Vol. 15, Karger, Basel 1969, p. 82.
112. Woodruff, M. F. A.: *Nature (London)* **195,** 727 (1962).

CHAPTER 19

# XENOGENEIC ANTILYMPHOCYTE SERUM

by

M. BENCZÚR, K. NOUZA and G. GY. PETRÁNYI



## INTRODUCTION

Immunization of animals with lymphocytes or thymocytes taken from animal of another species or from man leads to the production of xenogeneic anti-lymphocyte serum (ALS) and anti-thymocyte serum (ATS), respectively. In the clinical practice the globulin fractions of these antisera (ALG and ATG) are administered most frequently.

The successful clinical application of ALS was preceded by an explosion-like development of experimental studies in the field of tissue, cell and organ transplantation.

Metchnikoff immunized rabbits with lymphoid cells of rats and guinea pigs before 1899 already. The resulting sera significantly inhibited the activity of the rat and guinea pig lymphocytes and macrophages *in vitro*, but also appeared to be toxic for the granulocytes and mast cells of the respective species [95].

Subsequently, it was shown that the production of an effective ALS needs repeated immunizations. Antisera thus obtained usually killed lymphoid cells *in vitro* in the presence of complement or at least reduced their mobility. The agglutinating capacity was not lost during decomplementation by heat. In a few experiments *in vivo*, ALS treatment was accompanied by a transient lymphopenia and an initial involution of the lymphoid organs. These were, however, followed by a rapid lymphoid hyperplasia and a returning of the lymphocyte count to normal. These effects could not be attributed to cytotoxins, for the ALS remained effective even after cytotoxins had been absorbed [77*a*, 94, 117].

Early attempts to suppress the immune response to allografts and xenografts failed. Only after long experimentation, Woodruff and Anderson [170*a*] in 1963 were the first to prove that the allograft response may be efficiently suppressed by ALS. In their experiments rat skin allografts survived significantly longer in rats, treated with an ALS of rabbit origin. Further, Monaco's and Medawar's groups demonstrated that rabbit ALS is extremely immunosuppressive also in mice [23, 37, 45, 46, 87*a*, 99, 100].

Nevertheless, several years had to elapse until the clinical administration of ALS was accepted as an effective and safe immunosuppressive treatment. The first experience with renal transplantations showed that the survival of the grafts was better and prolonged if ALS treatment was combined with other immunosuppressive procedures; moreover, the dosage of immunosuppressive drugs (and thus the probability of their toxic effect) could be significantly reduced [146, 149]. Nowadays, ALG is used also in liver and heart transplantation [25] and for the pretreatment of bone marrow graft recipients [93].

Recently, ALS treatment has been found to be beneficial also in the therapy of numerous experimental as well as clinical immunopathological processes and autoimmune diseases [158].

## PREPARATION OF ALS

ALS is regularly produced by immunizing animals with lymphoid cells from xenogeneic donors. Experiments aimed at producing immunosuppressive allogeneic ALS have led so far to unsatisfactory results.

Cells for immunization are obtained from the thymus, lymph nodes, spleen, thoracic duct, or from the peripheral blood of normal donors or patients with chronic lymphoid leukaemia [65*a*, 92, 170*a*]. Some authors recommend the use of lymphoblasts, continuously produced in tissue culture [103, 106]. Thymocytes and thoracic duct cells seem to be most suitable. Subcellular fractions or cell membranes from lymphoid cells and from cultured fibroblasts [56, 77*c*, 78, 104, 159*a*] as well as antigen–antibody complexes (ALG–murine thymic cells [174]) have also been used for this purpose.

The production of ALS has so far been rather empirical [65*a*, 87*a*, 126, 127]. Immunization schedules have been developed for several animal species, e.g. for rabbit, horse, sheep, swine, goat, duck and dog. The activity of different pools may be variable even if the same immunization schedule is used. Recent experience seems to support the advantage of short immunization schedules, i.e. those consisting of two or three injections given 1–2 weeks apart [60, 87*a*, 123*a*, 131, 149].

For clinical use, ALS is usually produced in horses and the purified IgG fraction (ALG) of the antiserum is most frequently administered. Recently commercial preparations became available (Searle).

## GENERAL (HAEMATOLOGICAL AND MORPHOLOGICAL) EFFECTS OF ALS

Lymphopenia caused by ALS produced by different methods may be of varying degrees, but, irrespective of the degree of lymphopenia, the peripheral lymphocyte count soon returns to, or approximates the normal level, even after a prolonged course of ALS [1, 63, 72, 87*b*]. A sustained lymphopenia occurs only rarely [102].

There is no direct correlation between lymphopenia and the immunosuppressive effect (see below). Granulocytes do not decrease in number, whereas the platelet count may fall significantly [18, 19, 150].

The data shown in Table 19-I come from our own experiments. The selective effect of ALS on the peripheral lymphocytes is clearly seen.

TABLE 19-I

*Effect of ALS on the peripheral blood picture of mice**

| Animal no. | Changes in total lymphocyte count | Changes in granulocyte count | Changes in white cell count |
|---|---|---|---|
| 1 | −88 | +20 | −84 |
| 2 | −66 | +650 | −5 |
| 3 | −75 | +510 | −46 |
| 4 | −70 | +102 | −51 |
| 5 | −66 | +125 | −49 |
| 6 | −77 | +185 | −64 |
| 7 | −89 | −7 | −81 |
| 8 | −74 | −1 | −77 |
| 9 | −82 | −42 | −76 |

* CBA mice received 1 ml of ALG subcutaneously. Blood was examined before, and 24 h after, ALG treatment. The figures represent per cent changes related to the initial absolute cell numbers.

Similar effects are known from clinical experience. However, the clinical evaluation of the effect of the ALS is complicated by the usual combination of ALS treatment with other immunosuppressive procedures [149, 150].

The involution of the thymus in the course of ALS administration has been observed by several authors. The view that ALS exerts its effect *via* the thymus (see below) was based on these observations. At present, however, the thymus involution is mainly attributed to a stress effect and functional exhaustion due to ALS treatment. This is supported by the fact that the ALG molecules cannot pass the blood–thymus barrier and ALS-coated lymphocytes do not reach the thymus at all [33*b*] (see, coating of lymphocytes).

The picture in the peripheral lymphoid organs is variable. Obviously, different ALS preparations may exert different effects, but most of the divergencies are attributable to the fact that different observations reflect different phases of the same process. Thus, it is understandable that a severe depletion of the lymph-node follicles was observed by some authors [2, 102] and their hypertrophy was observed by others [87*d*, 111].

Many investigations have proved the intensive effect of ALS on lymphocytes in the paracortical region of the lymph node and on the periarteriolar sheet of the splenic white pulp. It should be mentioned that mainly thymus dependent lymphocytes, i.e. those responsible for cell-mediated immunity are located in these regions [154, 159*a*].

Special attention was paid to the renal aspects, because treatment with heterologous proteins may induce Masugi-like nephritis or serum sickness. In the former case, the ALS may damage the kidney due to the determinants common to the lymphocytes and glomerular basement membrane. In the latter case, the kidney damage may be due to lodging in the glomeruli of microprecipitates (immune complexes) consisting of anti-ALG and ALG. Such damage was mainly demonstrated in animals injected with ALS intravenously [63]. Two cases of Masugi nephritis occurred among 113 patients treated with ALS intravenously [24], deposition of immune complexes seems to be less dangerous.

## IMMUNOLOGICAL EFFECTS OF ALS *IN VIVO*

### EFFECTS ON HUMORAL ANTIBODY PRODUCTION

The experiments demonstrating the suppressive effect of ALS on antibody production to various antigens are summarized in Table 19-II.

TABLE 19-II

*Suppressive effect of ALS on the humoral immune response to various antigens*

| Experimental animal | Antigen | Reference No. |
|---|---|---|
| Mouse | Sheep RBC | 32, 77*a*, 87*b*, 100, 101*a*, *b* |
| | BCG | 16 |
| | Salmonella | 45 |
| | Tetanus toxoid | 128 |
| Rat | Sheep RBC | 29*a*, *b*, 66*a*, 163 |
| | Bovine serum albumin | 65*b*, 66*a*, 67 |
| Dog | Brucella | 124 |
| | Sheep RBC, salmonella | 12*a*, *b* |

Supposedly, the first stages of the immune response, i.e. the recognition of the antigen, triggering of immunocompetent cells, the first steps in cellular co-operation and differentiation, are the processes with which the ALG interferes. This is supported by the following experimental evidence: (*i*) it has been shown by means of 'normal lymphocyte transfer' [87*a*] that, in contrast to the other immunosuppressive agents, ALG inhibited the first phase of the response; (*ii*) according to Loewi et al. [88] and others [89], ALS is able to agglutinate and, in the presence of complement, to lyse macrophages; (*iii*) ALS is much more effective when administered before the antigen than if it is given thereafter [101*a*].

According to numerous authors [45, 66*a*, 67, 100, 129], the primary immune response is much more sensitive to ALS than the secondary response. Presensitized cells are resistant, therefore, the previously acquired immunity can be transmitted passively with sensitized cells in spite of ALS treatment [65*c*].

Recent findings, however, indicate, that also a processing immune response can be inhibited by ALS, produced with activated lymph node cells [151].

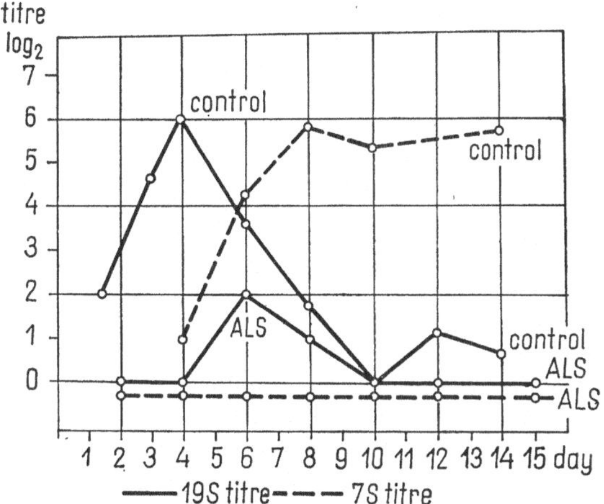


Fig. 19-1. Effect of ALG on haemolysin production in mice. Animals received 0.4 ml ALG on each of days −3, −2 and −1 and were immunized i. p. with $2.2 \times 10^8$ sheep erythrocytes on day 0. Differentiating of IgG- and IgM-type haemolysins was made by mercapto-ethanol inactivation

According to our own experiments, the 7S heterohaemolysin response was inhibited to a greater extent than the 19S heterohaemolysin response (Fig. 19-1). The selective blocking of the 7S production may be related to the different sensitivity of the systems producing the different classes of antibodies. Irradiation, some cytotoxic drugs (e.g. R-74) and hydrocortisone produce similar effects [119, 175]. It should be noted, however, that ALS preparations produced according to different immunization schedules need not manifest a specific anti-7S effect. In a recent experimental study [7] the synthesis of IgM-type antibodies was mainly inhibited.

In general, antibody formation is inhibited by ALS to a lesser degree than cell-mediated immunity [77*c*]. This is of practical advantage if ALS is used in organ transplantation, where the blocking or inhibition of the antibacterial, antiviral, antifungal and antihelminthic immunity is undesirable [62*a*, 75, 77*d*, 83, 116,

124, 125]. However, this property is not an absolute one and may vary from batch to batch; one of the preparations examined by us showed a reverse effect: it failed to influence the rejection reaction while intensively inhibited the humoral immune response. In *in vitro* tests some ALG preparations induced blast transformation of B lymphocytes without affecting T lymphocytes. Some controversial results can be explained on the basis of recently demonstrated cellular co-operation between T (thymus derived) and B [bone marrow (bursa) derived] cells in most humoral responses. ALS seems to affect more intensively recirculating T than sessile B cells. Therefore each ALS pool should be tested prior to use.

## EFFECTS ON CELL-MEDIATED IMMUNITY AND ON AUTOIMMUNE PROCESSES

The tuberculin-reaction-inhibiting effect of the ALS had already been known before Woodruff's experiments [60, 62*a*, *b*]. Recent investigations have shown that ALS exerts a suppressive effect on contact delayed-type hypersensitivity [164, 165], allergic skin reactions to fungal antigens [27, 101*c*, 147], and on the Arthus phenomenon [163], on experimental allergic encephalomyelitis [85, 165], the haemolytic anaemia of NZB mice [32, 33*a*], lymphocytic choriomeningitis [1, 6, 20, 42, 58], further on experimental allergic thyroiditis and adjuvant polyarthritis. On the basis of experimental evidence ALS has also been tested in clinical autoimmune diseases, such as myasthenia gravis, rheumatoid arthritis, arteritis temporalis, and dermatomyositis [124, 164], nephrotic syndrome, chronic hepatitis and multiple sclerosis. In myasthenia gravis, sympathetic ophthalmia and SLE, clinical remission was achieved [24].

The mechanism of action of ALS in these processes is not fully clear: the interference with the sensitization process as well as the suppression of effector mechanisms may be considered. Because of mysteries in the pathogenesis of autoimmune diseases and frequent spontaneous remissions, the value of ALS treatment is at present difficult to assess.

## EFFECTS ON THE TRANSPLANTATION REACTION

Because of the practical importance of the transplantation therapy, the analysis of ALS effect on allograft reaction has received particular attention. The most important results are summarized in Table 19-III.

The earliest observations in mice were published by two working teams: that of Medawar, Levey and Lance in England and that of Russell, Gray and Monaco in the USA. Their experiments showed that not only the allogenic skin reaction but, to a lesser extent, also the xenogeneic and second-set reactions are blocked by ALS. Besides, the development of cell-mediated immunological memory is significantly inhibited [45, 66*a*, 67, 87*a*, 100, 101*a*, *b*, 132].

In experiments on mice treated with rabbit ALS we have shown that the immunosuppressive effect of ALS depends on the genetic difference between donor and recipient. In the case of strong (H-2) barrier, very efficient ALS preparations are needed to exert a demonstrable effect; if the genetical difference is weak, even less potent antisera may be effective. On the other hand, ALS may help

TABLE 19-III

*Suppressive effect of ALS on transplantation immunity in experimental animals and in man*

| Recipient | Antigen used for immunization | Donor of ALS | Graft | Reference No. |
|---|---|---|---|---|
| **Mouse** | Thymus cells, thymus cell fraction, epidermis, lymphocytes | Rabbit | Skin | 87*b*, *c* |
| | Lymph node cells in Freund's adjuvant | Rabbit | Skin | 100, 136*a*, *b* |
| | Thymus cells | Horse | Skin | 68 |
| | Thymus cells | Rabbit | Skin | 30, 65*b*, 86 |
| | Thymus cell–ALG immune complex | Horse | Skin | 174 |
| **Rat** | Thoracic duct lymph cells | Rabbit | Skin | 170*a*, *b* |
| | Thoracic duct lymph cells | Horse | Skin | 67, 172*a* |
| | Thymic and lymph node cells in Freund's adjuvant | Rabbit | Skin | 105*a* |
| | Lymph node cells | Rabbit | Skin | 47, 48, 70*a*, *b*, *c* |
| | Thymus cells | Rabbit | Kidney | 49*a*, *b*, *c* |
| Dog | Thoracic duct lymph cells | Horse | Kidney | 1, 123*a*, 125 |
| | Lymph node cells in Freund's adjuvant | Horse | Kidney | 99, 138 |
| | Lymph node and spleen cells | Horse | Kidney | 61, 63, 148 |
| | Thymus cells | Rabbit | Kidney | 139 |
| | Thoracic duct lymph cells | Horse | Liver | 96, 112, 149 |
| | Lymphoid cells | Sheep | Heart | 50 |
| | Thoracic duct and lymph node cells | Rabbit | Kidney | 3, 12*a*, *b*, 40, 53, 82, 83 |
| | Thymus cells | Rabbit | Kidney | 55 |
| | Spleen cells | Sheep | Kidney | 97, 115 |
| Rabbit | Thymic and lymph node cells | Guinea pig | Skin | 44 |
| Swine | Lymph node cells | Horse | Skin | 90 |
| Monkey | Thymus cells and lymphocytes | Rabbit | Skin | 18 |
| | Thymus cells and lymphocytes | Horse | Skin | 19, 157 |
| | Thymus cells | Horse | Kidney | 34 |
| Man | Lymph node cells | Rabbit | Skin | 101*c*, 102 |
| | Lymph node, spleen and thymus cells, lymphocytes | Horse | Kidney | 74, 139, 144*b*, 147, 148, 149, 150 |
| | Lymph node cells, thymus cells, peripheral lymphocytes | Horse | Liver | 28 |
| | Thoracic duct lymph cells | Horse | Kidney | 155, 156 |
| | Lymphoid cells | Horse | Heart | 35 |
| | Lymphocytes | Horse | Heart, kidney, liver | 25 |
| | Lymphoid cells | Horse | Heart, kidney | 24 |

to differentiate the strength of allograft reactions, indistinguishable in non-suppressed recipients [30, 54, 108].

The survival time of mouse skin allografts was prolonged by pretreatment of the donor with ALS [121]; besides the inhibition of the donor lymphocytes present in the graft, a role of graft-protection-enhancing antibodies has been assumed [26*b*].

## EFFECTS ON THE GRAFT-VERSUS-HOST REACTION*

It has been shown, using various experimental models including the 'normal lymphocyte transfer' reaction, runt disease, acute secondary disease, etc. that the GVH reaction may be inhibited by ALS in various phases. So, the treatment of donors considerably reduce the reactivity of its lymphoid cells [110]. Also a suitable 'timed' treatment of the recipients may suppress the GVH reaction. The most effective seems to be the pretreatment of recipients two or three days before the administration of donor cells. In this situation, the suppression of the lymphoid component and simultaneous stimulation of the haemopoietic one was demonstrated [111]. This observation is highly relevant to clinical bone marrow transplantation, where the GVH reaction represents a serious stumbling block.

The ALS is effective also *in vitro*. After binding to the surface of lymphocytes, relevant ALS antibodies deprive these cells of their capacity to react against the recipient. If cell-bound ALG was removed by trypsin treatment, the cells regained their reactivity.

According to some recent investigations, different cell populations may differ in their sensitivity to ALS; e.g. murine lymphoid cells were found to be approximately ten times more sensitive than murine haemopoietic cells *in vitro* and perhaps also *in vivo* [84]. These findings are of great importance since a higher resistence of haemopoietic cells would facilitate the use of ALS in bone marrow therapy of aregenerative and neoplastic aplasias. Unfortunately, attempts to reproduce the results with simian and human cells have failed so far.

## ALS AND IANTTUMOUR IMMUNITY

Tumours, transplanted to syngeneic (genetically identical) recipients, contain specific antigens, foreign to the recipient; these mostly evoke an immune reaction, but unfortunately, this is not fully effective. Tumours, transplanted to allogeneic (or xenogeneic) recipients, are, on the other hand, regularly rejected by a strong allograft (xenograft) reaction. ALS treatment has been found to counteract all these responses to support tumour growth and to increase the number of metastases [4, 5, 9*a*, *b*, 10, 52, 76, 173]. If the ALS is strong, even the growth of heterologous tumours (human cells in mice) is stimulated [143].

* The graft-versus-host (GVH) reaction is a pathological immune process evoked by immunologically competent cells transplanted into, and reacting against a genetically non-identical hyporeactive recipient [109]. (Graft cells, recognizing the foreign antigenic structure, initiate an immune response against the recipient) (see Chapter 29).

Accidentally, tumour cells were transplanted together with the donor's kidney: the tumour grew vigorously in the immunosuppressed recipient and regressed when therapy was stopped [168]. Moreover, there are data suggesting that malignant tumours occur with increased frequency in patients, treated with ALS and immunosuppressive drugs [146, 169c]. A local application of ALS may lead to the malignant process in the adjacent tissue [81].

## ALS INVESTIGATIONS *IN VITRO*

Prior to studies *in vitro*, the complement has to be inactivated, otherwise the lymphoid cells would be lysed by cytotoxins in ALS. ALS also agglutinates the lymphocytes [171].

The suppressive effect was observed in various *in vitro* systems including immunoadherence [14, 15], PHA-induced cytotoxic effect [104*a*] and macrophage migration [153]. Also colony forming haematopoietic cells are sensitive [31, 113]. The blast transformation after addition of tuberculin and in mixed lymphocyte cultures was also inhibited with suitable doses of ALS [44, 135].

On the other hand, ALS has an activating effect on some lymphocytes: a non-specific blast transformation occurs in a high percentage (60–90 per cent) of cells. The peak of the blast transformation is reached about the 72nd h following the exposure to ALS. In this respect, it acts like antiglobulin serum [136*b*] and PHA [107]. However, as shown by experiments carried out in our laboratory, the stimulation curve of the ALS is different in shape from the PHA curve [114], even if the same lymphocyte population is used (Fig. 19-2).

Various lymphoid cells differ in their sensitivity to ALS *in vitro*: lymph node

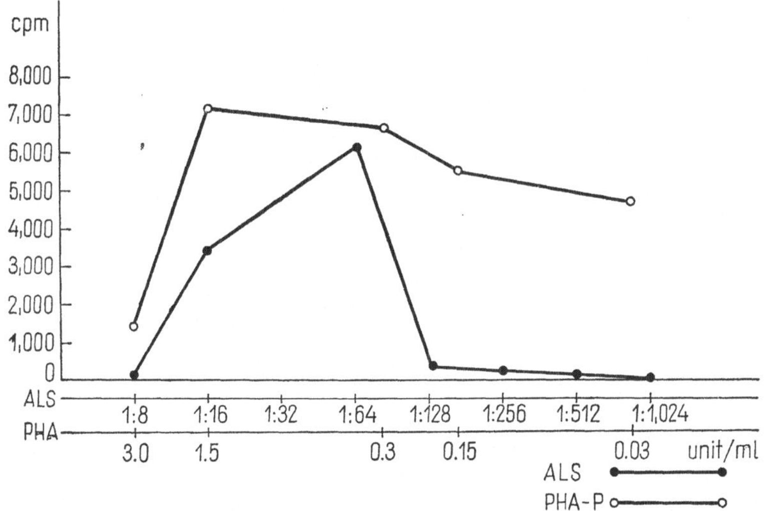


Fig. 19-2. Transformation of lymphocytes by anti-human ALS and by PHA-P. 12 h incorporation of $^{3}$H-thymidine into $1 \times 10^{6}$ lymphocytes per ml culture. The results were read at the 72nd h

cells are more resistant than spleen and thymus cells; thymus cells react by the most rapid blastogenic response. The effect of ALS also depends on the duration of the contact with cells: after short-term cultivation, the fragile and end-type cells disappear, whereas immunocompetent and haemopoietic cells develop from ALS non-sensitive precursors [112, 113].

The *in vitro* results described here served as a basis for the 'blind-folding' and 'sterile inactivation' hypotheses of ALS action (see below).

## RELATIONSHIP BETWEEN THE IMMUNOSUPPRESSIVE EFFECT OF ALS AND THE DIFFERENT FRAGMENTS OF THE ALS–IgG

Taking into consideration that the ALS is prepared by hyperimmunization, it is not surprising that the major component of its immunosuppressive potency is carried by IgG-type (7S) immunoglobulins [18, 66*a*, 77*a*]. The purified IgG fraction of the ALS (ALG) has leukoagglutinating, mitogenic, immunosuppressive and, partially, cytotoxic activities. The non-specific anti-inflammatory, haemolytic, anti-enzymatic, etc. activities are removed with the other fractions.

In the clinical practice, purified ALG preparations are used. However, only 1–3 per cent of the ALG binds to the lymphocyte surface specifically, indicating that only a very small proportion of the ALG may be considered as true anti-lymphocyte antibody. On the other hand, a large amount of the immunoglobulin binds to the lymphocytes ($10^6$–$10^7$ molecules per cell) non-specifically, i.e. by the Fc fragment, as demonstrated with $^{131}$I-labelled ALG molecules [169*d*]. The remaining mixture of antibodies, devoid of antilymphocyte activity, represents ballast as regards immunosuppression. Moreover, these antibodies may interfere with the effect of the active molecules by inducing anti-IgG antibody production. Experiments were therefore initiated to isolate the active fraction. As a result, true anti-lymphocyte antibodies were eluted from the surface of lymphocytes at low pH, and it was shown that the IgG fraction thus obtained induced blast transformation [169*b*]. It is, however, not quite clear whether the immunosuppressive activity of the eluted fraction remained intact [65*d*]. In some experiments, the substantial fraction of immunosuppressive activity was found in a T equine and IgM fraction, which throws some doubts on the suitability of preparing very pure ALS–IgG [64, 145].

The relationship between the molecular substructure and the immunosuppressive capacity of ALG have also been studied. The pepsin-digested ALG, containing $F(ab')_2$ fragments (Fig. 19-3*b*), gives rise to blast transformation and leukoagglutination and even suppresses the GVH reaction [49*d*]. However, efforts to reproduce the latter data have failed. The univalent Fab fragment, being less active biologically, induces practically no blast transformation and causes no immunosuppression (Fig. 19-3*c*). On the other hand, it is of interest that Sell et al. [137] have succeeded in inducing blast transformation with univalent Fab fragments isolated from antiglobulin serum. This is probably due to the fact that the Fab fragment of the ALG and that of the antiglobulin becomes bound to different receptors on the surface of lymphocytes. Data indicating that the Fab fragment of ALS may suppress MLC and GVH reaction *in vitro*, await confirmation.

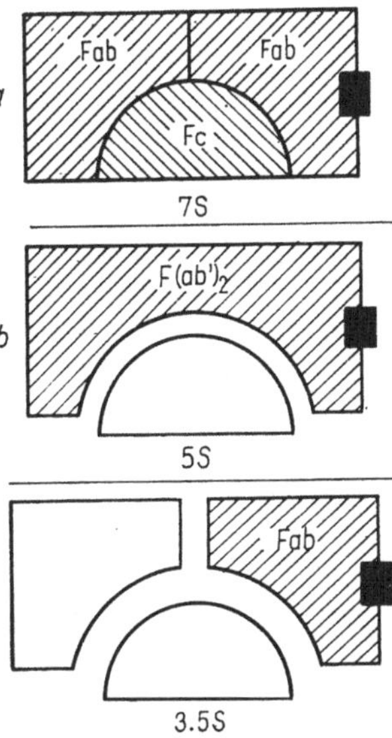

| | Biological activity | Effect | Reference |
|---|---|---|---|
| *a* (Fab, Fab, Fc; 7S) | Cytotoxicity | + + + | 63*a*, *b*, 165*a* |
| | Leukoagglutination | + + + | 63*a*, *b*, 165*a* |
| | Blast transformation | + + + | 165*a* |
| | Immunosupression | + + + | 8, 14, 61, 64, 65, 99*c* |
| *b* ($F(ab')_2$; 5S) | Cytotoxicity | – | 62*a*, 161*d* |
| | Leukoagglutination | + + | 161*d*, 163, 165*a* |
| | Blast transformation | + + | 161*d*, 163, 165*a* |
| | Immunosupression | – | 8, 62*a*, 63*a*, 165*a* |
| | | + | 48*a* |
| | GVH reaction | + | 48*d*, 87 |
| | | – | 106 |
| *c* (Fab; 3.5S) | Cytotoxicity | – | 8 |
| | Leukoagglutination | – | 165*a* |
| | Blast transformation | – | 165*a* |
| | | + | 131*a* |
| | Immunosupression | – | 8, 62*a*, 63*a*, 128 |
| | | + | 48*d* |

Fig. 19-3. Biological effects of the complete ALS–IgG molecule (*a*) and its fragments $F(ab')_2$ (*b*) and Fab (*c*).

The Fc fragment, obtained by papain digestion, is the carrier of a species-ecific marker and of the receptors necessary for binding to tissues and for mplement fixation. Figure 19-3*a* shows that its presence is also necessary for the imunosuppressive activity. This is supported by the finding that the anti-mouse ıck ALG, though active in the presence of fowl complement in experiments *vitro*, was ineffective *in vivo*, presumably because it was unable to bind mam-alian complement [133, 160].

## POSSIBLE MODE OF ALG ACTION

ALS has proved to act on all types of the cells participating in the humoral ımune response, i.e. T and B lymphocytes and macrophages [69, 118]. The role macrophages in the afferent arc of cell-mediated immune reaction is still dubi-ıs, but their participation with B lymphocytes in specific as well as non-specific fector mechanisms is highly probable [11]. Consequently, ALG may act through teraction with both kinds of lymphocytes and macrophages. Numerous hypo-ıeses on the mechanism of ALS action have been proposed, each having been ıpported by experimental evidence. Nevertheless, none of the hypotheses ex-ains in itself the manysided and complicated effects of ALG. It seems therefore ıstified to describe briefly the most important of these hypotheses.

## LYMPHOCYTOTOXIC EFFECT

Lymphocytes are lysed by ALG in the presence of complement and this process may participate in lymphocytopenia (Fig. 19-4*a*). Numerous authors have observed a parallelism between the cytotoxic titre of the ALS preparation and the degree of the lymphocytopenia [99, 100, 105*a*, 134, 167]. On the other hand, ALS preparations of quantitatively similar immunosuppressive activity have often shown different cytotoxic titres [26*b*] and sera of identical cytotoxic and/or leukoagglutinin titre may be of different immunosuppressive capacity [70*b*, 130]. The hypothesis based on the cytotoxic activity of the ALG has therefore become doubtful [1, 8, 18, 63, 70*c*, 83, 105*b*, 125]. Nevertheless, the fact that in our experiments the lymphocytes cultivated in diffusion chamber significantly decreased in number after ALS treatment suggests that the direct lymphocytotoxic effect may play some role even *in vivo* [21].

## COATING OR BLIND-FOLDING OF LYMPHOCYTES

According to this hypothesis, lymphocytes possess specific receptors for antigens and for ALG on their surface (Fig. 19-4*b*). The active ALG molecules bound to the surface of immunologically competent cells cover or mark the antigen receptors and thus make them unrecognizable. The blind-coated cells are also unable to take over information from macrophages [87*a*, 171, 172*b*]. The fixation of ALG to lymphoid cells has been demonstrated by immunofluorescence and radioisotope methods [87*a*]. Furthermore, it has been shown that lymphocytes, having been freed from the ALG molecules by digestion, may regain their activity [26*a*].

In spite of these arguments, there are some objections that weaken the validity of the blind-folding hypothesis: e.g. it does not explain why the progeny of the blind-folded lymphocytes are devoid of immunological activity [73, 87*c*].

## ENHANCEMENT OF THE TARGET ORGAN

Due to common antigenic determinants, ALG molecules may become bound not only to lymphoid, but also to other cells [23, 36], even to cells of the graft (Fig. 19-4*c*). For instance, ALG was found to be bound to the glomerular basement membrane of kidney allograft approximately ten times more intensively than normal globulin [49*a*]. Since the antigens of the graft coated by ALG are hardly recognizable by the host immune apparatus, the graft may survive for a prolonged period of time [49*a*, *c*].

However, some data are contradictory to this, 'enhancement' hypothesis: (*i*) the results obtained by Guttmann et al. [67] in rats could not be reproduced in dogs; (*ii*) the immune response to simple antigens (e.g. bovine albumin), which cannot bind ALG, was also reduced. However, some recent experiments indicate that ALS, suppressing more intensively the cell-mediated component of the allograft response, may favour the production of graft protecting—enhancing—antibodies by the host [112].

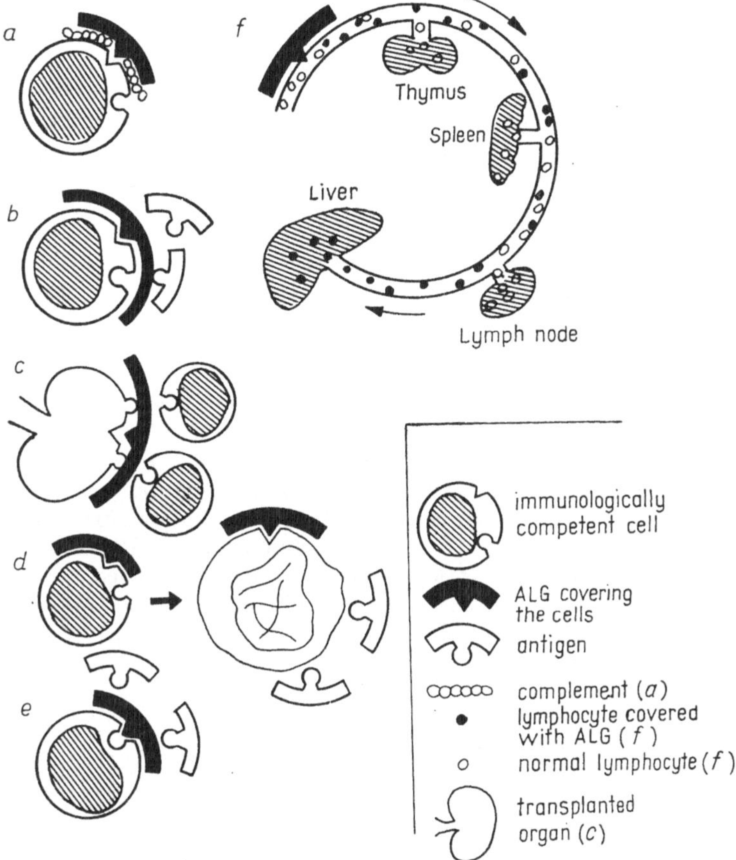


Fig. 19-4. Schematic illustration of the different hypotheses concerning ALG action. *a)* Lymphoid cells are lysed by ALG in the presence of complement (lympholytic effect). *b)* The receptors on the surface of lymphocytes are covered by the ALG (coating effect). The cells thus blind-folded do not recognize the antigen (blind-folding effect). *c)* The ALG molecules on the lymphocyte surface cover the antigenic structure of the transplanted cells, thus preventing the immunologically competent cells of the recipient from recognizing the antigen (enhancement). *d)* In the course of the ALG-induced blast transformation the antigen sensitive receptors become unable to recognize the antigen (sterile activation). *e)* ALG inhibits the immune reaction by competitive antagonism. *f)* ALG is bound to circulating lymphocytes; the cells covered by ALG are eliminated by the liver and reticulo-endothelial system instead of reaching the lymphoid organs

## STERILE ACTIVATION

Considering that ALG induces a non-specific blast transformation [43] and stimulates cell division in lymph nodes and in the blood, Levey and Medawar [87*a*, *b*] supposed that ALS would act by inducing non-specific cell activation. It should be noted that cells in the transformation or proliferation process are refractory to other stimuli. So, if the lymphoid cells transform and divide in a 'sterile' way under ALS influence, they are unable to react with specific antigens (Fig. 19-4*d*).

Numerous authors [171, 172*b*] have observed a parallelism between the transforming and immunosuppressive effects of ALG. In our studies the blast transformation test provided a relatively firm basis for estimation of the immunosuppressive potency of ALS preparations [142]. The sterile activation hypothesis seemed to be supported by the fact that PHA, another agent inducing blast transformation in a large proportion of lymphocytes may also be immunosuppressive [107]. However, as shown by Elves [36] and ourselves [123*a*], the immunosuppressive effect of PHA depends on strict conditions: e.g. PHA and antigen should be injected intraperitoneally. In other situations, the immune system is rather stimulated by the PHA. In our experiments, the cytokinetics of the immune response was accelerated by the intravenously administered PHA; supposedly, the cells treated with PHA did not loose their immunocompetence.

The importance of sterile activation is made doubtful by the observation that while the $F(ab')_2$ fragment of IgG induces blast transformation, it has no immunosuppressive effect [8, 65*a*].

## ANTIMACROPHAGE EFFECT

ALS as well as ATS inhibit the function of macrophages [39, 118]. In some experiments, immunosuppression induced by ALS was recovered more efficiently with spleen macrophages or Kupffer cells than with spleen lymphocytes or thymus cells [118]. Considering the well-known role of macrophages in cellular co-operation and the importance of cytophilic antibodies in allograft response [41], it has been proposed that the ALG effect is—at least partially—mediated by the suppression of macrophages. It is interesting that after anti-macrophage serum (AMS) treatment, an enhanced antibody production was observed [152].

## COMPETITION OF ANTIGENS

ALG, as a strong immunogen, is bound avidly to lymphocytes, and may in some way interfere with the specific immune response [65*a*]. There are, however, experimental data [7] suggesting that the effect of rabbit ALS is significantly enhanced in mice made tolerant to the normal rabbit serum proteins (Fig. 19-4*e*).

## ANTICOMPLEMENTARY EFFECT

Due to the intensive consumption of complement in the course of the binding of ALG to lymphocytes, a considerable part of the organism's complement reserve may be exhausted. The resulting low complement level may be accompanied by a decreased immunological reactivity. Also the anti-inflammatory effect of the ALG is thought to be mediated by its anticomplementary activity. This seems to be supported by the relatively high effectiveness of ALS in the mouse strains with low complement level [159*b*]. However, some experiments contradict this assumption [141].

## EFFECTS EXERTED ON THE THYMUS AND T LYMPHOCYTE POPULATION

Experimental data suggesting that ATS has a higher immunosuppressive effectiveness than ALS [105*a*] have raised the possibility that the effect of these antisera is mediated by the action on the thymus. However, the attempts to demonstrate ALG in the thymus by radioisotopes or immunofluorescence have failed [101*a*, 159*a*].

In ALS-treated animals, ALG molecules enter the circulation and get into contact with lymphocytes. Consequently, even small doses may affect peripheral lymphocytes and prevent them from taking up information from, and being sensitized by, antigens from skin, and organ allografts. The same doses of ALS do not interfere with the sensitization evoked by small doses of allogenic lymphoid cells, because these cells are transported to lymphoid organs which are reached by ALG molecules with difficulty [87*d*]. The fact that other procedures leading to a reduction in the number of lymphocytes—e.g. chronic drainage of thoracic duct lymph—are not accompanied by such immunosuppressive effect might be attributed to a selective damaging effect of ALG on T (thymus derived, dependent) population of lymphocytes which are unable to follow their recirculaton through lymphoid tissues and are sequestered in RES-rich tissues, e.g. lung and liver [33*a*, 66*b*, 77*b*, 91, 154]. This presumption can at best explain the pronounced immunosuppressive effectiveness of ALS on cell-mediated immune reactions. Helper T cells were selectively reduced in number after ALS treatment in the experiments carried out with hapten–carrier conjugates. The loss of helper function can be counterbalanced by lymphocytes obtained from animals immunized by the corresponding hapten [98*b*]. The immunological memory is reduced by ALS [141, 154].

However, it has been demonstrated recently that some of the ALS preparations, which appeared to be effective in skin transplantation experiments, stimulated the B lymphocytes selectively; others, in agreement with the hypothesis, exerted a selective stimulation on T cells [69]. The effect on B lymphocytes seems to be supported by cell electrophoresis experiments [22].

Generally, ALS and even ATS have an inherent anti-B activity. This must be removed for obtaining an agent with a pure anti-T effectiveness. On the other hand, also sera with a pronounced anti-B activity can be produced. In experimental animals, such sera may be produced easily, e.g. by immunization with chicken bursa cells, or with cells from mouse plasmacytomas [51, 57]. In man it may be possible to use for the immunization cells of B lymphatic leukaemias. Such sera may prove useful in suppressing production of tumour enhancing antibodies. Nevertheless, in our laboratory we were not able to detect anti-B activity of xenogeneic ALS produced with lymphocytes of chronic leukaemic xenogeneic patients [122].

## MAJOR PROBLEMS OF THE CLINICAL USE OF ALG

### MEASUREMENT OF IMMUNOSUPPRESSIVE POTENCY

In considering the great fluctuation in the immunosuppressive capacity of various ALG batches, it is necessary to estimate the immunosuppressive potency and the toxicity of each preparation. Unfortunately, none of the *in vitro* tests discussed above provides a clear-cut answer to this basic question. The inhibition of the spontaneous rosette formation of human or mouse lymphocytes *in vitro* has shown the best correlation with the immunosuppressive effectiveness *in vivo* [13, 15]. Other authors recommend to test the opsonizing or transforming activity, the titre of lymphocytophilic and anti-platelet antibody, adherability to macrophages and ability to suppress PHA or MLC responsiveness. The most precise method for the estimation of the immunosuppressive potency and safeness, is based on testing the survival of skin or organ allografts.

Fortunately, the immunosuppressive potency of anti-human ALG preparations may be determined in monkeys on the basis of prolonging the survival of skin allografts [17]. Monkeys have numerous transplantation antigens (HL-A) common with man [162]. The monkey test may provide also some information on the possible toxicity and other side-effects which may occur in the course of clinical use. It can, therefore, be considered as a step towards the standardization of ALG. This is the reason why the results of the monkey test have been accepted as a basis for a recent comparative study organized by the National Institute of Health (NIH) in Bethesda [157].

### DOSAGE OF ALG AND COMBINATION WITH OTHER IMMUNOSUPPRESSIVE PROCEDURES

It was shown in early studies that a combination of ALS therapy with other immunosuppressive procedures may be superior to the simple use of ALS. On the basis of favourable results in animal experiments Woodruff [169*a*] and subsequently, Starzl et al. [149] have introduced ALG treatment in human renal transplantations. ALG treatment was combined with the administration of standard immunosuppressive drugs, such as azathioprine (Imuran) and corticosteroids. Their results have shown that ALG pre- and post-treatment allow a substantial reduction of Imuran and prednisone dosage. The reduction of the corticosteroid therapy is accompanied by a reduction of numerous undesirable side-effects. Starzl and his co-workers have recommended the following dosage schedule:

| 1 week before surgery | 1st and 2nd weeks after surgery | 3rd and 4th weeks after surgery | 2nd months after surgery | 3rd and 4th months after surgery |
|---|---|---|---|---|
| every day | every day | every second day | twice a week | once a week |

Weekly doses of ALG: in the beginning 14–50 mg per kg; from the 2nd month onwards 2–6 mg per kg.

Other investigators have suggested to give much larger doses for shorter periods of time in a more intensive schedule. Taking also the body weight of the patient into account, the weekly dose varied from 700 to 14,000 mg per patient. However, the dosage schedule must be individualized from patient to patient and with various ALG preparations.

Surprisingly, the i.v. administration of ALG, a method believed to be highly dangerous on the principles of classical immunology ('foreign protein reactions'), proved to be a very effective and safe procedure probably because of the 'self antidotal effect' [134]. Another mode of reducing the side-effects might be the induction of immunotolerance to the ALG molecule by the administration of suitable doses of normal donor IgG [79, 123*b*]. The tolerance of ALG treatment is probably further improved by simultaneously applied immunosuppressive steroids and azathioprine. Brendel and Land [25] and Pichlmayr et al. [125] administered 500–1,000 mg of ALG as an i.v. infusion in 250–500 ml of saline, without serious complications. The intravenous administration of ALG has become more and more widely accepted [80].

TABLE 19-IV

*Combined ALS therapy*

| Additional therapy | Time of application | Experimental subject | Reference No. |
|---|---|---|---|
| *(a) Combinations stimulating immunosuppression* | | | |
| Drainage of thoracic duct | Before ALS | Rat | 170*a*, *b* |
| Whole body irradiation | Before ALS | Mouse | 87*a* |
| Hydrocortisone treatment | Before ALS | Mouse | 87*a* |
| Thymectomy | Before ALS | Rat | 70*a* |
| | | Mouse | 101*a*, *b*, *d* |
| Amethopterine, bromouridine, 6-thioguanine, prednisone | After ALS | Mouse | 59*a*, *b*, 14[illegible] |
| 6-mercaptopurine | After ALS | Mouse | 71 |
| Azathioprine | After ALS | Dog, man | 148, 166 |
| Azathioprine | After ALS | Monkey | 34 |
| *(b) Combinations weakening immunosuppression* | | | |
| Amethopterine + corticoid | Before ALS | Mouse | 140 |
| Whole-body irradiation + adrenalectomy | After ALS | Mouse | 87*b* |

To achieve a synergism between ALG and other immunosuppressive procedures, the suitable time relation must be respected. With an inadequate schedule the ALS effect may be depressed rather than potentiated. The advantageous and disadvantageous combination schedules are listed in Table 19-IV.

ALS is a potent agent in suitable dosage and timing for the induction of antigen-specific immunological unresponsiveness. In the transplantation systems, combination with donor cells or cellular antigens may facilitate a permanent survival of skin or organ (kidney) grafts. The participation of both immunological tolerance and immunological enhancement was demonstrated.

## SIDE-EFFECTS OF ALG TREATMENT

The early ALS preparations contained haemagglutinins, cytotoxins, precipitins to serum proteins and other undesirable antibodies. Consequently, anaemia, thrombocytopenia, haemorrhage, local necrosis, nephritis and anaphylactic reactions occurred frequently in the course of ALS treatment of experimental animals. All these reactions are attributable to common antigens shared by lymphocytes and other cells and to the fact that mainly spleen cells were used for the immunization [18, 38, 49*b*, 74, 147, 156].

It should be emphasized that the haemagglutinating activity of the ALS resides in the 19S (IgM) globulin, whereas the immunosuppressive activity is carried mostly by the 7S antibodies. The 19S globulins and other undesirable fractions responsible for the side-effects can be removed by salt fractionation, or DEAE cellulose chromatography and absorption with erythrocytes, plasma proteins and tissue (kidney) cells. The necessity of the purification of ALS is supported by the fact that dangerous host anti-ALS antibodies (precipitins) are predominantly directed against $\alpha$- and $\beta$-globulins contaminating crude ALS preparations [63]. Accordingly, purified ALS preparations contain less 'ballast' antigen. Much attention must also be paid to the anti-platelet activity which can lead to haemorrhagic as well as thrombotic complications and to anti-kidney activity. When absorption procedures fail, pools must be abandoned.

Some side-effects of ALG therapy cannot be fully eliminated. These include local phenomena (pain, oedema, inflammation) after i.m. application and systemic symptoms such as fever, shivering, allergic manifestations, generalized pruritus, urticaria, erythema, periorbital oedema and sometimes even typical anaphylactic reactions. The latter appeared 1 to 30 min after the injection of ALG; the patient was saved by a proper therapy [63, 74]. According to clinical experience, however, only very severe symptoms justified the interruption of ALG therapy. Here, ALG produced in animal of another species can be used. In the case of mild symptoms, the therapy was continued and the patients became more and more tolerant to ALG. These and other observations have shown that under favourable conditions immunological tolerance to ALG may develop [19, 63, 150, 155, 161].

## REFERENCES


1. Abaza, H. M., Nolan, B., Watt, J. G. and Woodruff, M. F. A: *Transplantation* **4,** 618 (1966).
2. Abaza, H. M. and Woodruff, M. F. A.: *Rev. franç. Ét. clin. biol.* **11,** 821 (1966).
3. Abbott, W. M., Otherson, H. B., Monaco, A. P., Simmons, R. L., Wood, M. A. and Russell, P. S.: *Surg. Forum* **17,** 228 (1966).
4. Allison, A. C., Berman, L. and Levey, R. H.: *Nature* **215,** 185 (1967).
5. Allison, A. C. and Law, L. W.: *Proc. Soc. exp. Biol. (N.Y.)* **127,** 207 (1968).
6. Anderlik, P.: In *Transplantációs Immunológia. (Immunology of Transplantation).* Ed. by Petrányi, Gy., Petrányi, G. Gy., Benczúr, M. and Jánossy, Gy. Akadémiai Kiadó, Budapest 1971, p. 235.
7. Anderson, H. R., Dresser, A. D., Iverson, G. M., Lance, E. M., Wortis, H. H. and Zebra, J.: *Immunology* **22,** 277 (1972).
8. Anderson, N. F., James, K. and Woodruff, M. F. A.: *Lancet* **i,** 1126 (1967).
9*a*. Anigstein, L., Anigstein, D. M. and Rennels, E. G.: *Texas Rep. Biol. Med.* **23,** 705 (1965).
9*b*. ibid., **25,** 214 (1967).
10. Anigstein, L., Anigstein, D. M., Rennels, E. G. and Ostsen, W. K.: *Cancer Res.* **26,** 1867 (1966).
11. Argyris, B.: *Transplantation* **8,** 538 (1969).
12*a*. Atai, M. and Kelly, W. D.: *Surg. Forum* **17,** 249 (1966).
12*b*. id., *Surg. Gynec. Obstet.* **125,** 13 (1967).
13. Bach, J. F.: *Transplant. Proc.* **3,** 27 (1971).
14. Bach, J. F. and Antoine, B.: *Nature* **217,** 258 (1968).
15. Bach, J. F. and Dormont, J.: *Transplantation* **11,** 97 (1971).
16. Badgett, B. A. and Tough, J. L.: *J. Immunol.* **99,** 1017 (1967).
17. Balner, H.: *Transplant. Proc.* **3,** 949 (1971).
18. Balner, H. and Dersjant, H.: In *CIBA Study Group 29. Antilymphocytic Serum.* Ed. by Wolstenholme, G. E. W. and O'Connor, M. Churchill, London 1967, p. 85.
19. Balner, H., van Bekkum, D. W., de Vries, M. J., Dersjant, H. and van Putten, L. M.: In *Advance in Transplantation.* Ed. by Dausset, J., Hamburger, J. and Mathé, G. Munksgaard, Copenhagen 1968, p. 449.
20. Bános, Zs., Anderlik, P. and Szeri, I.: Lecture delivered at the 23rd Meeting of the Section of Immunology, Hung. Assoc. Microbiol. Veszprém 1968.
21. Benczur, M.: Unpublished data (1972).
22. Bert, G., Forrester, J. A. and Davies, A. J. S.: *Nature* **234,** 86 (1971).
23. Bobory, J., Leövey, A., Petrányi, Gy. and Szegedi, Gy.: *Haematologia* **5,** 413 (1971).
24. Brendel, W.: *Transplant. Proc.* **3,** 280 (1971).
25. Brendel, W. and Land, W.: *Dtsch. med. Wschr.* **48,** 2309 (1968).
26*a*. Brent, L., Courtenay, T. and Gowland, G. *Nature* **215,** 1461 (1967).
26*b*. id., In *Advance in Transplantation.* Ed. by Dausset, J., Hamburger, J. and Mathé, G. Munksgaard, Copenhagen 1968, p. 117.
27. Brunstetter, F. H. and Claman, H. N.: *Transplantation* **6,** 485 (1968).
28. Calne, R. Y.: Personal communication (1968).
29*a*. Currey, H. L. F. and Ziff, M.: *Lancet* **ii,** 889 (1966).
29*b*. id., *J. exp. Med.* **127,** 185 (1968).
30. Démant, P. and Nouza, K.: *Folia biol. (Prague)* **17,** 410 (1971).
31. de Meester, T. R., Anderson, N. D. and Schaffer, Ch. F.: *J. exp. Med.* **127,** 731 (1968).
32. Denman, A. M., Denman, E. J. and Holborow, E. J.: *Lancet* **ii,** 841 (1966).
33*a*. Denman, A. and Frenkel, E. P.: *J. Immunol.* **99,** 498 (1967).
33*b*. id., *Immunology* **14,** 107 (1968).
34. Dicke, H. W., Marquet, R. L., Heystek, G. A. and Balner, H.: *Transplant. Proc.* **3,** 484 (1971).
35. Dubost, Ch. and Cachera, J. P.: *Presse méd.* **76,** 1713 (1968).
36. Elves, M. W.: *Int. Arch. Allergy* **37,** 353 (1968).
37. Fekete, B., Petrányi, Gy., Szegedi, Gy. and Szabó, G.: *Haematologia* **5,** 419 (1971).

38. Field, E. O. and Gibbs, J. E.: *Nature* **217,** 561 (1968).
39. Fishman, M. J. and Adler, F. L.: *J. exp. Med.* **117,** 595 (1963).
40. Fujimoto, Y., Miura, T., Uchida, H. and Inon, T.: *Jap. J. exp. Med.* **37,** 205 (1967).
41. Gill, P. G.: *Austr. J. exp. Biol. med. Sci.* **48,** 583 (1970).
42. Gledhill, A E.: *Nature* **214,** 178 (1967).
43. Gräsbeck, R., Nordman, C. T. and de la Chapelle, A.: *Acta med. scand.* **412** Suppl. 39 (1964).
44. Greaves, M. F., Roitt, I. M., Zamir, R. and Carnarghan, R. B. A.: *Lancet* **ii,** 1317 (1967).
45. Gray, J. G., Monaco, A. P. and Russell, P. S.: *Surg. Forum* **15,** 142 (1964).
46. Gray, J. G., Monaco, A. P., Wood, M. L. and Russell, P. S.: *J. Immunol.* **96** 217 (1966).
47. Grogan, J. B. and Hardy, J. D.: *Surgery* **62,** 352 (1967).
48. Grogan, J. B., Moynihan, P. C. and Hardy, J. D.: *Arch. Surg.* **97,** 144 (1968).
49*a*. Guttmann, R. D., Carpenter, C. B., Lindquist, R. R. and Merrill, J. P.: *Lancet* **i,** 248 (1967).
49*b*. id., *Transplantation* **5,** 1115 (1967).
49*c*. id., *J. exp. Med.* **126,** 1099 (1967).
49*d*. id., In *Advance in Transplantation*. Ed. by Dausset, J., Hamburger, J. and Mathé, G. Munksgaard, Copenhagen 1968, p. 141.
50. Halpern, B., Cachera, J. P., Lacombe, M., Hathway, A., Crepin, Y., Biu-Mong-Hung, Leandri, J., Laurent, D. and Dubost, Ch.: *C. R. Acad. Sci.* **266,** 963 (1968).
51. Harris, N. S., Jagarlamoody, S. M., McKhan, Ch. F. and Najarian, J. S.: *J. Immunol.* **108,** 958 (1972).
52. Hellmann, K., Hawkin, R. I. and Whitecross, S.: *Brit. med. J.* **2,** 533 (1968).
53. Herman, A. H. and Schloerb, P. R.: *Transplantation* **5,** 732 (1967).
54. Hilgert, I. and Nouza, K.: *Folia biol. (Prague)* **16,** 369 (1970).
55. Hinchey, E. J. and Bliss, J. G.: *Canad. med. Ass. J.* **95,** 1169 (1966).
56. Hintz, B. and Webber, M. M.: *Nature* **208,** 797 (1963).
57. Hirokawa, K., Nariuchi, M., Usui, M. and Matuhasi, T.: *Jap. J. exp. Med.* **42,** 239 (1972).
58. Hirsch, M. S., Murphy, F. A., Russe, H. P. and Hicklin, M. D.: *Proc. Soc. exp. Biol. (N.Y.)* **125,** 980 (1967).
59*a*. Hoehn, R. J. and Simmons, R. L.: *Surg. Forum* **17,** 251 (1966).
59*b*. id., *Transplantation* **5,** 1409 (1967).
60. Humphrey, J. H.: *Brit. J. exp. Path.* **36,** 283 (1955).
61. Huntley, R. T., Taylor, P. D., Iwasaki, Y., Marchioro, T. L., Jeejeebhoy, H., Porter, K. and Starzl, T. E.: *Surg. Forum* **17,** 230 (1966).
62*a*. Inderbitzin, T.: In *Mechanisms of Hypersensitivity*. Ed. by Shaffer, J. H., Lo Grippo, G. A. and Chase, M. W. *Henry Ford Hospital Int. Sympos. Detroit, 1959*. Churchill, London 1959, p. 495.
62*b*. id., *Int. Arch. Allergy* **8,** 150 (1966).
63. Iwasaki, Y., Porter, K. A., Amond, J. R., Marchioro, T. L., Zühlke, V. and Starzl, T. E.: *Surg. Gynec. Obstet.* **124,** 1 (1967).
64. Jacobsen, A. and Flatmark, A.: *Acta path. microbiol. scand. B.* **80,** 501 (1972).
65*a*. James, K.: *Clin. exp. Immunol.* **2,** 615 (1967).
65*b*. ibid., **2,** 685 (1967).
65*c*. id., *Nature* **217,** 261 (1968).
65*d*. id., Personal communication (1968).
66*a*. James, K. and Anderson, N. F.: *Nature* **213,** 1195 (1967).
66*b*. id., *Clin. exp. Immunol.* **3,** 227 (1968).
67. James, K. and Jubb, V. S.: *Nature* **215,** 367 (1967).
68. James, K. and Medawar, P. B.: *Nature* **214,** 1052 (1967).
69. Jánossy, G. and Greaves, M. F.: *Clin. exp. Immunol.* **10,** 525 (1972).
70*a*. Jeejeebhoy, H. F.: *Immunology* **9,** 417 (1965).
70*b*. id., *Transplantation* **5,** 273 (1967).
70*c*. ibid., **5,** 1121 (1967).
71. Jeejeebhoy, H. F., Rabbar, A. G. and Vela-Martinez, J.: *Transplantation* **6,** 765 (1968).
72. Jeejeebhoy, H. F. and Vela-Martinez, J. M.: *Transplantation* **6,** 149 (1968).

73. Jooste, S. V.: *Transplantation* **6,** 277 (1968).
74. Kashiwagi, I., Brantigan, C. O., Brettschneider, L., Groth, C. G. and Starzl, T. E.: *Ann. intern. Med.* **68,** 275 (1968).
75. Kassai, T., Szepes, G., Réthy, L. and Tóth, G.: *Ann. Immunol. Hung.* **11,** 207 (1968).
76. Kubista, T. P., Shorter, R. G. and Hallenbeck, G. A.: *Cancer Res.* **27,** 2072 (1967).
77*a*. Lance, E. M.: In *Cell-bound Immunity with Special Reference to Antilymphocyte Serum and Immunotherapy of Cancer.* Ed. by Bacq, Z. M., Castermans, A. and Lejeune, G. L'Université de Liège, Liège 1967, p. 103.
77*b*. id., In *Advance in Transplantation,* Ed. by Dausset, J., Hamburger, J. and Mathé, G. Munksgaard, Copenhagen 1968, p. 107.
77*c*. id., *Nature* **217,** 557 (1968).
77*d*. id., In *The Immune Response and its Suppression.* Ed. by Sorkin, E. Karger, Basel 1968, p. 310.
78. Lance, E. M., Ford, P. and Ruszkiewicz, M.: *Fed. Proc.* **29,** 106 (1970).
79. Land, W., Brendel, W., Hopf, U. and Seifert, J.: *Klin. Wschr.* **48,** 241 (1970).
80. Largiadèr, F., Linder, E., Senning, Å., Scheitlin, W., Wegmann, W. and van Rood, J.: *Schweiz. med. Wschr.* **100,** 18 (1970).
81. Law, L. W.: *Fed. Proc.* **29,** 171 (1970).
82. Lawson, R. K., Ellis, L. R. and Hodges, V. C.: *Surg. Forum* **17,** 515 (1966).
83. Lawson, R. K., Ellis, L. R., Kirchheim, D. and Hodges, C. V.: *Transplantation* **5,** 169 (1967).
84. Ledney, G. D. and van Bekkum, D. W.: In *Advance in Transplantation.* Ed. by Dausset, J., Hamburger, J. and Mathé, G., Munksgaard, Copenhagen 1968, p. 441.
85. Leibowitz, S., Lessof, M. H. and Kennedy, L. A.: *Clin. Exp. Immunol.* **3,** 753 (1968).
86. Leövey, A., Szegedi, Gy., Fekete, B., Bobory, J. and Petrányi, Gy.: *Haematologia* **5,** 407 (1971).
87*a*. Levey, R. H. and Medawar, P. B.: *Ann. N. Y. Acad. Sci.* **129,** 164 (1966).
87*b*. id., *Proc. nat. Acad. Sci. (Wash.)* **56,** 1130 (1966).
87*c*. ibid., **58,** 470 (1967).
87*d*. id., In *CIBA Study Group 29. Antilymphocytic Serum.* Ed. by Wolstenholme, G. E. W. and O'Connor, M. Churchill, London 1967, p. 72.
88. Loewi, G., Temple, A., Nind, A. P. P. and Axelrad, A.: *Immunology* **16,** 1 (1969).
89. Lónai, P., Köteles, Gy. and Antóni, P.: Lecture delivered at the 22nd Meeting of the Section of Immunology, Hungarian Assoc. Microbiol. Veszprém, 1968.
90. Mandel, M. A. and Asofsky, R.: *J. Immunol.* **100,** 1259 (1968).
91. Martin, W. J. and Miller, J. F. A. P.: *Lancet* **ii,** 1285 (1967).
92. Mathé, G.: Personal communication (1968).
93. Mathé, G., Amiel, J. L., Schwarzenberg, L., Choay, J., Trolard, P., Schneider, M., Hayat, M., Schlumberger, J. R. and Jasmin, C.: *Brit. med. J.*, **2,** 131 (1970).
94. Medawar, P. B.: In *CIBA Study Group 29. Antilymphocytic Serum.* Ed. by Wolstenholme, G. E. W. and O'Connor, M. Churchill, London 1967, p. 81.
95. Metchnikoff, I. I.: *Ann. Inst. Pasteur* **13,** 737 (1899).
96. Mikaeloff, Ph., Pichlmayr, R., Rassat, J.-P., Messmer, K., Bomel, J., Tidow, G., Étiennemartin, M., Malluret, J., Belleville, P., Jouvenceau, A., Falconnet, J., Descotes, J., and Brendel, W.: *Presse méd.* **75,** 1967 (1967).
97. Mitchell, R. M., Sheil, A. G. R., Slafsky, S. R. and Murray, J. E.: *Transplantation* **4,** 323 (1966).
98*a*. Mitchison, N. A.: *Bull. AIIMS.* **3,** 153 (1969).
98*b*. id., *Eur. J. Immunol.* **1,** 68 (1971).
99. Monaco, A. P., Abbott, W. M., Othersen, H. B., Simmons, R. L., Wood, M. L., Flax, M. H. and Russell, P. S.: *Science* **153,** 1264 (1966).
100. Monaco, A. P., Wood, M. L., Gray, J. G. and Russell, P. S.: *J. Immunol.* **96,** 229 (1966).
101*a*. Monaco, A. P., Wood, M. L. and Russell, P. S.: *Fed. Proc.* **24,** 377 (1965).
101*b*. id., *Science* **149,** 432 (1965).
101*c*. id., *Ann. N. Y. Acad. Sci.* **129,** 180 (1966).
101*d*. id., *Transplantation* **5,** 1106 (1967).

102. Monaco, A. P., Wood, M. L., vanWerf, B. A. and Russell, P. S.: In *CIBA Study Group* 29. *Antilymphocytic Serum*. Ed. by Wolstenholme, G. E. W. and O'Connor, M.: Churchill, London 1967, p. 111.
103. Moore, G. E., Hasenpusch, P., Gerner, R. E. and Burus, A.: *Biotech. Bioeng.* **10,** 625 (1968).
104. Moynihan, P. G., Grogan, J. Б. and Hardy, J. D.: *I. Int. Congr. Transplant. Soc.* (Abstracts) Paris 1967, p. 153.
104*a*. Möller, G., Lundgren, G. and Balner, H.: *Transplantation* **9,** 166 (1970).
105*a*. Nagaya, M. and Sieker, H. O.: *Science* **150,** 1181 (1965).
105*b*. id., *Proc. Soc. exp. Biol. (N.Y.)* **121,** 722 (1966).
106. Najarian, J. S., Merkel, F. K., Moore, G. E., Gord, R. A. and Aust, J. C.: *Transplant. Proc.* **1,** 460 (1969).
107. Naspitz, Ch. K. and Richter, M.: *Progr. Allergy* **12,** 1 (1968).
107*a*. Naysmith, J. D. and James, K.: *Nature* **217,** 260 (1968).
108. Němec, M., Nouza, K. and Démant, P.: *Transplant. Proc.* **5,** 275 (1973).
109. Nouza, K.: *Rev. franç. Ét. clin. biol.* **13,** 747 (1968).
110. Nouza, K. and Haśkovcová, H.: *Folia biol. (Prague)* **16,** 391 (1970).
111. Nouza, K., Haśkovcová, H. and Némec, M.: *Folia biol. (Prague)* **17,** 312 (1971).
112. Nouza, K., Němec, M., and Dráber, P.: Unpublished data.
113. Nouza, K., Sejkorová, J., Stoyanov, S., Haškovcová, H. and Křeček, M.: *Biomédicine* **18,** 23 (1973).
114. Onody, K.: Unpublished data (1972).
115. Otte, H., Grosjean, O. and Castermans, A.: *C. R. Soc. Biol. (Paris)* **161,** 959 (1967).
116. Padányi, M., Réthy, L., Bácskai, L. and Hegedüs, L.: *Ann. Immunol. Hung.* **13,** 147 (1969).
117. Pappenheimer, A. M.: *J. exp. Med.* **26,** 163 (1917).
118. Patterson, J. T., Pisano, J. C. and Di Luzio, N. R.: *Proc. Soc. exp. Biol. (N.Y.)* **135,** 831 (1970).
119. Petrányi, G. Gy., Benczúr, M. and Alföldy, P.: *Immunology* **21,** 151 (1971).
120. Petrányi, G. Gy., Jánossy, Gy. and Alföldy, P.: *Nature* **221,** 76 (1969).
121. Petrányi, Gy., Szegedi, Gy. and Fekete, B.: *Orv. Hetil.* **112,** 1852 (1971).
122. Phan, D. T. and Benczúr, M.: Unpublished data (1972).
123*a*. Pichlmayr, R.: *Z. ges. exp. Med.* **143,** 161 (1967).
123*b*. id., *Langenbeck's Arch. klin. Chirurgie* **329,** 723 (1971).
124. Pichlmayr, R., Brendel, W., Mikseloff, Ph., Wiebecke, B., Rassat, J. P., Pichlmayr, I., Bonnet, J., Fateh-Megdaham, A., Thierfelder, St., Messmer, K., Descoles, J. and Knedel, M.: In *Advance in Transplantation*. Ed. by Dausset, J., Hamburger, J. and Mathé, G. Munksgaard, Copenhagen 1968, p. 147.
125. Pichlmayr, R., Brendel, W. and Zenker, R.: *Surgery* **61,** 774 (1967).
126. Réthy, L.: *Ann. Immunol. Hung.* **13,** 106 (1969).
127. Réthy, L. and Bácskai, L.: *Ann. Immunol. Hung.* **11,** 199 (1968).
128. Réthy, L., Hegedüs, L., Bácskai, L. and Tóth, G.: *Ann. Immunol. Hung.* **11,** 203 (1968).
129. Réthy, L., Hegedüs, L., Padányi, M. and Bácskai, L.: *Ann. Immunol. Hung.* **13,** 141 (1969).
130. Réthy, L., Juhász, Vera, P. and Sulyok, S.: *Ann. Immunol. Hung.* **13,** 153 (1969).
131. Réthy, L., Ormai, I., Sulyok, S. and Kaiser, G.: *Ann. Immunol. Hung.* **13,** 127 (1969).
132. Réthy, L., Sulyok, S. and Bácskai, L.: *Ann. Immunol. Hung.* **13,** 135 (1969).
133. Riethmüller, G., Rieber, P., Riethmüller, D.: *I. Int. Congr. Transplant. Soc.* (Abstracts) Paris 1967, p. 155.
134. Sacks, J. H., Filippone, D. R. and Hume, D. M.: *Transplantation* **2,** 60 (1964).
135. Schwarz, R. M.: *J. Reticuloendoth. Soc.* **7,** 146 (1970).
136*a*. Sell, S.: *J. exp. Med.* **125,** 289 (1967).
136*b*. ibid., **127,** 1139 (1968).
137. Sell, S. and Gell, P. G. H.: *J. exp. Med.* **122,** 423 (1965).
138. Shanfield, I., Ladaga, L. G., Wren, S. F. G., Blennerhassett, J. B. and Max Lean, L. D.: *Surg. Gynec. Obstet.* **127,** 29 (1968).

139. Shorter, R. G., Hallenbeck, G. A., Nave, C., O'Kane, H. O., De Weerd, J. H. and Johnson, W. J.: *Arch. Surgery* **97,** 323 (1968).
140. Simmons, W. K.: *Transplantation* **5,** 1136 (1967).
141. Simons, M. J.: *Lancet* **ii,** 866 (1968).
142. Skamene, E., Sejkorová, J., Nouza, K. and Iványi, J.: *Folia biol. (Prague)* **14,** 289 (1968).
143. Stanbridge, E. J. and Perkins, F. T.: *Nature* **221,** 80 (1969).
144. Starzl, T. E.: In *CIBA Group* 29. *Antilymphocytic Serum.* Ed. by Wolstenholme, G. E. W. and O'Connor, M. Churchill, London 1967, p. 108.
145. Starzl, T. E., Brettschneider, L., Penn, I., Schmidt, R. W., Bell, P., Kashiwagi, N., Townsend, C. M. and Putnam, C. W.: *Transplant. Proc.* **1,** 448 (1969).
146. Starzl, T. E., Groth, C. G., Brettschneider, L., Smith, G. V., Penn, I. and Kashiwagi, N.: In *The Immune Response and its Suppression.* Ed. by Sorkin, E., Karger, Basel 1968, p. 349.
147. Starzl, T. E., Marchioro, T. L., Hutchison, D. K., Porter, K. A., Cerilli, G. J. and Brettschneider, L.: *Transplantation* **5,** 1100 (1967).
148. Starzl, T. E., Marchioro, T. L. and Iwasaki, Y.: *Fed. Proc.* **26,** 944 (1967).
149. Starzl, T. E., Marchioro, T. L., Porter, K. A., Iwasaki, Y. and Cerilli, G. J.: *Surg. Gynec. Obstet.* **124,** 301 (1967).
150. Starzl, T. E., Porter, K. A., Iwasaki, Y., Marchioro, T. L. and Kashiwagi, N.: In *CIBA Study Group 29. Antilymphocytic Serum.* Ed. by Wolstenholme, G. E. W. and O'Connor, M. Churchill, London 1967, p. 4.
151. Sundaresan, P., Sundaram, K. and Phondke, G. P.: *Immunology* **23,** 439 (1972).
152. Surján, M.: *Experientia (Basel)* **28,** 470 (1972).
153. Švejcar, J., Pekárek, J. and Johanovský, J.: *Z. Immun.-Forsch.* **142,** 166 (1971).
154. Taub, R. N. and Lance, E. M.: *Immunology* **15,** 633 (1968).
155. Traeger, J., Fries, D., Carraz, M., Brochier, J., Bernhardt, J. P., Veyssere, C., Prevost, R., Traeger-Fouillet, Y., Bryon, P. A. and Manuel, Y.: In *Cell-bound Immunity with Special Reference to Antilymphocyte Serum and Immunotherapy of Cancer.* Ed. by Bacq, Z. M., Castermans, A. and Lejeune, G. L'Université de Liège, Liège 1967.
156. Traeger, J., Rerrin, J., Fries, D., Saubier, E., Carraz, M., Bonnet, R., Archimand, J. P., Bernhardt, J. P., Brochier, J., Bateul, H., Veysseyre, C., Bryon, P. A. Prevost, J., Jouvenceau, A., Bansillon, V., Zech, P. and Rollet, A.: *Lyon méd.* **15,** 307 (1968).
157. *Transplantation and Immunology Catalog.* Suppl. NIH. Bethesda 1972. (Manuscript.)
158. Trepel, F., Pichlmayr, K., Kimura, I., Brendel, W. and Begemann, H.: *Klin. Wschr.* **46,** 856 (1968).
159*a*. Turk, J. L. and Willoughby, D. A.: *Lancet* **i,** 249 (1967).
159*b*. id., In *The Immune Response and its Suppression.* Ed. by Sorkin, E. Karger, Basel 1968, p. 267.
160. Unanue, E. and Dixon, F. J.: *J. exp. Med.* **119,** 965 (1964).
161. va.n Bekkum, D. W., Ledney, G. D., Balner, H., van Putten, L. M. and de Vries, M J.: In *CIBA Study Group 29. Antilymphocytic Serum.* Ed. by Wolstenholme, G. E. W. and O'Connor, M. Churchill, London 1967, p. 97.
162. van Rood, J. J., van Leeuwen, A. and Balner, H.: *Transplant. Proc.* **4,** 55 (1972).
163. Végh, P. and Kovács, T.: Lecture delivered at the 22nd Meeting of the Section of Immunology, Hungarian Assoc. Microbiol. Veszprém 1968.
164. Waksman, B. H. and Arbouys, S.: In *Mechanisms of Antibody Formation.* Ed. by Holub, M. and Jarošková, J. Publ. House Acad. Sci. Prague 1960, p. 165.
165. Waksman, B. H., Arbouys, S. and Arnason, B. G.: *J. exp. Med.* **114,** 997 (1961).
166. Weil, R. III. and Simmons, R. L.: *Ann. Surg.* **167,** 239 (1968).
167. Wilhelm, R. E., Fisher, J. P. and Cooke, R. A.: *J. Allergy* **29,** 493 (1958.)
168. Wilson, R. E., Hager, E. B., Hampers, C. L., Corson, J. M., Merrill, J. P. and Murray, J.: *New Engl. J. Med.* **278,** 479 (1968).
169*a*. Woodruff, M. F. A.: *Transplantation* **5,** 1127 (1967).
169*b*. id., *Nature* **217,** 821 (1968).
169*c*. id., In *The Immune Response and its Suppression.* Ed. by Sorkin, E. Karger, Basel 1968, p. 234.

169*d*. id., *Transplant. Proc.* **3**, 34 (1971).
170*a*. Woodruff, M. F. A. and Anderson, N. F.: *Nature* **200**, 702 (1963).
170*b*. id., *Ann. N. Y. Acad. Sci.* **120**, 119 (1964).
171. Woodruff, M. F. A., Anderson, N. F., James, K. and Reid, B. L.: In *CIBA Study Group* 29. *Antilymphocytic Serum.* Ed. by Wolstenholme, G. E. W. and O'Connor, M. Churchill, London 1967, p. 57.
172*a*. Woodruff, M. F. A., Reid, B. L. and James, K.: *Nature* **215**, 591 (1967).
172*b*. ibid., **216**, 758 (1967).
173. Yamanouchi, K. and Hayami, M.: *Jap. J. med. Sci. Biol.* **23**, 395 (1970).
174. Zola, H., Mosedale, T. and Mosedale, B.: *Experientia (Basel)* **28**, 192 (1972).
175. Zsebők, Z., Petrányi, G. Gy., Benczúr, M., Alföldy, P. and Kovács, L.: In *V. Conf. Hung. Ther. and Invest. Pharmacol.* Ed. by Leszkovszky, G. P. Akadémiai Kiadó, Budapest 1971, p. 543.

# INDEX